HEPATIC SURGERY

Edited by **Hesham Abdeldayem**

Hepatic Surgery

http://dx.doi.org/10.5772/3461

Edited by Hesham Abdeldayem

Contributors

Hesham Abdeldayem, Hiromichi Ishii, Atsushi Toma, Tsuyoshi Itoh, Kenji Nakamura, Shimpei Ogino, Koki Ikemoto, Kenichi Takemoto, Ronald Chamberlain, Carmen Peralta, Julio Cesar Wiederkehr, Barbara Wiederkehr, Henrique Wiederkehr, Izabel Coelho, Sylvio Avilla, Chunbao Guo, John Lang, Kun-Ming Chan, Ashok Thorat, Ahmad Sira, Mostafa Mohamed Sira, Hiroshi Sadamori, Bilal Aljiffry, Owaid Almalki, Wei-Chen Lee, Hideaki Uchiyama, Ling Lu, Lu Hao, Stuart Robinson, Steve White, Derek Manas, John Scott, Elsayed I. Salama, Mattia Garancini, Luca Gianotti, Fabrizio Romano, Franco Uggeri, Vittorio Giardini, Guido Torzilli, Samah Khayat, Rajan Jagad, Jan Stoot, Kees Dejong, Mirela Patricia Sîrbu Boeți, Hiroshi Yoshida, Mazen Hassanain, Ahmad Medkhali, Faisal Alsaif, Abdusalam Alsharabi, Murad Aljiffry, Fabio Uggeri, Luca Nespoli, Angelo Nespoli

Published by InTech

Janeza Trdine 9, 51000 Rijeka, Croatia

Publishing Process Manager Danijela Duric
Technical Editor InTech DTP team
Cover InTech Design team

Additional hard copies can be obtained from orders@intechopen.com

Hepatic Surgery, Edited by Hesham Abdeldayem
p. cm.
ISBN 978-953-51-0965-5

For EU product safety concerns:
IN TECH d.o.o., Prolaz Marije Krucifikse Kozulić 3, 51000 Rijeka, Croatia,
info@intechopen.com or visit our website at intechopen.com.

Meet the editor

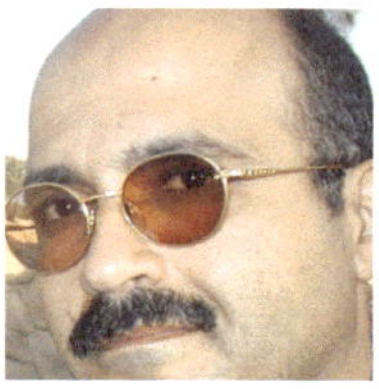

Dr Hesham Abdeldayem is a professor of surgery at the National Liver Institute, Egypt. He was trained at Starzl Transplantation Institute, University of Pittsburgh Medical Center, in USA. Dr Abdeldayem is a WHO-certified trainer in publishing medical journals. He published many papers and several books, both in English and Arabic, in the fields of liver transplantation and hepatobiliary and pancreatic surgery, like Liver Transplantation-basic issues ISBN 978-953-51-0016-4 and Liver Transplantation-technical issues and complications issues ISBN 978-953-51-0015-7.

Contents

Preface

Longmire, called it a "hostile" organ because it welcomes malignant cells and sepsis so warmly, bleeds so copiously, and is often the first organ to be injured in blunt abdominal trauma. To balance these negative factors, the liver has two great attributes: its ability to regenerate after massive loss of substance, and its ability, in many cases, to forgive insult.

This book covers a wide spectrum of topics including, history of liver surgery, surgical anatomy of the liver, techniques of liver resection, benign and malignant liver tumors, portal hypertension, and liver trauma. Some important topics were covered in more than one chapter like liver trauma, portal hypertension and pediatric liver tumors.

As the editor, I wish to thank my colleagues, the authors, for their co-operation and desire to share their precious experience with the medical community. They are well-known experts from many centers across the world. On their behalf, I wish to express the hope that our publication will facilitate access to the latest scientific achievements in the field of liver surgery all across the world.

This book is dedicated to our Patients without whose goodwill and trust, no progress in medicine would be possible. To all my colleagues at the National Liver Institute in Egypt who supported me, and embraced me with their warm feelings: I love you all. To professor, Amr Helmy, and all my professors who so generously guided me by their example, wisdom and insights: thank you. Finally, to Ms. Romana Vukelic, who shared me the birth of this book, and to Ms. Danijela Duric who completed the job as the publishing manager: thank you, Romana and Danijela...

Hesham Abdeldayem, MD.
Professor of Surgery
National Liver Institute
Menoufeyia University
Egypt

Chapter 1

General Introduction: Advances in Hepatic Surgery

J.H.M.B. Stoot, R.J.S. Coelen, J.L.A. van Vugt and
C.H.C. Dejong

Additional information is available at the end of the chapter

http://dx.doi.org/10.5772/54710

1. Introduction

Hepatic resection is a commonly performed procedure for a variety of malignant and benign hepatic tumours [1, 2]. Historically, liver resection, irrespective of the indication, was associated with a high morbidity and mortality [2-4]. During the last decades however, perioperative outcome after hepatic resection has improved, due to increased knowledge of liver anatomy and function, improvement of operating techniques and advances in anaesthesia and postoperative care [1, 3, 4].

Hepatic resectional surgery is possible since the liver has the ability to regenerate. Although it is doubtful whether the ancient Greeks already appreciated this unique quality of the liver, it was first described in the myth of Prometheus (Προμηθεύς): he enraged the Gods for his disrespect (ὕβρις) after climbing the Mount Olympus and stealing the torch in order to give fire to the humans. He was punished by Zeus and chained to a rock in the Kaukasus Mountains. Every couple of days, an eagle came and ate part of his liver. As the liver regenerated every time, the eagle returned again and again to eat the liver and thereby torture poor Prometheus (figure 1). With this ancient knowledge it was considered possible to take parts of the liver, as this organ has enough capacity to work with a smaller part and is able to regenerate.

Apart from the eagle, no human dared to remove a part of the liver. In the ancient period of the Assyrian and Babylonian cultures of 2000 - 3000 BC the liver played an important role to predict the future by reading the surface of sacrificed animals [5]. This was also common in the Etruscan society, where the haruspices predicted the future from sheep livers. Hippocrates (460-377 BD), one of the founding fathers of ancient medicine, produced not only an oath with ethical rules, which is still used in modern times for all doctors. His careful observations also led to the recommendation to incise and drain abscesses of the liver with a knife [5]. Celsus documented the treatment of exposed liver in war wounds. Although he was not a physician,

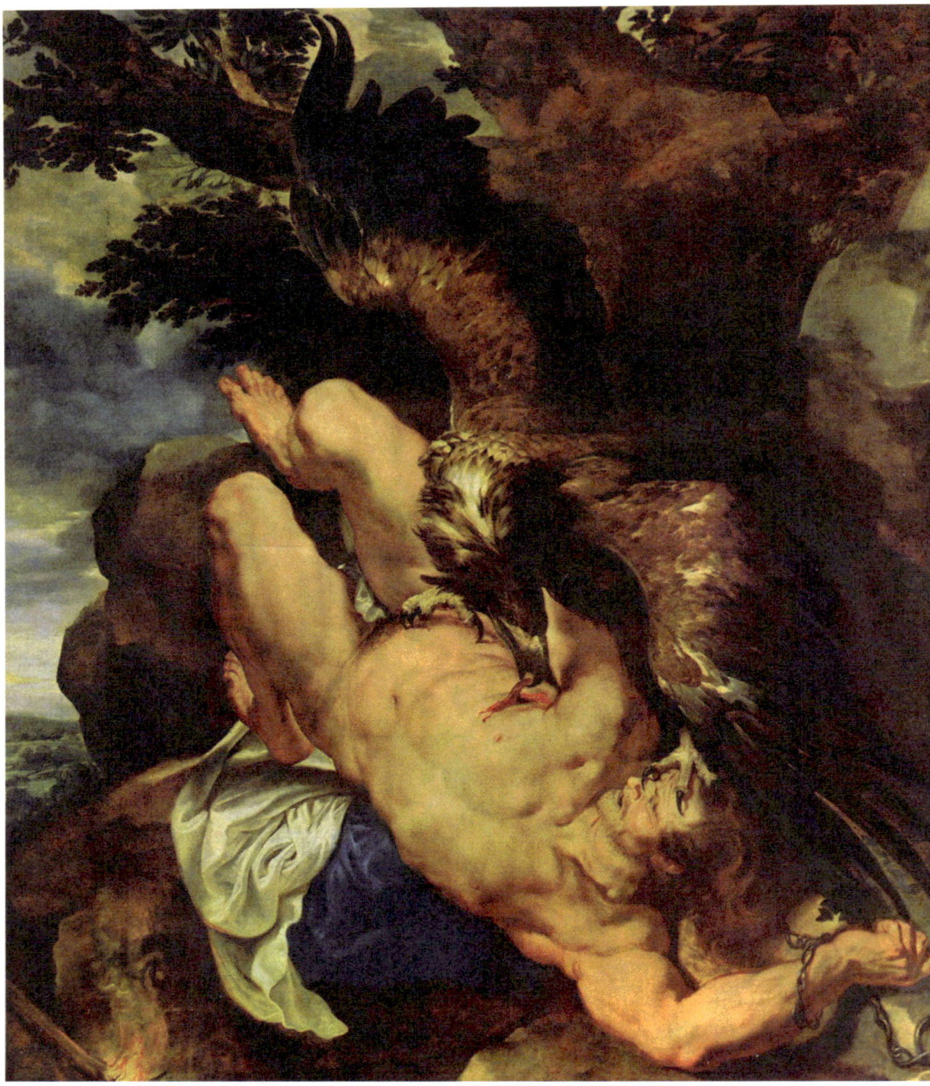

Figure 1. Prometheus chained (243 x 210 cm), Peter Paul Rubens, ca. 1611-1618, Philadelphia, Philadelphia Museum of Art.

he described his observations in the first century AD from the Alexandrian school led by Herophilus of Chalcedon and Erisastratus of Chios [5]. In the same era, the Greek Galen became one of the emperor's physicians in Rome and wrote reports about the dissection of many species of animals, including primates. He described the central role of the liver in absorption and digestion and his work remained of great importance for the coming centuries [5]. In the centuries thereafter many reports were produced describing the treatment of war or trauma wounds.

Glisson performed extensive investigations of the vascular anatomy in 1654 (figure 2) [6]. It took more than two centuries before his work was rediscovered and further clarified by Rex (1888) in Germany and Cantlie (1897) in England [5, 7]. These contributions led to the division of the liver in a left and right lobe [5].

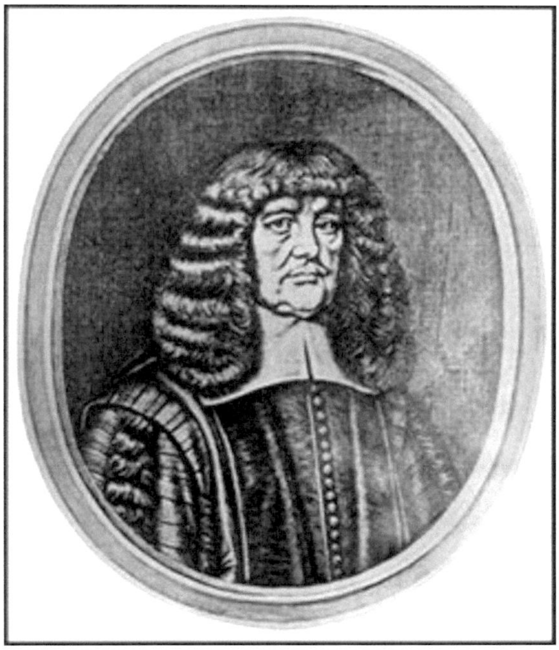

Figure 2. Francis Glisson (1599-1677).

2. History of hepatic surgery

It still took 17 centuries before Hildanus successfully performed the first partial liver resection for trauma [8]. The introduction of ether anaesthesia (1846) and the growing knowledge of antisepsis (1867) made successful elective abdominal operations possible (table 1) [5]. Langenbuch was the first to perform a successful elective liver resection in 1887 (figure 3) and Wendel did the first hemihepatectomy in 1911 [8]. The principles of liver haemostasis and regeneration were determined in the period 1880-1900 [8]. The knowledge of the principle of inflow and outflow of the liver and vascular control was one of the major advancements. Before that, wedge resections and mattress sutures were mostly used. This insight of inflow and outflow reduction was marked by the publication of James Hogart Pringle of Glasgow, Scotland (figure 4) [9]. He described the idea of digital control of the hilar ligament to reduce liver haemorrhage. In his famous report (1908) on liver haemorrhage after trauma, eight patients were included. Three died before the operation, one refused the operation and all four operated patients died; two died during the operation and two shortly thereafter [5, 9]. However, his idea of digital vascular control of the hilum was more successful in the laboratory setting, where he operated three rabbits with better results, which led to his publication. Nowadays, more than a century later, the 'Pringle manoeuvre' or 'Pringle's pinch' is still used worldwide in hepatic resectional surgery and taught to all young surgeons to control haemorrhage of the liver.

1846	Introduction of Ether anaesthesia	Morton
1863	Bacterial fermentation of wine	Pasteur
1867	Antisepsis	Lister
1870	First successful excision of section of the liver	Bruns
1880	Discovery of Streptococci, staphylococci and pneumococci	Pasteur
1881	First successful gastrectomy	Billroth
1882	First successful cholecystectomy	Langenbuch
1883	First human colon anastomosis	Billroth and Senn
1884	Pancreas excised for cancer	Billroth
1886	Report on appendicitis	Fitz
	Introduction of sterilisation by steam	Von Bergmann
	First elective liver resection for adenoma	Lius
1887	First successful elective liver resection	Langenbuch
1887	Successful packing of stabwound of liver	Burckhardt
1888	First successful laparotomy for traumatic liver injury	Willet

Table 1. Advances in the beginning of surgery [5].

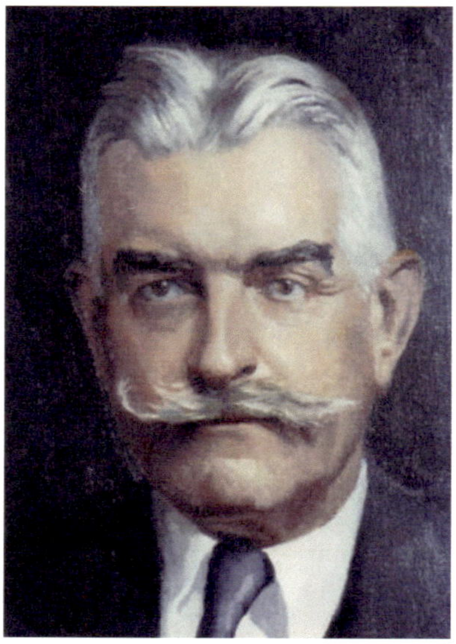

Figure 3. James Hogarth Pringle (1863-1941).

http://dx.doi.org/10.5772/54710

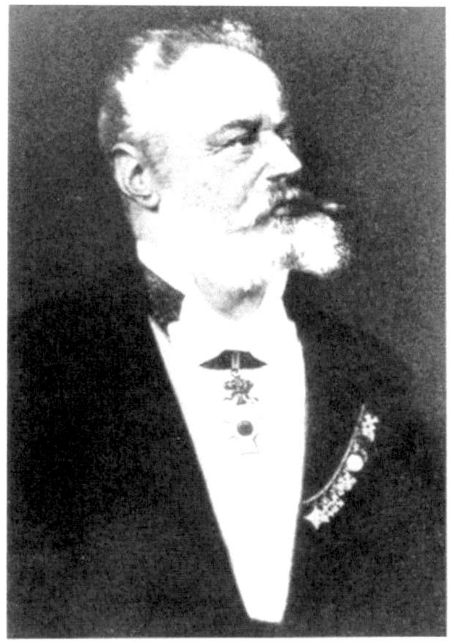

Figure 4. Carl Langenbuch (1846-1901).

Liver surgery became gradually more popular as a better understanding of anatomic segments was established after the work of Couinaud [10]. The classic morphological (outside) anatomy with two main lobes (left and right) was extended by the internal hepatic anatomy with several independent functional segments (figure 5). Each hepatic segment consists of liver parenchyma with an efferent hepatic vein branch and a portal triad; a hepatic artery branch, an afferent portal vein, and an efferent bile duct. The classic right lobe consists of four segments, the left lobe consists of three segments and the caudate lobe is segment 1.

With knowledge of the segmental anatomy of the liver, a safe transection plane could be chosen for resection without excessive blood loss and without necrosis of remnant liver. This specific anatomy of independent functional segments made it possible to resect parts of the liver without compromising the hepatic function of remnant segments. Moreover, as already described by the myth of Prometheus, the liver has regeneration capacity in contrast to other human organs. In other words after partial resections, the liver can recover its mass and function. The term 'function of the liver' is actually a collective term for a range of functions including amongst others ammonia detoxification, urea synthesis, bile synthesis and secretion, protein synthesis, gluconeogenesis and clearance or detoxification of drugs, bacterial toxins and bacteria [11]. As the liver is the main detoxifying organ in humans, adaptation of its function is crucial to survive. Regeneration however, takes time. After liver surgery with a reduction of the hepatic cell mass, a 'survival programme' may start for vital liver functions [12]. Some of these functions are increased rapidly in the remnant liver after resection [13]. In the light of major hepatic resections, it is conceivable that too little functional liver remnant may lead to liver failure, a lethal complication of liver surgery.

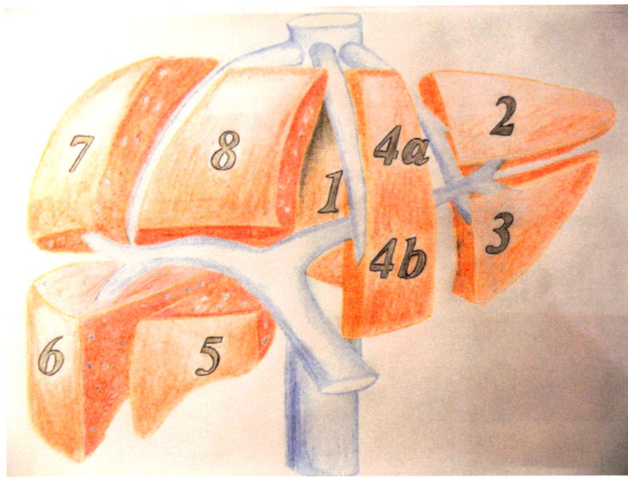

Figure 5. The anatomy of the liver with separate segments following Couinaud's classification. In this drawing only major venous vessels are displayed (portal vein, caval vein and hepatic veins).

3. Resectional hepatic surgery

Hepatobiliary surgery incorporates a wide range of indications for surgical treatment of the liver, varying from biopsy and resection to liver transplantation. The most important indications for surgical treatment are liver lesions: these comprise a wide range of both benign and malignant lesions, which can be either primary tumours (hepatocellular carcinoma) or secondary tumours (i.e. metastases). Also, some infectious diseases of the liver (such as echinococcosis) may be an indication for surgery. Irreversible liver dysfunction caused by acute or chronic liver diseases, may be an indication for transplantation of the liver. Other benign diseases of the liver such as symptomatic simple cysts and Polycystic Liver Disease (PCLD) may also warrant surgical treatment. Other reasons for surgery of the liver may be after severe injury or trauma of the liver. The latter indications are beyond the scope of this chapter. Since hepatic lesions form the main surgical indication for hepatic diseases, the focus will be on resectional liver surgery.

3.1. History of hepatic surgery for malignant lesions

The report of the first anatomical right hepatectomy for cancer by Lortat-Jacob in 1952 marked a new era in liver surgery [14]. In the beginning, however, blood loss and mortality were considerable. A multicentre analysis in 1977 of more than 600 hepatic resections for various indications showed an operative mortality of 13%, which rose to 20% for major resections [15]. Despite this, pioneers in liver surgery continued the quest for improving this challenging field of expertise and gradually mortality decreased to 5.6% [16]. The 5 year survival rates have increased from 20% in the beginning [16, 17] to as high as 67% in selected patients [18]. Earlier developments in liver surgery have been marked by major contributions of Starzl (USA), Bismuth (France) and Ton That Tung (Vietnam) [19-22]. With better knowledge of the segmental anatomy, it was shown that parenchyma-sparing segmental resections were equally effective as classic lobar resections, and in this way more functional remnant liver was preserved [3, 23, 24]. Also, anaesthetic care and liver transection techniques were modernized and improved over time [1, 3, 4, 25, 26].

Over the last decades, it was shown in several large series that perioperative results became more encouraging, with operative mortality rates less than 5% in high volume centres [3, 24, 25]. Due to these improvements in liver surgery which not only proved to prolong life but also to be a potentially curative treatment option for primary and metastatic cancers [27, 28], liver surgery became standard of care for selected patients with primary and secondary hepato-biliary malignancies. Moreover, with the increasing improvements in the safety of hepatic resections, this evolved to the most effective treatment for some benign diseases [29].

It is hard to pinpoint one discriminating factor that made the improvements in outcome possible [3]. Many factors contribute to the gradually improved outcome. Most important factors in this regard are probably the better knowledge of hepatic anatomy and thus anatomically based resections, better patient selection, general improvements in operative and anaesthetic care and the development of hepatobiliary surgery as a distinct area of specialisation [3].

3.2. Transection techniques in hepatic resection

Parenchymal transection is the most challenging part of liver resection. Due to the complicated vascular and biliary anatomy of the liver, haemorrhage is a great risk [30-35]. The firstly performed liver resections failed as a consequence of haemorrhage or patients died shortly after because of bleeding [31]. Before the 1980s, mortality after hepatic resection was 10 to 20% and haemorrhage was a common cause [30]. Moreover, blood transfusion in the perioperative period is associated with poorer outcome in the long term [33]. In contrast to patient- or tumour-related factors, surgical techniques can be changed in order to prevent blood loss and transfusion.

Parenchymal division was first described in 1958 when Lin and colleagues introduced the finger fracture technique (digitoclasy) in which liver tissue is crushed between the surgeon's fingers [30]. Vessels and bile ducts are exposed, identified and then divided. Soon this technique was improved by using surgical clamps (i.e. Kelly clamp) and called the crush-clamp technique [30, 31]. Division of the vessels and bile ducts can be achieved by suture ligation, bipolar electrocautery, vessel sealing devices or vascular clips. It is frequently combined with intermittent inflow occlusion by portal triad clamping (Pringle maneuver) [31].

Subsequently, many transection techniques have been developed in order to improve results. The Cavitron Ultrasonic Surgical Aspirator (CUSA, Tyco Healthcare, Mansfield, MA, USA) combines ultrasonic energy with aspiration and results in a more precise transection plane.

Vessels and bile ducts are exposed and can then be divided with a method according to the surgeon's preference [30, 31]. In a recent study, liver parenchyma transection using CUSA was associated with higher numbers of potentially dangerous air embolism although patients did not show clinical symptoms [36]. The Harmonic Scalpel (Ethicon Endo-Surgery, Cincinnati, OH, USA) is comparable to the CUSA, but it uses ultrasonic shears and vibration to cut through the parenchyma. It instantly coagulates blood vessels by protein denaturation and is mainly used in laparoscopic procedures, because of the difficulties using the other transection instruments in this setting. The hydro or water jet uses a high-pressure water jet to dissect liver parenchyma and expose vessels and bile ducts after which they can be divided. Like with the Harmonic Scalpel, less thermal damage is caused. In radiofrequency-assisted liver resection radiofrequent electrodes are inserted in the transection plane and radio frequent energy is applied for one to two minutes, followed by transection of the coagulated liver using a conventional scalpel. [30, 31].

In a review including seven randomized controlled trials with a total of 556 patients, the clamp-crush technique was quicker and associated with lower rates of blood loss and transfusion compared with CUSA, hydrojet and radiofrequency dissecting sealer. No significant differences in mortality, morbidity, liver dysfunction, ICU stay and length of hospital stay were found. The crush-clamp technique comes with low costs and does not need any extra advanced tools. However, not all techniques in the trials were combined with vascular occlusion. This may have led to a bias in favour of the clamp-crush technique [32, 34]. The CRUNSH trial will demonstrate whether vascular stapling is superior to the crush-clamp method in elective hepatic resection [37]. Palavecino and colleagues developed the so-called 'two-surgeon method', combining a saline-linked cautery and an ultrasonic dissector. Exposure of vessels and biliary ducts and haemostasis are performed simultaneously. Retrospectively, significantly lower transfusion rates were seen [33].

In conclusion, the clamp-crush technique seems to be superior especially as it is an easy method and comes with low costs. It might be regarded as the golden standard with which new devices or methods should be compared. However, high-quality randomized controlled trials are missing. Besides, the surgeon's experience plays an important role. Because of this, one could say that the method of choice is the clamp-crush technique and other techniques can be applied, or combined, dependent on the surgeon's experience and preference.

3.3. Malignant lesions

The liver has an important function as a detoxifying organ and due to the anatomical position in the abdomen; most gastro-intestinal organs drain their venous blood to the liver. This makes the liver a frequent location of metastases from a variety of intra-abdominal and sometimes even extra-peritoneal primary cancers. Also, primary cancers can arise in the liver. Of these the hepatocellular carcinoma is the most common malignancy. With a normal functioning liver, resection is the treatment of choice for most of these malignant lesions.

Metastases of colorectal origin are the most frequent malignant lesions in the liver. With nearly one million new cases diagnosed each year and around half a million deaths annually, colorectal cancer is one of the most common causes of cancer related death worldwide [38]. Over half of the patients with colorectal cancer will develop liver metastases [39]. Moreover, up to 25% of these patients present with liver metastases at the same time of the primary diagnosis [40]. Colorectal liver metastases may therefore be regarded as a major health problem [39].

The only chance of long-term survival in patients with liver metastases is provided by resection of these liver metastases, with 5-year survival rates around 30-40% [41]. Until recently, however, few patients with malignant liver lesions were considered for partial hepatic resection. Due to the restricted resection criteria, only 10-20% of the patients with malignant lesions were selected. Palliative chemotherapy was offered for the remaining proportion of the patients, resulting in a median survival of 6-12months [8, 42]. Due to the increased safety of liver surgery, liver resection is currently also used for other metastases such as neuroendocrine tumours [43], sarcoma's [44], melanoma [45-47], gastric cancer [48-50] and breast cancer [48, 51, 52].

The selection criteria for liver resections were initially fairly strict: unilobar distribution, less than four metastases, maximum tumour size of 5 cm and tumour free margin of 1 cm. These resection criteria have been evaluated over time and have gradually been abandoned, as these appeared to be not as important as previously assumed [53-55]. Even in elderly patients and poor prognostic groups, complete tumour resection results in a good long-term survival [56-58].

In the treatment of malignant liver disease, many improvements have been developed in recent years: new surgical strategies for safer resection (including two stage hepatectomy and portal vein embolisation), more effective chemotherapy, and additional techniques such as local ablation therapies to increase possible curative treatment [59-64]. The combination of these developments has led to an important progress and has resulted in more patients being considered suitable for liver resection to almost 30% [62]. Better survival of patients with primary or metastatic liver cancer has been reported in recent years and liver resection is currently the only potentially curative treatment option.

3.4. Benign hepatic lesions

In case of malignant hepatic disease, surgical resection is currently felt justified despite a morbidity and mortality, which may be as high as 42% and 6.5% respectively [1, 3, 65-67]. In case of benign hepatic disease, however, this decision remains more difficult. Due to the widespread use of imaging modalities such as ultrasonography, computed tomography (CT), and magnetic resonance imaging (MRI), benign hepatic masses are increasingly being identified. However, not all benign hepatic tumours require resection. Careful diagnosis with contrast enhanced CT or MRI needs to be performed first. Benign lesions can grossly be divided in solid and non-solid lesions (table 2).

Solid lesions	Symptoms	Treatment
Hepatocellular adenoma	Variable: from incidental finding to severe abdominal pain and shock in case of rupture	<5cm watchful waiting, stop oral contraceptives ≥5cm resection to prevent rupture and malignant degeneration
Focal Nodular Hyperplasia	Mostly incidental finding	Surgery rarely indicated
Angiomyolipoma	Mostly incidental finding	Surgery rarely indicated
Nodular regenerative hyperplasia	Mostly asymptomatic, should be considered in patients with clinical signs of portal hypertension without evidence of cirrhosis	No proven treatment
	Non-solid lesions	
Simple hepatic cyst	Variable: from incidental finding to abdominal pain	Surgery indicated only in case of symptoms
Biliary cystadenoma	Variable: from incidental finding to abdominal pain	Surgery may be indicated (malignant degeneration)
Biliary hamartoma	None	Surgery not indicated
Cavernous haemangioma	Variable, depending on size	Surgery rarely indicated
Hydatid disease	Variable: from incidental finding to severe abdominal pain and shock	Surgery indicated to relieve symptoms and to prevent rupture

Table 2. Most important benign liver lesions, divided in solid and non-solid lesions.

3.5. History of hepatic surgery for benign lesions

The first case of surgical resection for a presumably benign liver tumour was described in 1886 by Antonio Lius in Italy [68]. Lius was the assistant of Theodore Escher who excised a pedunculated adenoma with the size of a child's head (15.5 cm in greatest diameter) from the left liver lobe of 67-year-old women. An uncontrollable bleeding was encountered during the operation and the patient died several hours following surgery. The German surgeon Von Langenbuch was the first to perform a successful resection of a benign solid pedicled liver mass weighing 370 gram of the left liver in a 30-year-old woman who complained of abdominal discomfort in the years following her first child's birth in 1887 [69]. Postoperatively, secondary haemorrhage occurred due to a bleeding hilar vessel. This was managed at re-exploration and the patient survived. The course of symptoms and events in the latter case suggests the tumour was most likely a hepatocellular adenoma.

It is nowadays well established that small benign lesions compatible with a diagnosis of haemangioma, focal nodular hyperplasia (FNH) or hepatocelular adenomas (HCAs) are no indication for liver resection [53]. Hepatocellular adenomas are considered the most important, albeit uncommon, benign tumours of the liver that mostly occur in women. They are known for their increased risk of haemorrhage and malignant transformation into hepatocellular carcinoma (HCC) if size exceeds 5 cm. Therefore, surgical resection of HCAs is recommended for larger lesions [53, 54]. Focal nodular hyperplasia and haemangiomas have not been regarded as potentially premalignant lesions.

The first case report of malignant transformation of a HCA was published in 1981 by Tesluk and Lawrie [70]. The patient was a 34–year-old female with a large HCA measuring 16 cm in diameter. She first presented with tumour haemorrhage after which her oral contraceptive use was discontinued and the tumour subsequently shrank to a stable 5 cm. Three years later a partial hepatectomy was performed when the tumour had reverted to its size at first presentation. Histological analysis revealed a well-differentiated HCC. The patient died of sepsis five weeks postoperatively.

Foster and Berman were the first to report an estimated risk of malignant transformation in 1994, as they found a frequency of 13% in their series of 13 patients [71]. More recently, a systematic review of the literature of the past 40 years containing more than 1600 HCAs worldwide identified 68 reports of malignant transformation resulting in an overall frequency of 4.2% among all adenoma cases [72]. Nowadays several other risk factors for malignant potential of HCAs apart from size have been identified [73-84]. These are listed in table 3.

Risk factors
Tumour size ≥5 cm
Presence of β-catenin activating mutation
Presence of liver cell dysplasia within HCA
Patients with glycogen storage disease
History of androgen or anabolic steroid intake
Male sex
Obesity/overweight

Table 3. Risk factors for malignant transformation of hepatocellular adenomas.

3.6. Surgical treatment of hepatocellular adenomas

The identification of several risk factors for malignant potential of HCAs in recent years, provides better indications for surgical treatment of these presumably benign tumours. Also, the Bordeaux adenoma tumour markers (table 4) have greatly contributed to the subtype classification of HCAs and have given clearer insights into the pathological mechanism of malignant evolvement [79]. More recently, MR imaging techniques have been shown to be of value in identifying premalignant HCAs [85, 86]. These advances in risk factor stratification, together with tumour subtyping prior to hepatic surgery, might aid in selecting HCAs at high risk of malignant evolvement for surgical resection. Unfortunately, routine performance of biopsy of an HCA has not been implemented yet owing to the risk of sampling error, bleeding, needle-track tumour seeding and the difficult interpretation of β-catenin staining. However, a change towards a more stringent selection process in the near future is inevitable and may imply a major reduction of the number of liver resections, and thus morbidity and even mortality, in a selected group of predominantly young patients.

HCA type	Frequency (%)	Malignant transformation	Markers
β-catenin activated	10-15	Yes	β-catenin+/GS+
HNF1α inactivated	30-50	Rarely	LFABP-
Inflammatory	35	No	SAA+/CRP+
Unclassified	5-10	No	None

CRP, C-reactive protein; GS, glutamine synthetase; HCA, hepatocellular adenoma; HNF1a, hepatocyte nuclear factor 1a; LFABP, liver-fatty acid binding protein; SAA, serum amyloid A; +, positive; -, negative. Table adapted with permission from Stoot et al. 2010 [72].

Table 4. Types of HCAs and their immunohistochemical markers.

Concerning the management of ruptured HCAs, emergency surgery is associated with high morbidity and mortality rates [73, 85]. Although this treatment is still suggested by some authors [86], the maximally invasive therapy of immediate liver resection has gradually been abandoned. Many liver surgeons prefer conservative management of ruptured HCAs consisting of immediate resuscitation with laparotomy and gauze packing [74]. Selective arterial embolisation for ruptured HCAs may be a valuable alternative although it has rarely been reported [55, 63, 70, 72, 87].

In conclusion, hepatic resection for benign tumours is mainly reserved for HCAs at risk for malignant evolvement or haemorrhage. Advances in pathological subtyping, radiological imaging and risk stratification have led to new insights and aid in justifying hepatic resection in a more selected population.

4. Advances in the surgical treatment of benign cystic lesions: hydatid disease

Surgical treatment may also be indicated for infectious diseases of the liver such as benign lesions caused by the parasitic infection called Echinococcosis. Human echinococcosis is a zoonosis caused by larval forms (metacestodes) of Echinococcus (E.) tapeworms found in the small intestine of carnivores. Two species are of clinical importance – *E. granulosus* and *E. multilocularis* – causing cystic echinococcosis (CE) and alveolar echinococcosis (AE) in humans, respectively [87]. Besides, in the beginning of the 20th century the so-called neotropical echinococcosis species *E. oligarthrus* and *E. vogeli* were discovered to cause polycystic echinococcosis (PE). *E. vogeli* causes disease similar to AE and *E. oligharthrus* has a more benign character [88]. Echinococcosis is endemic worldwide in large sheep-raising areas including Africa, the Mediterranean region of Europe, the Middle East, Asia, South America, Australia and New Zealand [89-96]. Human cystic echinococcosis is one of the most neglected parasitic diseases in the world. In many endemic regions most infected patients suffer considerably from this disease, usually because of the lack of treatment possibilities due to poor infrastructure and shortage of equipment and drugs [97, 98]. The incidence of hydatid disease in Western industrial nations is relatively low [93, 94, 99]. Migration and travelling has led to an increase of the prevalence of this disease in Northern parts of Europe and North America [96, 100]. The diagnosis of hepatic echinococcosis can be made with a combination of patients' symptoms, liver imaging findings, detection of Echinococcis-specific antibodies and microscopic or molecular examination of cyst fluid. The most frequent site for cystic lesions is the liver (60% of patients), followed by the lungs in about 20% of patients. The remaining lesions are found throughout the body [92, 95, 99, 101, 102].

The natural course of this infection can be extremely variable [101]. The hepatic cysts can spontaneously collapse, calcify or even disappear. These patients can remain symptom-free for years. It is not uncommon that the cysts are detected when abdominal imaging is performed for a different reason. On the other hand, the cysts can also steadily grow about 1-3 cm in diameter per year [96, 99]. They do not tend to grow infiltratively or destructively, but pressure or mass effects of the cysts can displace healthy tissue and organs. Thus, most patients present with symptoms from mechanical effects on other organs or structures, which can lead to pain in the upper right quadrant, hepatomegaly and jaundice, depending on the location and nature of the cysts [91, 96, 99, 101]. Infection of the cysts can result in sepsis and/or the formation of liver abscesses. A feared complication is rupture of hepatic hydatid cysts into the peritoneal cavity. This can result in serious anaphylaxis, sepsis and/or peritoneal dissemination. The content of the ruptured cyst can disseminate into the biliary tract leading to cholangitis or cholestasis, but also to the pleurae or lungs leading to pleural hydatidosis or bronchial fistula, respectively [91, 92, 102].

4.1. History of hepatic surgery for hydatid disease

Hydatid disease was already recognized by Hippocrates more than two millennia ago. This benign disease has been shown to act as a malignant disease as it has the tendency to disseminate to other organs and to cause a devastating disease sometimes even leading to death. The serious effects of this disease were known in the late 1880s, when Loretta performed the first left lateral liver resection for echinococosis in Bologna [8]. Last years many developments have improved the course of hydatid disease: better medical therapy, improved surgical procedures and the development of minimally invasive techniques.

From a historical perspective, the main treatment option of hepatic hydatid disease was the open surgical approach with side packing and several radical or more conservative surgical techniques [96, 99]. This terminology in literature might be confusing. Conservative surgery means that tissue-sparing techniques are used; the hydatid cyst is evacuated and the pericyst is left in situ, while in radical procedures both the cyst and the pericyst are removed. The most common conservative techniques include simple tube drainage, marsupialization, capitonnage, deroofing, partial cystectomy or open or closed total cystectomy with or without omentoplasty. Conservative operations have good results regarding blood loss and length of hospital stay [103, 104]. In contrast, the cyst content and the entire pericystic membrane are removed in radical procedures; a total pericystectomy or liver resection (hemihepatectomy or lobectomy) is performed [90, 94, 101, 104].

In surgical interventions of hepatic hydatid cysts, complete removal of the parasite should be performed. Also, prevention of intraoperative spilling of cyst content and saving healthy hepatic issue is of utmost importance [91, 93, 96]. Spilling could not only lead to recurrence of hydatid disease, it could also lead to anaphylactic shock before the introduction of the antihelmintic drugs. Therefore, surgeons need to perform procedures with a focus on safe and complete exposure of the cyst, safe decompression of the cyst, safe evacuation of the cyst contents, sterilization of the cyst, treatment of biliary complications and management of the remaining cyst cavity. Especially in non-endemic areas where the number of operations is low, the technique needs to be safe and easily reproducible, with a low complication rate. In the former century, hydatid disease was operated with a high risk of morbidity and recurrence, possibly due to the spilling of cyst content during the operation. In the 1970s, Saidi developed a special cone, which was frozen to the cyst in order to reduce the risk of spilling cyst contents. This cone also simplified the disinfection of the cyst cavity [105]. Recently, this old treatment, also known as the 'frozen seal method', was evaluated in a non-endemic area and it was concluded to be an effective surgical treatment for hepatic hydatid disease [104]. In this retrospective study, 112 consecutive patients were treated surgically with the 'frozen seal' method for hydatid disease between 1981 and 2007. Recurrence rate was observed in 9 (8%) patients and morbidity occurred in twenty patients (17.9%). More importantly, no mortality was observed in this study of more than 25 years of surgically treated 'echinococcosis'. It was concluded that this surgical method used in the past century was still safe and effective in the new millennium. This technique is especially useful in non-endemic areas as it provides high efficacy and low morbidity rates.

Apart from the 'frozen-seal method', surgical treatment options may vary from conservative treatment (cystectomy) to radical treatment (complete open resection) to laparoscopic techniques. The debate on best surgical treatment is still ongoing: should this be conservative surgery or radical surgery in which the cyst is totally removed including the pericyst by total pericystectomy or partial hepatectomy or should it be the open or laparoscopic approach [101, 102].

4.2. Percutaneous treatments

With the introduction of antihelmintic drugs, new possibilities for treatment arose. By using this medication, the risk of anaphylaxis became smaller and percutaneous treatments were developed. One of these treatments for hydatid disease is PAIR: Percutaneous Aspiration, Injection and Re-aspiration. In a recent meta-analysis of operative versus non-operative treatment (PAIR) of hepatic echinococcosis [92], PAIR plus chemotherapy proved to be superior compared to surgery. The meta-analysis showed that PAIR was associated with improved efficacy, lower rates of morbidity, mortality, disease recurrence and shorter hospital stay [92].

In conclusion, the main treatment options for hepatic cystic echinococcosis are threefold: medical therapy, surgery and percutaneous drainage (Puncture Aspiration Injection and Reaspiration, also known as PAIR) or a combination of these therapies [91, 92, 100]. In the last revision of the WHO IWGE it was stated that surgery remains the cornerstone of treatment of hydatid disease, since it has the potential to remove the hydatid cyst and lead to complete cure. However, it is advised to evaluate surgical treatment carefully against other less invasive options such as percutaneous interventions. [88]

5. Improvements in pre-operative planning

An important way to improve the outcome in liver surgery is to prevent liver resection related complications. One of the main feared complications in liver surgery remains postresectional liver failure. This major complication may occur if the extent of tumour involvement requires major liver resection (3 or more segments), leaving a small postoperative remnant liver [3, 106, 107]. Due to impaired liver function this may even result in mortality. Obviously, limiting the liver resection, in order to leave enough liver remnant volume for proper function of the liver, can prevent this. However, major hepatectomies are performed increasingly often, mainly because indications for liver resection are continuously being extended. Former contraindications such as bilobar disease, number of metastases and even extrahepatic disease have been abandoned gradually and compromised liver function may be expected after aggressive induction chemotherapy. Consequently, postoperative remnant liver volume and function have become the main determinants of respectability [108-110]. In order to improve outcome in extended resections and thus to prevent postoperative liver failure after liver resection, a reliable volumetric assessment of the part of the liver to be resected as well as future residual liver volume should be a critical part of preoperative evaluation particularly. The safety of liver resection may increase if an estimate of minimal remnant liver volume is obtained via CT-volumetry [106, 111].

The utility of existing professional image-processing software is often limited by costs, lack of flexibility and specific hardware requirements such as coupling to a CT-scanner. In addition, the intended operation should be known to the investigator to predict the remnant liver volume accurately and requires the expertise of a liver surgeon. Therefore, CT-volumetry has hitherto been a multidisciplinary modality requiring the efforts of dedicated surgeons and radiologists and expensive software. Prospective CT-volumetric analysis of the liver on a Personal Computer performed by the operating surgeon in patients undergoing major liver would greatly enhance this preoperative assessment. ImageJ is a free, open-source Java-based image processing software programme developed by the National Institute of Health (NIH) and may be used for this purpose [112]. OsiriX® is Apple's version for image analysis and has been tested for CT volumetry of the liver [113]. It is also a freely available, user-friendly software system, which can be used for virtual liver resections and volumetric analysis [113].

As more major liver resections are performed, it is becoming more important to perform liver volumetry. Recently, these two open source image processing software packages were investigated to measure prospectively the remnant liver volume in order to reduce the risk of post-resectional liver failure. Volumes of total liver, tumour and future resection specimen of the included patients were measured preoperatively with ImageJ and OsiriX by two surgeons and a surgical trainee [114]. Results were compared with the actual weights of resected specimens and the measurements of the radiologist using professional CT scanner-linked Aquarius iNtuition® software. It was concluded that the prospective hepatic CT-volumetry with ImageJ or OsiriX® was reliable and can be accurately used on a Personal Computer by non-radiologists. ImageJ and OsiriX® yield results comparable to professional radiological software iNtuition®.

6. Minimally invasive surgery

To minimize the damage of treatment, laparoscopic surgery was introduced to avoid large incisions for many gastrointestinal operations in the previous century. After the first laparoscopic cholecystectomy in 1987 [115], the number of indications for this minimally invasive approach increased. The outcome has encouraged surgeons to develop a laparoscopic technique for many procedures including liver resections [116]. Although this type of surgery is technically more demanding and thereby time-consuming [117, 118], it proved to be beneficial for patients with less pain and better recovery compared to open liver surgery [119-121].

6.1. The history of laparoscopic surgery

The fundamentals of laparoscopic surgery were laid down in the early twentieth century when the German surgeon Kelling reported on the endoscopic visualization of the peritoneal cavity in an anesthetized dog using a Nitze cystoscope (1887) in 1902 [122]. Following the introduction of endoscopic inspection of the abdominal contents in an animal model, fellow countryman Jacobeus started experimenting with laparoscopy in human cadavers as well asliving humans. In 1911 he reported on 80 laparoscopic examinations of the abdominal cavity [123, 124]. In the years thereafter the laparoscopic approach was enhanced with the introduction of illumination techniques, advancement in lens systems, the use of more than one single trocar and induction of pneumoperitoneum (Goetze and Veress). The era of therapeutic laparoscopy was then born, making it possible to minimize damage of treatment and avoid large incisions for many gastrointestinal operations. However, it was not until 1987 that the first laparoscopic cholecystectomy was performed [115].

At first, liver surgery was thought to be unsuitable for laparoscopic techniques since it might impose the risk of gas embolisms and major blood loss during transection of the liver. Also, sceptics pointed out the suspected risk of trocar site metastases in skin incisions. Gradually, as some expert centres progressively reported feasibility and safety, it became more popular.

This novel approach for liver resections was introduced during the 1990s. At first the procedure was only used for diagnostic laparoscopies and liver biopsies, later indications were extended to fenestration of liver cysts and anatomic liver resections. In 1992, Gagner et al. reported the first laparoscopic wedge resection of the liver. Only three years later, Cuesta et al. were the first to perform two cases of limited laparoscopic liver surgery of segment II and IV in the Netherlands [125]. The first laparoscopic left lateral bisegmentectomy of the liver was performed by the group of Azagra [126]. Since then, several studies have reported the feasibility

http://dx.doi.org/10.5772/54710

and safety of laparoscopic resections for liver tumours in centres with extensive experience in both hepatobiliary surgery and laparoscopic surgery [116, 117, 127-130].

However, after its introduction, laparoscopic liver resection remained challenging because of the difficulties concerning safe mobilization and exposure of this fragile and heavy organ. Therefore, in the beginning only superficial and peripheral lesions in anterolateral segments were selected for the laparosopic approach. In recent times, centres with extensive experience in laparoscopy and hepatic surgery have also performed major hepatic resections laparoscopically with satisfactory outcomes. Importantly, no evidence of a compromised oncological clearance in laparoscopic liver resection has hitherto been found [120]

6.2. Advantages of the laparoscopic technique

The laparoscopic approach is said to have shifted the pain of the patient to the surgeon, as the latter had to obtain new operative skills and more demanding techniques. In fact laparoscopic surgery is a totally different concept of surgery. The conventional three-dimensional field is inherently two-dimensional, and the tactile feedback is impaired as compared to open surgery. Moreover, a full ambidexterity is required, as well as the skills to manipulate fragile structures with long instruments under minimal tactile feedback. Also, the surgeon becomes even more dependent on his team and instruments, as he will need experienced assistance for traction and camerawork and needs to trust the material even more compared to open surgery. For patients the most important presumed advantages of the laparoscopic procedure are reduced blood loss [119, 120], less postoperative pain [118, 127, 131], earlier functional recovery [127, 130], shorter postoperative hospital stay [118, 120, 121, 127, 130-132] and improved cosmetic aspects [127, 130]. Reoperations are reported to be easier due to reduced adhesions [127, 130-132]. Also, open-close procedures with large incisions can be avoided if peritoneal metastases are detected at laparoscopy.

However, up till now no randomised controlled trials comparing the open and laparoscopic liver resection technique have been reported. This may well be one of the reasons why many surgeons remained reluctant to incorporate this new laparoscopic approach. The currently available evidence is primarily based on case-series and identifies a technique that is reproducible with limited morbidity and mortality. In a consensus statement on laparoscopic liver resections, Buell J et al [133] concluded that resection of segments 2 and 3 by the laparoscopic approach should be the standard of care. In that same year a large international study reported comparable encouraging results concerning the superiority of laparoscopic liver resections in terms of complications from 109 patients: the complication rate was only 12% and there were no perioperative deaths [134]. Median hospital length of stay was 4 days. Negative margins were achieved in 94.4% of patients.

Overall survival rates and disease-free survival rates for the entire series were 50% and 43% at 5-year respectively. It was concluded that laparoscopic liver resection for colorectal metastases was safe, feasible and comparable to open liver resection for both minor and major liver resections in oncologic surgery. This is confirmed in a recent meta-analysis on short and long-term outcomes after laparoscopic and open resection. This study included a total of 26 studies, incorporating a population of 1678 patients [135]. Although laparoscopic liver resections resulted in longer operation time, most endpoints were superior for the laparoscopic approach compared with open resection, including reduced blood loss, portal clamp time, overall and liver specific complications, ileus and length of hospital stay. As for the long-term outcomes, no difference was found for oncologic outcomes between the laparoscopic and open surgical techniques. Therefore, it was concluded that the laparoscopic liver resection was a feasible alternative to open surgery in experienced hands [135].

7. Enhanced Recovery After Surgery (ERAS) or fast-track liver surgery

Another recent development in elective liver surgery is the introduction of Enhanced Recovery After Surgery (ERAS) programmes, also referred to as fast track perioperative care. These multimodal enhanced recovery programmes proved to be beneficial in open colonic and liver surgery [136, 137]. The multimodal recovery programme is evidence based and combines several interventions in perioperative care to reduce the stress response and organ dysfunction with a focus on enhancing recovery [137, 138]. In patients undergoing colorectal surgery, the ERAS® programme enabled earlier recovery and consequently shorter length of hospital stay [137-140]. Also, reduction of postoperative morbidity in patients undergoing intestinal resection was reported [141-144]. In other fields of elective surgery similar programmes have also shown a reduction in hospital stay of several days [145, 146].

One of the pioneers of the fast track colonic surgery is the Danish surgeon Henrik Kehlet. He treated 60 consecutive patients with colonic resection in a fast track surgery programme and reported a median postoperative hospital stay of 2 days. At that time, patients undergoing a colonic resection usually required 5 to 10 days postoperative hospital stay [147, 148]. Previously, he stressed the importance of a multimodal approach in order to improve rehabilitation after surgery (figure 6) [149]. This rehabilitation programme after surgery combined a number of interventions to reduce stress of the surgical intervention, risk of organ dysfunction and loss of functional capacity. Stress induced organ dysfunction, pain, nausea and vomiting, ileus, hypoxemia and sleep disturbances, immobilisation and semi-starvation had to be reduced.

Factors were identified that contribute to postoperative functional deterioration. These were actually traditional postoperative care principles such as use of drains, nasogastric tubes, fasting regimes and bed rest. Kehlet initiated a multimodal programme that abandoned the traditional care principles and introduced innovations such as: carbohydrate loading before surgery, regional anaesthetic techniques, maintenance of normal temperature during surgery, minimally invasive or laparoscopic surgical techniques, optimal treatment of postoperative pain and prophylaxis of nausea and vomiting [139, 150]. This programme improved postoperative recovery, physical performance and pulmonary function and reduced hospital length of stay [142].

In collaboration with Kehlet, the Enhanced Recovery After Surgery (ERAS) group was initiated to investigate the perioperative care in four other hospitals (Royal Infirmary, Edinburgh, UK, The Karolinska Institutet at Ersta Hospital, Stockholm, Sweden, the University Hospital of Nothern Norway, Tromso, Noway and Maastricht University Medical Centre) [151]. Thus,

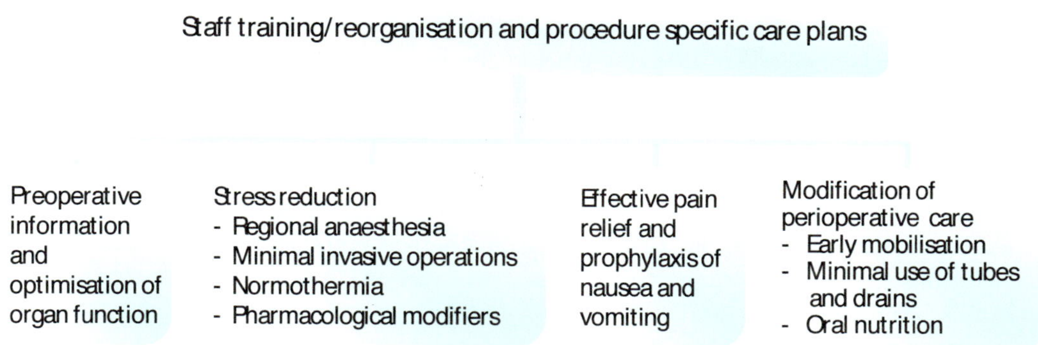

Figure 6. Multimodal interventions may lead to a reduction in postoperative morbidity and improved recovery. [149] Figure adapted with kind permission from Kehlet *et al.* 1997.

with Kehlet's programme as a starting point, a new evidence based programme was developed incorporating different aspects leading to faster recovery. Preoperative counselling, perioperative intravenous fluid restriction, optimal pain relief preferably without the use of opioid analgesia, early oral nutrition, enforced mobilisation, no nasogastric tubes and no drains are the key elements of this protocol (figure 7). Since the colonic programme showed improvements in recovery, the liver surgeons of the ERAS® group (Maastricht, Edinburgh and Tromso) set up an ERAS-programme for every patient undergoing open liver resection [136] (www.erassociety.org).

So far, the ERAS programmes have shown promising results with respect to improved recovery and outcome in open elective colorectal and liver surgery [136, 137]. One of the first studies on ERAS for liver surgery showed that the majority of patients treated within this multimodal enhanced recovery programme tolerated fluid within four hours of surgery and a normal diet one day after surgery. As an effect of the accelerated functional recovery, these patients were discharged two days earlier than the patients treated with traditional care, without significant differences in readmission, morbidity and mortality rates [136].

These results were confirmed in a recent systematic review including seven studies on fast-track programmes for hepatopancreatic resections, incorporating more than 550 patients treated in fast track setting [152]. This study showed that the primary hospital stay was reduced significantly after the introduction of a multimodal perioperative care programme for open liver surgery [152]. Moreover, there were no significant differences in rates of readmission, morbidity and mortality.

7.1. Synergy of ERAS and laparoscopic liver surgery

For solid tumours in the liver, the open approach for resection is gradually replaced by the laparoscopic technique in many expert centres worldwide. The results, mostly from cohort studies, suggest benefits with notably shorter postoperative stay [120]. Recently, the added value of a fast-track ERAS-programme in laparoscopic liver surgery specifically has been elucidated [153]. A group consisting of patients undergoing laparoscopic liver resections in an ERAS-setting was compared with historical data from consecutive laparoscopic liver resections performed either in that same centre before the introduction of the ERAS-programme or in other major liver centres in the Netherlands performing laparoscopic liver surgery in a traditional perioperative care programme.

- A significant difference with a median of two days in time to full functional recovery was observed between the ERAS-treated group and the traditional care group. The difference in median hospital length of stay (LOS) of two days between these two groups did not attain significance. The authors suggested that it was probably due to the small number of patients in this multicentre pilot-study. Apart from faster functional recovery in patients in the enhanced recovery group, this study also showed reduced blood loss in this group.
- As from a historical perspective, this multicentre fast-track laparoscopic liver resection study was the first study to explore the effect of ERAS and laparoscopic surgery. This small study suggests that a multimodal enhanced recovery programme for laparoscopic liver surgery is feasible, safe and may lead to accelerated functional recovery and reduction in length of hospital stay. With these findings it may be concluded that the additional effect of ERAS leads to an improvement of liver surgery and outcome.

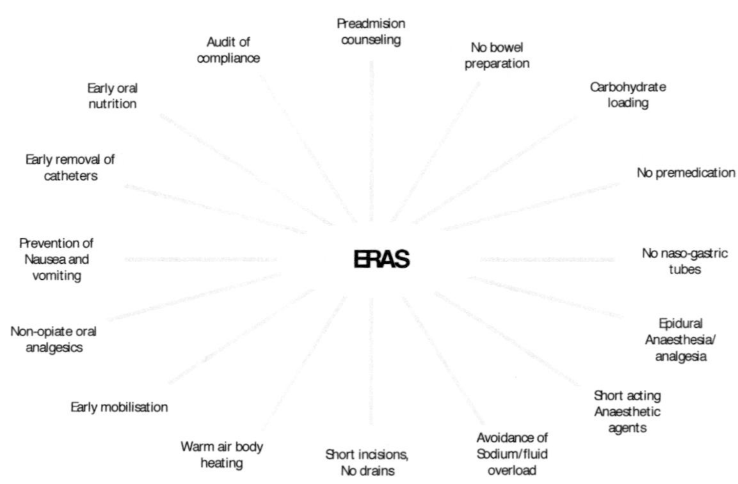

Figure 7. Important elements of the Enhanced Recovery After Surgery programme. [138] Figure adapted with kind permission from Fearon *et al.* 2005.

8. Recent developments in hepatic malignancies

As for the recent developments in the treatment of liver diseases, these can be mainly divided into surgical and non-surgical treatment modalities. Developments in surgical treatment can be divided in true surgical and perioperative care improvements. The focus is on the surgical treatments in this chapter, but some thoughts will also be spent on the non-surgical treatment modalities, an interesting and expanding field of expertise.

For malignant liver tumours, the majority of which are colorectal liver metastases, the main concern is the resectability if colorectal cancer is diagnosed. Colorectal cancer is one of the most common causes of cancer related death worldwide [38] and more than half of patients with colorectal cancer will develop liver metastases [39]. Unfortunately, only 20% of the patients can be treated with surgical resection of these liver metastases [154]. The remaining 80% of the patients present with lesions, which are not suitable for a safe resection. This can be caused by large diameters of the lesions, location of the lesion near vascular and biliary structures and extrahepatic disease. Also, the number of lesions can be the cause of non-resectability: resection can only be carried out safely if 25-30% of functioning liver remains after resection [155]. The non-surgical treatment by means of chemotherapy for the patients with unresected liver metastases has proven very successful in decreasing the size and number of liver lesions. It was shown that new chemotherapy regimens could change the previously unresectable liver metastases into resectable liver disease [156]. With neoadjuvant chemotherapy more patients with colorectal liver metastases can be offered a treatment with curative intent [156]. It was concluded that neoadjuvant chemotherapy enables liver resection in some patients with initially unresectable colorectal metastases. Long-term survival proved to be similar to that reported for a priori surgical candidates [56]. As for the future perspective of chemotherapy, neoadjuvant treatment will improve curability and long-term survival for selected patients.

Other non-surgical therapies for malignant liver disease are external irradiation (whole liver irradiation) [157, 158], stereotactic liver irradiation [159-162] and injectable small radioactive particles that irradiate the tumours within the liver (e.g. Yttrium-90(^{90}Y) radio-embolisation [163, 164], radioactive holmium microspheres [165, 166]). These modalities may have curative potential but future studies have to be awaited. Another attractive field of development are the thermal ablative therapies for unresectable liver metastases. These ablative thermal therapies can be used either percutaneously or in adjunct with surgery and have shown to decrease focal liver lesions [167-170]. Microwave ablation is a tumour destruction method to treat patients with unresectable liver lesions [169]. It can be used with a single insertion of the probe and it was shown to be a safe and effective method for treating unresectable hepatic tumours, with a low rate of local recurrence [170]. Overall survival is comparable to alternative ablation modalities [169].

8.1. Future perspectives

As for surgical treatments, different treatment strategies have been developed to increase the number of patients suitable for surgery as described earlier. Current research has focussed on improving resectability in terms of the quantity of resected liver tissue, but at the same time studies focussed on reducing perioperative distress in patients undergoing liver resections by multimodal perioperative treatment protocols and minimally invasive surgery. Since the introduction of laparoscopic liver surgery in 1992, more liver resections have been performed with this minimally invasive approach for primary and secondary malignant liver lesions [129,

134, 153]. For future perspectives, some gain might be expected from even less invasive modalities as the first reports on single incision laparoscopic resections have been presented [171-173]. Also, a two-stage laparoscopic approach for malignant liver disease and the robotic approach for liver resections have been published [174-176].

As discussed previously in this chapter, the recent developments in liver surgery include the introduction of laparoscopic surgery and enhanced recovery programmes, which focus on improvement of postoperative recovery and/or shorter hospital length of stay. A significantly accelerated recovery after open liver resection was previously reported if patients were managed within a multimodal ERAS protocol. Median hospital length of stay was reduced from 8 to 6 days (25%) [136]. Moreover, since there was a delay between recovery and discharge of the patients a further reduction of stay should be possible. Regarding the results of previous, non-randomised randomized studies and case series, it seems that laparoscopic left lateral liver sectionectomy is associated with shorter hospital length of stay, less postoperative pain, better quality of life and a faster recovery [177]. In most trials aiming at a reduction of hospital length of stay, surgery and/or perioperative management are not standardised. No randomised trials have hitherto been reported to study the added value of ERAS and/or laparoscopy for liver surgery. There is a need for a randomised controlled trial covering these aspects of improving the recovery and outcome of liver surgery.

9. Liver transplantation

Liver transplantation surgery is one of the main advances in hepatic surgery. Until recently, it was considered to be too complex, since artificial organ support, like haemodialysis in renal failure, was considered impossible. The term liver transplantation was first used in an article of Welch (NY, USA) in 1955 [178]. The first experimental liver transplantation surgery was performed on animals (dogs) in the 1950s and 1960s by Starzl (Denver, USA, figure 8) and Moore (Boston, USA). These transplantations failed as a result of the stagnation of blood in the mesenterial vessels and a lack of blood flow to the heart after clamping the inferior vena cava. Methods for a venovenous bypass to the superior vena cava were developed, whereupon transplantation seemed to be realizable. Despite the fact that immunosuppressive drugs became available at that time, most grafts were rejected though. As a result, only a few dogs survived [178-181].

9.1. The history of liver transplantation in humans

In 1963 the first three orthotropic liver transplantations in humans were performed by Starzl and colleagues. All livers came from non-heart beating donors (NHBDs). Although the first transplantation was performed in one session, the second and third took two sessions; the first session was designated for the preparation of the removal of the liver from the donor and in the second session the liver was removed and transplanted in the recipient after the donor died. In the donor patient extracorporeal perfusion was performed via the femoral vein and artery. The structures in the hepatoduodenal ligament were cut through and the liver was

http://dx.doi.org/10.5772/54710

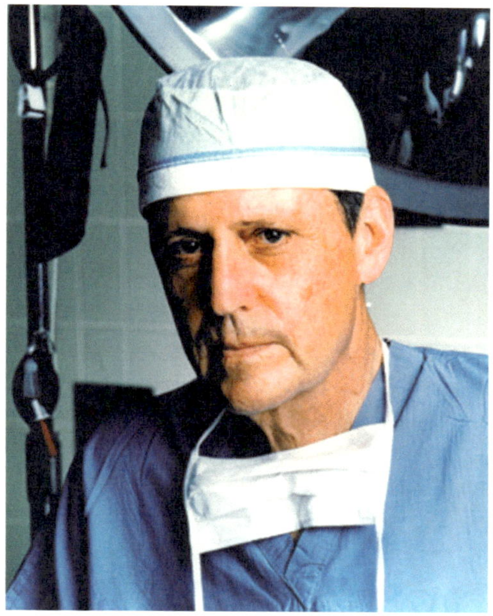

Figure 8. Thomas E. Starzl (1926).

taken out with the vena cava. In the recipient the liver was taken out likewise and a venovenous bypass was made to circumvent the hemodynamic effects of clamping the vena cava [182]. Immunosuppressive therapy, by ways of azathioprine and prednisone, was applied since these drugs were proven to be effective in renal transplantation [183]. The first patient was a three-year-old boy with biliary atresia who died during the operation due to haemorrhage, the second and third patient were adult males suffering from liver cancer who died 7 and 22 days postoperative, as a result of lung embolism [182]. Starzl then decided to take a break to have a period of reflection. Four years later, in 1967, he decided to try again and he then performed the first successful liver transplantation with a one-year-survival [184].

Infections were frequently occurring complications [185]. The most important complication of these early transplantations however, was severe blood loss. This was caused by manipulation of abdominal veins which had been under great pressures due to chronic liver diseases [179]. The first orthotropic liver transplantation in Europe was performed in Cambridge in 1968 by Calne [186]. In the same year consensus was achieved concerning the concept of cerebral death. From that moment on, heart-beating donation with donor organs originating from heart beating, brain dead donors was possible [184]. Nowadays the above described venovenous bypass has been abandoned in many centres in Europe. Since the beginning of the 1990's most centres use the so called 'piggyback' technique. The liver is exposed from the vena cava after which the vena cava is partially clamped longitudinally. After the liver has been flushed with albumin to remove ischemic waste products, a side-to-side cavocaval anastomosis is made. In doing so, the hemodynamic stability of the patient is guaranteed. Then, the portal liaison is made by an end-to-end anastomosis, the liver is perfused and the arterial anastomosis is made. Finally the biliary ducts are connected by way of end-to-end anastomosis and in case of sclerosis a Roux-en-Y-reconstruction [187, 188].

9.2. Immunsuppressive drugs

The discovery and appliance of immunosuppressive medication to prevent graft rejection has been an important development in transplantation surgery. Despite the fact that graft rejection has been a serious problem during the early years of liver transplantation, many transplanted patients survived more than 20 years as a result of this immunosuppressive therapy with an azathioprine-prednisone cocktail. Some time later, a third immunosuppressive drug, antilymphocyte-globulin (ALG), was added to the therapy [178, 189, 190]. Then Calne discovered the possibility to use cyclosporin A, a calcineurin inhibitor, as an immunosuppressive drug [191]. After cyclosporine A was first used in renal transplantations in 1980 [192], it was then applied in liver transplantation and the one-year-survival rate in liver transplantation turned out to have increased to 80% [193]. Currently Tacrolimus (FK 506), also a calcineurin inhibitor, is recommended [194-197]. A detailed overview of the development and the working mechanisms of immunosuppressive drugs is beyond the scope of this chapter.

9.3. Split liver transplantation

The concept of liver transplantation has been developed gradually, which made it a widely accepted treatment with an increasing number of indications and good survival rates. This caused a shortage of donor organs, especially among children, and long waiting lists. New techniques had to be developed to answer to this growing demand. In 1984 Bismuth developed the reduced-size adult liver transplantation; an adult left lobe was transplanted into a child. This is a unique method, only applicable in liver transplantation surgery because of its segmental anatomy with independently functioning parts [198]. Further development of segmental liver surgery resulted in the split liver transplantation (SLT); the donor liver is splitted, the left part (segment 2 and 3 with the common hepatic duct and common hepatic artery) is transplanted into a child and the right part (segment 1, 4-7 with the vena cava) into an adult. In the recipient of the left liver part, the vena cava is preserved and an anastomosis is made with the left hepatic vein. The other anastomoses are made in the usual way. In the recipient of the right liver part, an anastomosis is made between the right hepatic artery of the donor liver and the common hepatic artery of the recipient by means of a saphenous vein interposition graft. Two intrahepatic biliary ducts are connected with the jejunum through a Roux-en-Y loop, the other anastomosis are executed in the usual way [199]. There are two ways of splitting the liver, in situ and ex situ, both with its (dis)advantages. The main disadvantage of in situ splitting is a longer operation time and therefore the need for a haemodynamically stable patient. Splitting ex situ on the other hand, is done in blood vacuum. The time of cold ischemia is longer and it is harder to distinguish structures from each other. Hence, strict donor selection is essential and there is a trend to only select donors <50 years or who are heamodynamically stable. Bile spill is reported as the most common complication. Other complications are an insufficient hepatic artery, portal vein thrombosis, intra-abdominal haemorrhage and gastro-intestinal bleeding. Mortality rates of 11% have been reported [200, 201]. In Europe, in 2003, 89% of all liver transplantations consisted of full-size transplantations, 4% of SLT's and 5% of reduced-liver transplantations. In specialized centres, the survival rates of these techniques are comparable to the survival rates of regular transplantation [202].

9.4. Living-donor liver transplantation (LDLT)

In 1987 Raia (Brazil) developed the living-donor liver transplantation (LDLT) from an adult into a child. The operation itself was successful, but the recipient child died due to a transfusion reaction [203]. The first successful LDLT from mother to son with a left liver lobe was performed in Australia by Strong [204] after which this method was refined by many other pioneers. It is a very difficult operation technique in which precise knowledge of the anatomy is a prerequisite. Because of a great shortage of donor organs in Asia, most experience with the LDLT was gained there. Innovative surgery was the only possibility to tide over this shortage. These techniques seemed to be effective; waiting-list-related mortality among children was reduced to almost 0% [205, 206]. Since Fan (Honk Kong) introduced the adult-to-adult living liver transplantation with a hemi-liver (dependent on the size of donor and recipient either the right or left lobe is transplanted) in 1997, the availability of donor livers for adults increased [207].

The main advantage of LDLT is limitation of warm ischemia because operations can be planned simultaneously [208]. The results of LDLT are comparable to those of regular (orthotopic) liver transplantation. According to the Japanese Liver Transplantation Society the 5-year-survival rate in adults is 69%. In children this rate is significantly higher with 83% [205]. In the USA the reported survival rate in adults is 80% [209]. In Europe, a 5-year-survival of 75% (80% in children, 66% in adults) between 1991 and 2001 was reported [202, 205]. In Europe, in 2003, only 1.6% of all liver transplantations consisted of LDLT [202].

The main disadvantages of this technique are the potential complications in the healthy donor and the psychological impact [189, 210]. The number of postoperative complications in donors is reported to be 20%. Worldwide 10 (0.15%) donor deaths have been reported. The mortality rate in Europe, in 2010, was 0.2% (6/2906) [211]. The critical period for death and primary dysfunction is within 6 months from the operation. In a graft too small for the recipient, dysfunction will develop with hyperbilirubinemia, ascites and liver function failure resulting in coagulation disorders and renal failure. A graft which is too big for the recipient will result in necrosis because of shortage in blood supply. Besides good patient selection, proper calculation to determine the correct graft size has to be done to prevent these complications [189, 205].

9.5. Improving survival

In 1997 the Institute of Medicine (USA) declared NHBD-organs to be medically effective and ethically acceptable [178]. From that time on, the trend exists to use NHBD- and marginal organs (livers with steatosis) again to tide over the shortage of donor organs and shorten the waiting lists. Marginal livers are associated with primary non-function [212]. The main problem of NHBD's is the prolonged period of warm ischemia. A distinction between controlled NHBD's (Maastricht type I and II) and uncontrolled NHBD's (Maastricht type III and IV) is made. Controlled NHBD's provide organs with less chance on ischemic damage and a greater chance on good post-transplantation function. In this group of patients a controlled end of vital support takes place after which a circulation stop occurs. In most cases the patient is already in the operation theatre with a transplantation team on site. This way, the time of warm ischemia is minimalised. In uncontrolled NHBD's a non-foreseen circulation stop occurs, usually before arrival in the hospital, possibly followed by resuscitation. A variable period of warm ischemia occurs with a higher chance on complications [212, 213]. Cold ischemia causes damage of sinusoidal endothelial cells and warm ischemia of hepatocytes [214]. Besides, warm ischemia intensifies the effects of cold ischemia and predisposes for a higher incidence of ischemic biliary structures both on the short and the long term. In such cases, re-transplantation might be needed [215]. Since the University of Wisconsin Solution, introduced in 1988, has become the golden standard for cooling donor organs and the maximum period of cold ischemia has been limited to 12 hours, ischemic damage due to cold ischemia has been reduced drastically with increased graft survival [202]. However, as a consequence of warm ischemia graft survival is lower in NHBD's compared to heart-beating donors with a 3-year-survival of 63.3% versus 72.1%. The risk of primary non-function is also significantly higher among NHBD's: 11.8% versus 6.4% [189, 216]. For this reason NHBD's can be used to overcome organ shortage, on condition that strict criteria are maintained: strict donor (<60 years) and recipient (haemodynamically stable and not intubated) selection, minor warm (<30 minutes) and cold (<8 hours) ischemia, no extensive steatosis of the donor liver and the use of at most one inotropic drug (to prevent hypotension and thus hypoperfusion) [212].

With the gradual progression in surgical competences, management of postoperative complications and the development of immunosuppressive drugs to prevent graft rejection, liver transplantation has nowadays become a widely accepted treatment for an increasing number of indications and it has become the golden standard for patients with irreversible decompensated chronic liver failure (e.g. as a result of cirrhosis or hepatocellular cancer) and acute liver failure (e.g. as a result of hepatic viruses or intoxication with medication). In the early days cancer was the most common indication for liver transplantation. In Europe, however, with 50% the most important indication for liver transplantation was cirrhosis (of which 24% was caused by a virus (especially Hepatitis C) and 18% by alcohol abuse), followed by pathology of the biliary tract (13%), primary liver tumours (10%), of which hepatocellular cancer is the most common, and acute liver failure (9%), with fulminant viral hepatitis as the most important cause. The most important indications in children are biliary atresia (56%) and metabolic diseases (21%) [202]. Due to the development of different methods and techniques, organ shortage has been reduced and waiting lists have been shortened. Hence, one can conclude that liver transplantation is a recent and very important advancement, which has expanded in a short time. It is a perfect example of modern and innovative medical practice, in which the challenge remains to find solutions to new problems time after time.

http://dx.doi.org/10.5772/54710

Author details

J.H.M.B. Stoot[1,2,3*], R.J.S. Coelen[1,2], J.L.A. van Vugt[2] and C.H.C. Dejong[1,4]

*Address all correspondence to: jan@stoot.com

1 Department of Surgery, Maastricht University Medical Centre, Maastricht, The Netherlands

2 Department of Surgery, Orbis Medical Centre, Sittard, The Netherlands

3 Department of Surgery, Atrium Medical Centre, Heerlen, The Netherlands

4 NUTRIM School for Nutrition, Metabolism and Toxicology, Maastricht University Medical Centre, Maastricht, The Netherlands

References

[1] Poon, R. T, et al. Improving perioperative outcome expands the role of hepatectomy in management of benign and malignant hepatobiliary diseases: analysis of 1222 consecutive patients from a prospective database. Ann Surg, (2004). discussion 708-10., 698-708.

[2] Cescon, M, et al. Trends in perioperative outcome after hepatic resection: analysis of 1500 consecutive unselected cases over 20 years. Ann Surg, (2009). , 995-1002.

[3] Jarnagin, W. R, et al. Improvement in perioperative outcome after hepatic resection: analysis of 1,803 consecutive cases over the past decade. Ann Surg, (2002). discussion 406-7., 397-406.

[4] Tsao, J. I, et al. Trends in morbidity and mortality of hepatic resection for malignancy. A matched comparative analysis. Ann Surg, (1994). , 199-205.

[5] Foster, J. H. History of liver surgery. Arch Surg, (1991). , 381-387.

[6] Glisson, F. Anatomia Hepatis. London, England, 1654.

[7] Cantlie, J. On a new arrangement of the right and left lobes of the liver. J. Anat. Physiol., (1898). , 4-9.

[8] Hardy, K. J. Liver surgery: the past 2000 years. Aust N Z J Surg, (1990). , 811-817.

[9] Pringle, J. H. V. Notes on the Arrest of Hepatic Hemorrhage Due to Trauma. Ann Surg, (1908). , 541-549.

[10] Couinaud, C. Le Foie. Etudes anatomiques et chirurgicales. Paris: Masson, (1957).

[11] Guyton, A, & Hall, J. The liver as an organ, in Textbook of Medical Physiology(1996). Philadelphia: WB Saunders. , 883-888.

[12] Taub, R. Liver regeneration: from myth to mechanism. Nat Rev Mol Cell Biol, (2004). , 836-847.

[13] van de PollM.C., et al., Effect of major liver resection on hepatic ureagenesis in humans. Am J Physiol Gastrointest Liver Physiol, (2007). , G956-G962.

[14] Lortat-jacob, J. L, Robert, H. G, & Henry, C. Excision of the right lobe of the liver for a malignant secondary tumor]. Arch Mal Appar Dig Mal Nutr, (1952). , 662-667.

[15] Foster, J. H, & Berman, M. M. Solid liver tumors. Major Probl Clin Surg, (1977). , 1-342.

[16] Ekberg, H, et al. Determinants of survival in liver resection for colorectal secondaries. Br J Surg, (1986). , 727-731.

[17] Adson, M. A, et al. Resection of hepatic metastases from colorectal cancer. Arch Surg, (1984). , 647-651.

[18] Simmonds, P. C, et al. Surgical resection of hepatic metastases from colorectal cancer: a systematic review of published studies. Br J Cancer, (2006). , 982-999.

[19] Iwatsuki, S, Shaw, B. W, & Jr, T. E. Starzl, Experience with 150 liver resections. Ann Surg, (1983). , 247-253.

[20] Bismuth, H, Houssin, D, & Castaing, D. Major and minor segmentectomies "reglees" in liver surgery. World J Surg, (1982). , 10-24.

[21] Bismuth, H. Surgical anatomy and anatomical surgery of the liver. World J Surg, (1982). , 3-9.

[22] Tung, T. T. Les resections majeures et mineures du foie. Paris: Masson, (1979).

[23] Billingsley, K. G, et al. Segment-oriented hepatic resection in the management of malignant neoplasms of the liver. J Am Coll Surg, (1998). , 471-481.

[24] Fan, S. T, et al. Hepatectomy for hepatocellular carcinoma: toward zero hospital deaths. Ann Surg, (1999). , 322-330.

[25] Farid, H, & Connell, T. O. Hepatic resections: changing mortality and morbidity. Am Surg, (1994). , 748-752.

[26] Poon, R. T. Recent advances in techniques of liver resection. Surg Technol Int, (2004). , 71-77.

[27] Adam, R, et al. Patients with initially unresectable colorectal liver metastases: is there a possibility of cure? J Clin Oncol, (2009). , 1829-1835.

[28] Tomlinson, J. S, et al. Actual 10-year survival after resection of colorectal liver metastases defines cure. J Clin Oncol, (2007). , 4575-4580.

[29] Charny, C. K, et al. Management of 155 patients with benign liver tumours. Br J Surg, (2001). , 808-813.

[30] Poon, R. T. Current techniques of liver transection. HPB (Oxford), (2007). , 166-173.

[31] Aragon, R. J, & Solomon, N. L. Techniques of hepatic resection. J Gastrointest Oncol, (2012). , 28-40.

[32] Gurusamy, K. S, et al. Techniques for liver parenchymal transection in liver resection. Cochrane Database Syst Rev, (2009). , CD006880.

[33] Palavecino, M, et al. Two-surgeon technique of parenchymal transection contributes to reduced transfusion rate in patients undergoing major hepatectomy: analysis of 1,557 consecutive liver resections. Surgery, (2010). , 40-48.

[34] Pamecha, V, et al. Techniques for liver parenchymal transection: a meta-analysis of randomized controlled trials. HPB (Oxford), (2009). , 275-281.

[35] Rahbari, N. N, et al. Meta-analysis of the clamp-crushing technique for transection of the parenchyma in elective hepatic resection: back to where we started? Ann Surg Oncol, (2009). , 630-639.

[36] Koo, B. N, et al. Hepatic resection by the Cavitron Ultrasonic Surgical Aspirator increases the incidence and severity of venous air embolism. Anesth Analg, (2005). table of contents., 966-970.

[37] Rahbari, N. N, et al. Clamp-crushing versus stapler hepatectomy for transection of the parenchyma in elective hepatic resection (CRUNSH)--a randomized controlled trial (NCT01049607). BMC Surg, (2011). , 22.

[38] Boyle, P, & Leon, M. E. Epidemiology of colorectal cancer. Br Med Bull, (2002). , 1-25.

[39] Steele, G, & Jr, T. S. Ravikumar, Resection of hepatic metastases from colorectal cancer. Biologic perspective. Ann Surg, (1989). , 127-138.

[40] Manfredi, S, et al. Epidemiology and management of liver metastases from colorectal cancer. Ann Surg, (2006). , 254-259.

[41] Scheele, J, et al. Resection of colorectal liver metastases. World J Surg, (1995). , 59-71.

[42] Thirion, P, et al. Modulation of fluorouracil by leucovorin in patients with advanced colorectal cancer: an updated meta-analysis. J Clin Oncol, (2004). , 3766-3775.

[43] Mayo, S. C, et al. Surgical management of hepatic neuroendocrine tumor metastasis: results from an international multi-institutional analysis. Ann Surg Oncol, (2010). , 3129-3136.

[44] Rehders, A, et al. Hepatic metastasectomy for soft-tissue sarcomas: is it justified? World J Surg, (2009). , 111-117.

[45] Mondragon-sanchez, R, et al. Repeat hepatic resection for recurrent metastatic melanoma. Hepatogastroenterology, (1999). , 459-461.

[46] Pawlik, T. M, et al. Hepatic resection for metastatic melanoma: distinct patterns of recurrence and prognosis for ocular versus cutaneous disease. Ann Surg Oncol, (2006). , 712-720.

[47] Frenkel, S, et al. Long-term survival of uveal melanoma patients after surgery for liver metastases. Br J Ophthalmol, (2009). , 1042-1046.

[48] Karavias, D. D, et al. Liver resection for metastatic non-colorectal non-neuroendocrine hepatic neoplasms. Eur J Surg Oncol, (2002). , 135-139.

[49] Hirai, I, et al. Surgical management for metastatic liver tumors. Hepatogastroenterology, (2006). , 757-763.

[50] Makino, H, et al. Indication for hepatic resection in the treatment of liver metastasis from gastric cancer. Anticancer Res, (2010). , 2367-2376.

[51] Lermite, E, et al. Surgical resection of liver metastases from breast cancer. Surg Oncol, (2009). , e79-e84.

[52] Sakamoto, Y, et al. Hepatic resection for metastatic breast cancer: prognostic analysis of 34 patients. World J Surg, (2005). , 524-527.

[53] Figueras, J, et al. Effect of subcentimeter nonpositive resection margin on hepatic recurrence in patients undergoing hepatectomy for colorectal liver metastases. Evidences from 663 liver resections. Ann Oncol, (2007). , 1190-1195.

[54] Figueras, J, et al. Surgical resection of colorectal liver metastases in patients with expanded indications: a single-center experience with 501 patients. Dis Colon Rectum, (2007). , 478-488.

[55] Khatri, V. P, Petrelli, N. J, & Belghiti, J. Extending the frontiers of surgical therapy for hepatic colorectal metastases: is there a limit? J Clin Oncol, (2005). , 8490-8499.

[56] Adam, R, et al. Five-year survival following hepatic resection after neoadjuvant therapy for nonresectable colorectal. Ann Surg Oncol, (2001). , 347-353.

[57] Figueras, J, et al. Surgical treatment of liver metastases from colorectal carcinoma in elderly patients. When is it worthwhile? Clin Transl Oncol, (2007). , 392-400.

[58] Adam, R, et al. Liver resection of colorectal metastases in elderly patients. Br J Surg, (2010). , 366-376.

[59] De Haas, R. J, Wicherts, D. A, & Adam, R. Resection of colorectal liver metastases with extrahepatic disease. Dig Surg, (2008). , 461-466.

[60] Adam, R, et al. Is hepatic resection justified after chemotherapy in patients with colorectal liver metastases and lymph node involvement? J Clin Oncol, (2008). , 3672-3680.

[61] Wicherts, D. A, et al. Impact of portal vein embolization on long-term survival of patients with primarily unresectable colorectal liver metastases. Br J Surg, (2010). , 240-250.

[62] Choti, M. A, et al. Trends in long-term survival following liver resection for hepatic colorectal metastases. Ann Surg, (2002). , 759-766.

[63] De Haas, R. J, et al. R1 resection by necessity for colorectal liver metastases: is it still a contraindication to surgery? Ann Surg, (2008). , 626-637.

[64] Wicherts, D. A, et al. Long-term results of two-stage hepatectomy for irresectable colorectal cancer liver metastases. Ann Surg, (2008). , 994-1005.

[65] Virani, S, et al. Morbidity and mortality after liver resection: results of the patient safety in surgery study. J Am Coll Surg, (2007). , 1284-1292.

[66] Dixon, E, et al. Mortality following liver resection in US medicare patients: does the presence of a liver transplant program affect outcome? J Surg Oncol, (2007). , 194-200.

[67] Fong, Y, Blumgart, L. H, & Cohen, A. M. Surgical treatment of colorectal metastases to the liver. CA Cancer J Clin, (1995). , 50-62.

[68] Lius, A. Di un adenoma del fegato. Gazz delle cliniche, (1886).

[69] Langenbuch, C. Ein Fall von Resektion eines linksseitigen Schnurlappens der Leber. Berl Klin Woschenschr, (1888). , 37-38.

[70] Tesluk, H, & Lawrie, J. Hepatocellular adenoma. Its transformation to carcinoma in a user of oral contraceptives. Arch Pathol Lab Med, (1981). , 296-299.

[71] Foster, J. H, & Berman, M. M. The malignant transformation of liver cell adenomas. Arch Surg, (1994). , 712-717.

[72] Stoot, J. H, et al. Malignant transformation of hepatocellular adenomas into hepatocellular carcinomas: a systematic review including more than 1600 adenoma cases. HPB (Oxford), (2010). , 509-522.

[73] Bioulac-sage, P, et al. Hepatocellular adenoma subtypes: the impact of overweight and obesity. Liver Int, (2012).

[74] Dokmak, S, et al. A Single Center Surgical Experience of 122 Patients with Single and Multiple Hepatocellular Adenomas. Gastroenterology, (2009).

[75] Franco, L. M, et al. Hepatocellular carcinoma in glycogen storage disease type Ia: a case series. J Inherit Metab Dis, (2005). , 153-162.

[76] Gorayski, P, et al. Hepatocellular carcinoma associated with recreational anabolic steroid use. Br J Sports Med, (2008). discussion 75., 74-75.

[77] Labrune, P, et al. Hepatocellular adenomas in glycogen storage disease type I and III: a series of 43 patients and review of the literature. J Pediatr Gastroenterol Nutr, (1997). , 276-279.

[78] Velazquez, I, & Alter, B. P. Androgens and liver tumors: Fanconi's anemia and non-Fanconi's conditions. Am J Hematol, (2004). , 257-267.

[79] Zucman-rossi, J, et al. Genotype-phenotype correlation in hepatocellular adenoma: new classification and relationship with HCC. Hepatology, (2006). , 515-524.

[80] Anthony, P. P, Vogel, C. L, & Barker, L. F. Liver cell dysplasia: a premalignant condition. J Clin Pathol, (1973). , 217-223.

[81] Ho, J. C, Wu, P. C, & Mak, T. K. Liver cell dysplasia in association with hepatocellular carcinoma, cirrhosis and hepatitis B surface antigen in Hong Kong. Int J Cancer, (1981). , 571-574.

[82] Lee, R. G, Tsamandas, A. C, & Demetris, A. J. Large cell change (liver cell dysplasia) and hepatocellular carcinoma in cirrhosis: matched case-control study, pathological analysis, and pathogenetic hypothesis. Hepatology, (1997). , 1415-1422.

[83] Su, Q, et al. Human hepatic preneoplasia: phenotypes and proliferation kinetics of foci and nodules of altered hepatocytes and their relationship to liver cell dysplasia. Virchows Arch, (1997). , 391-406.

[84] Tao, L. C. Oral contraceptive-associated liver cell adenoma and hepatocellular carcinoma. Cytomorphology and mechanism of malignant transformation. Cancer, (1991). , 341-347.

[85] Van Aalten, S. M, et al. Hepatocellular adenomas: correlation of MR imaging findings with pathologic subtype classification. Radiology, (2011). , 172-181.

[86] Laumonier, H, et al. Hepatocellular adenomas: magnetic resonance imaging features as a function of molecular pathological classification. Hepatology, (2008). , 808-818.

[87] Brunetti, E, Kern, P, & Vuitton, D. A. Expert consensus for the diagnosis and treatment of cystic and alveolar echinococcosis in humans. Acta Trop, (2010). , 1-16.

[88] Tappe, D, Stich, A, & Frosch, M. Emergence of polycystic neotropical echinococcosis. Emerg Infect Dis, (2008). , 292-297.

[89] Ammann, R. W, & Eckert, J. Cestodes. Echinococcus. Gastroenterol Clin North Am, (1996). , 655-689.

[90] Dziri, C, Haouet, K, & Fingerhut, A. Treatment of hydatid cyst of the liver: where is the evidence? World J Surg, (2004). , 731-736.

[91] Gourgiotis, S, et al. Surgical techniques and treatment for hepatic hydatid cysts. Surg Today, (2007). , 389-395.

[92] Khuroo, M. S, et al. Percutaneous drainage compared with surgery for hepatic hydatid cysts. N Engl J Med, (1997). , 881-887.

[93] Smego, R. A, et al. Percutaneous aspiration-injection-reaspiration drainage plus albendazole or mebendazole for hepatic cystic echinococcosis: a meta-analysis. Clin Infect Dis, (2003). , 1073-1083.

[94] Smego, R. A, & Jr, P. Sebanego, Treatment options for hepatic cystic echinococcosis. Int J Infect Dis, (2005). , 69-76.

[95] Yagci, G, et al. Results of surgical, laparoscopic, and percutaneous treatment for hydatid disease of the liver: 10 years experience with 355 patients. World J Surg, (2005)., 1670-1679.

[96] Sayek, I, Tirnaksiz, M. B, & Dogan, R. Cystic hydatid disease: current trends in diagnosis and management. Surg Today, (2004)., 987-996.

[97] Seimenis, A. Overview of the epidemiological situation on echinococcosis in the Mediterranean region. Acta Trop, (2003)., 191-195.

[98] Menezes da SilvaA.M., Human echinococcosis: a neglected disease. Gastroenterol Res Pract, 2010. (2010). p. pii: 583297.

[99] Buttenschoen, K. and D. Carli Buttenschoen, Echinococcus granulosus infection: the challenge of surgical treatment. Langenbecks Arch Surg, (2003)., 218-230.

[100] Khuroo, M. S, et al. Percutaneous drainage versus albendazole therapy in hepatic hydatidosis: a prospective, randomized study. Gastroenterology, (1993)., 1452-1459.

[101] Dervenis, C, et al. Changing concepts in the management of liver hydatid disease. J Gastrointest Surg, (2005)., 869-877.

[102] Guidelines for treatment of cystic and alveolar echinococcosis in humansWHO Informal Working Group on Echinococcosis. Bull World Health Organ, (1996). , 231-242.

[103] Mueller, L, et al. A retrospective study comparing the different surgical procedures for the treatment of hydatid disease of the liver. Dig Surg, (2003)., 279-284.

[104] Stoot, J. H, et al. More than 25 years of surgical treatment of hydatid cysts in a nonendemic area using the "frozen seal" method. World J Surg, (2010)., 106-113.

[105] Saidi, F, & Nazarian, I. Surgical treatment of hydatid cysts by freezing of cyst wall and instillation of 0.5 per cent silver nitrate solution. N Engl J Med, (1971)., 1346-1350.

[106] Schindl, M. J, et al. The value of residual liver volume as a predictor of hepatic dysfunction and infection after major liver resection. Gut, (2005)., 289-296.

[107] Shoup, M, et al. Volumetric analysis predicts hepatic dysfunction in patients undergoing major liver resection. J Gastrointest Surg, (2003)., 325-330.

[108] Shah, S. A, et al. Surgical resection of hepatic and pulmonary metastases from colorectal carcinoma. J Am Coll Surg, (2006)., 468-475.

[109] Fusai, G, & Davidson, B. R. Management of colorectal liver metastases. Colorectal Dis, (2003)., 2-23.

[110] Scheele, J, et al. Resection of colorectal liver metastases. What prognostic factors determine patient selection?]. Chirurg, (2001)., 547-560.

[111] Karlo, C, et al. CT- and MRI-based volumetry of resected liver specimen: comparison to intraoperative volume and weight measurements and calculation of conversion factors. Eur J Radiol, (2010). , e107-e111.

[112] Dello, S. A, et al. Liver volumetry plug and play: do it yourself with ImageJ. World J Surg, (2007). , 2215-2221.

[113] Van Der Vorst, J. R, et al. Virtual liver resection and volumetric analysis of the future liver remnant using open source image processing software. World J Surg, (2010). , 2426-2433.

[114] Dello, S. A, et al. Prospective volumetric assessment of the liver on a personal computer by nonradiologists prior to partial hepatectomy. World J Surg, (2010). , 386-392.

[115] Dubois, F, Berthelot, G, & Levard, H. Laparoscopic cholecystectomy: historic perspective and personal experience. Surg Laparosc Endosc, (1991). , 52-57.

[116] Dagher, I, et al. Laparoscopic liver resection: results for 70 patients. Surg Endosc, (2007). , 619-624.

[117] Descottes, B, et al. Laparoscopic liver resection of benign liver tumors. Surg Endosc, (2003). , 23-30.

[118] Farges, O, et al. Prospective assessment of the safety and benefit of laparoscopic liver resections. J Hepatobiliary Pancreat Surg, (2002). , 242-248.

[119] Morino, M, et al. Laparoscopic vs open hepatic resection: a comparative study. Surg Endosc, (2003). , 1914-1918.

[120] Simillis, C, et al. Laparoscopic versus open hepatic resections for benign and malignant neoplasms--a meta-analysis. Surgery, (2007). , 203-211.

[121] Kaneko, H. Laparoscopic hepatectomy: indications and outcomes. J Hepatobiliary Pancreat Surg, (2005). , 438-443.

[122] Kelling, G. Ueber Oesophagoskopie, Gastroskopie und Kölioskopie. Münch Med Wochenschr, (1902). , 21-24.

[123] Jacobeus, H. Ueber die Möglichkeit die Zystoskopie bei Untersuchung seröser Höhlungen anzuwenden. Münch Med Wochenschr, (1910). , 2090-2092.

[124] Jacobeus, H. Kurze Uebersichtüber meine Erfahrungen mit der Laparo-thoraskopie. Münch Med Wochenschr, (1911). , 2017-2019.

[125] Cuesta, M. A, et al. Limited laparoscopic liver resection of benign tumors guided by laparoscopic ultrasonography: report of two cases. Surg Laparosc Endosc, (1995). , 396-401.

[126] Azagra, J. S, et al. Laparoscopic anatomical (hepatic) left lateral segmentectomy-technical aspects. Surg Endosc, (1996). , 758-761.

[127] Cherqui, D, et al. Laparoscopic liver resections: a feasibility study in 30 patients. Ann Surg, (2000). , 753-762.

[128] Cherqui, D. Laparoscopic liver resection. Br J Surg, (2003). , 644-646.

[129] Dagher, I, et al. Laparoscopic hepatectomy for hepatocellular carcinoma: a European experience. J Am Coll Surg, (2010). , 16-23.

[130] Gigot, J. F, et al. Laparoscopic liver resection for malignant liver tumors: preliminary results of a multicenter European study. Ann Surg, (2002). , 90-97.

[131] Buell, J. F, et al. An initial experience and evolution of laparoscopic hepatic resectional surgery. Surgery, (2004). , 804-811.

[132] Chang, S, et al. Laparoscopy as a routine approach for left lateral sectionectomy. Br J Surg, (2007). , 58-63.

[133] Buell, J. F, et al. The international position on laparoscopic liver surgery: The Louisville Statement, 2008. Ann Surg, (2009). , 825-830.

[134] Nguyen, K. T, et al. Minimally invasive liver resection for metastatic colorectal cancer: a multi-institutional, international report of safety, feasibility, and early outcomes. Ann Surg, (2009). , 842-848.

[135] Mirnezami, R, et al. Short- and long-term outcomes after laparoscopic and open hepatic resection: systematic review and meta-analysis. HPB (Oxford), (2011). , 295-308.

[136] Van Dam, R. M, et al. Initial experience with a multimodal enhanced recovery programme in patients undergoing liver resection. Br J Surg, (2008). , 969-975.

[137] Wind, J, et al. Systematic review of enhanced recovery programmes in colonic surgery. Br J Surg, (2006). , 800-809.

[138] Fearon, K. C, et al. Enhanced recovery after surgery: a consensus review of clinical care for patients undergoing colonic resection. Clin Nutr, (2005). , 466-477.

[139] Kehlet, H, & Wilmore, D. W. Multimodal strategies to improve surgical outcome. Am J Surg, (2002). , 630-641.

[140] Wilmore, D. W, & Kehlet, H. Management of patients in fast track surgery. Bmj, (2001). , 473-476.

[141] Basse, L, Madsen, J. L, & Kehlet, H. Normal gastrointestinal transit after colonic resection using epidural analgesia, enforced oral nutrition and laxative. Br J Surg, (2001). , 1498-1500.

[142] Basse, L, et al. Accelerated postoperative recovery programme after colonic resection improves physical performance, pulmonary function and body composition. Br J Surg, (2002). , 446-453.

[143] Delaney, C. P, et al. Prospective, randomized, controlled trial between a pathway of controlled rehabilitation with early ambulation and diet and traditional postoperative care after laparotomy and intestinal resection. Dis Colon Rectum, (2003). , 851-859.

[144] Zutshi, M, et al. Randomized controlled trial comparing the controlled rehabilitation with early ambulation and diet pathway versus the controlled rehabilitation with early ambulation and diet with preemptive epidural anesthesia/analgesia after laparotomy and intestinal resection. Am J Surg, (2005). , 268-272.

[145] Podore, P. C, & Throop, E. B. Infrarenal aortic surgery with a 3-day hospital stay: A report on success with a clinical pathway. J Vasc Surg, (1999). , 787-792.

[146] Trondsen, E, et al. Day-case laparoscopic fundoplication for gastro-oesophageal reflux disease. Br J Surg, (2000). , 1708-1711.

[147] Basse, L, et al. A clinical pathway to accelerate recovery after colonic resection. Ann Surg, (2000). , 51-57.

[148] Schoetz, D. J, et al. Ideal" length of stay after colectomy: whose ideal? Dis Colon Rectum, (1997). , 806-810.

[149] Kehlet, H. Multimodal approach to control postoperative pathophysiology and rehabilitation. Br J Anaesth, (1997). , 606-617.

[150] Kehlet, H, & Dahl, J. B. Anaesthesia, surgery, and challenges in postoperative recovery. Lancet, (2003). , 1921-1928.

[151] Nygren, J, et al. A comparison in five European Centres of case mix, clinical management and outcomes following either conventional or fast-track perioperative care in colorectal surgery. Clin Nutr, (2005). , 455-461.

[152] Spelt, L, et al. Fast-track programmes for hepatopancreatic resections: where do we stand? HPB (Oxford), (2011). , 833-838.

[153] Stoot, J. H, et al. The effect of a multimodal fast-track programme on outcomes in laparoscopic liver surgery: a multicentre pilot study. HPB (Oxford), (2009). , 140-144.

[154] Adam, R. Chemotherapy and surgery: new perspectives on the treatment of unresectable liver metastases. Ann Oncol, (2003). Suppl 2: , ii13-ii16.

[155] Abdalla, E. K, et al. Improving resectability of hepatic colorectal metastases: expert consensus statement. Ann Surg Oncol, (2006). , 1271-1280.

[156] Adam, R, et al. Rescue surgery for unresectable colorectal liver metastases downstaged by chemotherapy: a model to predict long-term survival. Ann Surg, (2004). discussion 657-8., 644-657.

[157] Yeo, S. G, et al. Whole-liver radiotherapy for end-stage colorectal cancer patients with massive liver metastases and advanced hepatic dysfunction. Radiat Oncol, (2010). , 97.

[158] Krishnan, S, et al. Conformal radiotherapy of the dominant liver metastasis: a viable strategy for treatment of unresectable chemotherapy refractory colorectal cancer liver metastases. Am J Clin Oncol, (2006). , 562-567.

[159] Schefter, T. E, & Kavanagh, B. D. Radiation therapy for liver metastases. Semin Radiat Oncol, (2011). , 264-270.

[160] Andolino, D. L, et al. Stereotactic body radiotherapy for primary hepatocellular carcinoma. Int J Radiat Oncol Biol Phys, (2011). , e447-e453.

[161] Minn, A. Y, Koong, A. C, & Chang, D. T. Stereotactic body radiation therapy for gastrointestinal malignancies. Front Radiat Ther Oncol, (2011). , 412-427.

[162] Chang, D. T, et al. Stereotactic body radiotherapy for colorectal liver metastases: a pooled analysis. Cancer, (2011). , 4060-4069.

[163] Saxena, A, et al. Factors predicting response and survival after yttrium-90 radioembolization of unresectable neuroendocrine tumor liver metastases: a critical appraisal of 48 cases. Ann Surg, (2010). , 910-916.

[164] Evans, K. A, et al. Survival outcomes of a salvage patient population after radioembolization of hepatic metastases with yttrium-90 microspheres. J Vasc Interv Radiol, (2010). , 1521-1526.

[165] Jakobs, T. F, et al. Hepatic yttrium-90 radioembolization of chemotherapy-refractory colorectal cancer liver metastases. J Vasc Interv Radiol, (2008). , 1187-1195.

[166] Smits, M. L, et al. Holmium-166 radioembolization for the treatment of patients with liver metastases: design of the phase I HEPAR trial. J Exp Clin Cancer Res, (2010). , 70.

[167] Mayo, S. C, & Pawlik, T. M. Thermal ablative therapies for secondary hepatic malignancies. Cancer J, (2010). , 111-117.

[168] Jiao, D, et al. Microwave ablation treatment of liver cancer with 2,450-MHz cooled-shaft antenna: an experimental and clinical study. J Cancer Res Clin Oncol, (2010). , 1507-1516.

[169] Bhardwaj, N, et al. Microwave ablation for unresectable hepatic tumours: clinical results using a novel microwave probe and generator. Eur J Surg Oncol, (2009). , 264-268.

[170] Martin, R. C, Scoggins, C. R, & Mcmasters, K. M. Safety and efficacy of microwave ablation of hepatic tumors: a prospective review of a 5-year experience. Ann Surg Oncol, (2009). , 171-178.

[171] Kobayashi, S, et al. A single-incision laparoscopic hepatectomy for hepatocellular carcinoma: initial experience in a Japanese patient. Minim Invasive Ther Allied Technol, (2010). , 367-371.

[172] Gaujoux, S, et al. Single-incision laparoscopic liver resection. Surg Endosc, (2010). , 1489-1494.

[173] Patel, A. G, et al. Video. Single-incision laparoscopic left lateral segmentectomy of colorectal liver metastasis. Surg Endosc, (2010). , 649-650.

[174] Giulianotti, P. C, et al. Robotic liver surgery: results for 70 resections. Surgery, (2010). , 29-39.

[175] Jain, G, et al. Stretching the limits of laparoscopic surgery": two-stage laparoscopic liver resection. J Laparoendosc Adv Surg Tech A, (2010). , 51-54.

[176] Machado, M. A, et al. Two-stage laparoscopic liver resection for bilateral colorectal liver metastasis. Surg Endosc, (2010). , 2044-2047.

[177] Alkari, B, Owera, A, & Ammori, B. J. Laparoscopic liver resection: preliminary results from a UK centre. Surg Endosc, (2008). , 2201-2207.

[178] Starzl, T. E, & Fung, J. J. Themes of liver transplantation. Hepatology, (2010). , 1869-1884.

[179] Calne, R. Y. Early days of liver transplantation. Am J Transplant, (2008). , 1775-1778.

[180] Starlz, T. E, et al. Reconstructive problems in canine liver homotransplantation with special reference to the postoperative role of hepatic venous flow. Surg Gynecol Obstet, (1960). , 733-743.

[181] Moore, F. D, et al. Experimental whole-organ transplantation of the liver and of the spleen. Ann Surg, (1960). , 374-387.

[182] Starzl, T. E, et al. HOMOTRANSPLANTATION OF THE LIVER IN HUMANS. Surg Gynecol Obstet, (1963). , 659-676.

[183] Starzl, T. E, Marchioro, T. L, & Waddell, W. R. THE REVERSAL OF REJECTION IN HUMAN RENAL HOMOGRAFTS WITH SUBSEQUENT DEVELOPMENT OF HOMOGRAFT TOLERANCE. Surg Gynecol Obstet, (1963). , 385-395.

[184] Starzl, T. E, et al. Orthotopic homotransplantation of the human liver. Ann Surg, (1968). , 392-415.

[185] Schroter, G. P, et al. Infections complicating orthotopic liver transplantation: a study emphasizing graft-related septicemia. Arch Surg, (1976). , 1337-1347.

[186] Calne, R. Y, et al. Liver transplantation in man. II. A report of two orthotopic liver transplants in adult recipients. Br Med J, (1968). , 541-546.

[187] GooszenLeerboek chirurgie. Bohn Stafleu van Loghum, (2006). , 425-426.

[188] Levi, D. M, et al. Liver transplantation with preservation of the inferior vena cava: lessons learned through 2,000 cases. J Am Coll Surg, (2012). discussion 698-9., 691-698.

[189] Abbasoglu, O. Liver transplantation: yesterday, today and tomorrow. World J Gastroenterol, (2008). , 3117-3122.

[190] Groth, C. G, et al. Historic landmarks in clinical transplantation: conclusions from the consensus conference at the University of California, Los Angeles. World J Surg, (2000). , 834-843.

[191] Calne, R. Y, et al. Cyclosporin A initially as the only immunosuppressant in 34 recipients of cadaveric organs: 32 kidneys, 2 pancreases, and 2 livers. Lancet, (1979). , 1033-1036.

[192] Starzl, T. E, et al. The use of cyclosporin A and prednisone in cadaver kidney transplantation. Surg Gynecol Obstet, (1980). , 17-26.

[193] Starzl, T. E, et al. Liver transplantation with use of cyclosporin a and prednisone. N Engl J Med, (1981). , 266-269.

[194] Starzl, T. E, et al. FK 506 for liver, kidney, and pancreas transplantation. Lancet, (1989). , 1000-1004.

[195] Todo, S, et al. Liver, kidney, and thoracic organ transplantation under FK 506. Ann Surg, (1990). discussion 306-7., 295-305.

[196] Grady, O, et al. Tacrolimus versus microemulsified ciclosporin in liver transplantation: the TMC randomised controlled trial. Lancet, (2002). , 1119-1125.

[197] Haddad, E. M, et al. Cyclosporin versus tacrolimus for liver transplanted patients. Cochrane Database Syst Rev, (2006). , CD005161.

[198] Bismuth, H, & Houssin, D. Reduced-sized orthotopic liver graft in hepatic transplantation in children. Surgery, (1984). , 367-370.

[199] Pichlmayr, R, et al. Transplantation of a donor liver to 2 recipients (splitting transplantation)--a new method in the further development of segmental liver transplantation]. Langenbecks Arch Chir, (1988). , 127-130.

[200] Ng, K. K, & Lo, C. M. Liver transplantation in Asia: past, present and future. Ann Acad Med Singapore, (2009). , 322-310.

[201] Chen, C. L, & De Villa, V. H. Split liver transplantation. Asian J Surg, (2002). , 285-290.

[202] Adam, R, et al. Evolution of liver transplantation in Europe: report of the European Liver Transplant Registry. Liver Transpl, (2003). , 1231-1243.

[203] Raia, S, Nery, J. R, & Mies, S. Liver transplantation from live donors. Lancet, (1989). , 497.

[204] Strong, R. W, et al. Successful liver transplantation from a living donor to her son. N Engl J Med, (1990). , 1505-1507.

[205] Sugawara, Y, & Makuuchi, M. Living donor liver transplantation: present status and recent advances. Br Med Bull, (2005). , 15-28.

[206] Broering, D. C, et al. Is there still a need for living-related liver transplantation in children? Ann Surg, (2001). discussion 721-2., 713-721.

[207] Lo, C. M, et al. Adult-to-adult living donor liver transplantation using extended right lobe grafts. Ann Surg, (1997). discussion 269-70., 261-269.

[208] Shimada, M, et al. Living-donor liver transplantation: present status and future perspective. J Med Invest, (2005). , 22-32.

[209] Brown, R. S, et al. A survey of liver transplantation from living adult donors in the United States. N Engl J Med, (2003). , 818-825.

[210] Malago, M, Burdelski, M, & Broelsch, C. E. Present and future challenges in living related liver transplantation. Transplant Proc, (1999). , 1777-1781.

[211] Dutkowski, P, et al. Current and future trends in liver transplantation in Europe. Gastroenterology, (2010). e1-4., 802-809.

[212] Busuttil, R. W, & Tanaka, K. The utility of marginal donors in liver transplantation. Liver Transpl, (2003). , 651-663.

[213] White, S. A, & Prasad, K. R. Liver transplantation from non-heart beating donors. BMJ, (2006). , 376-377.

[214] Ikeda, T, et al. Ischemic injury in liver transplantation: difference in injury sites between warm and cold ischemia in rats. Hepatology, (1992). , 454-461.

[215] Abt, P, et al. Liver transplantation from controlled non-heart-beating donors: an increased incidence of biliary complications. Transplantation, (2003). , 1659-1663.

[216] Abt, P. L, et al. Survival following liver transplantation from non-heart-beating donors. Ann Surg, (2004). , 87-92.

Chapter 2

Essential Functional Hepatic and Biliary Anatomy for the Surgeon

Ronald S. Chamberlain

Additional information is available at the end of the chapter

http://dx.doi.org/10.5772/53849

1. Introduction

That every surgeon will experience complications is a certainty. Indeed, it has been said that if one has no complications, one does not do enough surgery. Yet, major surgical complications are often avoidable and frequently the result of three tragic surgical errors. These errors are: 1) a failure to possess sufficient knowledge of normal anatomy and function, 2) a failure to recognize anatomic variants when they present, and 3) a failure to ask for help when uncertain or unsure. All but the last of these errors are remediable with study and effort. In regard to the last error, most surgeons learn humility through their failures and at the expense of their patients, while some never learn.

The importance of a precise knowledge of parenchymal structure, blood supply, lymphatic drainage, and variant anatomy on outcome is perhaps nowhere more apparent than in hepatobiliary surgery. Though the liver was historically an area where few brave men dared to tread, and even less returned a second time, recent advances in anesthetic technique and perioperative care now permit hepatic surgery to be performed with low morbidity and mortality in both academic and community hospitals. That said, surgeons are duly cautioned to inventory their own skills and knowledge before venturing forward into the right upper quadrant. This chapter will review functional biliary and hepatic anatomy necessary for the conduct of safe and successful hepatic operations.

2. The liver

2.1. Surface anatomy

The liver is situated primarily in the right upper quadrant, and usually benefits from complete protection by the lower ribs. Most of the liver substance resides on the right side, although it is not uncommon for the left lateral segment to arch over the spleen. The superior surface of the liver is molded to, and abuts the undersurface of the diaphragm on both the right and left side. During normal inspiration, the liver may rise as high as the 4th or 5th intercostal space on the right.

The liver itself is completely invested with a peritoneal layer except on the posterior surface where it reflects onto the undersurface of the diaphragm to form the right and left triangular ligaments. The liver is attached to the diaphragm and anterior abdominal wall by three separate ligamentous attachments, namely the falciform, round, and right and left triangular ligaments. (Figure 1) The falciform ligament, which is situated on the anterior surface of the liver, arises from the anterior leaflets of the right and left triangular ligaments and terminates inferiorly where the ligamentum teres enters the umbilical fissure. The gallbladder is normally attached to the undersurface of the right lobe and directed towards the umbilical fissure. At the base of the gallbladder fossa, is the hilar transverse fissure through which the main portal structures to the right lobe course. Additional important landmarks on the posterior liver surface include a deep vertical groove in which the inferior vena cava is situated, and a large bare area (i.e. no peritoneal coating) that is normally in contact with the right hemidiaphragm and right adrenal gland. The left lateral segment of the liver arches over the caudate lobe that is situated to the left of the vena cava. The caudate lobe is demarcated on the left by a fissure containing the ligamentum venosum (a remnant of the umbilical vein). Additional left-sided important surface features include the gastrohepatic omentum that is located between the left lateral segment and the stomach. The gastrohepatic omentum may contain replaced or accessory hepatic arteries. Finally, there is usually a thick fibrous band that envelops the vena cava high on the right side and runs posteriorly towards the lumbar vertebrae. This band, which is sometimes referred to as the vena caval ligament, must be divided to allow proper visualization of the suprahepatic cava and right hepatic veins.

2.2. Parenchyma (the liver substance)

The liver is comprised of two main lobes, a large right lobe, and a smaller left lobe. Although the falciform ligament is often thought to divide the liver into a right and left lobe, the true "anatomic" or "surgical" right and left lobes of the liver are defined by the course of the middle hepatic vein that runs through the main scissura of the liver. Although various descriptions of the internal anatomy of the liver have been proffered over the last century, Couinaud's (1957) segmental anatomy of the liver is the most useful for the surgeon.

Couinaud's classification system divides the liver into four unique sectors based upon the course of the three major hepatic veins. Each sector receives its blood supply from a separate portal pedicle. Within the *main scissura* lies the middle hepatic vein that courses from the left side of the suprahepatic vena cava to the middle of the gallbladder fossa. Functionally, the main scissura divides the liver into separate right and left lobes which have independent portal inflow, and biliary architecture. (Figures 2 and 3) An artificial line that divides the liver into right and left hemilivers is known as Cantlie's line. The right hepatic veins runs within the right segmental scissura and divides the right lobe into a right posterior and anterior sector,

http://dx.doi.org/10.5772/53849

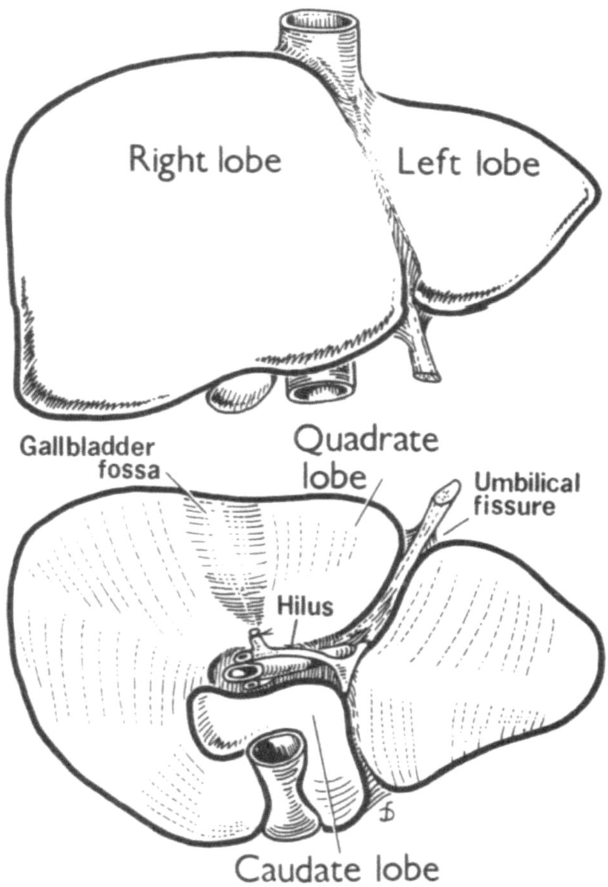

Figure 1. Surface anatomy of the liver. (A) Anterior surface, (B) Inferior surface of the liver. Reprinted with permission from Hahn and Blumgary, Functional Hepatic and Radiologic Anatomy in Surgery of the Liver and Biliary Tract (3rd Edition), Blumgart LH, Fong Y and WH Jarnigan (Eds.) Lippincott Williams, London, UK (2000).

while the left hepatic veins follows the path of the falciform ligament and divides the left lobe into a medial and lateral segment.

The right and left lobes of the liver are further divided into 8 segments based upon the distribution of the *portal scissurae*. At the hilus, the right portal vein pursues a very short course (1 – 1.5 cm) before entering the liver. Once entering the hepatic parenchyma, the portal vein divides into a right anterior sectoral branch that arches vertical in the frontal plane of the liver, and a posterior sectoral branch that follows a more posterolateral course. The right portal vein supplies the anterior (or anteriomedial) and posterior (or posterolateral) sectors of the right lobe. The branching pattern of these sectoral portal veins subdivides the right liver into 4 segments -- segments V (anterior and inferior) and VIII (anterior and superior) form the anterior sector, and segments VI (posterior and inferior) and VII (posterior and superior) form the posterior sector.

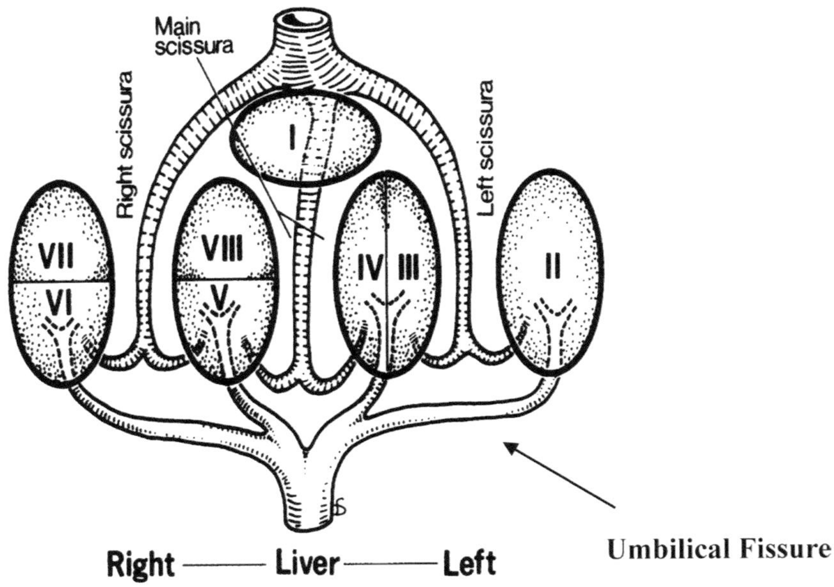

Figure 2. Segmental and sectoral anatomy of the liver. The liver is divided into three main scissura by the right, middle, and left hepatic vein branches. The middle hepatic courses through the main scissura (or Cantlie's line) and divides the liver into right and left lobes. The right hepatic vein divides the right liver into anterior (segments V and VIII) and posterior (segment VI and VII) sectors, while the left hepatic vein divides the left lobe into medial (segments IV A and B) and lateral segments (segments II and III). The intrahepatic branching of the right and left hepatic ducts, arteries and portal veins (shown) in the horizontal plane of the liver divides the liver into eight separate segments. The caudate lobe (segment I) is neither part or left lobe. Rather the caudate lobe receives venous and arterial branches from both the right and left side of the liver, and drains directly into the inferior vena cava.

In contrast to the right portal vein, the left portal vein has a long extrahepatic length (3 – 4 cm) coursing beneath the inferior portion of the quadrate lobe (segment 4B) enveloped in a peritoneal sheath (the hilar plate.) Upon reaching the umbilical fissure, the left portal vein runs anteriorly and superiorly within the liver substances, and gives off horizontal branches to the quadrate lobe medially (segments IV A (superior) and B (inferior)) and to the left lateral segment (segments III (inferior) and II (superior)) (Figure 3).

The caudate lobe (segment I) is neither part of the left nor right lobes, though it lies mostly on the left side (Figure 4). More precisely, it is the most dorsal portion of the liver situated behind the left lobe and embracing the retrohepatic vena cava from the hilum to the diaphragm. The portion of the caudate lobe that is within the right liver is usually quite small, and lies posterior to segment 4B. Figure 3 illustrates the location of the caudate lobe which lies between the left portal vein and vena cava on the far left, and the middle hepatic vein and vena cava within the right liver. The caudate lobe receives blood vessels and biliary tributaries from both the right and left hemilivers. The right side of the caudate lobe, and the caudate process, receives its blood supply from branches of the right or main portal vein, while the left side of the caudate receives a separate vessel from the left portal vein.

http://dx.doi.org/10.5772/53849

a

b

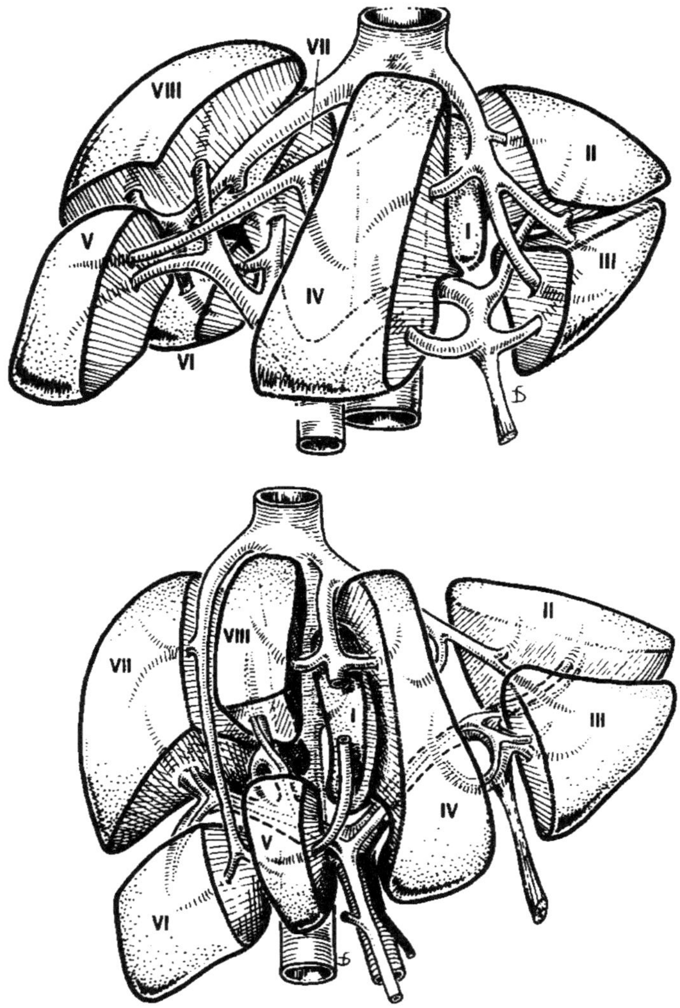

Figure 3. Couninaud's segmental anatomy of the liver. (a) *in vivo* appearance; (b) *ex vivo* appearance.

Aberrant segmental anatomy of the liver is uncommon. The presence of a diminutive left lobe is the most common anomaly reported, and is important only because it may serve as a limitation to the performance of extended right hepatectomies. Although reports of "accessory" hepatic lobes are not uncommon, these do not represent separate segments with independent intrahepatic vascular supply, but rather elongated tongues of normal liver tissue. Riedel's lobe is the most common of these "accessory" lobes, and is reality, an extended piece of liver tissue hanging inferiorly off segments 5 and 6.

3. Hepatic veins (Outflow)

The three major hepatic veins (the right, middle and left) comprise the main outflow tract for the liver, although additional veins (5 – 20) of varying size are always present as direct communications between the vena cava and the posterior surface of the right lobe. Uniquely, the caudate lobe (segment I) drains principally through direct communications with the retrohepatic cava.

The hepatic veins lie within the three major scissura of the liver dividing the parenchyma into the right anterior and posterior sectors, and the right and left lobes. (Fig 2 and 3) The right hepatic vein lies within the right scissura (or segmental fissure) and divides the right lobe into a posterior (segments VI and VII) and anterior (segments V and VIII) sector. The middle hepatic veins lies within the main hepatic scissura (or main lobar fissure) separating the right anterior sector (segments V and VIII) from the quadrate lobe (segment IV). Anatomically, the main scissura separates the liver into right and left lobes. The left hepatic vein lies within the left scissura (or the left segmental fissure) in line with or just to the right of the falciform ligament. The right hepatic vein drains directly into the suprahepatic cava, while the middle and left hepatic vein coalesce to form a short common trunk prior to entry. The umbilical vein represents an additional alternative site of venous efflux. It is located beneath the falciform ligament and eventually terminates in the left hepatic vein, or less commonly in the confluence of the middle and left hepatic veins.

4. Hepatic venous anomalies

Although the outline above should suffice as cursory knowledge of hepatic venous anatomy, it is far from exhaustive. For example, large accessory right hepatic veins are commonly found, and an appreciation of these structures on axial imaging can be important to operative planning. If a large accessory right hepatic vein is present, it may be possible to divide all three major hepatic veins in the performance of an extended left hepatectomy. Most importantly, the surgeon embarking on hepatic resection should have a thorough knowledge of the internal course of the hepatic veins, as the danger posed by hepatic venous bleeding cannot be overestimated.

5. Hepatic arteries (Inflow)

5.1. Extrahepatic arterial anatomy

"Normal" hepatic arterial anatomy is anything but normal. Indeed standard celiac arterial anatomy as described in most major anatomic treatise is found in only 60% of cases. An *accessory* hepatic artery refers to a vessel that supplies a segment of liver that also receives blood supply from a normal hepatic artery. An aberrant hepatic artery is called a *replaced*

http://dx.doi.org/10.5772/53849

hepatic artery as it represents the only blood supply to a specific hepatic segment. Precise knowledge of normal hepatic arterial anatomy is necessary to appreciate abnormal anatomy and will be the focus of this section.

The celiac artery arises from the aorta shortly after it emerges through the diaphragmatic hiatus. The celiac trunk itself is typically very short and divides into the left gastric, splenic, and common hepatic artery shortly after its origin. (Figure 5). The common hepatic artery typically passes forward for a short distance in the retroperitoneum where it them emerges at the superior border of the pancreas and left side of the common hepatic duct. The common hepatic artery supplies 25% of the liver's blood supply, with the portal vein supplying the remaining 75%.

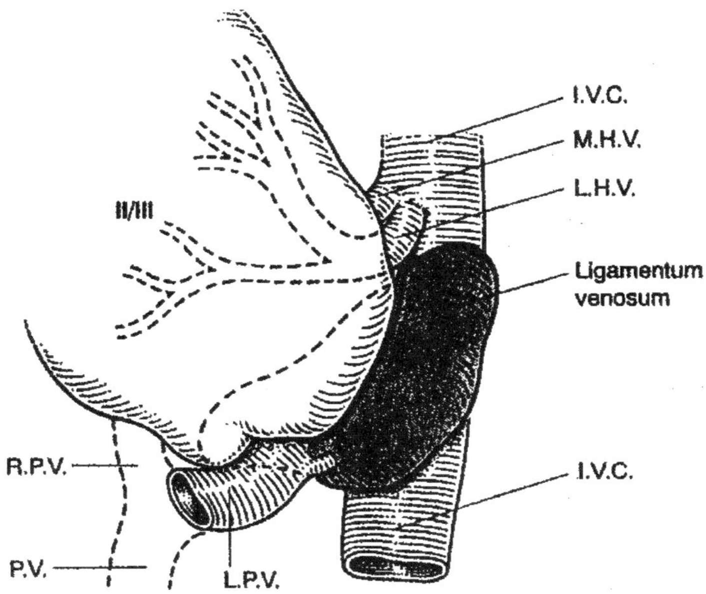

Figure 4. Caudate lobe anatomy. The caudate lobe is situated to the left of the inferior vena cava (I.V.C). Superiorly the caudate lobe is covered by segments II and III which are reflected laterally in this diagram. The ligamentum venousm, a remnant of the fetal umbilical vein, courses across the anterior surface of the caudate lobe to enter the left hepatic vein. The caudate lobe runs along the retrohepatic vena cava from the common trunk of the middle and left hepatic veins (M.H.V., L.H.V.) to the portal vein (P.V.) inferiorly. (Left (L.P.V.) and right portal vein (R.P.V.)). Small venous tributaries drain the caudate lobe directly into to the I.V.C. On its medial surface, the caudate lobe is attached to the right liver by the caudate process.

After arising from the celiac axis, the common hepatic artery turns upward and runs lateral and adjacent to the common bile duct. The gastroduodenal artery that supplies the proximal duodenum and pancreas is typically the first branch of the common hepatic artery. The right gastric artery takes off shortly thereafter and continues within the lesser omentum along the lesser curve of the stomach. At this point the common hepatic artery is referred to as the proper hepatic artery. The proper hepatic artery courses towards the hilum, and soon divides into the right and left hepatic arteries. Prior to the bifurcation, a small cystic artery branches off to

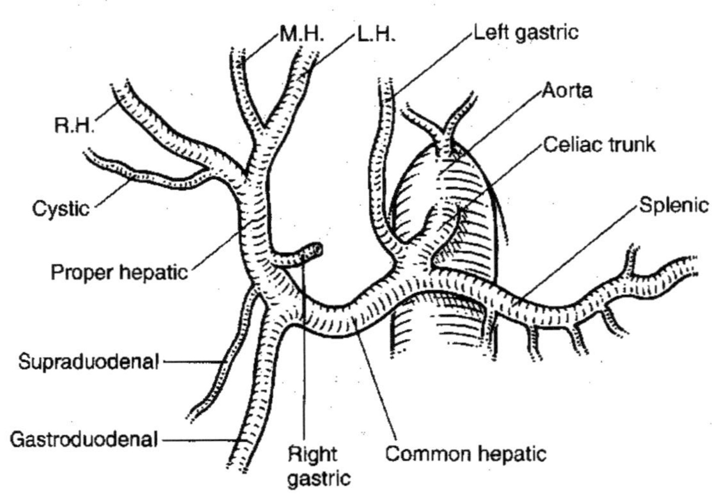

Figure 5. Normal celiac axis anatomy. The presence of the right hepatic (R.H.), middle hepatic (M.H.) to segment IV, and left hepatic (L.H.) artery are demonstrated.

provide blood supply to the gallbladder. While coursing through the hepatoduodenal ligament, the proper hepatic artery, common bile duct, and portal vein are enveloped in a peritoneal sheath within the hepatoduodenal ligament. The proper hepatic artery bifurcates earlier than the common bile duct and portal vein. In 80% of cases the right hepatic artery courses posterior to the common hepatic duct before entering the hepatic parenchyma. In 20% of cases, the right hepatic artery may lie anterior to the common hepatic duct. Upon reaching the hepatic parenchyma, the right hepatic artery branches into right anterior (Segments V and VIII), and right posterior sectoral branches (Segments VI and VII). The posterior sectoral branch initially runs horizontally through the hilar transverse fissure (of Gunz), normally present at the base of Segment V and adjacent to the caudate process. The left hepatic artery runs vertically towards the umbilical fissure where it gives off a small branch (often called the middle hepatic artery) to segment IV, before continuing on to supply Segments II and III. Additional small branches of the left hepatic artery supply the caudate lobe (segment I), although caudate arterial branches may also arise from the right hepatic artery. The sectoral and segmental bile ducts and portal veins follow the course of the hepatic artery branches. Intrahepatic branching of these structures will be discussed in more detail below.

The blood supply to the common bile duct is varied and multiple. Branches of the common hepatic, gastroduodenal, and pancreaticoduodenal arteries have all been shown to provide arterial supply at various levels.

5.2. Hepatic arterial anomalies

Variations in the arterial blood supply to the liver are common. Although the hepatic artery typically arises from the celiac axis, complete replacement of the main hepatic artery or its'

http://dx.doi.org/10.5772/53849

branches occur with variable frequency. Similarly, duplication or accessory hepatic arterial branches, particularly an accessory left hepatic artery, may be more the norm than an anomaly. The most common hepatic arterial anomaly involving a replaced vessel is a replaced right hepatic artery (25%). In this situation, the replaced right hepatic artery usually arises from the superior mesenteric artery and runs lateral and posterior to the portal vein within the hepatoduodenal ligament. (Figure 6). In rare instances, the entire common hepatic artery, or its' individual branches may arise directly off the celiac trunk or aorta.

6. Portal venous anatomy

The portal vein is formed by a union of the superior mesenteric vein (SMV) and splenic vein behind the neck and body of the pancreas. In up to one third of all individuals, the inferior mesenteric vein may also join this confluence. Venous tributaries from the pancreas may also drain directly into the portal vein, and generally correspond to the arterial supply. More precisely, there are anterior, posterior, superior and inferior pancreatic vessels. In addition, the left gastric vein and inferior mesenteric vein typically drain into the splenic vein, but in rare instances these vessels may enter the portal vein directly. Surgical dogma states that there are no venous branches on the anterior surface of the portal vein and, for the most part this is true – most veins enter the portal vein tangentially from the side. However, having paid homage to surgical dogma, the reality is that small anterior venous branches may exist, and any manipulation posterior to the pancreatic neck and anterior to the portal vein should be performed with maximum operative exposure and care.

Access to the portal vein is typically obtained by identifying the superior mesenteric vein on the inferior surface of the pancreas. In some circumstances it is necessary to first locate the middle colic vein within the transverse mesocolon and follow it inferiorly to the SMV. The length of the SMV is highly variable, and may range from only a few millimeters up to 4 cm. In many circumstances the SMV is made up of 2 to 4 venous branches that coalesce shortly before joining the portal vein rather than a single dominant vein. The inferior pancreaticoduodenal vein, which can be quite prominent, is the only vein that normally enters the SMV directly. Proper identification of this vein is necessary to avoid injury (and often substantial blood loss). All other pancreatic venous tributaries enter the portal vein, rather than the SMV.

In the performance of a pancreaticoduodenal resection, early division of the common bile duct (CBD) provides great exposure to the right lateral side of the portal vein, and facilitates the creation of a "tunnel" above the portal vein, and beneath the pancreas. Once a determination has been made regarding the resectability of the pancreatic lesion, we favor early transection of the common bile duct. If the tumor later proves unresectable, a palliative end to side bilioenteric bypass can be performed.

In addition to those variants described above, there are additional (but rare) congenital anomalies of the portal vein with which the surgeon should be aware. The two most common are an anterior portal vein that lies above the pancreas and duodenum, and a direct entry of the portal vein into the inferior vena cava-- a congenital "portocaval" shunt. The importance

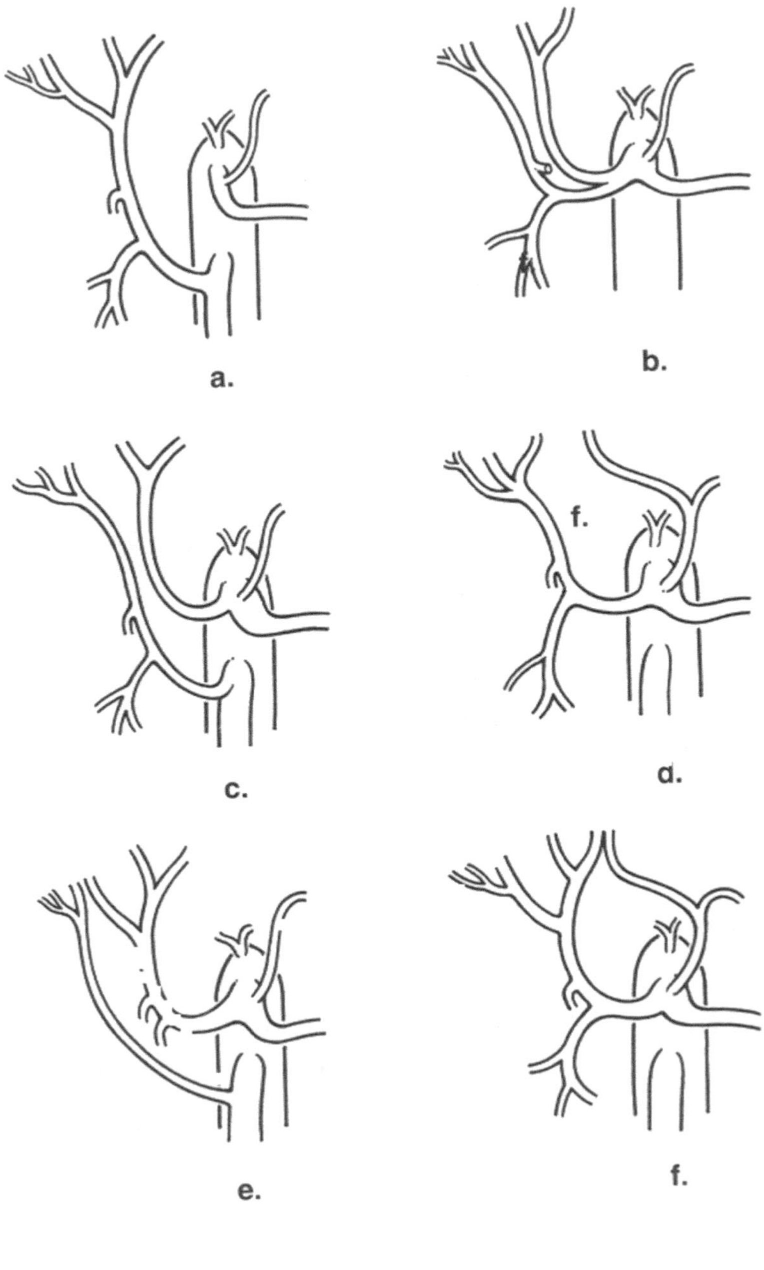

Figure 6. Hepatic arterial anomalies. (a) Replaced main hepatic artery arising from the superior mesenteric artery (SMA), (b) Independent origin of the right and left hepatic artery from the celiac axis, (c) Replaced right hepatic artery arising from the SMA, (d) Replaced left hepatic artery arising from the left gastric artery (LGA), (e) Accessory right hepatic artery arising from the SMA, (f) Accessory left hepatic artery arising from the LGA.

http://dx.doi.org/10.5772/53849

of careful dissection around the portal vein cannot be overemphasized. Inadvertent injury or transection of the portal vein or a main tributary is difficult to correct, and remains among the most lethal of surgical errors.

7. Intrahepatic arterial and portal venous anatomy

Throughout the course of the liver, the sectoral and segmental bile ducts, hepatic arteries and portal venous branches run together. (Figure 7) Whereas knowledge of precise intrahepatic biliary anatomy is of most practical value to the operating surgeon, further detail about intrahepatic anatomy will be discussed in that section below.

8. The biliary tract

Extrahepatic hepatic biliary anatomy

The extrahepatic biliary system consists of the extrahepatic portions of the right and left bile ducts that join to form a single biliary channel coursing through the posterior head of the pancreas to enter the medial wall of the second portion of the duodenum. The gallbladder and cystic duct form an additional portion of this extrahepatic biliary system that typically joins with the terminal portion of the common hepatic duct to form the common bile duct. In most instances, the confluence of the right and left bile ducts lies to the right of the umbilical fissure and anterior to the right branch of the portal vein. The right hepatic duct is typically short (< 1cm) and branches into a right posterior sectoral duct (segments VI/VII) and a right anterior sectoral duct (segments V/VIII) shortly after entering the hepatic parenchyma. In contrast, the left hepatic duct has a relatively long extrahepatic course (2- 3 cm) along the base of the quadrate lobe (segment IV) and enters the hepatic parenchyma at the umbilical fissure. Lowering the hilar plate (i.e., connective tissue enclosing the left hepatic elements and Glisson's capsule) at the base of the quadrate lobe provides great exposure to both the biliary hilum and the extrahepatic portion of the left hepatic duct. (Figure 8)

9. The common bile duct

By convention, the entry point of the cystic duct divides the main extrahepatic biliary channel into the common hepatic duct (above) and the common bile duct (below). The common bile duct continues inferiorly positioned anterior to the portal vein, and lateral to the common hepatic artery. If the hepatic artery bifurcates early, the right hepatic artery may be seen coursing below (80% of the time) the common bile duct (see details above). At the junction of the 1st and 2nd portion of the duodenum, the common bile duct ducks behind the duodenum posterior to the pancreatic head, in order to enter the medial wall of the duodenum (2nd portion) at the sphincter of Oddi.

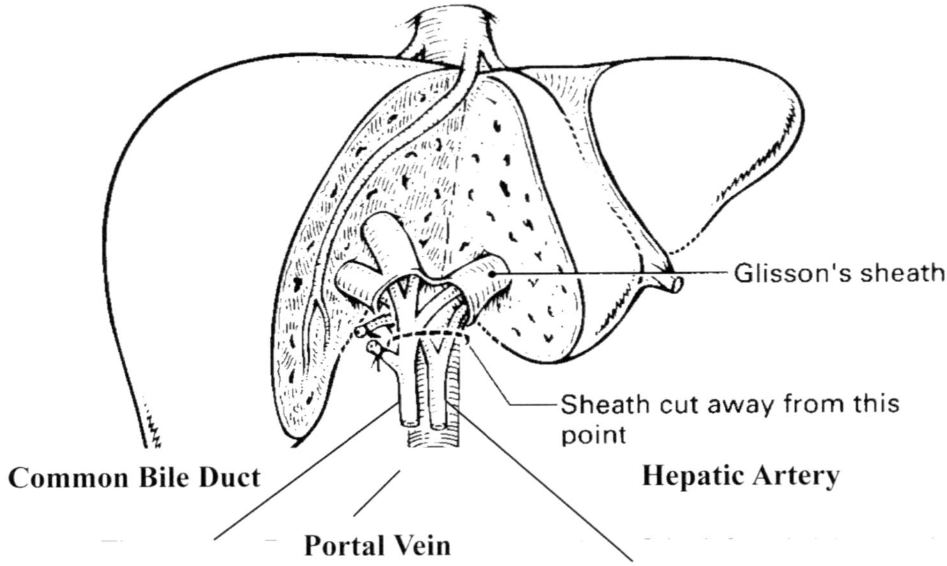

Figure 7. Portal pedicles. This cutaway view of the right and left portal pedicles demonstrate the course of the right and left portal veins, hepatic ducts, and hepatic arteries as they enter the hepatic parenchyma

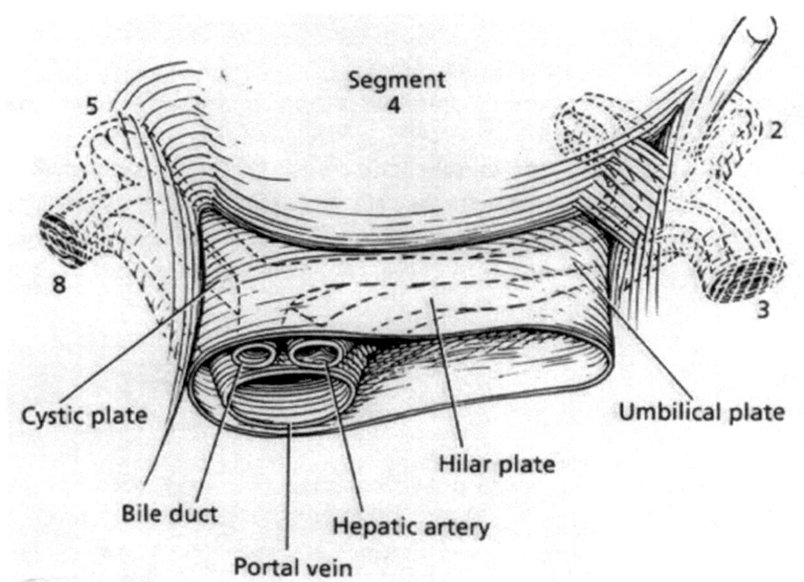

Figure 8. Lowering of the hilar plate and exposure of the left hepatic duct. The left hepatic duct runs at the base of the quadrate lobe (segment 4) and is covered by the hilar plate (a layer of connective tissue running between the hepatoduodenal ligament and the Glissonian capsule of the liver. Dividing this layer demonstrates the extrahepatic portion of the left hepatic duct arising from the umbilical fissure. (Numbers 2,3,4 and refer to segmental liver anatomy).

http://dx.doi.org/10.5772/53849

10. Gallbladder and cystic duct

The gallbladder is situated on the undersurface of the anterior inferior sector (segment V) of the right lobe of the liver. Though often densely adherent, it is separated from the liver parenchyma by the cystic plate, a layer of connective tissue arising from Glisson's capsule and in continuity with the hilar plate at the base of segment IV. In rare instances, the gallbladder is only loosely attached to the undersurface of the liver by a thinly veiled mesentery and may be prone to volvulus. Variations in gallbladder anatomy are rare. These variations include (a) bilobed or double gallbladders, (b) septated gallbladders, or (c) gallbladder diverticulums.

The cystic duct arises from the infindibulum of the gallbladder and runs medial and inferior to join the common hepatic duct. The cystic duct is typically 1-3 mm in diameter, and can range from 1 mm to 6 cm in length depending upon its union with the common hepatic duct. Spiral mucosal folds, referred to as valves of Heister, are present in the mucosa of the cystic duct. Cystic duct abnormalities are uncommon and include (a) double cystic ducts (very rare), (b) aberrant cystic duct entry sites, and (c) aberrant cystic duct union with the common hepatic duct. Aberrant entry points for the cystic duct include a low entry into the common hepatic duct retroduodenal or retropancreatic, and anomalous entry into the main right hepatic duct or sectoral duct. Aberrant union of the cystic duct and common hepatic duct can take multiple forms including (a) absence of a cystic duct (< 1%), (b) parallel course of the cystic duct and common hepatic artery with a shared septum (20%), and (c) an anomalous passage of the cystic duct posterior to the common hepatic duct with entry on the medial wall (5%). (Figure 9)

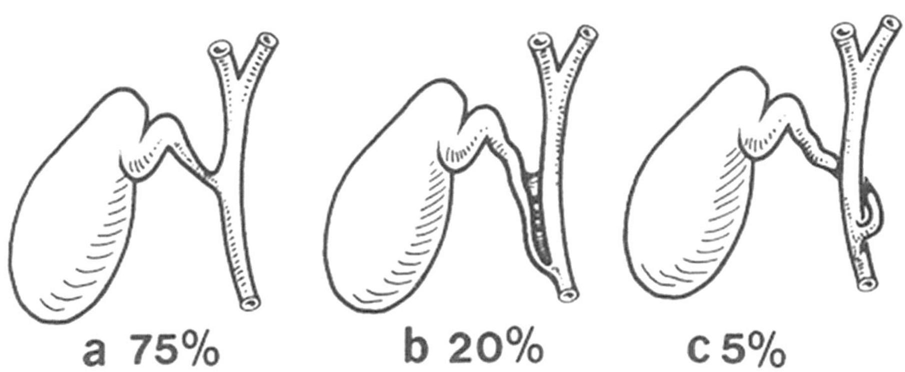

Figure 9. Variations in cystic ductal anatomy.

Typically, the cystic artery is a single vessel that courses lateral and posterior to the cystic duct. However, variations in the anatomy of the cystic artery are common. (Figure 10) Multiple cystic arteries, origin of the cystic artery from a segmental or lobar hepatic artery, aberrant course of the cystic artery over the cystic duct, and various other anomalies have been reported. A careful intra-operative determination of cystic artery anatomy is important to prevent unnecessary hemorrhage during cholecystectomy.

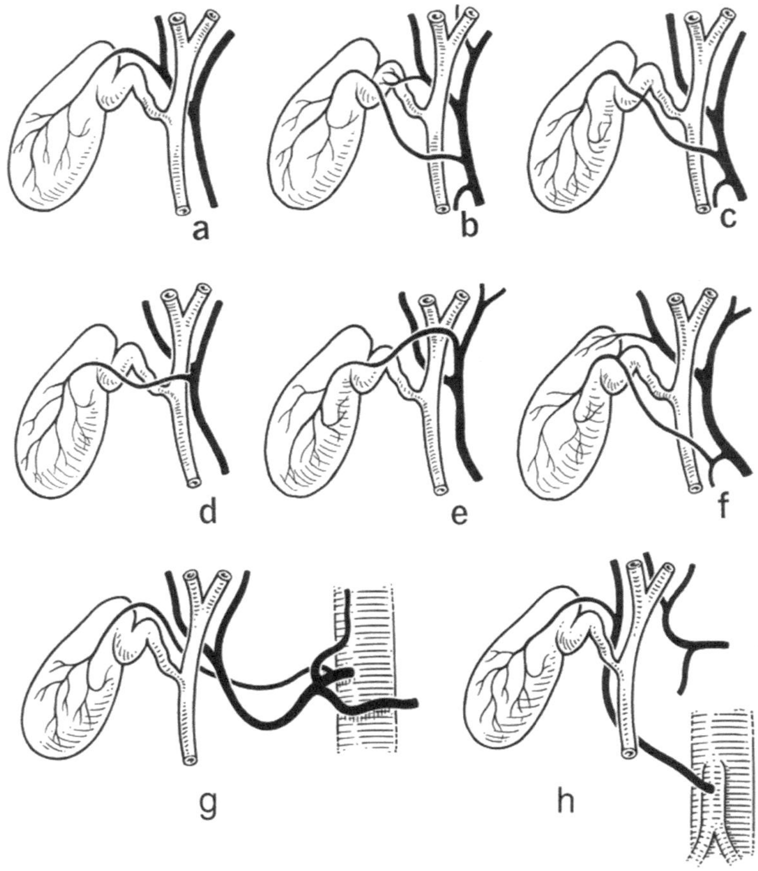

Figure 10. Cystic artery anomalies. (A) Typical course, (B) Double cystic artery, (C) cystic artery crossing anterior to the main bile duct, (D) cystic artery originating from the right branch of the hepatic artery and crossing the common hepatic duct anteriorly, (E) cystic artery originating from the left branch of the hepatic artery, (F) cystic artery originating from the gastroduodenal artery, (G) the cystic artery may arise from the celiac axis, (H) cystic artery originating from a replaced right hepatic artery.

10. Intrahepatic bile duct anatomy

An understanding of intrahepatic ductal anatomy is obviously important and vital to the performance of a high biliary anastomoses for cholangiocarcinoma (Klatskin tumors), an intrahepatic bilioenteric bypass, and complex hepatic resections such as caudate lobectomy, and left and right trisegmentectomy. The right and left lobes of the liver are drained separately by the right and left hepatic ducts. In contrast, 1 – 4 smaller ducts from either the right or left hepatic ducts drain the caudate lobe. Within the liver parenchyma, the intrahepatic biliary radicals parallel the major portal triad tributaries directed toward each hepatic segment of the liver. More specifically, bile ducts are usually situated superior to its complementary portal vein branch, while the hepatic artery lies inferiorly.

The left hepatic duct drains all 3 segments of the left liver. (Segment II, III, and IV). In some textbooks, segment IV, the quadrate lobe, is futher sub-divided into sub-segments (4A, superior, and 4B, inferior). So conceptually, both the right and left hepatic ducts each drains 4 segments. Although the left hepatic duct originates within the liver and terminates in the common hepatic duct, it is easier to describe its' path in reverse since the extrahepatic areas are readily visible to the operating surgeon. After the bifurcation into the right and left hepatic ducts, the left duct courses towards the umbilical fissure along the under surface of segment IVB above and behind the left branch of the portal vein. Access to this area can be gained by lowering the hilar plate (described above). Several small branches from the quadrate lobe (Segment 4) and the caudate lobe (Segment 1) may enter the left duct at this location. The left hepatic duct is formed within the umbilical fissure by the segment III (lateral), and segment IVB (medial) ducts. Following the course of the umbilical fissure vertically towards the falciform ligament, the segment II (lateral), and segment IVA (medial) branches are formed. Although a careful and tedious dissection is required to access the segmental biliary ducts for anastomoses, (e.g., a segment III bypass), control of the segmental portal triads to all areas of left lobe is readily achievable within the umbilical fissure. (see Figure 11)

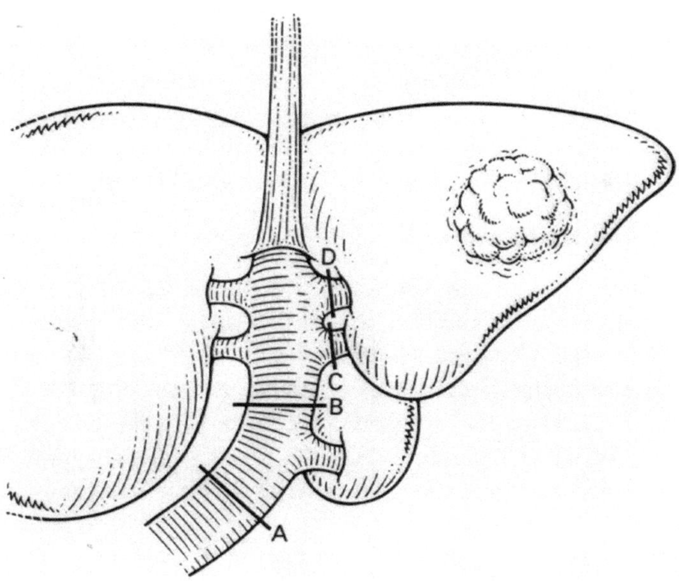

Figure 11. Left portal vein pedicle. The union of the segment IV, II, and III portal veins within the umbilical fissure forms the left portal vein. A separate segment I portal vein also enters the left portal vein before it coalesces with the right portal vein at the hilus. Lines A, B, C, D demonstrate various lines of portal vein transection which are required to complete various hepatic resections. Line A is the line of transection for completion of a left hepectecomy and caudate lobectomy. Line B is the line of transection for completion of a left hepatectomy. Line C is the line of transection for a segment II resection. Line D is the line of transection for a segment III resection.

The right hepatic duct emerges from the liver at the base of segment V just to right of the caudate process. This duct drains segments V, VI, VII, and VIII and originates at the junction of the right posterior (segments VI and VII), and anterior (segments V and VIII) sectoral ducts. The right posterior sectoral duct follows an almost horizontal course at the base of segments V and VI that can often been seen lying within a transverse fissure on the superficial surface of the liver. Segmental biliary branches from segments VI (inferior) and VII (superior) converge to form the main right posterior sectoral duct. Segmental branches from segments V and VIII form the right anterior sectoral duct. While the right posterior sectoral duct follows a horizontal course, the right anterior sectoral duct runs almost vertical within segment V, and receives branches from both segment V (inferior) and VIII (superior).

Biliary drainage of the caudate lobe is less predictable. Conceptually, the caudate lobe has three distinct areas -- a right part, a left part, and the caudate process. In some instances three separate bile ducts may be present. The caudate process represents a narrow bridge of tissue that connects the caudate to the right lobe (segment V). In more than 75% of cases the caudate drains into both the right and left hepatic ductal system, but isolated drainage into the right (< 10%), or left hepatic duct (~15%) can occur.

11. Anomalous biliary drainage

Normal intra- and extrahepatic biliary anatomy is present in approximately 75 percent of cases. (Figure 12) Every effort should be made to define existing intrahepatic anatomy based on pre-operative imaging, since failure to do so may result in devastating complications. Anomalies in both sectoral and segmental anatomy may exist together or separately. The more common type of each of the anomalies will be described in more detail below.

Anomalous sectoral biliary anatomy

Although the union of the right and left hepatic duct typically occurs at the hilum, a triple confluence of the right posterior and anterior sectoral ducts with the left hepatic duct may, exist in up to ~15% of cases. (Figure 12) In 20% of cases, one of the right sectoral ducts, more commonly the anterior sectoral duct, may enter the common hepatic duct distal to the confluence. If this situation is not recognized it can be very dangerous, and represents a common cause of injury during laparoscopic cholecystectomy. Less commonly (~5%), the right posterior sectoral duct (and rarely the right anterior sectoral duct) may cross to enter the intrahepatic portion of the left hepatic duct. Failure to appreciate this anomaly prior to right or left hepatectomy, can lead to significant post-operative problems. Note some authorities believe that this anomaly represents the most common intrahepatic biliary variations.

Anomalous segmental biliary anatomy

A large number of segmental biliary anomalies have been reported. Most are unimportant to the surgeon and of anatomical interest only. Figure 13 illustrates the more common anomalies that have been reported within the right lobe and the medial segment of the left lobe.

http://dx.doi.org/10.5772/53849

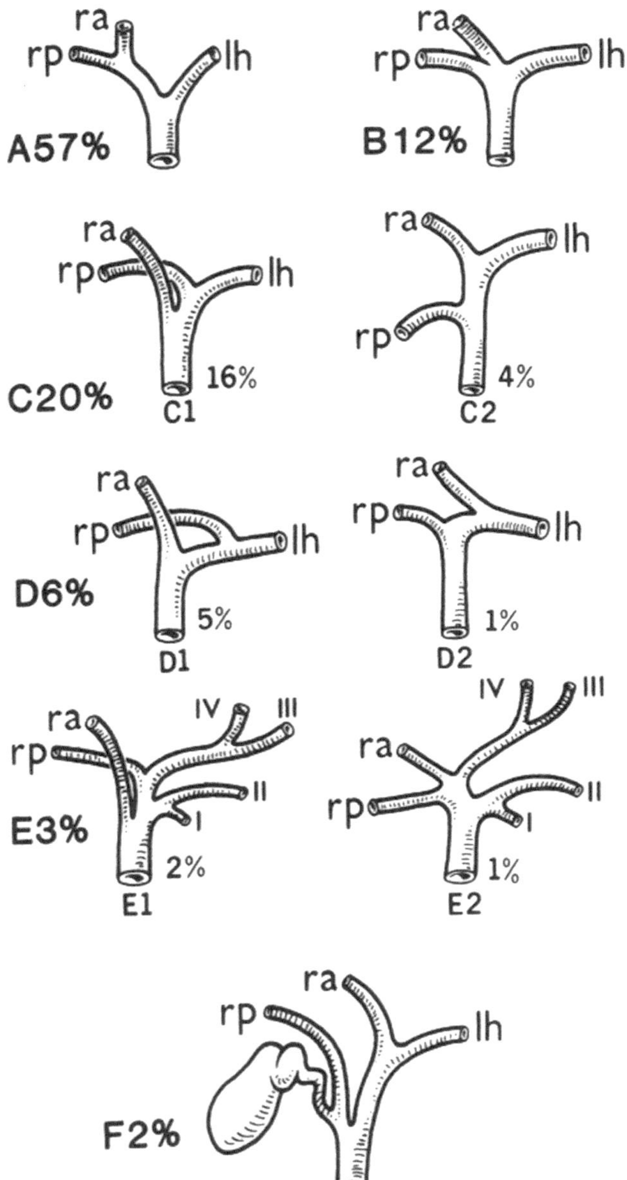

Figure 12. Normal and aberrant sectoral ductal anatomy. (A) Typical ductal anatomy, (B) triple confluence, (C) Ectopic drainage of a right sectoral duct into the common hepatic duct (C1, right anterior duct draining into the common hepatic duct; C2, right posterior duct draining into the common hepatic duct), (D) ectopic drainage of a right sectoral duct into the left hepatic ductal system (D1, right posterior sectoral duct draining into the left hepatic ductal system; D2, right anterior sectoral duct draining into the left hepatic ductal system, (E) absence of the hepatic duct confluence, (F) absence of right hepatic duct and ectopic drainage of the right posterior duct into the cystic duct.

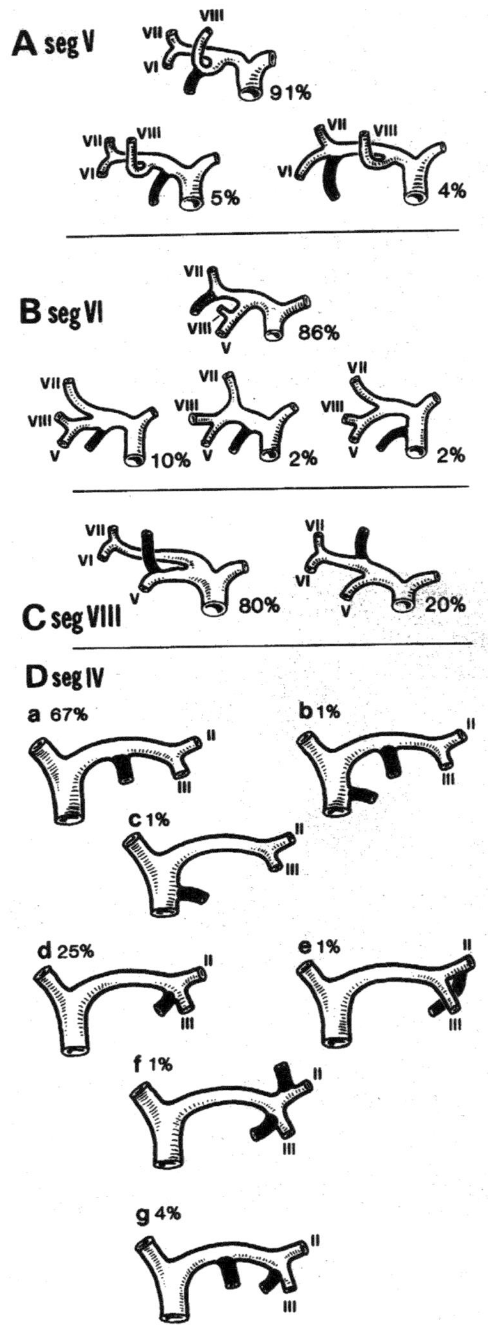

Figure 13. Normal and aberrant segmental ductal anatomy. (A), variations of segment V, (B) variations of segment VI, (C) variations of segment VIII, (D) variations of segment IV. Note there is no variation of drainage of segments II, III, and VII.

12. Summary

A comprehensive understanding of normal and aberrant anatomy is the cornerstone of surgery. The truth of this statement is nowhere more apparent than in the performance of complex hepatobiliary surgery. Mastery of the segmental anatomy of the liver, as well as a comprehensive understanding of both normal and anomalous arterial, venous and biliary anatomy, are the *sine qua non* for performing safe hepatic resections. Recent advances in peri-operative management of patients with hepatobiliary diseases (detailed elsewhere in this book), permit the surgeon to perform increasingly radical hepatic procedures (upon sicker patients.) Although the expertise offered by our radiology and anesthesiology colleagues is important, it is incumbent upon every surgeon who performs liver resection to be well prepared. An age-old surgical axiom states "98% of the surgical outcome is determined in the operating room." A good outcome in the performance of hepatic resections requires one to become a student of the game.

Author details

Ronald S. Chamberlain[1,2,3]

1 Department of Surgery, Saint Barnabas Medical Center, Livingston, NJ, USA

2 Department of Surgery, University of Medicine and Dentistry of New Jersey, Newark, NJ, USA

3 Saint George's University School of Medicine, Grenada, West Indies

References

[1] Abdalla, E. K, Vauthey, J. N, & Couinaud, C. The caudate lobe of the liver: implications of embryology and anatomy for surgery. Surg Oncol Clin N Am (2002). , 11, 835-48.

[2] Bismuth, H. Surgical anatomy and anatomical surgery of the liver. World J Surg (1982). , 6, 3-9.

[3] Bismuth, H. Surgical anatomy and anatomical surgery of the liver. In: Blumgart LH, editor. Surgery of the liver and biliary tract. Edinburgh (UK): Churchill Livingstone; (1988). , 3-10.

[4] Couinaud, C. Lobes et segments hepatiques: note sur l'architecture anatomique et chirurgicale du foie. Presse Med (1954).

[5] Ger, R. Surgical anatomy of the liver. Surg Clin N Am (1989). , 69, 179-93.

[6] Goldsmith, N. A, & Woodburne, R. T. Surgical anatomy pertaining to liver resection. Surg Gynecol Obstet (1957).

[7] Healey JE JrSchroy PC. Anatomy of the biliary ducts within the human liver: analysis of the prevailing pattern of branchings and the major variations of the biliary ducts. Arch Surg (1953).

[8] Healey JE JrVascular anatomy of the liver. Ann N Y Acad Sci (1970).

[9] Healey JE JrClinical anatomic aspects of radical hepatic surgery. J Int Coll Surg (1954).

[10] Hjortsjo, C. H. The topography of the intrahepatic duct system. Acta Anat (1951). , 11, 599-615.

[11] Longmire, W. P. Historic landmarks in biliary surgery. South Med J (1982). , 75, 1548-50.

[12] Meyers, W. C, Ricciardi, R, & Chiari, R. S. Liver. Anatomy and development. In: Townsend CM, editor. Sabiston textbook of surgery. 16th edition. Philadelphia: WB Saunders; (2001). , 997-1034.

[13] Mizumoto, R, & Suzuki, H. Surgical anatomy of the hepatic hilum with special reference to the caudate lobes. World J Surg (1988). , 12, 2-10.

[14] Nakamura, S, & Tsuzuki, T. Surgical anatomy of the hepatic veins and the inferior vena cava. Surg Gynecol Obstet (1981). , 152, 43-50.

[15] Skandalakis, L. J, Colborn, G. L, Gray, S. W, et al. Surgical anatomy of the liver and extrahepatic biliary tract. In: Nyhus LM, Baker RJ, editors. Mastery of surgery. 2nd edition. Boston: Little, Brown and Co; (1992). , 775-805.

[16] Skandalaki, J. E, Skandalakis, L. J, Skandalakis, P. N, & Mirilas, P. Hepatic Anatomy. Surg Clinc N Am 84 ((2004).

[17] Smith, R. In: Suzuki T, Nakayusu A, Kauabe K, et al, editors. Surgical significance of anatomic variations of the hepatic artery. Am J Surg (1971). , 122, 505-12.

Chapter 3

Anesthetic Considerations for Patients with Liver Disease

Aparna Dalal and John D. Jr. Lang

Additional information is available at the end of the chapter

http://dx.doi.org/10.5772/54222

1. Introduction

The liver is the largest gland in the body. The average human liver weighs approximately 1.5-1.7 kg, and holds a blood volume of approximately 500 ml. It receives approximately 25% of the cardiac output, of which 75% is supplied by the portal vein and the other 25% by the hepatic artery. Its venous drainage is to the inferior vena cava via the hepatic veins. The hepatic ductal system produces the bile which is then stored in the gall bladder.

The liver synthesizes most proteins, with the exception of gamma globulins and factor VIII. It is also responsible for protein degradation, glucose homeostasis, fatty acid β-oxidation, bilirubin production and excretion. Hepatocytes are embryologically less differentiated; hence the liver is the only organ capable of regeneration after surgical resection or trauma.

Hepatic blood flow is predominantly dependent upon systemic blood flow and pressure-based on pressure flow regulation and hepatic arterial buffer response. There is also central nervous system control of the hepatic blood flow via the thoracic sympathetic fibers. Sympathetic stimulation may cause the blood volume which is present in the liver to be expelled into the circulation, thus providing additional circulatory volume if needed.

Hepatic blood flow is reduced by all anesthetic agents and techniques via reductions in hepatic blood flow and hepatic oxygen uptake. The volatile agents, desflurane and sevoflurane have the least significant effect on total hepatic blood flow. Other perioperative causes of a reduction of hepatic blood flow include mechanical ventilation, hypercarbia, positive end-expiratory pressure, hypotension, hemorrhage, hypoxemia and surgery. A significant decrease in hepatic blood flow can result in parenchymal centrilobular necrosis when extreme resulting in further worsening of perioperative liver dysfunction.

In liver disease, anesthetic drug distribution, metabolism and elimination may be altered. Uptake and onset of anesthetic drug action is usually unaffected. Hepatic clearance of an agent is dependent upon volume of distribution, functional hepatic blood flow, hepatic extraction ratio and hepatic microsomal activity. As a result, opioids may accumulate and the pharmacological actions of drugs such as benzodiazepines maybe prolonged. In extreme situations, actions of non-depolarizing muscle relaxants such as vecuronium and rocuronium maybe also be prolonged.

The liver plays a critical role in coagulation as it is the principal site of synthesis for the majority of clotting factors: II, V, VII, IX, X, XI, and XII. All coagulation factors except for VIII, which is mainly produced by the endothelium, are markedly reduced in patients with liver disease. Patients with chronic liver disease may also develop thrombocytopenia secondary to splenomegaly caused by prolonged portal hypertension. Additionally, reduced levels of thrombopoietin, which regulates platelet production in the liver, may also further contribute to platelet counts in more advanced disease. Also, antithrombin-III (AT-III) levels fall due to reduced synthesis and/or increased consumption due to fibrinolysis. All of the proteins involved in fibrinolysis except for tissue plasminogen activator (tPA) and plasminogen activator inhibitor (PAI-1) are synthesized in the liver. However, tPA levels can be increased due to decreased clearance by the liver predisposing patients to further risks of intra- and perioperative hemorrhage. Hemostatic changes associated with surgical bleeding are thrombocytopenia, platelet function defects, inhibition of platelet aggregation and adhesion by nitric oxide and prostacyclin, decreased levels of coagulation factors: II, V, VII, IX, X, XI, quantitative and qualitative abnormalities of fibrinogen, low levels of α2-antiplasmin, Factor XIII and thrombin activatable fibrinolysis inhibitor, and elevated tPA. Hemostatic changes associated with thrombosis are elevated vWF, decreased levels of ADAMTS-13 (a vWF cleaving protease), and decreased levels of anti-coagulants: ATIII, Protein C and S, α2 macroglobulin, elevated levels of heparin cofactor II, elevated VIII, decreased levels of plasminogen, normal or increased PAI-1. Hypercoagulability can occur in patients with liver disease, especially those with cholestatic disease.

In the setting of acute liver failure (ALF), the coagulopathy encountered can be much more severe. Plasma concentrations of coagulation factors with the shortest half-life fall first; factors V and VII (12 hrs and 4-6hrs respectively) and factors II,VII and X subsequently. In a review of over 1000 patients with ALF by the US Acute Liver Failure Study Group, the mean international normalization ratio (INR) in ALF was 3.8 +/- 4.0 (range 1.5 - >10) with most having a moderately prolonged INR (1.5 to 5) and only 19% with an INR >5. Moreover, thrombocytopenia is common with 40% of patients having platelet counts < 90,000 on admission. [1]

2. Pathophysiology of End Stage Liver Disease

Liver disease can be acute or chronic. Common causes of chronic liver disease are viral hepatitis (B & C), autoimmune hepatitis, non-alcoholic steatohepatitis (NASH), Laennec's cirrhosis, cryptogenic cirrhosis, and metabolic diseases such as hemachromatosis and Wilson's disease. Cholestatic causes of liver disease include primary biliary cirrhosis and primary sclerosing cholangitis.

Predominant pathophysiological manifestation of liver disease is portal hypertension. There is increased resistance to portal blood flow due to hepatic parenchymal scarring and fibrosis, and splanchnic hyperemic resulting in hypersplenism, thrombocytopenia and the progression formation of varices. Normal portal pressures are usually in the range of 5-12 mmHg. Portal hypertension is generally defined when any 2 of the following 3 criteria are met: splenomegaly, ascites or bleeding esophageal varices. Portal pressures at this time are usually > 20 mmHg.

The combination of decreased production of albumin and portal hypertension results in the accumulation of ascites. It also occurs due to renal retention of sodium and water, and localization of this excess fluid in the peritoneal cavity. Tense ascites may decrease functional residual capacity (FRC), adversely affect pulmonary gas exchange and increase risk of aspiration. Hydrothorax or pleural effusions may produce atelectasis. Secondary hyperaldosteronism may manifest as hypokalemic metabolic alkalosis. Additionally, there is intra- and extra-pulmonary shunting, elevated mixed venous oxygen saturation (SvO2), altered lactate metabolism. The hyperdynamic circulation is a result of decreased systemic vascular resistance (SVR) and compensatory increased cardiac output to maintain tissue perfusion. Inadequate synthesis of coagulation factors produces coagulopathy. There is delayed gastric emptying creating putting the patient at-risk for aspiration. Increased ammonia levels (hyperammonemia) can result in hepatic encephalopathy.

3. Other clinically relevant associations with patients with liver disease includes

Portopulmonary hypertension (POPH) is a pulmonary hypertension syndrome with vascular obstruction and increased resistance to pulmonary arterial flow due to varying degrees of pulmonary endothelial/smooth muscle proliferation, vasoconstriction and in-situ thrombosis. The development of POPH has not been demonstrated to correlate with the severity of liver disease.

Hepatopulmonary syndrome (HPS) is characterized by arterial hypoxemia caused by intrapulmonary vascular dilatations. The clinical triad of 1) portal hypertension; 2) hypoxemia; and 3) pulmonary vascular dilatations characterizes the clinical presentation of HPS [2].

Hepatorenal syndrome is a form of pre-renal acute kidney injury that occurs in decompensated cirrhosis. The syndrome is classified into two types: Type 1 is characterized by a doubling of the serum creatinine level to greater than 2.5 mg/dl in less than 2 weeks while Type 2 is characterized by a stable or slower progressive course of renal failure [3].

Hepatic encephalopathy occurs due to accumulation of circulating neurotoxins such as unmetabolized ammonia, gamma aminobutyric acid, gut-derived false neurotransmitters leading to altered neurotransmission by glutamate or altered cerebral energy homeostatsis. [4] Clinically, it is manifested by neuropsychiatric abnormalities and generalized clonus on clinical examination.

4. Assessing perioperative risk

Patient operative risk is dictated by severity of liver disease, co-existing medical diseases and type of surgery (i.e., upper abdominal, emergent, cardiac etc.) It may also be dependent on s on the anesthetic conducted and ability to maintain of hepatic blood flow.

An important measure for assessing mortality risk is the Child-Pugh Classification. Though this was first used to stratify risk for surgical correction of portal hypertension, it is also found to be predictive of survival in cirrhosis. The score is assigned based upon bilirubin, albumin, prothrombin time (PT), ascites and encephalopathy. One point is given for each of the following: albumin > 3.5 g/dl, INR < 1.7, bilirubin <2mg/dl, no ascites, no encephalopathy. 2 points are given for each of the following: Albumin 1.8- 3.5 g/dl, INR between1.7-2.3, bilirubin 2-3 mg/dl, slight to moderate ascites, grade 1-2 encephalopathy. 3 points are given for each of the following: albumin < 1.8 g/dl, INR >2.3, bilirubin > 3 mg/dl, tense ascites, grade 3-4 encephalopathy. Class A = 5-6 points, Class B = 7-9 points, Class C = 10-15 points. [5] Child Pugh A, B, C predicts a perioperative mortality risk of 10, 30 and 80 % respectively. [6]

Other measures for predicting mortality include ascites, increased serum creatinine, preoperative GI bleed, high ASA physical status score and previous abdominal surgery. Steatosis and steatohepatitis may also be considered as risk factors for postoperative complications, especially after abdominal procedures. The Model of End Liver Disease (MELD) score predicts severity based upon serum creatinine, total bilirubin, and PT INR. It is used to estimate long term survival, as well as list patients for liver transplantation with the United network of Organ Sharing (UNOS). (need a reference here)

Elective surgery is contraindicated when the patient has acute viral hepatitis, alcoholic hepatitis, fulminant hepatic failure, severe chronic hepatitis, is a Child Pugh C patient or has other manifestations of end stage liver disease.

Patients with advanced liver disease should be effectively managed so that hepatic perfusion and hepatic oxygen delivery are maximized l and sequelae of their liver disease such as hepatic encephalopathy, cerebral edema, coagulopathy, hepatopulmonary syndrome, portopulmonary hypertension and portal hypertension has been identified and treated accordingly if possible.

5. Preoperative evaluation of patients with liver disease

Assessment of hepatic function includes evaluating risks for aggravating underlying liver disease, extra-hepatic complications, alterations of hepatic synthetic function and altered drug disposition.

http://dx.doi.org/10.5772/54222

Liver function tests do not measure hepatic function. They represent release of damaged or dead hepatocyte intracellular contents into the systemic circulation, hence provide a snapshot at that point in time only. Actual liver function is represented by albumin, prothrombin time and pseudocholinesterase concentrations. Obtaining liver function tests in healthy patients is not recommended as abnormal liver function tests (LFTs) exist in about 1 in 700 patients, and a vast majority of these patients do not have advanced liver disease. Thus, patients with asymptomatic elevations in serum transaminase levels (less than two times normal values) may undergo anesthesia and surgery with good outcomes.

Patients with chronic hepatitis should be screened prior to elective surgery even if they are asymptomatic. The INR is the most sensitive indicator of hepatocellular dysfunction. At present, though it is accepted that abnormal hemostasis is a result of liver disease, it is debatable whether the abnormal tests really predict bleeding risk [7]. Moreover, the relationship of coagulation profiles to the risk of bleeding with chronic as well as acute liver disease is uncertain [8]. Low platelet count may not be solely responsible for an increased risk of bleeding as the platelet function is also important. Bleeding time is no longer recommended as a test of platelet function. The current consensus is for a pre-procedure platelet count > 50,000, since it appears that a platelet count above 50,000 is likely to be adequate based on previous studies [9].

It is also important to assess the patient for extra-hepatic pathophysiology related to liver disease. The diagnostic criteria for POPH include a mean pulmonary artery pressure (mPAP) greater than 25 mmHg at rest and a pulmonary vascular resistance (PVR) of > 240 dynes.s.cm^{-5} [10]. A better measure is a transpulmonary gradient > 12 mmHg (mPAP-PAOP) as this reflects the obstruction to flow (PVR) and also distinguishes the contribution of intravascular volume and flow to the mPAP [11].

The European Respiratory Society (ERS)/European Association for Study of the Liver (EASL) Task Force have certain set diagnostic criteria for hepatopulmonary syndrome (HPS). These include diagnosis of liver disease, an A-a oxygen gradient > 15 mmHg, pulmonary vascular dilatation documented by "positive" delayed, contrast-enhanced echocardiography with left heart, detection of microbubbles for > 4 cardiac cycles after right heart opacification of microbubbles and brain uptake > 6% following 99mTc macroaggregated albumin (MAA) lung perfusion scanning. HPS can be diagnosed when there is a cirrhosis with ascites, serum creatinine of >1.5 mg/dL, no improvement of serum creatinine after at least 2 days with diuretic withdrawal and volume expansion with albumin, absence of shock, no current or recent treatment with nephrotoxic drugs and absence of parenchymal kidney disease as indicated by proteinuria > 500 mg/day, microhematuria, and/or abnormal renal ultrasonography. [12]

6. Cardiac assessment of End Stage Liver Disease (ESLD) patients

Cirrhotic patients with ESLD may suffer from cirrhotic cardiomyopathy. This is comprised of increased cardiac output and compromised ventricular response to stress. This entity is likely mediated by decreased beta-agonist transduction, increased circulating inflammatory mediators resulting in cardiac depression, and accompanying repolarization abnormalities [13-18]. Low systemic vascular resistance and bradycardia are also commonly seen in ESLD. Patients with ESLD may also demonstrate diastolic dysfunction. [19]. The electrophysiologic abnormalities found in cirrhotic cardiomyopathy include QT-interval prolongation, electrical and mechanical dyssynchrony and chronotropic incompetence [20-22]. Carvedilol administered to patients with ESLD has been demonstrated to reduce portal pressures by decreasing net splanchnic blood flow. [23].

Additionally, ESLD are also at risk for the development of coronary artery disease (CAD), however the liver itself has not been implicated. Approximately 25 % of these patients have at least one moderate or severe coronary artery with critical stenosis. Obstructive CAD was most common among patients with 2 traditional cardiac risk factors such as smoking, diabetes mellitus (DM),and/or hyperlipidemia [24]. Left ventricular hypertrophy and hyperdynamic systolic function in ESLD may result in hemodynamically significant left ventricular outflow tract obstruction (LVOTO). One retrospective review of 106 transplant recipients found inducible LVOTO on pre-operative dobutamine stress echocardiography (DSE) in 40% of patients [25]. In this study, an outflow gradient of 36 mm Hg was significantly associated with intraoperative hypotension. Many ESLD patients also have prolonged corrected QT interval (QTc) on an electrocardiogram which can be associated with an increased risk of ventricular arrhythmias. Though it is not a contraindication to surgery and anesthesia, one should look for electrolyte disturbances or the use of QT interval-prolonging drugs. All patients with ESLD should undergo a preoperative echocardiography to assess ventricular function, ventricular size, valvular function, pulmonary artery pressure, and to exclude the presence of a significant LVOTO or pericardial effusion. Pre-operative echocardiography is useful to calculate pulmonary artery systolic pressure. Pulmonary artery systolic pressures (PASP) values of 45-50 mmHg and /or right ventricular dysfunction are usually used for screening POPH. Right heart catheterization should be performed to gauge the mean pulmonary artery pressure (PAP), pulmonary capillary wedge pressure (PCWP) and transpulmonary gradient (TPG) as 5% to 10% of ESLD candidates have POPH [26],. A preoperative mPAP of 35 to 50 mm Hg has been associated with a 50% risk of mortality after liver transplantation in patients with POPH [26], and mortality approached 100% among patients with POPH and mPAP ≥50 mm Hg [27]. Thus, POPH warrants perioperative treatment with vasodilators such as epoprosterenol, sildenafil or nitric oxide. Stress testing of ESLD patients can be done to detect CAD. Dobutamine stress echocardiography has been found to have a negative predictive value in ESLD patients to be 85%.[28,29]. The predictive value of nuclear single-photon emission computed tomography (SPECT) stress imaging is limited by the chronic vasodilatory state exhibited by patients with ESLD [30]. The specificity of abnormal SPECT findings for obstructive CAD by coronary angiography is only 61% [31]. Coronary angiography is the gold standard for detecting CAD. When possible, it is important make an assessment of CAD risk in the ESLD patient before revascularization becomes contraindicated (usually an excessive bleeding risk due to coagulopathy and/or thrombocytopenia). Transesophageal echocardiography (TEE) and/or pulmonary artery catheterization may be used intraoperatively to allow for real-time hemodynamic monitoring and volume management..

7. Anesthetic agents

All volatile anesthetics decrease the mean arterial pressure and portal blood flow. Halothane has consistently the most dramatic effect in reducing hepatic arterial blood flow. [32,33]. On the other hand, sevoflurane, desflurane and isoflurane have been consistently shown to better preserve hepatic blood flow and function. Intravenous anesthetics have a modest impact on hepatic blood flow, and no meaningful adverse impact on postoperative liver function if the mean arterial pressure is adequately maintained throughout the time anesthetized. Induction agents such as etomidate and thiopental decrease hepatic blood flow, either from increased hepatic arterial vascular resistance or from reduced cardiac output and/or blood pressure. [34]. Ketamine has little impact on hepatic blood flow. [35] Propofol increases total hepatic blood flow in both hepatic arterial and portal venous circulation, suggesting a significant vasodilator effect. [36,37].

Opioids such as morphine have significantly reduced metabolism in patients with advanced cirrhosis. The elimination half-life of morphine is prolonged, potentially exaggerating sedative and respiratory depressant effects. Fentanyl is highly lipid soluble with a short duration of action, which is also metabolized in the liver. Fentanyl elimination is not appreciably altered in patients with cirrhosis. [38,39]. However, unlike fentanyl, the half-life of alfentanil is almost doubled in patients with cirrhosis. [40]. Remifentanil is a synthetic opioid with an ester linkage that allows for rapid hydrolysis by blood and tissue esterases. It elimination is unaltered in patients with severe liver disease. [41].

Thiopental has a small hepatic extraction ratio. However, its elimination half-life is unchanged in cirrhotics, as it has a large volume of distribution. The clearance of etomidate is unchanged in cirrhotic patients, but its clinical recovery time maybe unpredictable due to increased volumes of distribution [42]. The elimination kinetic profile of propofol is similar in cirrhotic patients as well as normal patients, but the mean clinical recovery times maybe longer after discontinuation of infusions. [43]. The half-life of midazolam is prolonged due to reduced clearance, reduced protein binding, resulting in a prolonged duration of action and an enhanced sedative effect, especially after multiple doses or prolonged infusions. [44] Dexmedetomidine, an $\alpha 2$-adrenergic agonist, with sedative and analgesic properties, is primarily metabolized in the liver. Dose adjustments are therefore indicated when used in patients with significant hepatic dysfunction. [45].

Vecuronium and rocuronium are steroidal muscle relaxants which undergo hepatic metabolism, hence have decreased clearance, prolonged half-lives, and prolonged neuromuscular blockade in patients with cirrhosis. [46,47]. Atracurium and cisatracurium which undergo Hofmann elimination and ester hydrolysis respectively, have clinical duration of actions similar to those in normal patients. [48,49]

8. Intraoperative considerations

For liver surgery where major bleeding is anticipated, it is prudent to secure intravenous access using large bore peripheral catheters as well as central venous access catheters. Rapid sequence induction is recommended in patients with tense ascites to minimize the risk of aspiration. Circulatory collapse should be prevented by concomitant administration of intravenous colloid solutions because intravascular volume re-equilibrium occurs 6 to 8 hrs after removal of larger volumes of ascitic fluid. [50]. Large volumes of colloids and crystalloids maybe given within a few minutes with the assistance of commercially available rapid infusion devices. Red cell salvage should be facilitated with use of Cell savers with/without leukocyte filters. Blood administration may be associated with hyperkalemia and hypocalcemia.

Bleeding during liver surgery could be either surgical, due to previous or acquired coagulation disturbances, or both. The preoperative INR has no predictive value in relation to intraoperative blood loss and the value of fresh frozen plasma (FFP) administration to correct abnormal INR values is debatable and may even increase bleeding due to the volume load [51]. Intraoperative hemostasis panels consisting of INR, fibrinogen and platelet count, and platelet function assays for both platelet count and function, may help to differentiate between the above. A very useful intraoperative test for coagulation is the thromboelastograph (TEG). This test denotes the net effect of pro and anti-coagulants and pro and anti-fibrinolytic factors and the resulting clot tensile strength. It provides information on the rate and strength of clot formation and also clot stability/fibrinolysis. (Table 1)

Parameter	Interpretation	Preferred therapy for abnormal values
R	R is the time of latency from the time that the blood was placed in the TEG® analyzer until the initial fibrin formation.	FFP
α	The α-value measures the rapidity (kinetics) of fibrin build-up and cross-linking and the speed of clot strengthening.	Cryoprecipitate
K	K time is a measure of the rapidity to reach a certain level of clot strength.	FFP
MA	MA, or Maximum Amplitude, is a direct function of the maximum dynamic properties of fibrin and platelet bonding and represents the ultimate strength of the fibrin clot.	Platelet

Table 1. TEG Parameters

http://dx.doi.org/10.5772/54222

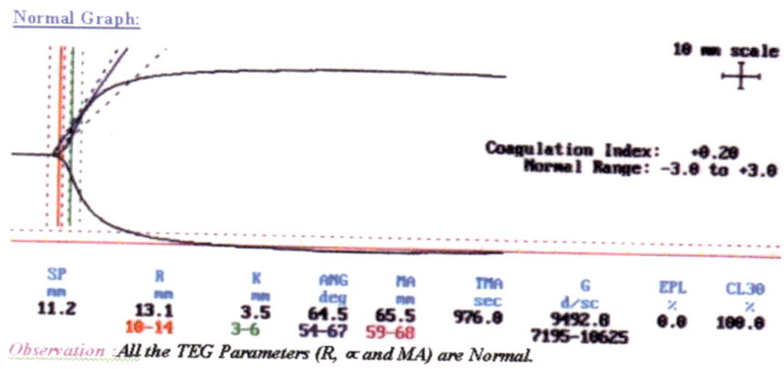

Figure 1. The Normal TEG Graph

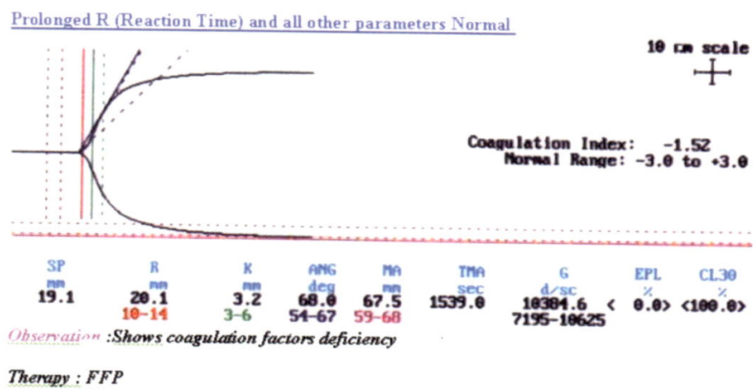

Figure 2. Prolonged Reaction Time

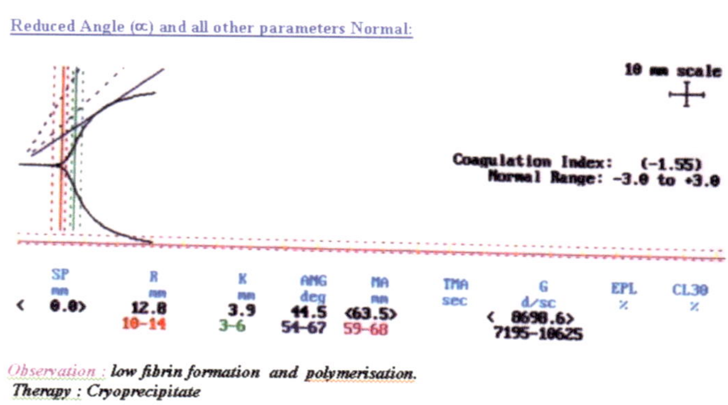

Figure 3. Reduced Angle

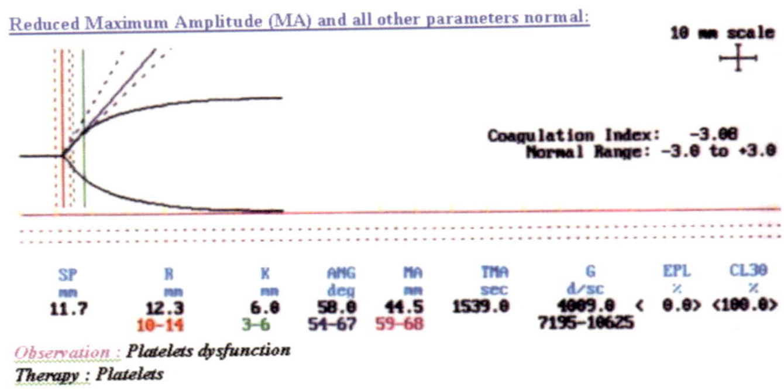

Figure 4. Reduced Maximum Amplitude.

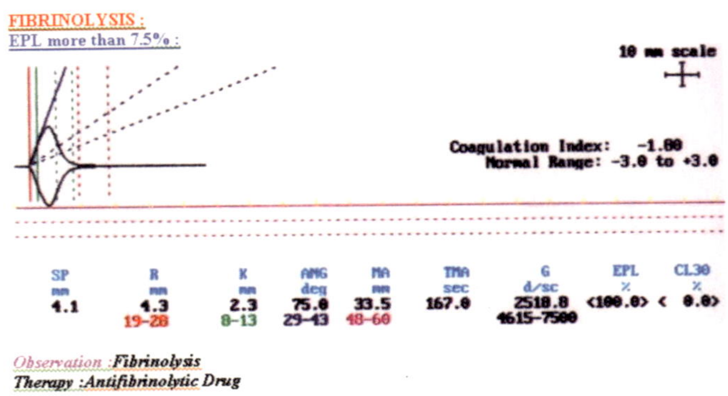

Figure 5. Fibrinolysis

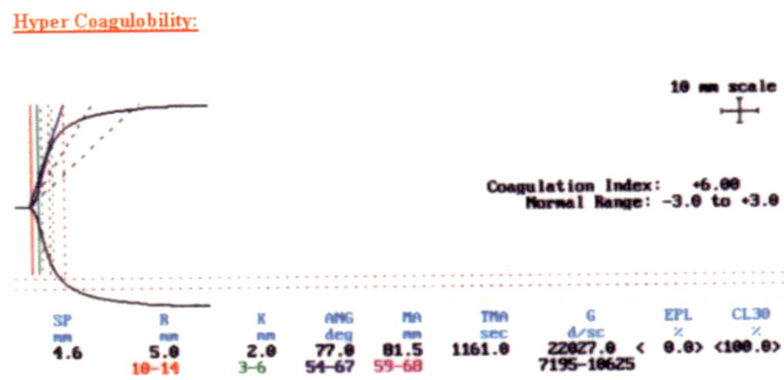

Figure 6. Hypercoagubility.

In addition, it is possible to detect heparin-like activity and to measure functional fibrinogen.(Figure 1-5,) Moreover, the only way to currently detect intraoperative hypercoagubility is via TEG. (Figure 6) Thus, TEG may act to facilitate specific goal directed therapy. If fibrinolysis is diagnosed on the TEG and it is causing clinically significant microvascular ooze, small doses of epsilon aminocaproic acid (EACA) or tranexamic acid (TA) are suitable antifibrinolytics. Factor VII has been used to control massive bleeding during liver surgery; however, it has not proved to be consistently effective to control bleeding and is associated with significant side effects. [52]

Transesophageal echocardiography (TEE) is a very useful cardiac monitoring tool to monitor function of the ventricles and assess intraoperative regional wall motion abnormalities (RWMAs), especially in patients with CAD. The monitoring of right heart systolic function is essential in patients with POPH. Moreover, it can be used effectively to assess volume status and guide fluid therapy.

9. Post-operative considerations

Surgery and anesthesia can further worsen hepatic function. Moreover, undiagnosed preexisting liver disease is often the cause of hepatic dysfunction postoperatively. Depending upon the surgical procedure, one may observe continued "third space" losses.. Potential for renal dysfunction or failure as a result of surgery is exacerbated with preexisting liver disease. As well, preoperative or intraoperative coagulopathy can continue postoperatively or can develop during first 24-48 hrs after surgery secondary to worsening hepatic dysfunction.

Postoperative jaundice occurs as a result of overproduction and under excretion of bilirubin, direct hepatocellular injury, or extra-hepatic obstruction. [53] Multiple blood transfusions can increase the levels of unconjugated bilirubin because approximately 10 % of stored whole blood undergoes hemolysis within 24 hours of transfusion. Each 0.5 – 1 unit of blood stored in CPDA-1 yields 7.5 g of hemoglobin, which is then converted to approximately 250 mg of bilirubin. [54] This may overwhelm the liver's ability to conjugate and excrete bilirubin. Immediate postoperative jaundice (< 3wks) can also occur due for multiple reasons including but not exclusive to hemolysis, anesthesia, hypotension, hypovolemia, drugs, infection, sepsis, bleeding, resorption of hematoma, bile duct ligation or injury, hepatic artery ligation, retained common bile duct stone, postoperative pancreatitis, Gilbert's syndrome, Dubin-Johnson Syndrome, inflammatory bowel syndrome, heart failure. [53] Delayed postoperative jaundice (>3 wks) can be a result of drugs, blood transfusion, post-intestinal bypass status and total parenteral nutrition. [53]

10. Postoperative pain relief role of epidural analgesia

Thoracic epidural analgesia provides excellent analgesia for liver resections. [55] The catheter is usually inserted at the T6-T9 space. Ropivacaine or bupivacaine are common local anesthetics used with or without the addition of small amounts of opioids such as fentanyl, sufentanil, hydromorphone or morphine. It also reduces the gastrointestinal paralysis compared with systemic opioids. [56]. There is benefit of using combined general and epidural anesthesia in patients with high-risk surgery, but this has not been extensively studied in hepatic surgery. The reasons are probably associated with the concerns with coagulation issues in this group. Additional concerns maybe harbored as neuroaxial blocks themselves are associated with risks. Estimated risk of having serious neurological injury may be as high as 0.08 %.[57, 58]. Moreover, direct spinal cord injury can occur without paraesthesias, whereas pain is more common in lesions affecting nerve roots. [59]. The incidence of persistent neurological deficit has been reported as 0.005-0.07 %. [60,61]. At our institution, we follow a practice where time from anticoagulant drug administration to epidural catheter placement is 3-5 days for warfarin, INR < 1.5, 4 hrs for heparin low dose subcutaneously, 12 hrs for low molecular weight heparin (LMWH), 5 days for clopidogrel and zero for aspirin. The time from epidural catheter removal to anticoagulant drug administration is at least 24 hrs for warfarin, 2 hrs for low dose heparin and 6-8 hrs for LMWH.

It is essential to understand that the degree of underlying parenchymal disease is not the only factor which is responsible for perioperative coagulopathy. Other important factors include amount of blood loss, dilution coagulopathy, amount and quality of residual liver parenchyma, its exposure to ischemia to name a few. [62-64]. Persistent pain or transient coagulopathy may cause delayed epidural catheter removal in patients undergoing partial hepatectomy [65]. The risk of meningitis or epidural abscess is in the range of 0.0004-0.05% [66,67].

11. Liver – specific surgical procedures

Transjugular Intrahepatic Portosystemic Shunt Procedure (TIPS)

TIPS is a procedure used in patients with end stage liver disease to decrease portal pressure and attenuate complications related to portal hypertension. It is usually done in the interventional radiology suite. The goal of this procedure is diversion of portal blood flow into the hepatic vein. The stent is passed through the internal jugular vein over a wire into the hepatic vein, which is located using fluoroscopic guidance. This stent is then advanced through the hepatic parenchyma into the portal vein. This will decompress the portal circulation. Usually, general anesthesia is requested for this procedure, as the radiologists prefer that the patients do not move during this procedure and it may be prolonged. Sedation is usually not preferred as there maybe potential respiratory depression in cirrhotic patients with underlying pulmonary dysfunction or hypoxemia from hepatopulmonary syndrome. Additionally, the presence of ascites may produce risk of aspiration. For this procedure, the central venous pressure (CVP) is monitored. After the stent is placed, the portal pressures are measured. Reduction of the difference between the two reflects the effectiveness of TIPS. Potential complications of this procedure include pneumothorax with internal jugular vein (IJV) cannulation, hematoma formation, inadvertent carotid puncture, cardiac arrhythmia

http://dx.doi.org/10.5772/54222

with intracardiac catheter passage, acute life threatening hemorrhage with hepatic artery puncture, hepatic capsular tear, extrahepatic portal venous puncture, development of pulmonary edema and congestive cardiac failure.

12. Radiofrequency Ablation (RFA) of hepatic tumors

Radiofrequency ablation of tumors up to 3 cm in size is currently used to treat non-resectable malignant tumors. During this procedure, a high-frequency, alternating current is delivered through a needle-like probe into the tumor, which induces coagulative necrosis of the tumor and surrounding tissue.[68,69]. PFA is done either percutaneously or laparoscopically. In a study which analyzed nationwide RFAs, it was found that procedure-specific complications were frequent (18.2 %), with transfusion requirements (10.7 %), intraoperative bleeding (4.3 %), and hepatic failure (2.8 %) being the most common. Postoperative complications were also common (12.0 %), with arrhythmias, heart failure, coagulopathy, and open surgical approach acting as significant predictors. [70]

Transarterial Chemoembolization (TACE)

Usually, an adequate amount of emulsion containing oil-based contrast agent Lipiodol and anticancer agents is injected through a catheter then the selected arteries are embolized by embolic agents. Superselective TACE is generally used to minimize damage to non-tumorous areas by using a microcatheter to embolize only the cancerous subsegment.[71-73] Epirubicin and cisplatin are commonly used as anticancer agents, and miriplatin, a new platinum drug, came into use in 2010.[74,75]. Indications for TACE are wide-ranging, and the procedure is generally performed in patients with hypervascular hepatocellular cancer (HCC) who are not indicated for surgery or local therapy for reasons such as multiple bilobar HCC, liver dysfunction, old age or co-morbidity, and in whom the first branch from the main portal vein is not occluded. In practice, this technique is commonly indicated for patients who are Child–Pugh class A or B with multiple tumors with a diameter of 3 cm or more or with four or more HCC. [76,77]. When TACE is combined with RFA, there may be several advantages. For example, TACE decreases the blood flow which in turn reduces the heat loss, thus increasing the size of the RFA ablative zone. In addition, the inclusion of TACE makes the evaluation of ablative margins easier, and enhances the control of satellite lesions.

Hepatic Resections

Liver resections can be done either open or robotic/laparoscopic. Hepatic resection procedures include partial resection, subsegmental resection, segmental resection, two segment resection, extended two-segment resection or three-segment resections. Pre-operative assessment should include the evaluation of the risk assessment using the CTP or MELD score, hepatic parenchymal function, and correction of severe anemia or coagulopathy, management of severe esophageal varices. The choice of anesthetic drugs as well as their doses should be based on the above assessment. There is a risk of significant blood loss. Therefore, it may be prudent to secure large bore intravenous access and be prepared for rapid infusion of colloids and crystalloids. Blood and blood products should be made available for perioperative use. Control of bleeding during resection is usually done with pressure, coagulation and hilar clamping or via the Pringle maneuver. Hilar occlusion produces a minimal increase in systemic arterial pressure, increase in systemic vascular resistance and a minimal decrease in cardiac index. There may be risk of air embolism with extensive resection and disruption of hepatic veins. Most surgeons request a low central venous pressure to facilitate dissection and minimize blood loss from the hepatic vessels and vena cava. Postoperative concerns are similar to those in major abdominal surgery. Central neuroaxial analgesia is not recommended if there is risk of coagulopathy which may result in hematoma formation in the epidural or spinal space.

Donor Liver Hepatectomy

One method of expanding donor pool for liver transplantation is the use of living donor grafts. Adult-to-adult living donor liver transplantation (LDLT) is a complex procedure that poses serious health risks to and provides no direct health benefit for the donor. Because of this uneven risk-benefit ratio, ensuring donor autonomy through informed consent is critical. However, informed consent for LDLT is sub-optimal as donors do not adequately appreciate disclosed information during the informed consent process, despite United Network for Organ Sharing/CMS regulations requiring formal psychological evaluation of donor candidates. [78] Types of donor liver grafts can be left lobe, left lobe and caudate, right lobe, extended right lobe and right lateral sector. After preoperative evaluation and screening, a virtual resection and volume analysis is done using contrast enhanced computed tomography (CT). These not only estimate SLV but can also determine segmental volume, delineate surgical planes, define anatomical landmarks of hepatic vasculature and biliary structures and calculate anticipated graft and remnant liver volumes post resection. It is essential that the minimal donor remnant volume be at least 30% of the original volume. Additionally, when right-lobe LDLT is planned, whether the middle hepatic vein (MHV) should remain in the donor or be resected is controversial. The MHV primarily provides various drainage of the right anterior lobe and segment IV. Most transplant surgeons prefer to leave the MHV in the donor to avoid congestion of segment IV and reduce the risk of liver failure in the donor.[79] The anesthesia management is similar to that of hepatectomy. In donors, several complications have been reported. In one study, right hepatectomy (resection of segments 5–8) was done in 101 donors, left lobectomy (resection of segments 2–3) in 11 donors, and left hepatectomy (resection of segments 2–4) in one donor. Minor anesthetic complications were shoulder pain, pruritus and urinary retention related to epidural morphine, and major morbidity included central venous catheter-induced thrombosis of the brachial and subclavian vein, neuropraxia, foot drop and prolonged postdural puncture headache. One of 113 donors died from pulmonary embolism on the 11th postoperative day. [80]. It was also observed that donor patients experienced significant postoperative pain despite the use of thoracic patient-controlled epidural analgesia (PCEA) infusion catheters as compared to patients who had undergone major hepatic resection. This was attributed to the longer surgical duration for donor hepatectomy and neuroplasticity which may play a role in exaggerated postoperative pain perception along with various psychological factors.[81]. It is also interesting to note that approximately 10% of donors had a platelet count < 150,000 x 10^9/liter, 2 to 3 years post-donation. [82]

13. Conclusion

Patients with liver disease are at increased risk for both perioperative morbidity and mortality. They require delineation of the degree of liver dysfunction present prior to undergoing surgery and have outcomes that are primarily dictated by the degree of hepatic dysfunction and type of surgery performed. They can certainly pose significant challenges for perioperative care.

Author details

Aparna Dalal* and John D. Jr. Lang

*Address all correspondence to: dalala1@uw.edu

The University of Washington School of Medicine, Department of Anesthesiology & Pain Medicine, NE Pacific, Seattle, WA, USA

References

[1] Munoz S, Reddy R, Lee W et al. Coagulopathy in acute liver failure. Neurocrit Care 2008;9:103-7

[2] Rodriguez-Roisin, R, Krowka MJ, Hepatopulmonary syndrome: a liver–induced lung vascular disorder. N Eng J Med 2008; 358: 2378-2387.

[3] Gines P, Schrier RW. Renal failure in cirrhosis. N Engl J Med, 2009; 361: 1279-90.

[4] Riordan SM, Williams R: Treatment of hepatic encephalopathy. N Engl J Med 1997; 337:473-479.

[5] Pugh RHN, Murray-Lyon IM, Dawson JL, et al. Transection of oesophagus for bleeding of oesophageal varices. Br J Surg 60:646-649,1973.

[6] Mansour A, Watson W, Shayani V, Pickelman J: Abdominal operations in patients with cirrhosis: Still a major surgical challenge. Surgery 1997; 22:730-736.

[7] Agarwal B, Shaw S, Hari MS et al. Continuous renal replacement therapy in patients with liver disease. J. Hepatol 2009;51:504-9

[8] Rockey DC, Caldwell SH, Goodman ZD et al. Liver Biopsy (AASLD Position Paper) Hepatology, 2009;3:1017- 1044.

[9] Tripodi A, Primignsni M, Chantarangkul V et al. Thrombin generation in patients with cirrhosis: the role of platelets. Hepatology 2006;44:440-445.

[10] Rodriguez-Roisin R, Krowka M, Hervé P, Fallon M. Pulmonary-hepatic vascular disorders (PHD). Eur Respir J 2004; 24:861-880.

[11] Ramsay M. Portopulmonary Hypertension and Right Heart failure in Patients with Cirrhosis. Curr Opin Anaesthesiol 2010;

[12] Salerno F, Gerbes A, Gines P et al. Diagnosis, prevention and treatment of hepatorenal syndrome in cirrhosis. Gut, 2007; 56: 1310-8.

[13] Alqahtani SA, Fouad TR, Lee SS. Cirrhotic cardiomyopathy. Semin Liver Dis 2008; 28:59–69.

[14] Baik SK, Fouad TR, Lee SS. Cirrhotic cardiomyopathy. Orphanet J Rare Dis 2007; 2:15.

[15] Gaskari SA, Honar H, Lee SS. Therapy insight: cirrhotic cardiomyopathy. Nat Clin Pract Gastroenterol Hepatol 2006;3:329 –37.

[16] Liu H, Song D, Lee SS. Cirrhotic cardiomyopathy. Gastroenterol Clin Biol 2002; 26:842–7.

[17] Moller S, Henriksen JH. Cirrhotic cardiomyopathy: a pathophysiological review of circulatory dysfunction in liver disease. Heart 2002;87:9 –15.

[18] Myers RP, Lee SS. Cirrhotic cardiomyopathy and liver transplantation. Liver Transpl 2000;6 Suppl 1:44 –52.

[19] Ward CA, Liu H, Lee SS. Altered cellular calcium regulatory systems in a rat model of cirrhotic cardiomyopathy. Gastroenterology 2001;121:1209–8.

[20] Bernardi M, Calandra S, Colantoni A, et al. Q-T interval prolongation in cirrhosis: prevalence, relationship with severity, and etiology of the disease and possible pathogenetic factors. Hepatology 1998;27: 28–34.

[21] Henriksen JH, Fuglsang S, Bendtsen F, Christensen E, Moller S. Dyssynchronous electrical and mechanical systole in patients with cirrhosis. J Hepatol 2002;36:513–20.

[22] Kelbaek H, Rabol A, Brynjolf I, et al. Haemodynamic response to exercise in patients with alcoholic liver cirrhosis. Clin Physiol 1987;7:35– 41.

[23] Tripathi D, Hayes PC. The role of carvedilol in the management of portal hypertension. Eur J Gastroenterol Hepatol 2010;22:905–11.

[24] Tiukinhoy-Laing SD, Rossi JS, Bayram M, et al. Cardiac hemodynamic and coronary angiographic characteristics of patients being evaluated for liver transplantation. Am J Cardiol 2006;98:178–81

[25] Maraj S, Jacobs LE, Maraj R, et al. Inducible left ventricular outflow tract gradient during dobutamine stress echocardiography: an association with intraoperative hypotension but not a contraindication to liver transplantation. Echocardiography 2004;21:681–5.

[26] Swanson KL, Wiesner RH, Nyberg SL, Rosen CB, Krowka MJ. Survival in portopulmonary hypertension: Mayo Clinic experience categorized by treatment subgroups. Am J Transplant 2008;8: 2445–53.

[27] Martinez-Palli G, Taura P, Balust J, Beltran J, Zavala E, Garcia- Valdecasas JC. Liver transplantation in high-risk patients: hepatopulmonary syndrome and portopulmonary hypertension. Transplant Proc 2005;37:3861– 4.

[28] Williams K, Lewis JF, Davis G, Geiser EA. Dobutamine stress echocardiography in patients undergoing liver transplantation evaluation. Transplantation 2000;69:2354–6.

[29] Donovan CL, Marcovitz PA, Punch JD, et al. Two-dimensional and dobutamine stress echocardiography in the preoperative assessment of patients with end-stage liver disease prior to orthotopic liver transplantation. Transplantation 1996;61:1180–8.

[30] Davidson CJ, Gheorghiade M, Flaherty JD, et al. Predictive value of stress myocardial perfusion imaging in liver transplant candidates. Am J Cardiol 2002;89:359–60.

[31] Aydinalp A, Bal U, Atar I, et al. Value of stress myocardial perfusion scanning in diagnosis of severe coronary artery disease in liver transplantation candidates. Transplant Proc 2009;41:3757– 60.

[32] Gatacel C, Losser MR, Payen D: The postoperative effects of halothane versus isoflurane on hepatic artery and portal vein blood flow in humans. Anesth Analg 2003; 96:740-745.

[33] Grundmann U, Zizzis A, Bauer C, Bauer M: In vivo effects of halothane, enflurane, and isoflurane on hepatic sinusoidal microcirculation. Acta Anaesthiol Scand 1997; 41:760-765.

[34] Thomson IA, Fitch W, Hughes RL, et al: Effects of certain I.V. anaesthetics on liver blood flow and hepatic oxygen consumption in the greyhound. Br J Anaesth 1986; 58:69-80.

[35] Thomson IA, Fitch W, Campbell D, et al: Effects of ketamine on liver blood flow and hepatic oxygen consumption: Studies in the anaesthetized greyhound. Acta Anaesthesiol Scand 1988; 32:10-14.

[36] Carmichael FJ, Crawford MW, Khayyam N: Effect of propofol infusion on splanchnic hemodynamics and liver oxygen consumption in the rat. Anesthesiology 1993; 79:1051-1060.

[37] Wouters PF, Van de Velde MA, Marcus MAE, et al: Hemodynamic changes during induction of anesthesia with eltanolone and propofol in dogs. Anesth Analg 1995; 81:125-131.

[38] Tegeder I, Lötsch J, Geisslinger G: Pharmacokinetics of opioids in liver disease. Clin Pharmacokinet 1999; 37:17-40.

[39] Haberer JP, Schoeffler P, Couderc E, et al: Fentanyl pharmacokinetics in anaesthetized patients with cirrhosis. Br J Anaesth 1982; 54:1267-1270.

[40] Ferrier C, Marty J, Bouffard Y, et al: Alfentanil pharmacokinetics in patients with cirrhosis. Anesthesiology 1985; 62:480-484.

[41] Dershwitz M, Hoke JF, Rosow CE, et al: Pharmacokinetics and pharmacodynamics of remifentanil in volunteer subjects with severe liver disease. Anesthesiology 1996; 84:812-820

[42] Van Beem H, Manger FW, Van Boxtel C, et al: Etomidate anaesthesia in patients with cirrhosis of the liver: Pharmacokinetic data. Anaesthesia 1983; 38:61-62

[43] Servin F, Cockshott ID, Farinotti R, et al: Pharmacokinetics of propofol infusions in patients with cirrhosis. Br J Anaesth 1990; 65:177-183.

[44] Trouvin JH, Farinotti R, Haberer JP, et al: Pharmacokinetics of midazolam in anaesthetized cirrhotic patients. Br J Anaesth 1988; 60:762-767.

[45] Baughman VL, Cunningham FE, Layden T: Pharmacokinetic/pharmacodynamic effects of dexmedetomidine in patients with hepatic failure. Anesth Analg 2000; 90(Suppl):S391.

[46] Arden JR, Lynam DP, Castagnoli KP, et al: Vecuronium in alcoholic liver disease: A pharmacokinetic and pharmacodynamic analysis. Anesthesiology 1988; 68:771-776.

[47] Magorian T, Wood P, Caldwell J, et al: The pharmacokinetics and neuromuscular effects of rocuronium bromide in patients with liver disease. Anesth Analg 1995; 80:754-759.

[48] De Wolf AM, Freeman JA, Scott VL, et al: Pharmacokinetics and pharmacodynamics of cisatracurium in patients with end-stage liver disease undergoing liver transplantation. Br J Anaesth 1996; 76:624-628.

[49] Ward S, Neill EA: Pharmacokinetics of atracurium in acute hepatic failure (with acute renal failure). Br J Anaesth 1983; 55:1169-1172.

[50] Menon KVN, Kamath PS: Managing the complications of cirrhosis. Mayo Clin Proc 2000; 75:501-509.

[51] Massicotte L, Capitanio U, Beaulieu D et al. Independent validation of a model predicting the need for RBC transfusion in liver transplantation. Transplantation 2009;88:386-91.

[52] Shami VM, Caldwell SH, Hespenheidee E. Recombinant factor VIIa for coagulopathy in fulminant hepatic failure compared to conventional therapy. Liver Transplant 2003.9:138-143.

[53] Nyberg LM, Pockros PJ: Postoperative jaundice. In Schiff ER, Sorrell MF, Maddrey WC, ed. Schiff's Diseases of the Liver, 8th ed. Philadelphia: Lippincott-Raven; 1999:599-605.

[54] Zuck TF, Basinger TA, Peck CC, et al: The in vivo survival of red blood cells stored in modified CDP with adenine: Report of a multi-institutional cooperative effort. Transfusion 1972; 17:374-382.

[55] Werawatganon T, Charuluxanun S. Patient controlled intravenous opioid analgesia versus continuous epidural analgesia for pain after intra-abdominal surgery. The Cochrane Database of Systematic Reviews 2005, Issue 1. Art. No.: CD004088.pub2. DOI: 10.1002/14651858.CD004088.pub2.

[56] Jørgensen H, Wetterslev J, Møiniche S, Dahl JB. Epidural local anaesthetics versus opioid-based analgesic regimens for postoperative gastrointestinal paralysis, PONV and pain after abdominal surgery. The Cochrane Database of Systematic Reviews 2001, Issue 1. Art. No.: CD001893. DOI: 10.1002/14651858.CD00001893.

[57] Horlocker TT, Abel MD, Messick JM Jr, Schroeder DR. Small risk of serious neurologic complications related to lumbar epidural catheter placement in anesthetized patients. Anesth Analg 2003;96:1547-52

[58] Rosenquist RW, Birnbach DJ. Editorial Epidural insertion in anesthetized adults: will your patients thank you? Anesth Analg 2003;96:1545-6.

[59] Tsui BC, Armstrong K. Can direct spinal cord injury occur without paresthesia? A report of delayed spinal cord injury after epidural placement in an awake patient. A nesth Analg 2005;101:1212-4.

[60] Wheatley RG, Schug SA, Watson D. Safety and efficacy of postoperative epidural analgesia. Br J Anaesth 2001;87:47-61.

[61] Horlocker TT, Wedel DJ. Neurologic complications os spinal and epidural anesthesia. Reg Anesth Pain Med. 2000;25(1):83-98. Review.

[62] Borromeo CJ, Stix MS, Lally A, Pomfret EA. Epidural catheter and increased prothrombin time after right lobe hepatectomy for living donor transplantation. Anesth Analg. 2000 Nov;91(5):1139-41.

[63] Schumann R, Zabala L, Angelis M, Bonney I, Tighiouart H, Carr DB. Altered hematologic profiles following donor right hepatectomy and implications for perioperative analgesic management. Liver Transpl. 2004 Mar;10(3):363-8.

[64] Siniscalchi A, Begliomini B, De Pietri L, Braglia V, Gazzi M, Masetti M, Di Benedetto F, Pinna AD, Miller CM, Pasetto A. Increased prothrombin time and platelet counts

in living donor right hepatectomy: implications for epidural anesthesia. Liver Transpl. 2004 Sep;10(9):1144-9.

[65] Tsui S L, Young B H, NG KFJ, et al.Delayed epidural catheter removal: the impact of postoperative coagulopathy. Anaesth Intensive Care 2004;32:630-6

[66] Moen V, Dahlgren N, Irestedt L. Severe neurological complications after central neuraxial blockades in Sweden 1990-1999. Anesthesiology 2004;101:950-9.

[67] Wang LP, Hauerberg J, Schmidt JF. Incidence of spinal epidural abscess after epidural analgesia. Anesthesiology 1999;91:1928-36.

[68] Curley SA, Marra P, Beaty K, Ellis LM, Vauthey JN, Abdalla EK, et al. Early and late complications after radiofrequency ablation of malignant liver tumors in 608 patients. Ann Surg. ;239:450–8.

[69] Krishnamurthy VN, Casillas J, Latorre L. Radiofrequency ablation of hepatic lesions: A review. Appl Radiol. 2003:32:11–26.

[70] Justin P. Fox, MD 1, Joshua Gustafson, MD2, Mayur M. Desai, PhD MPH1,3, Minia Hellan, MD4, Thav Thambi-Pillai, MD5, and James Ouellette, DO4. Short-Term Outcomes of Ablation Therapy for Hepatic Tumors: Evidence from the 2006–2009 Nationwide Inpatient Sample Ann Surg Oncol DOI 10.1245/s10434-012-2397-0.

[71] Matsui O, Kadoya M, Yoshikawa J et al. Small hepatocellular carcinoma: treatment with subsegmental transcatheter arterial embolization. Radiology 1993; 188: 79–83.

[72] Matsui O, Kadoya M, Yoshikawa J, Gabata T, Takashima T,Demachi H. Subsegmental transcatheter arterial embolization for small hepatocellular carcinomas: local therapeutic effect and 5-year survival rate. Cancer Chemother Pharmacol 1994; 33 (Suppl): S84–8.35

[73] Takayasu K, Arii S, Kudo M et al. Superselective transarterial chemoembolization for hepatocellular carcinoma. Validation of treatment algorithm proposed by Japanese guidelines. J Hepatol 2012; 56: 886–92.

[74] Okabe K, Beppu T, Haraoka K et al. Safety and short-term therapeutic effects of miriplatin-lipiodol suspension in transarterial chemoembolization (TACE) for hepatocellular carcinoma. Anticancer Res 2011; 31: 2983–8.

[75] Okusaka T, Kasugai H, Ishii H et al. A randomized phase II trial of intra-arterial chemotherapy using SM-11355 (Miriplatin) for hepatocellular carcinoma. Invest New Drugs 2011; doi. 10.1007/s10637-011-9776-4.

[76] Kudo M, Izumi N, Kokudo N et al. Management of hepatocellular carcinoma in Japan: Consensus-Based Clinical Practice Guidelines proposed by the Japan Society of Hepatology (JSH) 2010 updated version. Dig Dis 2011; 29: 339–64.

[77] Clinical Practice Guidelines for hepatocellular carcinoma – The Japan Society of Hepatology 2009 update. Hepatol Res 2010; 40 (Suppl 1): 2–144.

[78] Elisa J. Gordon,1,2,5 Amna Daud,et al. Informed Consent and Decision-Making About Adult-to-Adult Living Donor Liver Transplantation: A Systematic Review of Empirical Research (Transplantation 2011;92: 1285–1296)

[79] Hertl M, Cosimi AB: Living donor liver transplantation: how can we better protect the donors? Transplantation 83:263, 2007

[80] S. Ozkardeslera, D. Ozzeybeka, et al. Anesthesia-Related Complications in Living Liver Donors: The Experience from One Center and the Reporting of One Death American Journal of Transplantation 2008; 8: 2106–2110

[81] Jacek B. Cywinski, MD, Brian M. Parker, MD, Meng Xu, Samuel A. Irefin, MD. A Comparison of Postoperative Pain Control in Patients After Right Lobe Donor Hepatectomy and Major Hepatic Resection for Tumor. Anesth Analg 2004;99:1747–52.

[82] James F. Trotter, et al. Laboratory Test Results After Living Liver Donation in the Adult-to-Adult Living Donor Liver Transplantation Cohort Study LIVER TRANSPLANTATION 17:409-417, 2011

Chapter 4

Critical Care Issues After Major Hepatic Surgery

Ashok Thorat and Wei-Chen Lee

Additional information is available at the end of the chapter

http://dx.doi.org/10.5772/51767

1. Introduction

Major hepatic resections have become the routine aspect of managing certain liver conditions such as primary liver malignancies and certain secondaries. Five-year survival is negligible in un-treated patients compared with around 30% in those receiving hepatic resection [1]. Patients with liver disease who require surgery are at greater risk for surgical and anesthesia related complications than those with a healthy liver [2, 3, 4]. The magnitude of the risk depends upon the type of liver disease and its severity, the surgical procedure, and the type of anesthesia.

The first few days after major hepatic surgery are critical to successful outcome of the procedure. Metabolic and functional changes after hepatic resection are unique and cause significant challenges in management. A multidisciplinary approach is required along with effective communication among all caregivers. With attentive, anticipatory care, many potential problems can be averted and new problems can be detected early and treated appropriately. Contemporary critical care management after major hepatic surgery doesn't differ from standard intensive care which includes invasive hemodynamic monitoring, mechanical ventilation, vital parameter monitoring, strict antisepsis measures, metabolic control with due attention to the glycemic control and nutritional aspect which more or less always affected in the patients with cirrhosis.

The post-operative management after hepatic surgery is greatly influenced by hemodynamic monitoring intraoperatively. Patient's intra-operative course, blood loss, requirement of blood products during surgery largely defines the outcome in post-operative period along with patient's nutritional status, liver functions and associated comorbidities. Hence close co-operation with the anesthesiologist and surgeon is necessary.

Majority of postoperative management issues after liver resection are unique and require a thorough understanding of liver metabolism and the pathophysiology of liver disease. The purpose of this review is to elaborate on specific early postoperative management issues after liver resection, examine current evidence and present the management options.

2. Hepatic resections and general considerations

Through the recent surgical advances, hepatic resection could be carried out under the condition of liver cirrhosis or obstructive jaundice, but there are many complications and associated mortality in these cases. Hepatic cirrhosis limits the ability of the liver to regenerate. Fortunately, it appears that most of the advanced cirrhotic livers can tolerate even major resections, and the presence of cirrhosis should not preclude potentially curative or life-prolonging surgery [5]. Careful patient selection based on preoperative Child-Pugh score and ICG test, resections can be limited leaving behind enough liver parenchyma to avoid postoperative liver dysfunction. But such patients are more vulnerable to perioperative insults secondary to ischemia and hypoperfusion, which is reflected in perioperative morbidity and mortality [6]. The Child-Pugh clinical scoring system has been used as a reliable, validated prognostic tool for patients with chronic liver disease undergoing general or porto-caval shunt surgery and has gained widespread use in hepato-biliary surgery. It has recently been suggested that patients with scores of B or C should not receive liver resection surgery [7].

The associated cirrhosis greatly increases the risk for partial hepatectomy. In normal liver. even up to 70% of resection of liver is well tolerated. With underlying liver cirrhosis, partial hepatectomy is only offered to patients who are Pugh-Child's A and the most favorable class B patients [8]. While in Child C patients even minor hepatic surgery or even locoregional therapy can cause hepatic dysfunction. Post-operative outcome and level of post-operative care largely influenced by the underlying cirrhosis and post cirrhotic complications present at the time of surgery. Hence, even enucleation of hepatocellular carcinoma in Child C patients is a major surgery and procedure related mortality is present in one-third of patients [9].

3. Post-operative care

Variables such as severity of underlying cirrhosis, degree of debility before surgery, associated co-morbid diseases and operative complexity appear to have a significant influence on the rapidity at which patients progress through their early postoperative recovery phase.

Attributed to regenerating capacity of the liver, most of the major liver resections are well tolerated and seldom patients have significant biochemical abnormalities. Patients with compensated liver cirrhosis and its complications are more prone for intraoperative blood loss causing deterioration of organ functions and loss of reserve capacity to withstand even minor stress causing life-threatening complications. The disturbances in cardio-respiratory function should be carefully monitored in high Dependency unit. The complications are more in elderly patients. The condition of older patients can change rapidly and therapy may need to be adjusted every few hours if optimum cardio-respiratory function is to be maintained.

- Planning of intensive monitoring for high risk patients with associated co-morbidities should be done during surgery and in postoperative wards
- Diagnose and treat complications quickly
- Institute invasive monitoring and elective ventilation when required
- Continue postoperative care to increase the rate of recovery.

3.1. Immediate post operative

Initial postoperative assessment begins in operating room. Most patients with pre-operative normal liver functions and child A patients recover without any systemic effects. Such patients may not need intensive care unit and can directly be transferred to inpatient wards after an appropriate period of extremely close observation in recovery unit. Many centers usually monitor the patients in ICU for 24 hours before being transferred to inpatient setting after major liver resections.

Most of the patients are awakened in operating room after surgery, and if extubation criteria are fulfilled, the patient is extubated [10, 11]. It is advised that not all patients are candidates of early extubation and each case should be judged on its own merits. But prolonged intubation and mechanical ventilation in postoperative period associated with more pulmonary complications that further prolongs patient's recovery and increases the mortality & morbidity [12]. In addition, Mandell et al. demonstrated that immediately extubated patients experienced a shorter stay in the ICU, resulting in a significant reduction in ICU services and associated costs for extubated patients [13].

After arrival in ICU, initial vital assessment should be done. Most centers follow more or less same protocol. Fluid management is strictly based on patient's present hemodynamic conditions and blood products are administered as per the present condition requires. Input and output fluid charts are maintained with due attention to hourly urine output which should be minimum 0.5 ml/kg/min. Any renal dysfunction in the form of oliguria should be treated immediately because optimum renal function is of paramount importance as a determinant of good outcome [14].

Routine blood investigations, coagulation profile and organ specific tests are ordered. Patients still on ventilatory support, baseline arterial blood gas estimation is done at the arrival. Serum lactate level is determined as it depicts the imbalance between tissue oxygen supply and consumption, thus an indirect measure of tissue perfusion and cardiac output [15]. Postoperative aminotransferase and alanine aminotransferase and total bilirubin levels are not routinely measured after trauma-related surgery. However, in postoperative liver resection and living donor hepatectomy, these values are to be followed to ensure recovery of liver function [16]. A transient early increase in serum hepatic transaminase and alkaline phosphatase levels as a result of hepatocellular damage is common, but a persisting elevation suggests ongoing hepatic ischemia.

Hypothermia in postoperative period is prevented and core body temperature is maintained above 37°C. Hypothermia can cause vaso-constriction and coagulopathy. Core temperature should be monitored and normothermia maintained using warmed fluids and forced warm air blankets. The abdominal drains are examined for the color and content as postoperative hemorrhage is not uncommon after major liver resections and may require re-exploration. In liver transplant setting, due to underlying coagulopathy, ongoing hemorrhage must be detected at earliest. Gross blood stained drain fluid with acute fall in hemoglobin level should alarm surgeon and patient should be re-explored at earliest.

All patients receive broad spectrum antibiotics. The choice of antibiotics is usually center dependent. In our center, we usually administer single broad spectrum antibiotic, mostly third generation cephalosporin in stable patients with Child A score. But in high risk patients, defined by Child score & nutritional status, and patients who are on ventilator support postoperatively, we prefer to use combination broad spectrum antibiotics. In presence of fever, blood culture and antibiotics sensitivity defines the course of antibiotics administered.

3.2. Monitoring of vital parameters

Monitoring the vital parameters like pulse, blood pressure, respiratory rate, ECG, oxygen saturation and the urine output and immediate intervention are instituted to prevent postoperative complications. Vital organ functioning is monitored as follow:

1. Blood pressure, temperature, pulse, respiratory rate.
2. Electrolytes, glycemic control, liver and renal functions
3. Fluid balance and urine output
4. Drain and wound status and appropriate care
5. Medication for pain relief
6. Neurological and cardiac functions
7. Good nutritional intake and bowel movement

3.2.1. Cardiac Monitoring

Central venous line, arterial blood pressure monitoring, continuous record of pulse rate and heart rate are routine standards for monitoring the patients after major hepatic surgery. Arterial blood pressure monitoring accurately measures blood pressure even in presence of hypotension and hypovolemia. In addition, repeated blood sampling can be obtained for routine laboratory investigations and arterial blood gas monitoring. Patients are usually tachycardic postoperatively. But heart rate >100/min should be thoroughly checked for ongoing insults such as persistent hypovolemia, pain, ongoing hemorrhage (drain fluid & falling HB level are indicators) or cardiac arrhythmias. Sinus tachycardia is common after major surgery and should revert without any complications. If tachycardia increases, persistent infection, hypovolemia, pain or presence of cardiac arrhythmia are detected and treated promptly.

At least two large-bore intravenous cannulas are inserted. Although rapid infusion devices are seldom needed, they are available and primed in the ICU at all times. Pulmonary artery

http://dx.doi.org/10.5772/51767

catheterization is reserved for patients with known preoperative left-ventricular dysfunction. This allows continuous measurement of cardiac output and instantaneous calculation of systemic vascular resistance. Real-time ECG monitoring is carried out routinely on most critically ill patients. Changes in rate, rhythm, and character can be identified rapidly by physicians and nurses and acted on immediately.

Monitoring of central venous pressure (CVP) is an important aspect in patients after major liver resections. Measurement of CVP acts as guide for fluid management and hemodynamic manipulation. Liver resections usually carried out under low CVP, usually between 2-5 mm of Hg, to prevent blood loss. This especially an important strategy in patients with underlying liver cirrhosis with child score B & C. CVP is usually kept in same range after surgery and excess fluid administration is restricted. If patient is normotensive and urine output is adequate (>0.5 mL/kg/hr), any attempt to administer extra fluid to elevate CVP is avoided especially in first 48 hours. But after major liver resection, a hyperdynamic state with increased cardiac index and augmented splanchnic blood flow persists for at least 3 days postoperatively [17]. This increased blood supply to the residual liver parenchyma ensures rapid growth.

Signs and symptoms of the heart failure can easily be overlooked as they mimic those of cirrhosis and liver failure. Transthoracic echocardiography is a useful modality in such patients which can measure right ventricular systolic pressure and also shows the cardiac changes.

3.2.2. Pulmonary monitoring

Pulmonary functions are assessed by continuous pulse oximetry, intermittent arterial blood gas analysis, respiratory rate and if patient is on ventilator support, patients are observed via end-tidal carbon dioxide monitoring in addition to the standard ventilatory monitoring and alarm systems.

The course of extubated patients is fairly predictable and most of them recover without any complications. However, after major resections pulmonary complications such as pleural effusion, right sub-diaphragmatic collection causing right lung collapse and pulmonary edema are frequent. edema. These complications range from 50% to over 80% according to literature [18, 19]. Atelectasis is most common amongst these. Atelectasis can be reduced by early mobilization, aggressive chest physiotherapy, adequate pain control and incentive spirometry. Extubated patients should be given chest physiotherapy and incentive spirometry exercises as early as 8 hours post operatively. This will help the expansion of lung and prevent accumulation of the secretions causing atelectasis. Nebulisation with saline with or without anti-cholinergics is given daily 2-3 times and continued till patients are ambulatory.

If the patient is admitted to the ICU while intubated after reversal of the paralytic agents, the ventilatory settings are adjusted according to the patient's respiratory status and arterial blood gases. Patients with good cough and gag reflex, respiratory rate <30 breaths per minute, tidal volume >5ml/kg and aterial PO2 >70mmHg can be extubated. But in presence of pulmonary complications (described later), in very ill, malnourished patients weaning is not possible and may require prolonged ventilation. Metabolic abnormalities such as hypophosphatemia, hypomagnesemia, hypocalcemia and hypokalemia may lead to respiratory muscle dysfunction and inability to wean from ventilator [20]. Such patients in whom prolonged mechanical ventilation is needed for more than 1 week, tracheostomy should be considered to clear airway secretions and reduce the resistance that accompanies the use of standard long endotracheal tubes.

Extubated patients with postoperative hypoxemia are benefited by continuous positive airway pressure (CPAP) that increases the lung expansion and improves fair gas exchange across alveolar capillary membrane. Appropriate analgesia is essential to prevent pulmonary complications, but oversedation needs to be carefully avoided. In absence of coagulopathy and other contraindications, epidural analgesia should be considered and it has been shown to reduce the pulmonary complications [21]. Deep vein thrombosis prophylaxis is strongly encouraged after major liver surgery to prevent any thromboembolic complications.

However, in absence of complications in relatively stable postoperative patients, recovery is smooth and extubation is possible within 12 hours.

3.2.3. *Renal function monitoring*

Maintenance of effective renal function is a critical factor after major hepatic surgery including liver transplantation [22]. 3% of patients experience permanent and 10% transient renal dysfunction following major liver surgery [23]. Hence every attempt must be made to prevent and control renal failure in perioperative period.

Renal autoregulation effectively ceases below renal perfusion pressures of 70 mmHg to 75 mmHg, below which flow becomes pressure dependent. In cirrhotic patients, the concomitant sympathetic activation results in a rightward shift of the autoregulation curve; thus these patients have even less tolerance of reductions in renal perfusion pressure [24]. Adequate fluid management is imperative for both adequate renal perfusion pressure and flow throughout the entire post-operative period to prevent renal impairment.

Hourly monitoring of urine output and laboratory values such as blood urea and serum creatinine are good measures of adequate renal functioning. Urine output is monitored with as indwelling catheter and urine output is maintained at more than 1-2 ml/kg. Any decrease in urinary output should be assessed for the intravascular volume and hypovolemia if any should be corrected.

In presence of normal blood pressure and satisfactory intravascular volume, diuretics are used to improve the urine output. 1 to 2 mg/kg furosemide is given intravenously as bolus followed by a furosemide infusion of 0.2-0.4 mg/kg/hr titrated to maintain adequate urine flow. Continuous infusion results in increased urine output without much alteration in volume status often seen with intermittent bolus therapy.

Intraoperative hemodynamic instability and clamping of major vessels during major liver resections are the main causes of postoperative renal failure. Intraoperative blood loss can lead to renal perfusion problems leading to acute tubular necrosis (ATN) especially in cirrhotic patients with marginal renal functions from the outset. Drug induced nephrotoxicity is another cause of post-operative renal insufficiency.

Renal insufficiency, probably the most ominous perioperative complication in patients with liver disease, is usually a predictor of markedly reduced survival and a sign that hepatorenal syndrome may have developed.

3.2.4. Neurological assessment

Postoperative drowsiness and confusion are commonly caused by neuraxial or systemic opioid administration, which responds to simple changes in administration. However, these patients should be carefully assessed for more serious pathology. Most of the patients show normal neurological recovery. The patients who are extubated immediately after surgery, neurological recovery is complete and not associated with any morbidity. The intubated patients who require mechanical ventilation are usually sedated and neurological assessment in such patients is difficult and usually misleading.

Assessment of the patient's neurological status is done by Glasgow coma scale (GCS) scoring system that records the conscious state of the patient. Patients with GCS score 12 or more are fully conscious and if with endotracheal tube, can be extubated if other pulmonary criteria for extubation are met. Mechanically ventilated patients with sedation and under effect of paralyzing drugs are difficult to assess neurologically and assessment should be performed after wearing of effects of these drugs.

In patients undergoing liver transplantation, the marginal metabolism of anesthetic agents can cause delayed emergence from surgery, as well as residual hepatic encephalopathy [9]. Many patients usually resolve without any neurological aftereffects after major hepatic resections, but prolonged ICU stay due to postoperative complications can result in neurological dysfunction that range from anxiety, depression and sleep deprivation to frank hallucinations and delusional states. ICU psychosis is not uncommon. Patients developing postoperative hepatic dysfunction may develop hepatic encephalopathy which reflects a spectrum of neuropsychiatric abnormalities seen in patients with altered liver functions after exclusion of other known central nervous system disorders [25]. Drugs such as narcotics and sedatives should be avoided in patients with postoperative impairment of liver functions and used cautiously with underlying liver cirrhosis as they may cause prolonged depression of consciousness and precipitate hepatic encephalopathy [4]. Encephalopathy must be considered in a patient with deteriorating liver function and unexplained neurological symptoms. Measurement of blood ammonia may be useful if the diagnosis is unclear. Encephalopathy is treated with cardio-respiratory optimization, further lactulose and may require invasive ventilation.

3.3. Fluid and electrolyte management

Optimizing perioperative fluid management is essential in reducing the risk of postoperative complications and mortality as the cirrhotic patients tend to have limited physiologic reserve. Adequate fluid administration may reduce the stress response to surgical trauma and support recovery [26].

The immediate postoperative period after hepatic resection is characterized by fluid and electrolyte imbalances that are further accentuated by derangements of liver function. Maintenance of adequate fluid balance and normal renal function is critical. Cirrhotics are prone to fluid shifts, vasodilation and resultant hypotension. In this setting, colloids rather than crystalloids should be administered to restore intravascular volume. 50% of patients will also develop significant but self-limiting ascites during the first 48 h, which can cause hypovolemia. Management with sodium restriction and judicious use of diuretic therapy is recommended. Paracentesis may be necessary to prevent tense ascites [27].

At present, no widely accepted recommendations are available for the optimal peri-operative fluid regimen to be used in major non-thoracic surgery. The exact balance of fluid transfusion will be determined by the size of resection, plasma electrolytes and glucose measurements, and volaemic status of the patient. In liver transplantation, fluid overload has been shown to be a predictor of poor graft function and increased postoperative morbidity [28]. In liver resection it has been shown repeatedly that keeping the CVP low results in reduced blood loss and blood transfusion requirements [29-33].

Crystalloids mainly, 0.9% saline and lactated ringer, usually are used postoperatively as replacement and maintenance fluid. Colloids act as plasma expander and can be added as maintenance fluid, but should not be used as resuscitation fluid in case of shock.

Electrolyte abnormalities are common after major hepatic resections, especially beyond Child A patients. Hyponatremia is often seen in patients with cirrhosis and ascites. However, asymptomatic patients treated with normal saline and serum sodium is monitored. Sodium deficit is corrected gradually. In symptomatic patients, a goal increase of sodium with 1.5-2 mEq/L/hr for 3-4 hours until symptoms resolve appears to be safe. But it should not exceed 10 mEq/L in first 24 hours [34]. Rapid correction in any patients is avoided as it may result in central pontine myelinosis.

Hyperlactemia and hypophosphatemia are common derangements in patients undergoing liver resection. Due to the additive effects of lactate-containing intravenous solution, non-lactate containing solutions are recommended for postoperative use [35]. Hypophosphatemia is encountered in nearly all patients after major hepatic resection is believed to be due to increased phosphate uptake by regenerating hepatocytes. It may cause impaired energy metabolism in many organs and may lead to respiratory failure, cardiac arrhythmias, hematologic dysfunction, insulin resistance, and neuromuscular dysfunction [36, 37]. Standard liver resection management includes adequate replacement of phosphate with supplementation of maintenance fluids with potassium phosphate and oral/parenteral replacement.

Correction of potassium is an ongoing process after major liver resections. Patients with high urine output may have hypokalemia which should be corrected. In most cases supplementation is administered by the intravenous route, but it can also be given orally via nasogastric tube. Patients who have received multiple transfusions tend to have hyperkalemia. Before potassium correction underlying metabolic acidosis must be treated first. Severe hyperkalemia in patients with renal dysfunction or failure requires urgent treatment with pharmacological agents or early dialysis. In presence electrocardiographic changes, intravenous calcium to stabilize the cardiac membrane, intravenous insulin and glucose can be given to decrease serum potassium levels. However associated hypomagnesemia should be corrected as it is commonly seen in association with hypokalemia and hypercalcemia.

3.4. Glycemic control

Strict control of blood glucose in surgical patients admitted to intensive care unit has been shown to reduce morbidity and mortality [38]. Hyperglycemia may be induced by surgical stress causing dysregulation of liver metabolism and immune function, resulting in adverse postoperative outcomes [39]. Insulin therapy is particularly important and blood glucose levels are monitored serially to keep glucose levels in target range of 90-120 mg/dl. But development of insulin resistance after the liver resection makes adequate blood glucose control challenging. Some centers use insulin-sliding scale to keep blood glucose in target range, in which blood glucose levels are monitored at regular intervals and doses of insulin changed accordingly while some centers use continuous insulin infusion to control glucose levels. The doses of insulin are to be modified depending on the blood sugar levels.

Okabayashi et al. [40] examined the safety and effectiveness of closed loop insulin administration system, a type of artificial pancreas (STG-22, Nikkiso, Tokyo, Japan) in patients undergoing hepatic resection, but the mean sugar level was above the target levels 90-120 mg/dl. Hypoglycemia after insulin therapy is not uncommon. Hypoglycaemia may as well occur in postoperative due to result of impaired hepatic mobilization of glucose is in high-risk patients or large resections and may necessitate glucose infusion. Dextrose solutions are used to restore normal sugar level. If patients can take orally, or no contraindications for enteral feeding, oral or nasogastric feeding is always preferred.

3.5. Nutrition

Malnutrition is common in patients with liver disease and it may increase risk of postoperative complications after major liver surgeries [41].

The post-hepatic resection period the high demand of the regenerating liver is characterized by a catabolic state and often has glucose and electrolyte imbalances. Nutritional support during this critical period is of paramount importance to ensure adequate hepatic regeneration and postoperative-recovery. Non-cirrhotic patients with adequate preoperative nutritional status may not require any special intervention and should be started on early oral/enteral diet.

But patients who have poor nutritional intake, with or without compromised liver functions (cirrhosis or steatosis), after major liver resections the short-term outcome in such patients may be improved with the use of supplemental enteral nutrition. This may as well improve the child class of patients and reduce the mortality in patients with cirrhosis and malnutrition. If oral feeding can be tolerated, enteral feeding is always preferred over parenteral as it also maintains the intestinal integrity.

Richter, et al. [42] evaluated five randomized controlled studies that compared enteral versus parenteral nutrition in the post-hepatic resection patients [43-45] and concluded that the postoperative complications were significantly low in patients with enteral feeding. In addition, supplementation of branched chain amino acids has got immunomodulating role. Liver disease alters the metabolism of amino acids resulting in low levels of branched chain amino acids such as leucine, isoleucine and valine. Branched chain amino acids (BCAA) supplementation in patients with advanced cirrhosis is associated with improved nutritional status and decreased frequency of complications of cirrhosis. Okabayashi et al. showed improved quality of life in patients supplemented with BCAA after they underwent major hepatic resections [46]. Ishikawa et al. demonstrated increased levels of erythropoietin after short term supplementation with BCAA in non-hepatitis patients undergoing curative resection [47]. Erythropoietin has got protective effects on liver cells from ischemic injury.

Thus, adequate perioperative nutritional support and institution of early enteral nutrition are crucial. Protein restriction is advised only in presence of neurological complications like encephalopathy.

3.6. Correction of coagulopathy

Derangements in conventional markers of coagulation such as prothrombin time/ international ratio (PT/INR), partial thromboplastin time (PTT) and platelet count are common post hepatectomy and correlates with the extent of resection. Postoperative coagulopathy peaks 2-5 days post surgery. Decreased synthetic functions of the liver remnant and consumption of coagulation factors postoperatively can cause increase in INR postoperatively between 1 to 5 days with corresponding decrease in platelets and fibrinogen [48, 49].

Prolongation of PT/INR is often self-limited and usually resolves without the need for transfusion of fresh frozen plasma (FFP) in non-cirrhotics. In patients with cirrhosis, decreased hepatic protein synthesis contributes to a prolonged prothrombin time and partial thromboplastin time, both of which are prolonged usually in direct proportion to the impairment of hepatic reserve. Administration of fresh frozen plasma provides all necessary clotting factors and can correct underlying coagulopathy.

Patients having preoperative obstructive jaundice should receive vitamin K injection both before and after surgery. Sometimes determination of the precise cause of coagulopathy may be difficult in some patients with advanced liver disease, both vitamin K and fresh frozen plasma given together in such patients. In case of postoperative drop in hemoglobin and hematocrit, fresh whole blood transfusion is ideal replacement. A platelet count of 50,000/μl is acceptable. Administration of platelets in the absence of bleeding often results in platelet antibodies, even if type-specific platelets are used. Thrombocytopenia should be treated with platelet transfusion only if platelet count is less than 10,000/ μl or between 10,000-30,000/ μl in presence of active bleeding.

Currently, there is no consensus regarding the criteria for prophylactic FFP transfusion after hepatic resection. Cirrhotics are at increased risk of bleeding after resection. A combination of FFP transfusions, vitamin K, octreotide and human r-FVIIa may be utilized to correct coagulopathy and prevent bleeding.

http://dx.doi.org/10.5772/51767

4. Pain management

Postoperative pain following liver surgery is significant, and adequate analgesia remains a challenge for the caregivers. It helps in early mobilization, improves respiratory functions, permits smooth extubation and decreases systemic blood pressure [50]. Opioids are mainstay of postoperative pain management, morphine and fentanyl being most commonly used analgesics. However, opioids can certainly cause sedation, respiratory depression and exacerbation of hepatic encephalopathy. Due to decreased metabolism of opioids in cirrhotic patients, the bioavailability of these drugs is increased. Size of liver resection has been correlated with impaired opioid metabolism, larger volume resections result in greater impairment of opioid metabolism [51]. Hence, patients should be closely monitored for any signs of respiratory depression. In presence of renal dysfunction, fentanyl is better choice as it is less affected by renal impairment [52].

Epidural analgesia has emerged as an important pain management option in major surgeries and with adjunct to intravenous analgesics provides better pain control & less sedation. But many patients presenting for hepatic surgery have a coagulopathy or thrombocytopenia that makes them ineligible for an epidural or intrathecal therapy. The prolonged prothrombin time potentially predisposes these patients to spinal hematoma and cord compression. In our institute we use epidural analgesia only in patients with normal coagulation profile and good hepatic functions. Intrathecal morphine in doses of 0.5 mg to 0.7 mg can be used as an alternative in patients without coagulopathy. This significantly reduces systemic morphine requirements postoperatively.

Patient controlled analgesia (PCA) is newly emerged concept of self administration of analgesics in controlled doses by patient himself with a pump. This is preferred mode of administrating opioids for moderate to severe pain. Randomized controlled trials have shown the effectiveness of PCA over conventional parenteral analgesia in providing better pain control and increased patient satisfaction [53].

The use of NSAIDs is not recommended post hepatectomy in cirrhotic patients and in renal insufficiency due to risk of hemorrhage and hepatorenal syndrome. However, intravenous acetaminophen can be used in doses not exceeding more than 2 g/day in patients with liver impairment [54].

5. Postoperative complications

Approximately 20% of otherwise healthy patients may experience postoperative complications after elective liver resections [6]. Postoperative complications included surgical complications (bleeding from the surgical site and bile leak), hepatic dysfunction, cardiovascular, respiratory, and renal system dysfunction, and infection. Preoperative American Society of Anesthesiologists (ASA) classification [55], presence of steatosis, extent of resection, simultaneous extrahepatic resection, and perioperative blood transfusion [56] have been found to be independent predictors for the development of postoperative complications.

5.1. Infections

Infection after hepatic resection is a major contributor of postoperative morbidity and mortality and might be predictive of long-term outcomes [57]. Obesity, preoperative biliary drainage, extent of hepatic resection, operative blood loss, comorbid conditions and postoperative bile leak are the risk factors predictive of postoperative infectious complications [58, 59]. Standard measures to reduce the incidence of postoperative infectious complications such as early mobilization, strict antiseptic measures during patient care, changing or removing the urinary catheters within 10 days, removal of central venous catheters earliest possible and aggressive chest physiotherapy should be routine in the postoperative period.

Most frequent complications are pulmonary infection and intra-abdominal infections with abscess formation. Both of these complications are well responsive to the antibiotics. Intra-abdominal collections either biloma or frank abscesses should be drained under radiologic guidance. Septic shock is rare and associated mortality is high if develops. Early recognition of postoperative infection, prompt institution of broad-spectrum antibiotics and aggressive source control is of utmost importance.

Early enteral feeding has protective role in maintaining gut mucosal barrier function. Disruption of this barrier results in translocation of intestinal organisms that is the source of postoperative infections especially in malnourished patients. Strategies such as early enteral nutrition are aimed to protect the gut-barrier function and reduce infectious complication.

5.2. Post operative hemorrhage

Less frequent complications include post-operative hemorrhage that is associated with increased mortality. Underlying coagulopathy is the main reason. Patients with cirrhosis, steatosis, and after chemotherapy are at especially increased risk of coagulopathy and bleeding. Postoperative coagulopathy is at its peak 2-5 days post surgery may act as another contributory factor. Immediate re-exploration and hemostasis is the treatment. This may necessitate the blood transfusion.

5.3. Pulmonary complications

Pulmonary complications are not uncommon after major hepatic resections. Pulmonary complications are a major cause of morbidity and mortality during the postoperative period [60]. Common pulmonary complications occurring in the postoperative period include pulmonary atelectasis, pleural effusion, pulmonary edema and pneumonia.

5.3.1. Atelectasis

Atelectasis is one of the most common postoperative pulmonary complications, particularly following abdominal and thoraco-abdominal procedures [(61). Postoperative atelectasis is usually caused by decreased compliance of lung tissue, impaired regional ventilation, retained airway secretions, and/or postoperative pain that interferes with spontaneous deep breathing and coughing [62]. After major hepatic resections right sub-diaphragmatic collections and postoperative pain are the major causes. Continuous positive airway pressure (CPAP) is beneficial to patients who develop hypoxemia and/or increased respiratory effort due to postoperative atelectasis in the setting of few secretions. Patients with abundant respiratory secretions receive frequent chest physiotherapy such as postural drainage & percussion and oral suctioning. Flexible bronchoscopy should be performed for the patients who are unresponsive to chest physiotherapy and oral suctioning.

Any accumulation in right sub-diaphragmatic space should be drained under radiologic guidance. Atelectasis can be reduced by early mobilization, incentive spirometry, aggressive chest physiotherapy and adequate postoperative analgesia.

5.3.2. Pneumonia

Pneumonia is uncommon complication but may prove life threatening. It usually tends to occur within first five postoperative days [63]. It presents with fever, leukocytosis, increased secretions, and pulmonary infiltrates on chest radiographs. Patients develop hypoxemia and eventually respiratory distress. Postoperative pneumonia should be suspected in presence of fever, leukocytosis and development of new pulmonary infiltrates on chest radiographs. Empiric antibiotic treatment must be started and tailored as per the microbiological analysis of sputum samples.

5.3.3. Pleural effusion

Pleural effusion occurs mostly on right side and related to surgical manipulation or hepatic hydrothorax. Minimal pleural effusion is common during the immediate postoperative period and disappears within few days. However, larger collections and persistent pleural effusion affecting respiratory functions must be drained.

Subphrenic abscess is a complication of surgery that may induce pleural effusions; however, the effusions associated with a subphrenic abscess are distinct from the usual postoperative pleural effusion in that they usually become apparent about 10 days after surgery and are typically associated with signs and symptoms of systemic infection [64]. Subphrenic abscess must be drained and appropriate antibiotic treatment should be started.

5.3.4. Pulmonary edema

Extravascular lung-water accumulation, indicating mild to moderate pulmonary edema following liver resection, has been reported; however, this does not appear to affect oxygenation significantly in the postoperative period [65]. Early onset may be related to transfusion-related acute lung injury or overzealous fluid administration. It is due to increased permeability across alveolar capillary membrane [66]. Other causes include sepsis and acute respiratory distress syndrome. Treatment of pulmonary edema includes fluid restriction, diuretics and continuous positive airway pressure. Most cases resolve spontaneously in a relatively short period of time with no long-term sequelae [67]

5.3.5. Hepatic dysfunction

Postoperative hepatic failure remains a significant challenge. Liver dysfunction is common after liver surgery and anesthesia. It can range from mild enzyme elevations to fulminant hepatic failure. The abnormalities of liver functions noted postoperatively are mostly due to surgery itself or anaesthetic agents used. Although increased serum bilirubin is common postoperatively especially in cirrhotic patients (upto 20%), jaundice is infrequent (<1%) and its presence should prompt a thorough evaluation of the cause.

Although low residual liver volume was found to be associated with postoperative liver failure, the regenerative ability of the liver is remarkable, and the residual, otherwise healthy liver is expected to double in size within the first week following the resection. Increase in hepatic parenchymal mass does not necessarily result in full restoration of functional ability. Pre-existing cirrhosis or positive virus carrier status limits liver regeneration, and these patients are more susceptible to developing postoperative hepatic failure. Liver regenerating is also reduced in diabetic patients predisposing them for the liver failure after major resections [68].

But liver dysfunction can also occur in absence of any pre-existing liver disease. The hepatocellular dysfunction may occur due to drugs including anaesthetic agents, ischemia, shock, iatrogenic injury or viral hepatitis. Known causes of cholestatic dysfunction include sepsis, prolonged blood transfusions, drugs, biliary tract injury, choledocholithiasis and total parenteral nutrition [4]. Even if abnormalities are not noted on computed tomography or ultrasonography, choalngiographic studies are warranted in presence of strong suspicion of biliary obstruction.

Most cases of benign postoperative jaundice (without any obvious cause) eventually resolve spontaneously with supportive treatment only. Usually all cases of hepatic dysfunction are managed in ICU and liver functions are monitored serially along with the coagulation parameters. Hepatic failure is a life threatening complications. Presence of hepatic encephalopathy increases mortality. Increased ammonia due to underlying hepatic failure is a key element in the pathogenesis of encephalopathy. Coagulation parameters are often deranged with underlying liver failure and should be corrected with blood transfusion and fresh frozen plasma transfusion. If patient doesn't respond to the supportive medical management, liver transplantation must be considered. However, hepatic failure is rare complication after major resection and presence of underlying liver dysfunction should prompt specialized management of underlying cause to prevent progression of liver failure.

5.3.6. Other complications

In-hospital mortality following liver resection has been associated with perioperative myocardial infarction, sepsis with multiple organ failure and pulmonary embolism. After major abdominal surgeries, the risk of deep venous thrombosis and pulmonary embolism is 15-40% that increases the mortality, morbidity and length of hospital stay significantly [69].

Early mobilization, intermittent pneumatic compression devices and pharmacologic agents have important role in prevention of venous thromboembolism (VTE). While pharmacologic thromboprophylaxis is widely accepted for most general surgery procedures, the fear of bleeding after major hepatectomy has limited its use. But venous thromboembolism can still occur even in presence of deranged coagulation parameters (prolonged INR & aPTT [70]. A higher incidence of VTE has been noted in patients not receiving thromboprophylaxis and should be administered starting the day of surgery unless high risk of bleeding exists.

6. Summary

The expansion of major liver surgery as a treatment option for various liver tumours has presented new challenges to surgeons and physicians in terms of the assessment and management of postoperative complications, particularly those involving hepatic insufficiency and susceptibility to infection. Understanding of hepatic pathophysiology is important for optimal perioperative care. Multiple factors contribute to increased mortality in patients with underlying liver disease. But due to advances in surgery, anesthesia and improved critical care management, there is progressive improvement in survival even in complex situations. Patient selection with evaluation of the risk factors in various liver conditions is needed. Reduction in mortality in patients with liver disease undergoing resection depends on close attention to coagulation, intravascular volume, renal function, electrolyte levels, cardiovascular status and nutrition. patient selection, appropriate monitoring, and multidisciplinary postoperative management are the key elements in improved survival among patients undergoing liver resections.

Author details

Ashok Thorat and Wei-Chen Lee*

*Address all correspondence to: weichen@cgmh.org.tw

Division of Liver and Transplantation Surgery, Department of General Surgery, Chang-Gung Memorial Hospital at Linkou, Chang-Gung University College of Medicine, Taiwan

References

[1] Simmonds, P. C., Primrose, N. J., Colquitt, J. L., Garden, O. J., Poston, G. J., & Rees, M. (2006). Surgical resection of hepatic metastases from colorectal cancer: a systematic review of published studies. *Br J Cancer*, 94, 982-99.

[2] O'Leary, J. G., Yachimski, P. S., & Friedman, L. S. (2009). Surgery in the patient with liver disease. *Clin Liver Dis*, 13(2), 211-231.

[3] Friedman, L. S. (1999). The risk of surgery in patients with liver disease. *Hepatology*.

[4] Patel, T. (1999). Surgery in the patient with liver disease. *Mayo Clin Proc*, 593-9.

[5] Redai, I., Emond, J., & Brentjens, T. (2004). Anesthetic considerations during liver surgery. *Surg Clin N Am*, 84, 401-411.

[6] Belghiti, J. , Hiramatsu, K., Benoist, S., Massault, P. P., Sauvanet, A., & Farges, O. (2000). Seven hundred forty-seven hepatectomies in the 1990s: an update to evaluate the actual risk of liver resection. *J Am Coll Surg*, 191(1), 38-46.

[7] Clavien, P. A., Petrowsky, H., De Oliveira, M. L., & Graf, R. (2007). Strategies for safer liver surgery and partial liver transplantation. *N Engl J Med*, 356, 1545-59.

[8] Franco, D., & Borgonovo, G. (1994). Liver resection in cirrhosis of the liver. In: Blumgart LH (ed). *Surgeryof the Liver and Biliary Tract, 1st ed. Edinburgh: Churchill Livingstone*, 1539-1555.

[9] Bismuth, H., Chiche, L., Adam, R., et al. (1993). Liver resection versus transplantation for hepatocellular carcinoma in cirrhotic patients. *Ann Surg*, 218(2), 145-151.

[10] Mandell, S., Lockrem, J., & Kelley, S. (1997). Immediate tracheal extubation after liver transplantation: Experience of two transplant centers. *Anesth Analg*, 84, 249-253.

[11] Wong, D., Cheng, D., Kustra, R., et al. (1999). Risk factors of delayed extubation, prolonged length of stay in intensive care unit, and mortality in patients undergoing coronary artery bypass graft with fast-track cardiac anesthesia: A new cardiac risk score. *Anesthesiology*, 91, 936-950.

[12] Krowka, M. J., & Cortese, D. A. (1985). Pulmonary aspects of chronic liver disease and liver transplantation. *Mayo Clin Proc*, 60, 407-418.

[13] Neelakanta, G., Sopher, M., Chan, S., Pregler, J., Steadman, R., Braunfeld, M., et al. (1997). Early tracheal extubation after liver transplantation. *J Cardiothorac Vasc Anesth*, 11, 165-167.

[14] Bilbao, I., Armadans, L., Lazaro, J. L., Hidalgo, E., Castells, L., & Margarit, C. (2003). Predictive factors for early mortality following liver transplantation. *Clin Transplant*, 17, 401-11.

[15] Basaran, M., Sever, K., Ugurlucan, M., et al. (2006). Serum Lactate Level Has Prognostic Significance After Pediatric Cardiac Surgery. 20(1), 43-47.

[16] Imamura, H., Kokudo, N., Sugawara, Y., Sano, K., Kaneko, J., & Takayama, T. (2004). Pringle's manoeuvre and selective inflow occlusion in living donor liver hepatectomy. *Liver Transpl*, 10(6), 771-8.

[17] Thasler, W. E., Bein, T., & Jauch, K. H. (2002). Perioperative effects of hepatic resection surgery on hemodynamics, pulmonary fluid balance, and indocyanine green clearance. *Langenbecks Arch Surg*, 387(2), 271-5.

[18] Pirate, A., Ozgur, S., Torgay, A., Arslan, G., et al. (2004). Risk factors for postoperative respiratory complications in adult liver transplant recipients. *Transplant Proc*, 36, 218-220.

[19] Duran, F. G., Piqueras, B., Romero, M., Clemente, G., et al. (1998). Pulmonary complications following orthotopic liver transplant. *Transplant Int*, 11(1), 255-259.

[20] Aubeir, M., Murciano, D., Lecocguic, Y., et al. (1985). Effect of hypophosphatemia on diaphragmatic contractibility in patients with acute respiratory failure. *N Engl J Med*, 313-420.

[21] Lawrence, V. A., Cornell, J. E., & Smetana, G. W. (2006). Strategies to reduce postoperative pulmonary complications after noncardiothoracic surgery: systematic review for the American College of Physicians. *Ann Int Med*, 144, 596-608.

[22] Nair, S., Verma, S., & Thuluvath, P. J. (2002). Pretransplant renal function predicts survival in patients undergoing orthotopic liver transplantation. *Hepatology*, 35, 1179-1185.

[23] Melendez, J. A., Arslan, V., Fisher, M. E., Wuest, D., Jarnagin, W. R., Fong, Y., et al. (1998). Perioperative outcomes of major hepatic resections under low central venous pressure anesthesia: blood loss, blood transfusion, and the risk of postoperative renal dysfunction. *J Am Coll Surg*, 187(6), 620-5.

[24] Dagher, L., & Moore, K. (2001). The hepatorenal syndrome. *Gut*, 49(5), 729-737.

[25] Ferenci, P., Lockwood, A. , Mullen, K. , et al. (2002, 1998). Hepatic encephalopathy-definition, nomenclature, diagnosis and qualification: final report of the working party at the 11th World Congresses of Gastroenterology. Vienna. *Hepatology*, 35, 716-721.

[26] Hamilton, M. A. (2009). Perioperative fluid management: Progress despite lingering controversies. *Cleveland clinic journal of Medicine*, 28-31.

[27] Wrighton, L. J., O'Bosky, K. R., Namm, J. P., & Senthil, M. (2012). Postoperative management after hepatic resection. *J Gastrointest Oncol*, 3, 41-47.

[28] Bennett-Guerrero, E., Feierman, D. E., Winfree, W. J., et al. (2001). Preoperative and intraoperative predictors of postoperative morbidity, poor graft function, and early rejection in 190 patients undergoing liver transplantation. *Arch Surg*, 136, 1177-83.

[29] Furrer, K., Deoliveira, M. L., Graf, R., & Clavien, P. A. (2007). Improving outcome in patients undergoing liver surgery. *Liver Int*, 27, 26-39.

[30] Vassilios, S., Georgia, K., Kassiani, T., Dimitrios, T., & Contis, J. C. (2004). The role of central venous pressure and type of vascular control in blood loss during major liver resections. *Am J Surg*, 187, 398-402.

[31] Jones, R., Moulton, C. E., & Hardy, K. J. (1998). Central venous pressure and its effect on blood loss during liver resection. *Br J Surg*, 85, 1058-60.

[32] Melendez, J. A., Arslan, V., Blumgart, L. H., et al. (1998). Perioperative outcomes of major hepatic resections under low central venous pressure anesthesia: blood loss, blood transfusion, and the risk of postoperative renal dysfunction. *Am Coll Surg*, 187, 620-5.

[33] Wang, W. D., Liang, L. J., Huang, X. Q., & Yin, X. Y. (2006). Low central venous pressure reduces blood loss in hepatectomy. *World J Gastroenterol*, 12, 935-9.

[34] Sterns, R., Cappuccino, J., Silver, S., et al. (1994). Neurologic sequelae after treatment of severe Hyponatremia: a multicenter prospective. *J Am Soc Nephrol*, 4, 1522.

[35] Watanabe, I., Mayumi, T., Arishima, T., Nakao, A., et al. (2007). Hyperlactemia can predict the prognosis of liver resection. *Shock*, 28, 35-8.

[36] Geerse, D. A., Bindels, A. J., Kuiper, M. A., Roos, A. N., Spronk, P. E., & Schultz, M. J. (2010). Treatment of hypophosphatemia in the intensive care unit: a review. *Crit Care*, 14, R147.

[37] Shor, R., Halabe, A., Rishver, S., Tilis, Y., Matas, Z., Fux, A., et al. (2006). Severe hypophosphatemia in sepsis as a mortality predictor. *Ann Clin Lab Sci*, 36, 67-72.

[38] Van den Berghe, G., Wouters, P., Weekers, F., Verwaest, C., Bruyninckx, F., Schetz, M., et al. (2001). Intensive insulin therapy in the critically ill patients. *N Engl J Med*, 345, 1359-67.

[39] Huo, T. I., Lui, W. Y., Huang, Y. H., Chau, G. Y., Wu, J. C., Lee, P. C., et al. (2003). Diabetes mellitus is a risk factor for hepatic decompensation in patients with hepatocellular carcinoma undergoing resection: a longitudinal study. *Am J Gastroenterol*, 98, 2293-8.

[40] Okabayashi, T., Hnazaki, K., Nishimori, I., Sugimoto, T., Maeda, H., Yatabe, T., et al. (2008). Continuous post-operative blood glucose monitoring and control using a closed-loop system in patients undergoing hepatic resection. *Dig Dis Sci*, 53, 1405-10.

[41] Dicecco, S. R., Wieners, E. J., Weisner, R. H., et al. (1989). Assessment of nutritional status of patients with end-stage liver disease undergoing liver transplantation. *Mayo Clin Proc*, 64, 95-102.

[42] Richter, B., Schmandra, T. C., Golling, M., & Bechstein, W. O. (2006). Nutritional support after open liver resection: a systematic review. *Dig Surg*, 23, 139-45.

[43] Shirabe, K., Matsumata, T., Shimada, M., Takenaka, K., Kawahara, N., Yamamoto, K., et al. (1997). A comparison of parenteral hyperalimentation and early enteral feeding regarding systemic immunity after major hepatic resection--the results of a randomized prospective study. *Hepatogastroenterology*, 44, 205-9.

[44] Mochizuki, H., Togo, S., Tanaka, K., Endo, I., & Shimada, H. (2000). Early enteral nutrition after hepatectomy to prevent postoperative infection. *hepatogastroenterology*, 47, 1407-10.

[45] Hu, Q. G., & Zheng, Q. C. (2003). The influence of Enteral Nutrition in postoperative patients with poor liver function. *World J Gastroenterol*, 9, 843-6.

[46] Okabayashi, T., Iyoki, M., Sugimoto, T., Kobayashi, M., & Hanazaki, K. (2011). Oral supplementation with carbohydrate- and branched-chain amino acidenriched nutrients improves postoperative quality of life in patients undergoing hepatic resection. *Amino Acids*, 40, 1213-20.

[47] Ishikawa, Y., Yoshida, H., Mamada, Y., Taniai, N., Matsumoto, S., Bando, K., et al. (2010). Prospective randomized controlled study of short-term perioperative oral nutrition with branched chain amino acids in patients undergoing liver surgery. *Hepatogastroenterology*, 57, 583-90.

[48] De Pietri, L., Montalti, R., Begliomini, B., Scaglioni, G., Marconi, G., Reggiani, A., et al. (2010). Thromboelastographic changes in liver and pancreatic cancer surgery: hypercoagulability, hypocoagulability or normocoagulability? *Eur J Anaesthesiol*, 27, 608-16.

[49] Shontz, R., Karuparthy, V., Temple, R., & Brennan, T. J. (2009). Prevalence and risk factors predisposing to coagulopathy in patients receiving epidural analgesia for hepatic surgery. *Reg Anesth Pain Med*, 34, 308-11.

[50] Recart, A., Duchene, D., White, P. F., Thomas, T., Johnson, D. B., & Cadeddu, J. A. (2005). Efficacy and safety of fast-track recovery strategy for patients undergoing laparoscopic nephrectomy. *J Endourol*, 19(10), 1165.

[51] Rudin, A., Lundberg, J. F., Hammarlund-Udenaes, M., Flisberg, P., & Werner, M. U. (2007). Morphine metabolism after major liver surgery. *Anesth Analg*, 104, 1409-14.

[52] Chandok, N., & Watt, K. D. (2010). Pain management in the cirrhotic patient: the clinical challenge. *Mayo Clin Proc*, 85, 451-8.

[53] Hudcova, J., Mc Nicol, E., Quah, C., Lau, J., & Carr, D. B. (2006). Patient controlled opioid analgesia versus conventional opioid analgesia for postoperative pain. *Cochrane Database Syst Rev.*

[54] Mimoz, O., Incagnoli, P., Josse, C., Gillon, M. C., Kuhlman, L., Mirand, A., et al. (2001). Analgesic efficacy and safety of nefopam vs. propacetamol following hepatic resection. *Anaesthesia*, 56, 520-5.

[55] Wolters, U., Wolf, T., Stutzer, H., & Schroder, T. (1996). ASA classification and perioperative variables as predictors of postoperative outcome. *British Journal of Anaesthesia*, 77, 217-222.

[56] Melendez, J., Ferri, E., Zwillman, M., Fischer, M., De Matteo, R., Leung, D., et al. (2001). Extended hepatic resection: A 6-year retrospective study of risk factors for perioperative mortality. *J Am Coll Surg*, 192(1), 47-53.

[57] Neal, C. P., Mann, C. D., Garcea, G., Briggs, C. D., Dennison, A. R., & Berry, D. P. (2011). Preoperative systemic inflammation and infectious complications after resection of colorectal liver metastases. *Arch Surg*, 146, 471-8.

[58] Kaibori, M., Ishizaki, M., Matsui, K., & Kwon, A. H. (2011). Postoperative infectious and non-infectious complications after hepatectomy for hepatocellular carcinoma. *Hepatogastroenterology*, 58, 1747-56.

[59] Okabayashi, T., Nishimori, I., Yamashita, K., Sugimoto, T., Yatabe, T., Maeda, H., et al. (2009). Risk factors and predictors for surgical site infection after hepatic resection. *J Hosp Infect*, 73, 47-53.

[60] Lawrence, V. A., Hilsenbeck, S. G., Mulrow, C. D., Dhanda, R., Sapp, J., & Page, C. P. (1995). Incidence and hospital stay for cardiac and pulmonary complications after abdominal surgery. *J Gen Intern Med*, 10(12), 671.

[61] Xue, F. S., Li, B. W., Zhang, G. S., et al. (1999). The influence of surgical sites on early postoperative hypoxemia in adults undergoing elective surgery. *Anesth Analg*, 88, 213.

[62] Platell, C., & Hall, J. C. (1997). Atelectasis after abdominal surgery. *J Am Coll Surg*, 185, 584.

[63] Montravers, P., Veber, B., Auboyer, C., et al. (2002). Diagnostic and therapeutic management of nosocomial pneumonia in surgical patients: results of the Eole study. *Crit Care Med*, 30, 368.

[64] Goodman, L. R. (1980). Postoperative chest radiograph: I. Alterations after abdominal surgery. *AJR Am J Roentgenol*, 134, 533.

[65] Thasler, W. E., Bein, T., & Jauch, K. H. (2002). Perioperative effects of hepatic resection surgery on hemodynamics, pulmonary fluid balance, and indocyanine green clearance. *Langenbecks Arch Surg*, 387(2), 271-5.

[66] Barrett, N. A., & Kam, P. C. (2006). Transfusion-related acute lung injury: a literature review. *Anaesthesia*, 61, 777-785.

[67] Mulkey, Z., Yarbrough, S., Guerra, D., et al. (2008). Postextubation pulmonary edema: a case series and review. *Respir Med*, 102, 1659.

[68] Shirabe, K., Shimada, M., Gion, T., Hasegawa, H., Takenaka, K., Utsunomiya, T., et al. (1999). Postoperative liver failure after major hepatic resection for hepatocellular carcinoma in the modern era with special reference to remnant liver volume. *J Am Coll Surg*, 188(3), 304-7.

[69] Geerts, W. H., Bergqvist, D., Pineo, G. F., Heit, J. A., Samama, C. M., Lassen, M. R., et al. (2008). Prevention of venous thromboembolism: American College of Chest Physicians Evidence-Based Clinical Practice Guidelines. 8th Edition, *Chest*, 133, 381S-453S.

http://dx.doi.org/10.5772/51767

[70] Lesmana, C. R., Inggriani, S., Cahyadinata, L., & Lesmana, L. A. (2010). Deep vein thrombosis in patients with advanced liver cirrhosis: a rare condition? *Hepatol Int*, 4, 433-8.

Chapter 5

Strategies to Decrease Morbidity After Hepatectomy for Hepatocellular Carcinoma

Hiroshi Sadamori, Takahito Yagi and
Toshiyoshi Fujiwara

Additional information is available at the end of the chapter

http://dx.doi.org/10.5772/51765

1. Introduction

In-hospital mortality rates after hepatectomy for HCC have been greatly improved due to advances in surgical techniques and perioperative management [1-4]. However, relatively high morbidity rates remain problematic, and bile leakage and organ/space surgical site infection (SSI) are still common causes of major morbidity after hepatectomy for HCC [5-13].

Various types of hepatectomy in many centres have recently been performed based on the degree of hepatic functional reserve and the location of the HCC. Anatomic hepatectomy for HCC, including subsegmentectomy, reportedly contributes to the prognosis for patients with HCC [14-16]. In addition, the rate of repeat hepatectomy for recurrent HCC has recently increased from 10% to 31% as the prognosis for patients with HCC has improved [17-22].

In our institution, anatomic and repeat hepatectomies for HCC have been performed aggressively [12, 16, 22]. We investigated risk factors for bile leakage and organ/space SSI following hepatectomies for HCC in the present series, which included a large number of patients with a high proportion of anatomic or repeat hepatectomy. Furthermore, causes, management and outcomes of intractable bile leakage and organ/space SSI were investigated and strategies to reduce major morbidity were considered.

2. Methods

2.1. Patients

Medical records of 359 patients who underwent hepatectomy without biliary reconstruction for HCC in our department between January 1, 2001 and March 31, 2010 were studied retrospectively. Patients comprised 292 men and 67 women, with a mean age of 65 years (range, 32-89 years). The aetiology of liver disease was hepatitis C virus in 163 patients, hepatitis B virus in 122 patients, both hepatitis C virus and hepatitis B virus in 31 patients, and alcoholic liver disease in 16 patients. Child-Pugh class was A in 332 patients and B in 27 patients. A total of 296 patients (82.5%) underwent anatomic hepatectomy including subsegmentectomy. Repeat hepatectomy was performed for 59 patients (16.4%). Repeat hepatectomy was indicated when all tumours detected on preoperative imaging could be resected within the hepatic functional reserve. When recurrent HCC tumours were 2 cm in maximum diameter and 3 were present, percutaneous ablation therapies were selected despite the feasibility of repeat hepatectomy, depending on tumour location in the liver.

2.2. Surgical procedure

Laparotomy was performed through a J incision in 287 patients, a Mercedes incision in 33 patients, a midline incision in 23 patients, and a thoraco-abdominal incision in 16 patients. Preoperative cholangiography was not usually performed. Intraoperative ultrasonography was performed to determine the extent of HCC and the line of parenchymal transection. Parenchymal transection was performed using an ultrasonic dissector (Sonop 5000; Aloka, Tokyo, Japan) combined with bipolar electrocautery. Glisson's pedicles in livers dissected by the ultrasonic dissector were ligated and small pedicles were resected using metallic surgical clips. For hemihepatectomies or extended operations, hilar dissection was performed to divide the ipsilateral branches of the hepatic artery and portal vein. The hepatic duct was exposed inside the liver during parenchymal transection and was ligated or oversewn using fine non-absorbable sutures. Parenchymal transection in hemihepatectomy or extended operations was performed largely without occlusion of vascular inflow. For segmentectomies or subsegmentectomies, Glisson's pedicle was transected at the hepatic hilus and an intermittent Pringle manoeuvre was applied during parenchymal transection.

Intraoperative cholangiography was undertaken for selected patients when the integrity of the bile duct was in doubt. A bile leakage test using a cholangiography catheter was also performed for selected patients when many Glisson's pedicles were exposed in the plane of hepatic resection. In principle, two abdominal drainage tubes were systematically positioned and the method of placing the drainage tubes was changed according to the type of hepatectomy. In hemihepatectomy, one drainage tube was placed on the cut surface of the liver and another was positioned at the Winslow hiatus. In subsegmentectomy and segmentectomy, one drainage tube was placed on the cut surface of the liver and another was positioned in the right subphrenic space. From 2001 to 2005, an open drainage system was employed using 12-mm silicone Penrose drains (Kaneka, Osaka, Japan). From 2006 to 2010, a closed drainage system was used with 24-Fr BLAKE silicone drains (Johnson & Johnson, Somerville, NJ, USA). Drains were removed when the drainage was serous and contained no bile, usually around postoperative day (POD) 5.

http://dx.doi.org/10.5772/51765

2.3. Definition of bile leakage

Postoperative bile leakage was defined as the drainage of macroscopic bile from surgical drains for more than 7 days after surgery. Major bile leakage was defined as macroscopic bile discharge >100 ml/day that did not decrease from one day to the next. Minor bile leakage was defined as bile leakage that did not fulfil the definition for major bile leakage. Intractable bile leakage was defined as bile leakage requiring endoscopic retrograde biliary drainage (ERBD) or percutaneous transhepatic biliary drainage (PTBD) during postoperative management.

2.4. Definition of SSIs

SSIs were defined according to the National Infections Surveillance system [23]. Using these criteria, SSIs are classified as either incisional (superficial or deep) or organ/space. Criteria for superficial incisional SSI included infection occurring at the incision site within 30 days after surgery that involved only the skin and subcutaneous tissue and at least one of the following: 1) pus discharge from the incision; 2) bacteria isolated from a sample culture from the superficial incision; 3) localized pain, tenderness, swelling, redness, or heat; and 4) wound dehiscence. Criteria for deep incisional SSI included infection of the fascia or muscle related to the surgical procedure occurring within 30 days after surgery and at least one of the following: 1) pus discharge from the deep incision; 2) spontaneous dehiscence of the incision; or 3) deliberate opening of the incision when the patient displayed the previously described signs and symptoms of infection. The definition of organ/space SSI was based on postoperative findings of at least one of the following: 1) purulent drainage from a drain without macroscopic bile discharge; or 2) intra-abdominal collection of purulent fluid confirmed at the time of reoperation or percutaneous drainage. If intra-abdominal collection at the time of reoperation or percutaneous drainage contained macroscopic bile discharge, bile leakage was considered present. If purulent fluid was drained first and macroscopic bile leakage subsequently became apparent, this was defined as bile leakage. In contrast, if drainage of purulent fluid was still observed after the cessation of macroscopic bile leakage, this was defined as organ/space SSI.

2.5. Antimicrobial prophylaxis

Prophylactic antibiotics regimens were as follows. With initial hepatectomy, a first-generation cephalosporin was injected intravenously within 30 min prior to skin incision. In patients who underwent operations lasting longer than 3 h, additional antimicrobial agents were injected intravenously every 3 h, as recommended by the Center for Disease Control guidelines [23]. These agents were also administered up to POD 2. In repeat hepatectomy, second-generation cephalosporin was injected intravenously in the same manner as in the initial hepatectomy and continued until POD 3.

2.6. Intervention for methicillin-resistant *Staphylococcus aureus* (MRSA)

With the exception of two emergency cases, all patients underwent preoperative evaluation for MRSA, including nasal culture. As a result, 9 of the 359 patients (2.5%) showed colonisation with MRSA on admission to our institution. In those 9 patients with detection of MRSA colonisation from preoperative nasal cultures, decolonisation was performed using intranasal mupirocin therapy (administered twice daily for 3-5 days preoperatively). Prophylactic intravenous infusion of vancomycin was not applied in the 9 patients with intranasal MRSA colonisation.

2.7. Analysis of risk factors for bile leakage and SSIs

Patient demographics, operative and tumour factors, and preoperative liver function were evaluated to determine impacts on the occurrence of bile leakage and organ/space SSI. Preoperative factors included patient age, sex, aetiology of liver disease, Child-Pugh classification, indocyanine green dye retention rate at 15 min (ICG-R15), serum albumin, history of diabetes mellitus, previous radiofrequency ablation (RFA) and previous transarterial chemoembolisation (TACE). The cut-off level for ICG-R15 was set at 20%, because ICG-R15 <20% has been reported as the safe range for bisegmentectomy [3,5,9]. Surgical factors were evaluated for the type of skin incision, type of hepatectomy, number of hepatectomies, blood loss, operative time, blood transfusion, and method of abdominal drainage. With regard to the type of hepatectomy, anterior segmentectomies and medial (S4) segmentectomies were sub-grouped for analysis. The cut-off point for operative time was determined by an analysis of the receiver operating characteristics curve for bile leakage. The optimal cut-off for operative time was 306 min; sensitivity and specificity were 0.696 and 0.728, respectively. We thus set 300 min as the cut-off level for operative time. Tumour factors included the number of HCC lesions and the maximum diameter of HCC. Cut-off level for HCC diameter was determined according to results from previous reports that analysed risk factors for morbidity after hepatectomy for HCC [3,5,9,12].

2.8. Investigation of intractable bile leakage

Management and outcomes were investigated for 46 patients with postoperative bile leakage. Indications for ERBD to treat postoperative bile leakage were based on postoperative findings of at least one of the following: 1) amount of macroscopic bile discharge from surgical drains >200 ml/day at 2 weeks after surgery; 2) amount of macroscopic bile discharge from surgical drains >100 ml/day at 4 weeks after surgery; or 3) macroscopic bile discharge from surgical drains still continuing at 6 weeks after surgery. PTBD was indicated when postoperative cholangiography and biliary drainage by ERBD were considered impractical. Intractable bile leakage necessitating ERBD or PTBD was encountered in 8 patients. The operative procedure, number of hepatectomies, timing of biliary procedures, sites of bile leakage and possible causes of bile leakage were evaluated in these 8 patients with intractable bile leakage.

2.9. Investigation of characteristics in organ/space SSI

Organ/space SSI was classified according to the modified Clavien system [24]: grade I, minor risk events not requiring special treatment; grade II, potentially life-threatening complications requiring pharmacological treatment; grade III, complications requiring surgical, endoscopic or radiological intervention, either with (III-b) or without (III-a) general anaesthesia; grade IV,

http://dx.doi.org/10.5772/51765

life-threatening complications involving dysfunction of one (IV-a) or multiple (IV-b) major organs; and grade V, complications resulting in the death of the patient. Management and outcomes were investigated for 31 patients with organ/space SSI. In addition, the causative bacterium was identified for both incisional and organ/space SSIs. Furthermore, pre- and intraoperative parameters, causative bacteria and hospitalisation were compared between groups classified by the number of hepatectomies in patients with organ/space SSI.

2.10. Statistical analysis

Operative time, blood loss and postoperative hospital stay are presented as mean ± standard error of the mean. Differences in qualitative variables were assessed using Fisher's exact test or the ^{2} test, while differences in quantitative variables were analysed using the Mann-Whitney test. Uni- and multivariate logistic regression analyses were used to identify risk factors for bile leakage and organ/space SSI based on the 18 above-mentioned clinical factors. Relative risk was described by the estimated odds ratio (OR) with a 95% confidence interval. Two-sided *P*-values were computed and an effect was considered significant at the level of *P* 0.05. All statistical analyses were performed using SPSS II statistical software (SPSS, Tokyo, Japan).

3. Results

3.1. Risk factors for bile leakage (Tables 1, 3)

Univariate logistic regression analysis revealed several factors associated with increased risk of developing bile leakage. Repeat hepatectomy influenced the risk of developing bile leakage, with an OR of 3.78 compared to the initial hepatectomy. In contrast, neither previous RFA nor TACE had any significant impact on the occurrence of bile leakage. Operative time 300 min was associated with increased risk (OR, 5.32; *P*< 0.001), as was blood loss 2 000 ml (OR, 4.12; *P*< 0.001). Multivariate analysis regarding bile leakage confirmed operative time 300 min as an independent risk factor.

Variable	OR	95%CI	*P*
Bile leakage			
Operative time (<300 min vs. ≧300 min)	5.32	2.71–10.4	<0.001
Blood loss (<2000 ml vs. ≧2000 ml)	4.12	2.07–3.20	<0.001
Number of hepatectomies (initial vs. repeat)	3.78	1.91–7.48	<0.001

Table 1. Univariate analysis of risk factors for bile leakage.

3.2. Risk factors for SSIs (Tables 2, 3)

SSIs developed in 14.5% of patients (n=52), and 3 patients showed both incisional and organ/space SSIs. Univariate logistic regression analysis revealed several factors associated with increased risk of developing SSIs. Repeat hepatectomy influenced the risk of developing SSIs, with an OR of 8.27 for initial hepatectomy. Operative time 300 min was associated with increased risk (OR, 4.46; P<0.001). The presence of blood transfusion influenced the risk of developing SSIs. Presence of bile leakage was associated with increased risk of SSIs (OR, 6.40; P=0.002). Multivariate analysis regarding SSIs confirmed both repeat hepatectomy and operative time 300 min as independent risk factors.

3.3. Risk factor for incisional SSI (Tables 2, 3)

Incidence of incisional SSI was 6.7% (n=24). Univariate logistic regression analysis revealed that the presence of blood transfusion was associated with increased risk of developing incisional SSI. Type of skin incision classified according to the presence or absence of transverse incision showed no significant influence on the occurrence of incisional SSI in this series. Multivariate analysis regarding incisional SSI confirmed the presence of blood transfusion as an independent risk factor.

3.4. Risk factors for organ/space SSI (Tables 2, 3)

Organ/space SSI developed in 8.6% of patients (n = 31). Univariate logistic regression analysis revealed several factors associated with increased risk of developing organ/space SSI. Repeat hepatectomy influenced the risk of developing organ/space SSI, with an OR of 4.29 compared to initial hepatectomy. In contrast, neither previous RFA nor TACE exerted any significant impact on occurrence of organ/space SSI.

Variable	OR	95%CI	P
SSIs			
Operative time (<300 min vs. ≧300 min)	4.46	1.64–5.46	<0.001
Number of hepatectomies (initial vs. repeat)	8.27	2.24–8.24	<0.001
Bile leakage (absence vs. presence)	6.40	1.55–6.46	0.002
Blood transfusion (absence vs. presence)	2.05	1.37–4.55	0.003
Incisional SSI			
Blood transfusion (absence vs. presence)	4.38	1.85–10.4	<0.001
Organ/space SSI			
Number of hepatectomies (initial vs. repeat)	4.29	3.79–18.0	<0.001
Bile leakage (absence vs. presence)	3.16	2.90–14.3	<0.001
Operative time (<300 min vs. ≧300 min)	2.99	2.03–9.81	<0.001
Blood loss (<2000 ml vs. ≧2000 ml)	2.63	0.73–6.59	0.010

Table 2. Univariate analysis of risk factors for SSIs.

The method of abdominal drainage (open Penrose drains or closed suction drains) showed no significant influence. Operative time 300 min was associated with increased risk of organ/space SSI (OR, 2.99; P< 0.001). Presence of bile leakage was likewise associated with increased risk (OR, 3.16; P = 0.01). Blood loss 2 000 ml was associated with increased risk (OR, 2.63; P< 0.001). Multivariate analysis confirmed both repeat hepatectomies and presence of bile leakage as independent risk factors for organ/space SSI.

Variable	OR	95%CI	P
Bile leakage			
Operative time (<300 min vs. ≧ 300 min)	25.9	2.28 – 29.4	0.009
SSIs			
Number of hepatectomies (initial vs. repeat)	3.43	1.73 – 6.80	<0.001
Operative time (<280 min vs. ≧ 280 min)	2.32	1.22 – 4.43	0.011
Incisional SSI			
Blood transfusion (absence vs. presence)	7.56	2.58 – 22.1	<0.001
Organ/space SSI			
Number of hepatectomies (initial vs. repeat)	6.15	2.69 – 14.1	<0.001
Bile leakage (absence vs. presence)	3.01	1.20 – 7.56	0.018

Table 3. Multivariate analysis of risk factors for bile leakage and SSIs.

3.5. Management and outcomes of bile leakage (Figure 1)

Management and outcomes of the 46 patients with bile leakage are shown in Figure 1.

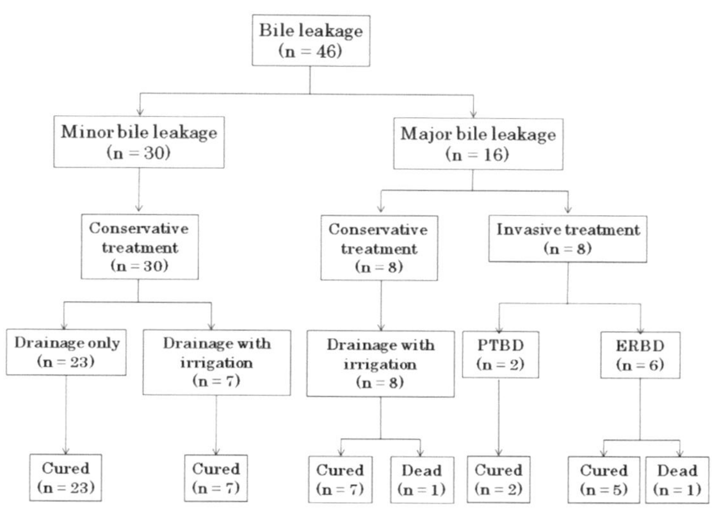

Figure 1. Medical management and outcomes for patients with postoperative bile leakage.

Minor bile leakage in 30 patients (65%) was controllable and cured by conservative therapies comprising drainage alone in 23 patients and drainage with irrigation in 7 patients. Sixteen patients (35%) showed complications of major bile leakage. In 8 of these patients, the major bile leakage was treated using drainage with irrigation. One patient died due to subsequent intractable ascites and liver failure during drainage with irrigation, while the other 7 patients healed. The remaining 8 patients with major bile leakage needed either ERBD or PTBD.

3.6. Characteristics of 8 patients with intractable bile leakage (Table 4)

We investigated the characteristics of the 8 patients who needed either ERBD or PTBD for bile leakage. High-risk surgical procedures were performed in most of these cases and repeat hepatectomy was performed in 6 of the 8 patients. The median timing of biliary procedures was POD 21.5 (range, POD 2-45). Bile leakage sites identified on postoperative cholangiography included the hepatic duct in 2 patients and the raw surface of the liver in 6 patients. Possible causes of bile leakage as assessed by postoperative cholangiography were as follows: stricture of the hepatic duct that existed preoperatively, possibly due to previous treatments for HCC in 4 patients (2 patients due to previous hepatectomies, 1 patient due to previous TACE, 1 patient due to previous RFA), stricture of the hepato-jejunostomy from previous pancreatoduodenectomy in 1 patient, dyskinesis of the papilla of Vater in 1 patient and intraoperative injury of the left hepatic duct related to repeat hepatectomy in 2 patients. Three of these 8 patients subsequently showed complications of intractable ascites. In 2 patients, both bile leakage and intractable ascites were cured without intra-abdominal septic complications. The other patient with stricture and injury of the left hepatic duct caused by a previous RFA died due to intractable ascites, uncontrollable biliary infection and liver failure. Bile leakage in the other 5 patients healed after either ERBD or PTBD, with no other major morbidities.

Age/Sex	Operative procedure	Number of hepatectomies	Biliary procedure (Timing)	Site of bile leakage	Cause of bile leakage	Outcome
62/M	Caudate lob.	Repeat	Endoscopic (14POD)	Lt. hepatic duct	Stricture and injury of lt. hepatic duct due to previous RFA	Died (Biliary infection and liver failure)
53/M	Anterior seg.	Repeat	Endoscopic (10POD)	Lt. hepatic duct	Intra-operative injury of lt. hepatic duct	Cured
72/M	S5 subseg.	Initial	PTBD (43POD)	Raw surface of liver	Stricture of hepato-jejunostomy of previous pancreatoduodenectomy	Cured
60/M	S6 subseg.	Repeat	Endosopic (30POD)	Raw surface of liver	Stricture of rt. hepatic duct due to previous hepatectomy	Cured
62/M	S8 partial hep.	Initial	Endosopic (2POD)	Raw surface of liver	Dyskinesis of the papilla of Vater	Cured
67/F	Central biseg.	Repeat	PTBD (45POD)	Raw surface of liver	Stricture of rt. hepatic duct due to intra-operative injury	Cured
50/M	Posterior seg.	Repeat	Endoscopic (15POD)	Raw surface of liver	Stricture of rt. hepatic duct due to previous TACE	Cured
70/F	S4 seg.	Repeat	Endoscopic (28POD)	Raw surface of liver	Stricture of lt. hepatic duct due to previous hepatectomy	Cured

lob = lobectomy; seg = segmentectomy; hep = hepatectomy; PTBD = percutaneous transhepatic biliary drainage; RFA = radiofrequency ablation; TACE = transcatheter arterial chemoembolization; POD = postoperative day

Table 4. Characteristic and management of 8 patients with intractable bile leakage.

3.7. Management and outcome of organ/space SSI

Organ/space SSI in 31 patients was classified as follows: abscess on the cut surface of the liver in 26 patients; right subphrenic abscess in 4 patients; and liver abscess in 1 patient. One of the 31 patients with organ/space SSI was treated by reoperation due to right subphrenic abscess, but died due to myocardial infarction. Eleven patients needed percutaneous drainage of organ/space SSI and all of them were cured. Organ/space SSI in 19 patients healed with irrigation of the pre-existing drain. As a result, 31 patients with organ/space SSI were stratified according to the modified Clavien system as follows: grade I, 0 patients; II, 13 patients; III-a, 15 patients; III-b, 2 patients; IV-a, 1 patient; IV-b, 0 patients; and V, 0 patients. No mortality was associated with organ/space SSI in this series, but the postoperative hospital stay was significantly longer for patients with organ/space SSI (53 7.2 days) than for patients without organ/space SSI (27 0.9 days, P = 0.001).

3.8. Bacteria causing incisional and organ/space SSI (Table 5)

Causative bacteria for incisional and organ/space SSI comprised gram-positive cocci in 17 patients (70.8%) and 19 patients (61.3%), and gram-negative rods in 6 patients (25.0%) and 9 patients (29.0%), respectively, indicating similar proportions of gram-positive cocci and gram-negative rods in both incisional and organ/space SSI. MRSA was the causative bacteria in 12 of 19 patients with organ/space SSI caused by gram-positive cocci.

Causative bacteria	Incisional (n = 24)	Organ/space (n = 31)
Gram-positive cocci		
MRSA	8	12
MSSA	0	1
S. epidermidis	4	2
Enterococcus sp.	4	4
Steptococcus sp.	1	0
Total	17 (70.8%)	19 (61.3%)
Gram-negative bacilli		
Escherichia coli	1	2
Klebsiella sp.	2	1
Pseudomonas sp.	2	4
Enterobacter sp.	1	1
Bacteroides sp.	0	1
Total	6 (25.0%)	9 (29.0%)
Negative	1	3

MRSA: Methicillin-resistant Staphylococcus aureus
MSSA: Methicillin-sensitive Staphylococcus aureus

Table 5. Causative bacteria of incisional and organ/space SSI.

3.9. Comparison between initial and repeat hepatectomies in patients with organ/space SSI (Table 6)

We compared clinical parameters between initial and repeat hepatectomies in patients with organ/space SSI (Table 6). HCC diameter was significantly larger in patients with organ/space SSI who underwent initial hepatectomy than in patients who underwent repeat hepatectomy. No significant differences were seen between groups in any other preoperative parameters, including patient demographics and preoperative liver function. No significant differences were identified between groups in operative parameters, including blood loss, operative time and blood transfusion. Rates of bile leakage were similar between groups. In contrast, in terms of bacteria causing organ/space SSI, detection of MRSA was significantly more frequent in the repeat hepatectomy group than in the initial group.

	Number of hepatectomies		
	Initial (n=14)	Repeat (n=17)	*P value*
Age	59.6 ± 3.2	62.2 ± 2.5	0.523
Etiology of liver disease			
HCV-related	5	5	0.713
HBV-related	6	11	0.231
HCV+HBV	2	0	0.113
Child-Pugh class			
A / B	14 / 0	15 / 2	0.192
ICG R15 (%)	12.7 ± 1.7	18.5 ± 3.4	0.149
Albumin (g/dl)	4.0 ± 0.1	3.9 ± 0.1	0.610
Diabetes mellitus			
Negative / Positive	12 / 2	13 / 4	0.524
Number of HCC lesions			
1 / >1	11 / 3	8 / 9	0.078
Diameter of HCC (cm)	4.5 ± 0.9	2.4 ± 0.3	< 0.05
Type of hepatectomy			
Partial hepatectomy	0	3	0.104
Subsegmentectomy	3	5	0.619
Segmentectomy	4	5	0.960
Hemihepatectomy	7	4	0.132
Trisegmentectomy	0	0	
Blood loss (ml)	1833 ± 511	1697 ± 307	0.822
Operative time (min)	333 ± 11	343 ± 29	0.767
Blood transfusion			
Absence / Presence	9 / 5	8 / 9	0.345
Bile leakage			
Absence / Presence	9 / 5	10 / 7	0.531
MRSA			
Negative / Positive	12 / 2	7 / 10	< 0.05
Hospital stay (days)	41 ± 7	63 ± 11	0.111

HCV: hepatitis C virus, HBV: hepatitis B virus, ICG R-15: indocyanine green dye retension rate at 15 min, MRSA: Methicillin-resistant Staphylococcus aureus

Table 6. Comparison between initial nad repeat hepatectomies in patients with organ/space SSI.

http://dx.doi.org/10.5772/51765

4. Discussion

In-hospital mortality rates after hepatectomy for HCC have been greatly improved due to advances in surgical techniques and perioperative management [1-4]. However, relatively high morbidity rates remain problematic. The overall morbidity rates after hepatectomy for liver tumors have been reported to be 22.6 – 47.7%, and bile leakage and organ/space surgical site infection (SSI) are still common causes of major morbidity after hepatectomy for HCC [5-13]. Various types of hepatectomy in many centres have recently been performed based on the degree of hepatic functional reserve and the location of the HCC. In addition, the rate of repeat hepatectomy for recurrent HCC has recently increased from 10% to 31% as the prognosis for patients with HCC has improved [17-22]. The characteristic of our study is that this series consisted of a large number and percentage of both anatomic and repeat hepatectomies for HCC.

Rates of bile leakage after hepatectomy for liver tumours and benign lesions have been reported as 3.6%-12.0%, varying widely among different studies [6, 7, 11, 12, 25-30]. However, no standardised definition of bile leakage after hepatectomy has been established. In previous reports [6, 8, 11, 13, 30], the definition based on the drainage of macroscopic bile has been adopted. Several studies has proposed the definition on quantitative basis using the bilirubin concentration within the drain [26, 28], but these cut-off values varied. Currently, the International Study Group of Liver Surgery has proposed a consensus definition of bile leakage based on the postoperative course of bilirubin concentration in serum and drainage fluid [31]. Application of a uniform definition of bile leakage is indispensable to enabling standardised comparison of the results of different clinical reports and to facilitating objective evaluation of therapeutic modalities in the field of hepatectomies.

In the present study, prolonged operative time was identified as an independent risk factor for bile leakage and the type of hepatectomy had no significant impact on the rate of bile leakage. Several groups have reported that hepatectomies in which the cut surface exposed the major Glisson's sheath (i.e., central bisegmentectomy, S4 segmentectomy, and S8 subsegmentectomy) were independent risk factors for bile leakage [8, 28-30]. However, our results indicate that the standard types of hepatectomy were not risk factors for bile leakage, even if a wide cut surface with an exposed major Glisson's sheath was necessary, when assessment of liver function was appropriate and surgical procedures were performed carefully during transection of the liver parenchyma. We assume that the prolongation of operative time in this study was related to the extended duration of liver parenchymal transection and/or resection for severe intra-abdominal adhesions around the liver.

Our results revealed latent stricture of the biliary anatomy and intraoperative injury of the hepatic duct related to repeat hepatectomy as the main causes of intractable bile leakage requiring invasive treatment. Preoperative assessment of the biliary anatomy should therefore be considered for selected patients at high risk of intractable bile leakage. Various measures could also be applied during surgery to diminish the incidence of major and intractable bile leakage. First, intraoperative cholangiography should be used, particularly in repeat hepatectomies and in patients who have been treated with RFA or TACE for HCC located in the hepatic hilar region, as the identification of bile duct injury or stricture could allow immediate correction. Second, T-tube drainage or trans-cystic duct drainage of the common bile duct could be indicated in patients needing decompression of the biliary tree, such as patients with dyskinesis of the papilla of Vater. Third, particularly in repeat systematised hepatectomies, division of the bile ducts could be performed inside the liver during parenchymal transection, as this procedure could decrease the risk of injury to the bile ducts compared to division of the bile ducts at the liver hilum.

In the 1980s and 1990s, organ/space SSI formation after hepatectomy was reported as a fatal complication causing liver failure and death [32-34]. Although rates of organ/space SSI after hepatectomy have been reported as 4.7%-25% [35-42], hospital mortality rates caused by organ/space SSI have declined [7-10, 36, 40]. Several groups have reported high patient age and presence of diabetes mellitus as independent risk factors for organ/space SSI [36, 39]. However, these variables were not identified as independent risk factors for organ/space SSI in the present study. Our key result was the identification of repeat hepatectomy as an independent risk factor for organ/space SSI, suggesting that treatment strategies need to be established to reduce the high rate of organ/space SSI after repeat hepatectomy.

Repeat hepatectomy was identified as an independent risk factor for SSI and organ/space SSI, but previous RFA and TACE were not. Repeat hepatectomy for recurrent HCC is useful in establishing the good long-term outcomes. Cumulative 5-year survival rates after second hepatectomy have been reported as 41-69% [17-22]. RFA has recently been confirmed as a safe and promising therapy for recurrent HCC after hepatectomy. However, sufficient evidence does not exist to confirm whether RFA actually improves long-term outcomes. Cumulative 5-year survival rates after RFA for recurrent HCC after hepatectomy have been reported as 18-51.6% [43-45]. RFA is sometimes ineffective for HCC on the liver surface or near large vessels. In addition, postoperative adhesions between the remnant liver and gastrointestinal tract may prevent safe percutaneous RFA in patients with recurrent HCC.

In this study, MRSA was detected more frequently in organ/space SSI after repeat hepatectomy compared with after initial hepatectomy. We assume that most organ/space SSIs with MRSA after repeat hepatectomy develop as a result of contamination when the surgical procedure comes into contact with intra-abdominal colonisation or micro-abscesses of MRSA that had formed after the initial hepatectomy. This assumption might be partially supported by our result that the method of abdominal drainage (open or closed) had no significant influence on the occurrence of organ/space SSI. If this assumption is valid, preoperative interventions for MRSA, consisting of nasal culture and decolonisation of nasal MRSA, will not greatly reduce the occurrence of organ/space SSI involving MRSA after repeat hepatectomy. Walsh et al. recently reported that an MRSA intervention program, in which all patients received intranasal mupirocin and those patients colonised with MRSA received prophylactic intravenous infusion of vancomycin, resulted in near-complete and sustained elimination of MRSA SSIs after cardiac surgery [46]. Regarding patients who undergo repeat hepatectomies, preoperative detection of intra-abdominal colonisation or micro-abscess containing MRSA is difficult. MRSA intervention programs thus need to be improved, particularly for patients who undergo repeat hepatectomies, by considering the prophylactic intravenous administration of vancomycin.

In conclusion, our results reveal prolonged operative time as an independent risk factor for bile leakage, and latent stricture of the biliary anatomy and intraoperative injury of the hepatic duct related to repeat hepatectomy as the main causes of intractable bile leakage necessitating invasive treatment. Repeat hepatectomy was also identified as an independent risk factor for organ/space SSI, with MRSA as the main causative bacteria in organ/space SSI after repeat hepatectomy for HCC. Establishment of treatment strategies is thus important for reducing the high rate of organ/space SSI after repeat hepatectomy. In addition, preoperative assessment of the biliary anatomy and surgical procedures to decrease the incidence of major bile leakage should be considered for selected patients at high risk of intractable bile leakage.

Author details

Hiroshi Sadamori*, Takahito Yagi and Toshiyoshi Fujiwara

*Address all correspondence to: sada@md.okayama-u.ac.jp

Department of Gastroenterological Surgery, Okayama University Graduate School of Medicine, Dentistry and Pharmaceutical Sciences, Okayama, Japan

References

[1] Fan, S. T., Lo, C. M., Liu, C. L., et al. (1999). Hepatectomy for hepatocellular carcinoma: toward zero hospital deaths. *Ann Surg*, 229, 323-330.

[2] Fong, Y., Sun, R. L., Jarnagin, W., & Blumgart, L. H. (1999). An analysis of 412 cases of hepatocellular carcinoma at a Western center. *Ann Surg*, 229, 790-800.

[3] Torzilli, G., Makuuchi, M., Inoue, K., et al. (2007). No mortality liver resection for hepatocellular carcinoma in cirrhotic and noncirrhotic patients. *Arch Surg*, 134, 984-992.

[4] Sadamori, H., Yagi, T., Matsuda, H., et al. (2010). Risk factors for major morbidity after hepatectomy for hepatocellular carcinoma in 293 recent cases. *J Hepatobiliary Pancreat Sci*, 17, 709-718.

[5] Shimada, M., Takenaka, K., Fujiwara, Y., et al. (1998). Risk factors linked to postoperative morbidity in patients with hepatocellular carcinoma. *Br J Surg*, 85, 195-198.

[6] Lo, C. M., Fan, S. T., Liu, C. L., Lai, E. C. S., & Wong, J. (1998). Biliary complication after hepatic resection-Risk factors, management, and outcome. *Arch Surg*, 133, 156-161.

[7] Belghiti, J., Hiramatsu, K., Benoist, S., Massault, P., Sauvanet, A., & Farges, O. (2000). Seven hundred forty-seven hepatectomies in the 1990s: an update to evaluate the actual risk of liver resection. *J Am Coll Surg*, 191, 38-46.

[8] Yamashita, Y., Hamatsu, T., Rikimaru, T., et al. (2001). Bile leakage after hepatic resection. *Ann Surg*, 233, 45-50.

[9] Capussotti, L., Muratore, A., Amisano, M., Polastri, R., Bouzari, H., & Massucco, P. (2005). Liver resection for hepatocellular carcinoma on cirrhosis: analysis of mortality, morbidity and survival-a European single center experience. *Eur J Surg Oncol*, 31, 986-993.

[10] Taketomi, A., Kitagawa, D., Itoh, S., et al. (2007). Trends in morbidity and mortality after hepatic resection for hepatocellular carcinoma: An institute's experience with 625 patients. *J Am Coll Surg*, 204, 580-587.

[11] Virani, S., Michaelson, J., Hutter, M., et al. (2007). Morbidity and mortality after liver resection: Results of the patient safety in surgery study. *J Am Coll Surg*, 204, 1284-1292.

[12] Sadamori, H., Yagi, T., Shinoura, S., et al. (2012). Risk factors of organ/space surgical site infection after hepatectomy for hepatocellular carcinoma in 359 recent cases. *J Hepatobiliary Pancreat Sci*, Jan 25. [Epub ahead of print]. PMID: 22273719.

[13] Sadamori, H., Yagi, T., Shinoura, S., et al. (2012). Intractable bile leakage after hepatectomy for hepatocellular carcinoma in 359 recent cases. *Dig Surg*, 29, 149-156.

[14] Hasegawa, K., Kokudo, N., Imamura, H., et al. (2005). Prognostic impact of anatomic resection for hepatocellular carcinoma. *Ann Surg*, 242, 252-259.

[15] Eguchi, S., Kanematsu, T., Arii, S., et al. (2008). Liver Cancer Study Group of Japan. Comparison of the outcomes between an anatomical subsegmentectomy and a non-anatomical minor hepatectomy for single hepatocellular carcinomas based on a Japanese nationwide survey. *Surgery*, 143, 469-475.

[16] Sadamori, H., Matsuda, H., Shinoura, S., et al. (2009). Anatomical subsegmentectomy in the lateral segment for hepatocellular carcinoma. *Hepatogastroenterology*, 56, 971-977.

[17] Farges, O., Regimbeau, J. M., & Belghiti, J. (1998). Aggressive management of recurrence following surgical resection of hepatocellular carcinoma. *Hepatogastroenterology*, 45, 1275-1280.

[18] Shimada, M., Takenaka, K., Taguchi, K., et al. (1998). Prognostic factors after repeat hepatectomy for recurrent hepatocellular carcinoma. *Ann Surg*, 227, 80-85.

[19] Poon, R. T., Fan, S. T., Lo, C. M., Liu, C. L., & Wong, J. (1999). Intrahepatic recurrence after curative resection of hepatocellular carcinoma: long-term results of treatment and prognostic factors. *Ann Surg*, 229, 216-222.

[20] Minagawa, M., Makuuchi, M., Takayama, T., & Kokudo, N. (2003). Selection criteria for repeat hepatectomy in patients with recurrence hepatocellular carcinoma. *Ann Surg*, 238, 703-710.

[21] Itamoto, T., Nakahara, H., Amano, H., et al. (2007). Repeat hepatectomy for recurrent hepatocellular carcinoma. *Surgery*, 141, 589-597.

[22] Umeda, Y., Matsuda, H., Sadamori, H., Matsukawa, H., Yagi, T., & Fujiwara, T. (2011). A prognostic model and treatment strategy for intrahepatic recurrence of hepatocellular carcinoma after curative resection. *World J Surg*, 35, 170-177.

[23] CDC NNIS System. (2004). National Infections Surveillance (NNIS) system report, data summary from January 1992 to June 2004, issued October 2004. *Am J Infect Control*, 32, 470-485.

[24] Dindo, D., Demartines, N., & Clavien, P. A. (2004). Classification of surgical complications: a new proposal with evaluation in a cohort of 6336 patients and results of a survey. *Ann Surg*, 240, 205-213.

[25] Benzoni, E., Cojutti, A., Lorenzin, D., et al. (2007). Liver resective surgery: a multivariate analysis of postoperative outcome and complication. *Langenbecks Arch Surg*, 392, 45-54.

[26] Tanaka, S., Hirohashi, K., Tanaka, H., et al. (2002). Incidence and management of bile leakage after hepatic resection for malignant hepatic tumors. *J Am Coll Surg*, 195, 484-489.

[27] Reed, D. N., Jr Vitale, G. C., Wrightson, W. R., Edwards, M., & Mc Masters, K. (2003). Decreasing mortality of bile leaks after elective hepatic surgery. *Am J Surg*, 185, 316-318.

[28] Nagano, Y., Togo, S., Tanaka, K., et al. (2003). Risk factors and management of bile leakage after hepatic resection. *World J Surg*, 27, 695-698.

[29] Lee, C. C., Chau, G. Y., Lui, W. Y., et al. (2005). Risk factors associated with bile leakage after hepatic resection for hepatocellular carcinoma. *Hepatogastroenterology*, 52, 1168-1171.

[30] Capussotti, L., Ferrero, A., Vigano, L., Sgotto, E., Muratore, A., & Polastri, R. (2006). Bile leakage and liver resection: Where in the risk? *Langenbecks Arch Surg*, 141, 690-694.

[31] Koch, M., Garden, O. J., Padbury, R., et al. (2011). Bile leakage after hepatobiliary and pancreatic surgery: A definition and grading of severity by the International Study Group of Liver Surgery. *Surgery*, 149, 680-688.

[32] Yanaga, K., Kanematsu, T., Takenaka, K., & Sugimachi, K. (1986). Intraperitoneal septic complications after hepatectomy. *Ann Surg*, 203, 148-152.

[33] Anderson, R., Saarela, A., Tranberg, K. G., & Bengmark, S. (1990). Intraabdominal abscess formation after major liver resection. *Acta Chir Scand*, 156, 707-710.

[34] Nagasue, N., Kohno, H., Tachibana, M., Yamanoi, A., Ohmori, H., & El-Assai, O. (1999). Prognostic factors after hepatic resection for hepatocellular carcinoma associated with Child-Turcotte class B and C cirrhosis. *Ann Surg*, 229, 84-90.

[35] Wu, C. C., Yeh, D. C., Lin, M. C., Liu, T. J., & P'eng, F. K. (1998). Prospective randomized trial of systemic antibiotics in patients undergoing liver resection. *Br J Surg*, 85, 489-493.

[36] Togo, S., Matsuo, K., Tanaka, K., et al. (2007). Perioperative infection control and its effectiveness in hepatectomy. *J Gastroenterol Hepatol*, 22, 1942-1948.

[37] Shiba, H., Ishii, Y., Ishida, Y., et al. (2009). Assessment of blood-products use as predictor of pulmonary complications and surgical infection after hepatectomy for hepatocellular carcinoma. *J Hepatobiliary Pancreat Surg*, 16, 69-74.

[38] Okabayashi, T., Nishimori, I., Yamashita, K., et al. (2009). Risk factors and predictors for surgical site infection after hepatic resection. *J Hospital Infect*, 73, 47-53.

[39] Kobayashi, S., Gotohda, N., Nakagohri, T., Takahashi, S., Konishi, M., & Kinoshita, T. (2009). Risk factors of surgical site infection after hepatectomy for liver cancers. *World J Surg*, 33, 312-317.

[40] Uchiyama, K., Ueno, M., Ozawa, S., et al. (2011). Risk factors for postoperative infectious complications after hepatectomy. *J Hepatobiliary Pancreat Sci*, 18, 67-73.

[41] Togo, S., Kubota, T., Takahashi, T., et al. (2008). Usefulness of absorbable sutures in preventing surgical site infection in hepatectomy. *J Gastrointest Surg*, 12, 1041-1046.

[42] Arikawa, T., Kurokawa, T., Ohwa, Y., et al. (2011). Risk factors for surgical site infection after hepatectomy for hepatocellular carcinoma. *Hepatogastroenterology*, 58, 143-146.

[43] Lau, W. Y., & Lai, E. C. (2009). The current role of radiofrequency ablation in the management of hepatocellular carcinoma: a systemic review. *Ann Surg*, 249, 20-5.

[44] Choi, D., Lim, H. K., Rhim, H., Kim, Y. S., Yoo, B. C., Paik, S. W., et al. (2007). Percutaneous radiofrequency ablation for recurrent hepatocellular carcinoma after hepatectomy: long-term results and prognostic factors. *Ann Surg Oncol*, 14, 2319-9.

[45] Taura, K., Ikai, I., Hatano, E., Fujii, H., Uyama, N., & Shimahara, Y. (2006). Implication of frequent local ablation therapy for intrahepatic recurrence in prolonged survival of patients with hepatocellular carcinoma undergoing hepatic resection: an analysis of 610 patients over 16 years old. *Ann Surg*, 244, 265-73.

[46] Walsh, E. E., Greene, L., & Kirshner, R. (2011). Sustained reduction in methicillin-resistant Staphylococcus aureus wound infections after cardiothoracic surgery. *Arch Intern Med*, 171, 68-73.

Chapter 6

Experimental Models in Liver Surgery

M.B. Jiménez-Castro, M. Elias-Miró,
A. Casillas-Ramírez and C. Peralta

Additional information is available at the end of the chapter

http://dx.doi.org/10.5772/51829

1. Introduction

Ischemia-Reperfusion (I/R) injury is an important cause of liver damage occurring during surgical procedures including hepatic resections and liver transplantation (LT) [1-3]. The shortage of organs has led centers to expand their criteria for the acceptance of marginal grafts that exhibit poor tolerance to I/R [4]. Some of these include the use of organs from older donors and grafts such as small-for-size or steatotic livers. However, I/R injury is the underlying cause of graft dysfunction in marginal organs [4]. Indeed, the use of steatotic livers for transplantation is associated with an increased risk of primary nonfunction or dysfunction after surgery [5]. In addition, the occurrence of postoperative liver failure after hepatic resection in a steatotic liver exposed to normothermic ischemia has been reported [6]. A large number of factors and mediators play a part in liver I/R injury. The relationships between the signalling pathways involved are highly complex and it is not yet possible to describe, with absolute certainty, the events that occur between the beginning of reperfusion and the final outcome of either poor function or a non-functional liver graft. We will show that the mechanisms responsible for hepatic I/R injury depends on the experimental model used, who are valuable tool for understanding the physiopathology of hepatic I/R injury and discovering novel therapeutic targets and drugs. Several strategies to protect the liver from I/R injury have been developed in animal models and, some of these, might find their way into clinical practice. The species used for experimental investigation of hepatic I/R injury range from mice to pigs. The book chapter will discuss the numerous experimental models used to study the complexity of hepatic I/R injury, data reported in choice of the animal model, when selecting an animal species, the age, the sex, the degree of steatosis…etc. Thus, the different strengths and limitations of the different experimental models will be discussed. Also the standardized experimental conditions, such as anesthetic and analgesic procedures will be described. We also attempt to highlight the fact that the types of ischemia (cold and warm ischemia) play an important role in experimental liver surgery. The most existing reviews concerning about mechanisms responsible of I/R does not make a distinction between cold and warm ischemia. We will discuss the different experimental models of normothermic ischemia including global hepatic ischemia with portocaval decompression, global liver ischemia with spleen transposition and partial liver ischemia. Among the different experimental models of cold hepatic I/R injury, we will described the different experimental models used, including a section on orthotopic liver transplantation (OLT) because it is a common yet and complex microsurgical technique. In an attempt to expand the size of the donor pool, the different surgical techniques including reduced-size liver transplantation (RSLT), split liver transplantation (SLT) and living donor liver transplantation (LDLT) will be mentioned in the book chapter. In line with this, the optimization of graft function and survival through the static organ preservation and machine perfusion will also discused. Static organ preservation was a breakthrough and remains the conventional method of preservation. The machine perfusion has emerged as a suitable strategy for preserving liver grafts with promising data over the past decade, especially when marginal organs such as steatotic liver are used for transplantation. The strengths and disadvantages of the different types of machine perfusion (normothermic, hypothermic and subnormothermic machine perfusion) will be discussed. Furthermore some factors, including the duration and extent of hepatic ischemia, starvation, graft, age, and steatosis-which must be considered before the selection of an experimental model of hepatic I/R-will be mentioned. All of these factors contribute to enhancing liver susceptibility to I/R injury. In line with this, we will focused on the negative effects of ischemia on liver regeneration in both normal and marginal livers when they are subjected to liver surgery associated with hepatic resections or LT. The different experimental models of hepatic I/R in which both conditions-ischemia and resection- are present will be described.

2. Hepatic ischemia-reperfusion injury

Due to the complexity of hepatic I/R injury, the present review summarizes the established basic concepts of the mechanisms and cell types involved in this process (Fig. 1). The imbalance between nitric oxide (NO) and endothelin production, contributes to microcirculatory diseases associated with I/R. Concomitantly, the activation of Kupffer cells (KC) releases reactive oxygen species (ROS) and proinflammatory cytokines, including tumour necrosis factor-α (TNF-α) and interleukin-1 (IL-1) [7-9]. ROS can also derive from mitochondria and the xanthine dehydrogenase/xanthine oxidase (XDH/XOD) pathway in activated SEC and hepatocytes. Cytokines promote neutrophil activation and accumulation, thereby contributing to the progression of parenchymal injury by releasing ROS and proteases [7,10]. Capillary narrowing also contributes to hepatic neutrophil accumulation [11]. Besides, IL-1 and TNF-α recruit and activate CD4+ T-lymphocytes, which produce granulocyte-macrophage colony-stimulating factor (GM-CSF), interferon gamma (INF-γ) and TNF-β. These cytokines amplify KC activation and TNF-α and IL-1 secretion and promote neutrophil recruitment and adherente into the liver sinusoids [12]. Platelet activating factor can prime neutrophils for ROS generation, whereas leukotriene B4 (LTB4) contributes to the amplification of the neutrophil response [7,10]. In addition, I/R initiates protein misfolding in the endoplasmic reticulum (ER), which can activate a highly conserved unfolded protein response (UPR) signal transduction pathway. The UPR is characterized by coordinated activation of three ER transmembrane proteins, inositol-requiring enzyme 1 (IRE1), PKR-like ER kinase (PERK) and activating transcription factor (ATF)-6. If the damage is so severe that homeostasis cannot be restored, ER stress signal transduction pathways ultimately initiate apoptosis and necrosis [9]. In addition to the high ROS level–generating system found in liver grafts shows low levels of antioxidants such as glutathione (GSH) and superoxide dismutase (SOD) [1,9]. Alterations in the renin-angiotensin system (RAS), retinol binding protein 4 (RBP4), adiponectin and peroxisome proliferator activated receptor gamma (PPARγ) contribute to oxidative stress. Toll like receptor (TLR4) signaling pathway is also responsible for the hepatic I/R damage. Myeloid differentiation primary response gene 88 (MyD88) and TIR-domain-containing adapter-inducing interferon-β (TRIF) activate intracellular signaling cascades that ultimately trigger an inflammatory response [9,13].

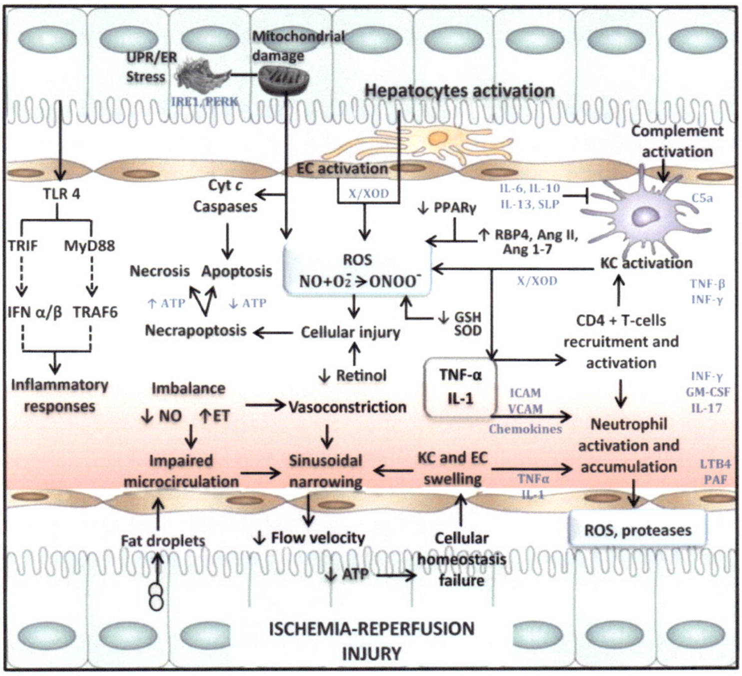

Figure 1. *Mechanisms involved in hepatic ischemia-reperfusion injury*. ATP, adenosine triphosphate; Cyt c: cytochrome c; EC, endothelial cell; ET, endothelin; GM-CSF, granulocyte-macrophage colony-stimulating factor; GSH, glutathione; ICAM, intracellular cell adhesion molecule; IFN α/β, interferon α/β; IL, interleukin; INF, interferon; IRE1, inositol-requiring enzyme 1; KC, kupffer cell; LTB4, leucotriene B4; MyD88, myeloid differentiation primary response gene 88; NO, nitric oxide; $ONOO^-$, peroxynitrite; PAF, platelet activating factor; PERK, protein kinase-like endoplasmic reticulum kinase; PPARγ, peroxisome proliferator-activated receptor γ; RBP4, retinol binding protein 4; Renin-Angiotensin system (RAS): Ang II and Ang 1-7, angiotensin; ROS, reactive oxygen species; SLP, secretory leukocyte protease inhibitor; SOD, superoxide dismutase; TLR4, toll-like receptor 4; TNF, tumor necrosis factor; TRAF6, TNF receptor-associated factor 6; TRIF, TIR-domain-containing adapter-inducing interferon- β; UPR/ER, unfolded protein response/endoplasmic reticulum; VCAM, vascular cell adhesion molecule; X/XOD, xanthine/xanthine oxidase

3. Experimental models

Experimental surgery is an activity within the scientific development, offering a wide range of possibilities for the progress of medicine. As a discipline can be accessed from various branches of science and allows testing and development of surgical procedures and learning the scientific method, so that, working with laboratory animals has been and is required prelude to innovation and development of advances in clinical surgery. The reproduction and validation of experimental models has facilitated the extrapolation of the knowledge acquired to Medicine [16]. The animals used in research models have been divided into four groups: spontaneous, induced, negative and orphans. 1) The spontaneous or non-manipulated models are obtained by selection of inbred animals that express a variable or among populations in which a large number of animals that express variable; 2) Induced or manipulated models are obtained by an experimental challenge that can be classified into five groups: A. Administration of biologically active substances, eg., induction of steatosis after alcohol ingestion. B. Surgical manipulation, such as partial hepatectomy (PH) for the study of liver regeneration. C. Administration of modified diets, lack or surplus components, e.g., in the study of hyperlipidemia. D. Genetic manipulation and transgenic animals which produce special models that are being helpful in understanding mechanisms of pathogenesis and therapy. 3) The negative patterns are those in which a given variable does not develop. The interest is in studying the mechanisms that provide resistance. 4) Orphan models are those expressing an unknown variable in humans [16].

The speed of human studies is slow, the majority of human tissues are not routinely accessible for research purposes, and there is a very limited opportunity for interventional studies. Although scientific research has always relied on the use of cell cultures, information that is obtained through *in vitro* studies can be extrapolated to biomedical research only when analyzed within a complex organism with metabolic functioning. Therefore, one avenue holding tremendous potential in the search for therapies against I/R damage is the use of intact living systems, in which complex biological processes can be examined. There are many advantages of animal studies: large numbers of animals (especially rodents) can be bred and studied, interventional studies can be performed, and established and emerging tools for targeted manipulation of gene expression levels provide insight into the function of mediators in hepatic I/R injury.

Comparison of the results of animal studies and their extrapolation to human beings is feasible, but with limitations. Among the primary obstacles are differences in hypothermia and ischemia tolerance, differences in the anatomy of the livers of various species and subspecies, differences between and within the experimental models used, and differences in the modes of administration, dosage, and metabolic breakdown of the drugs under investigation. Thus, it is very important to choose the animal species and the experimental model and to standardize the protocol according to the clinical question under study.

Small and large animals have their own advantages and disadvantages but the ultimate choice of animal species depends essentially on the scientific problema in question. Small animals such as mice and rats are exceptionally useful because they are easy to manage, present minimal logistical, financial, or ethical problems, and provide the potential for genetic alterations (e.g., transgenic and knockout animals). However, an important drawback is that the results of studies performed in small animals are of limited applicability to human beings due to their varying size and anatomy of the liver and their faster metabolism [17]. Large animals such as pigs, sheep, and dogs exhibit greater similarity in their anatomy and physiology to human beings. Thus, they are more suited for the study of problems of direct clinical relevance. However, their use is restricted by serious logistical and financial difficulties and often by ethical concerns. Furthermore, the technical possibilities of blood and tissue processing are extremely restricted because of the limited availability of immunological tools for use in large animal species [17].

Extensive data exist on liver anatomy in various species of animals, but a few examples of species variations will suffice to prove that caution is warranted in the extrapolation of this data to humans. Mice and rats each have 4 liver lobes: median (or middle), left, right, and caudate and all, except the left, are further subdivided into 2 or more parts. Human liver lobes can be subdivided into 9 segments based on the vascular and ductal branching patterns to the right and lefts sides. The hepatic lobes of the rat appear to have similar fundamental portal and hepatic venous systems, and thus segments, comparable to that of human liver. The vascular systems to or from lobes show individual variations in humans as well as in rats. In humans and other mammals, sinusoids drain only into the terminal hepatic veins whereas in the rat sinusoids enter the hepatic venous system at all levels of the hepatic venous tree. In rats, unlike humans, the sinusoids are supplied not only by the terminal portal venules but also directly from larger venous branches. In addition, rat livers lack the septal vein branches, which are present both in humans and pigs [18]. The presence of arterio-portal anastomosis is very frecuent in rats but not in hamsters and humans. The rat is unique in possessing a perihilar biliary plexus, which is present from the large hiliar portal tracts to smaller portal tracts. An equivalent, less developed structure exists in humans only in large portal tracts. The biliary system in pigs lacks this plexus altogether, but contains numerous side pouches throughout the course of the bile duct [18,19]. Mice and humans have a gall bladder, but not the rat. Significant difference is present among the species with respect to the extent of hepatic parenchymal innervation and the human has the most abundant supply of autonomic nerves in the intraparenchymal region [20]. Differences in hepatic cell types have been reported depending of species evaluated. For example, regarding to endothelial cells, rats have relatively higher fenestrae compared to some other species. Defenestration is though to play a role in some liver diseases [18]. Intrinsic biochemical differences between the hepatocytes of the various species have been also reported. Rats and mice are extremely sensitive to the response of peroxisome proliferators, hamsters show a less marked response while primates and humans are insensitive or non-responsive [21]. There are two principle hypotheses to explain species differences in response to PPs: quantity of PPARa and/or the quality of the PPARα-mediated response [22].

When selecting an animal species, the age and sex of the animals should be considered. Depending on the duration of ischemia, young (35–50 g) and older rats (250–400 g) exhibit significant differences in their hepatic microcirculation [23]. A mature rat weighing more than 250 g (14–16 weeks old) is the most suitable because younger rats can present technical problems, whereas older rats are more prone to respiratory infections and fat accumulation. Sex selection also affects experimental results, as hormone levels in female animals are dependent on the estrous cycle, which certainly affects the ischemia tolerance of the liver. For instance, a study demonstrated that after normothermic liver ischemia, male rats were less sensitive to reperfusion injury than female rats.

Considering the relevancy of hepatic steatosis in surgery, experimental models of hepatic I/R injury in the presence of steatosis have been developed. However, the mechanisms involved in hepatic I/R injury, as it will be described in following sections, are different depending on the method used to induce steatosis. The different models of steatosis include 1) induced genetic models; 2) animals fed diets with high levels of saturated fat and/or carbohydrates and/or proteins; 3) animals fed diets deficient in methyl groups (choline, methionine, folates); and 4) animals fed modified high-fat diets (lower methionine and choline and higher-fat content).

The induction of I/R injury must be performed under standardized experimental conditions. Of primary importance are the conditions under which the animals are kept such as adequate acclimatization time, maintenance under climatized conditions with 12 hours light / 12 hours darkness, and standardized diets. The anesthetic method and postoperative analgesic regimen must also be standardized. When choosing the anesthetic and analgesic procedures, possible interactions with liver metabolism must be considered. Attention must be paid to adequate monitoring of blood pressure, heart rate, and body temperature.

4. Normothermic hepatic ischemia

4.1. Global hepatic ischemia with portocaval decompression

The model of global liver ischemia with portal decompression ideally simulates the clinical situation of warm ischemia after the Pringle maneuver for liver resection and LT. The first successful shunt operation in humans was performed by Vidal in 1903 [24]. Blakemore was one of the first workers to report successful portal-systemic anastomosis in rats working principally with endothelium-lined tubes [25]. Burnett et al., modified this technique to form a portocaval shunt [26]. In 1959 Bernstein and Cheiker developed the portosystemic shunt that conducted the portal blood after functional hepatectomy into one of the iliac veins [27]. In small animals, in addition to many other shunt techniques such as the portofemoral shunt and the mesentericocaval shunt via the jugular vein, in 1995, Spiegel et al., developed the splenocaval shunt [28] (Figure 2).

http://dx.doi.org/10.5772/51829

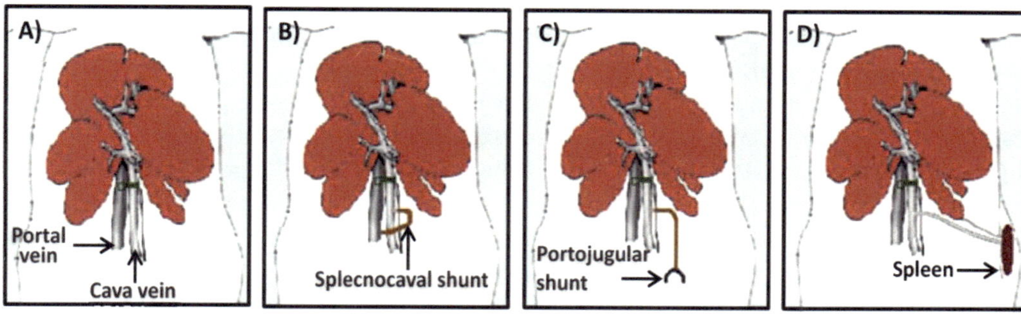

Figure 2. Models of global normotermic liver ischemia. A) Pringle-maneuver. B) Splecnocaval shunt. C) Portojugular shunt. D) Spleen transposition.

4.2. Global liver ischemia with spleen transposition

Bengmark et al., developed this model in 1970 for the surgical treatment of portal hypertension [29]. In 1981 Meredith and Wade presented a rat model that by transposition of the spleen produced a portosystemic shunt in the anhepatic rat [30]. A small incision is made in the left hypochondrium. After transposition of the spleen into a subcutaneous pouch, adequate portosystemic anastomoses arise after two to three weeks (Figure 2). Reversal of blood flow in the splenic vein, induced by the transposition, stimulates angiogenesis. In the second step 2 weeks later, the surgeon performs a median laparotomy and temporary occlusion of the hepatoduodenal ligament. This decompression by spleen transposition does not require microsurgical technique and is therefore easy to perform. Two-to-three weeks postoperatively, the spleen will have been encapsulated without any signs of bleeding or inflammation. One disadvantage of this model is the long time lapse (3 weeks) until the formation of adequate portosystemic collaterals. Not until this point in time are the collaterals sufficiently large to take over portal vein flow completely. Furthermore, it is uncertain how the changes in hepatic inflow will react upon the collaterals [31].

4.3. Partial liver ischemia and liver regeneration

In 1982, Yamauchi et al., described a model of hepatic ischemia [32]. In this technique, ischemia is induced by occlusion of the hepatic artery, the portal vein, and the bile duct of the left and median lobes. An extracorporeal shunt is not necessary because blood flow continues through the right and caudal liver lobes. This model of 70% partial ischemia has been widely used in experimental studies of hepatic I/R [13,33]. Additionally, an experimental model of 30% partial liver ischemia has been used in which blood supply to the right lobe of the liver is interrupted by occlusion at the level of the hepatic artery and portal vein [34]. It is known that, in clinical situations, PH under I/R is usually performed to control bleeding during parenchymal dissection. *In vitro* studies, although they have proved helpful in disclosing the signal transmission pathways of various hepatocyte mitogens, need to be supplemented by *in vivo* studies with experimental animals so as to simulate the interactions between the various cell populations of the liver. Different strategies have been adopted for the experimental induction of liver regeneration as follow below [35]. On the other hand, the use of an experimental model including both hepatic regeneration and I/R injury is advisable to simulate the clinical situation of selective or hemihepatic vascular occlusion for liver resections. In experimental model, after resection of left hepatic lobe, a microvascular clamp is placed across the portal triad supplying the median lobe (30%). Congestion of the bowel is avoided during the clamping period by preserving the portal flow through the right and caudate lobes. At the end of ischemia time, the right lobe and caudate lobes are resected, and reperfusion of the median lobe is achieved by releasing the clamp. This model of hepatic resection does not require any portal decompression and also fulfills certain important criteria such as reversibility, good reproducibility, and simple performance [36].

4.4. Other experimental models of liver regeneration – Regeneration after liver injury

There are large numbers of toxins that can cause liver damage and cell death in the liver parenchyma followed by liver regeneration. Carbon tetrachloride, d-galactosamine, ethanol, thioacetamide and acetaminophen are the hepatotoxins that have been most frequently employed to induce experimental liver regeneration in the hope of answering various questions [35]. In contrast to PH, these so-called hepatotoxic models of liver regeneration are easier to perform and of greater clinical relevance. Whereas PH leaves all the remaining hepatic acini intact, hepatotoxins can be used selectively to induce centrilobular or periportal necrotic lesions and can thus better simulate certain liver diseases. One serious weakness of toxin-induced liver regeneration is the por reproducibility and standardisability of the models, because the local and systemic effects of the toxin depend on the dose, the mode of administration, the species of animals, their age and nutritional status and other factors, and the extent of the liver injury and the regeneration can vary accordingly. The regenerative response of the liver is often determined by the dose and mode of administration. Furthermore, the toxins can directly interfere with the cellular and molecular mechanisms of liver regeneration, e.g., by damaging membranes (interruption of the interaction between growth factors and membrane receptors), impairment of gene expression and protein synthesis, inflammatory reactions (increased production of cytokines and oxygen radicals) or activation of nonparenchymal cells [37]. Finally, in these toxic models the processes of liver injury and repair are closely interwoven, a fact that adds to the difficulties of investigating liver regeneration. It is therefore difficult to predict the extent of liver damage and liver regeneration and to avoid significant variability between individual experiments [35].

5. Liver transplantation

The development and implementation of different surgical techniques in LT have been based upon animal experimental studies. LT in larger laboratory animals such as dogs and pigs is technically easier. However, the rat has become the most important subject for experimental LT because of, among other factors, the availability of genetically defined animals [38]. The first experimental liver replacement with OLT was reported by Cannon in 1956,

http://dx.doi.org/10.5772/51829

but none of those dogs survived [39]. Surgical techniques for experimental OLT on pigs were started by Garnier et al., in 1965 [40]. OLT in mice is technically very difficult, even without reconstruction of the hepatic artery. By contrast, OLT in rats is technically accessible, producing more clinically relevant and reliable data [41]. The development of clinically relevant OLT models in rats [41] has advanced clinical knowledge in LT. These experimental models facilitate the study of new preservation methods, tolerance induction, rejection mechanisms, and novel immunosuppressor therapies [42].

The first model of OLT in the rat was described by Lee et al., in 1973 using hand-suture techniques [43]. This technique includes standard microvascular suture technique for venous anastomoses and a miniaturized extracorporeal portal-tojugular shunt ("microsuture model"). Rearterialization of the graft is performed by anastomosing the donor aorta end-to-side to the host aorta, and the donor bile duct is implanted into the duodenum [43]. Two years later, in 1975, Lee reported a modified model without hepatic artery reconstruction and temporal shunt of the portojugular venovenous bypass [44]. However, these models were not widely used due to the prolonged surgical time and technical demand. In 1979, Zimmermann introduced a microsuture model [45] that is similar to the simplified model of Lee [44]. He developed a new technique for bile duct reconstruction that preserves the sphincter of ampulla "splint technique". In the same year, Kamada and Calne [46] developed a cuff technique for anastomoses of portal vein and bile duct to simplify Lee's model and especially to shorten the anhepatic time and reduce biliary complications. With the cuff method being introduced by Kamada and Calne [46], OLT in rats without hepatic artery reconstruction became globally accepted [41]. Other models introduced by later investigators contain for the most part only a few modifications. In 1980 Miyata introduced the "three-cuff model" [47] with cuff technique for the three venous anastomoses. Bile duct anastomosis is performed by using the splint technique first described by Zimmermann [45], in which reestablishment of hepatic blood flow is not carried out. Anastomosis of the portal vein is done by the method of Kamada and Calne [46]. For connecting the bile duct, splint technique was used [47]. In 1982 Engemann [48] devised a microsuture model that corresponds closely to the model of Lee [43]. During the anhepatic time he dispensed with portosystemic bypass and used an aortic-celiac segment for rearterialization. This had been already prepared in the donor operation, and anastomosed end-toside to the infrarenal aorta of the recipient. Bile duct anastomosis is performed using the splint technique [48]. Portal vein clamping causes a rise of endotoxin in the portal vein, which could lead to disturbances in hepatic microcirculation. Lee was the first to use a portosystemic shunt, but in further models it has not been established because the acceleration of the transplantation procedure by improved anastomotic techniques was expected to preclude the need for this complicated operative procedure [38]. Kitakado completed the "two-cuff model" in 1992 by developing a bioabsorbable material (synthesis of D, L-lactic acid and glycolic acid). Its *in vivo* degradation time is about 4 months when used for cuff anastomosis of portal vein and infrahepatic vein cava [49]. He established a longterm model in OLT in rat. This surgical procedure is usually performed according to the procedure described by Kamada and Calne [46]. After arterial and portal perfusion, the suprahepatic vena cava is dissected free from the diaphragmatic ring, and the intrathoracic vena cava is transected. The aorta is cut around the celiac axis to form the aortic patch. Finally, the inferior vena cava, the portal vein, and the bile duct are cut, and the graft is placed in a cold preservation solution (Figure 3). OLT is then performed by suture or mechanical microvascular anastomoses. Sutured vascular anastomosis reduces the incidence of thrombosis but takes a long time to perform. Suprahepatic vena cava anastomosis is performed by the continuous suturing technique. Then, portal vein and infrahepatic vena cava anastomosis is performed in the same manner. Hepatic artery reconstruction in rat LT can prevent bile duct ischemia and preserve the structure of the liver [50]. Several techniques of rearterialization by suture have been proposed [50], the best being the aortic segment anastomosis technique. After rearterialization, the common bile duct is anastomosed. OLT by hand-sewn microanastomosis is a very useful method because this technique comes closest to the techniques used in human transplantation surgery. Alternatively, livers can be satisfactorily allografted in rats by using the rapid cuff-ligature technique for anastomosis [46]. In the simplified technique, the donor hepatic artery can be ligated because it will not be anastomosed [42].

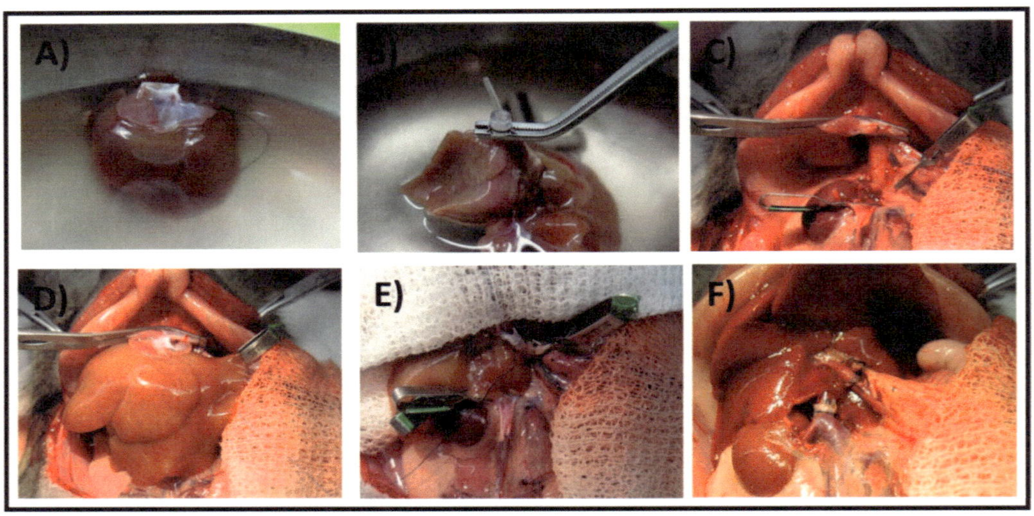

Figure 3. Liver transplantation procedure. A) Suprahepatic cava vein prepared for the anastomosis. B) Inferior vein cava cuff attachment. C) Anhepatic phase in the recipient rat. D) Anastomosis of suprahepatic cava vein by continuous suture. E) Portal vein anastomosis trhough the cuff method. F) Anastomosis of the bile duct.

6. Strategies to expand the size of the donor pool

In an attempt to expand the size of the donor pool, a number of surgical techniques have been developed over the past 15 years, including reduced-size liver transplantation (RSLT), split liver transplantation (SLT) and living donor liver transplantation (LDLT) [51]. For children and small adult recipients, RSLT has been developed to maximize the use of donor organs. Bismuth and Houssin in 1984, transplanted the left lateral segment of the left liver lobe from a cadaveric donor into a small child and discarded the remainder of the donor liver [52]. Couinaud's anatomical classification permits the creation of partial liver allografts from either deceased or living donors. Couinaud's classification divides the liver into eight independent segments, each of which has its own vascular inflow, outflow, and biliary drainage [53]. Segments IV to VIII are used for adults, whereas left lateral lobes (Segments II and III) or left lobes (Segments II, III, and IV) are used for pediatric recipients. Bleeding, bilomas, and portal vein thrombosis are complications related to the procedure itself, which are associated with an increased number of re-operation. SLT, first performed in 1988, allows the division of the adult donor liver, together with its vascular and biliary structures, into two or more functional grafts, which can be transplanted into two or more recipients [54]. Liver splitting is performed either *ex situ* or *in situ*. So far, there is no consensus on which technique is superior because both techniques demonstrate similar patient and graft survival rates compared with whole liver grafting [54]. Biliary complications occur in 22% of recipients. In 1990, Broelsch et al., reported the first 20 series of LDLT in the USA [55]. In 1996, Lo et al., [56] performed the first successful LDLT using an extended right lobe from a living donor for an adult recipient. One of the benefits of reduced-size grafts from living donors is a graft of good quality with a short ischemic time, this latter being possible because live donor procurements can be electively timed with the recipient procedure. Conversely, the major concern over the application of LDLT for adults is graft-size disparity. Small grafts require posterior regeneration to restore the liver/body ratio. A small graft may result in malfunction or the small for size syndrome in which the recipient fails to sustain adequate metabolic function. It is well known that I/R significantly reduce liver regeneration after hepatectomy. Thus, the identification and subsequent modulation of mechanism that are involved in liver injury and regeneration might favor the recovery and functioning of the transplanted organ.

To mimic some of the pathophysiological events that occur during such clinical situations, several experimental models of RSLT have been developed. For example, OLT with the implantation of liver grafts that approximated 30%–70% of the normal mass of a rat liver has been performed. Graft size is important for normal liver function and host survival [51]. It has been reported that 100% of recipient rats that were implanted with 40%, 50%, 60%, or 70% of the liver survived regardless of the duration of preservation. This suggests that graft sizes of 40% or greater are sufficient to meet the metabolic demands of the recipients. The transplantation of a graft of 30% of the normal liver mass provides an extreme model of hepatic reduction that presumably stimulated a maximal regenerative response [51]. Three possibilities exist with respect to the timing of the graft reduction: in the donor before perfusion, in the container (ex situ), or in the recipient after reperfusion. If the reduction is done *in vivo* prior to the removal of the donor liver, then two concerns exist: 1) excessive bleeding might stimulate systemic responses that could alter the liver and 2) the immediate phase of the regeneration response could be initiated in the donor animal. The second choice, ex situ reduction, can be done without the risk of damaging the graft by manipulation or affecting anastomosis after reperfusion. Finally, resection of the graft after implantation in the recipient adds surgical stress and the risk of bleeding.

7. Modes of organ preservation and optimizing the graft

The ideal method of organ preservation should: 1) Reverse injury sustained during donor death and organ procurement; 2) Provide viability testing; 3) Prolong safe preservation time and 4) Improve the graft quality [57]. There are currently 2 modes of preservation methods for livers: static and dynamic (Figure 4). Simple cold storage is the main method for static storage while hypothermic machine perfusion (HMP) and normothermic machine perfusion (NMP) comprise some of the methods for dynamic preservation. Of these methods, only simple cold store is roved clinically for livers. The remaining methods are in various stages of pre-clinical and early clinical studies. Dynamic preservation methods require some dynamic movement of either fluid or gas to facilitate preservation. The advantage of these methods over simple cold storage is that they all have been shown to improve recovery of donor after cardiac death organs. These organs have the potential to increase the donor pool by 20–40%.

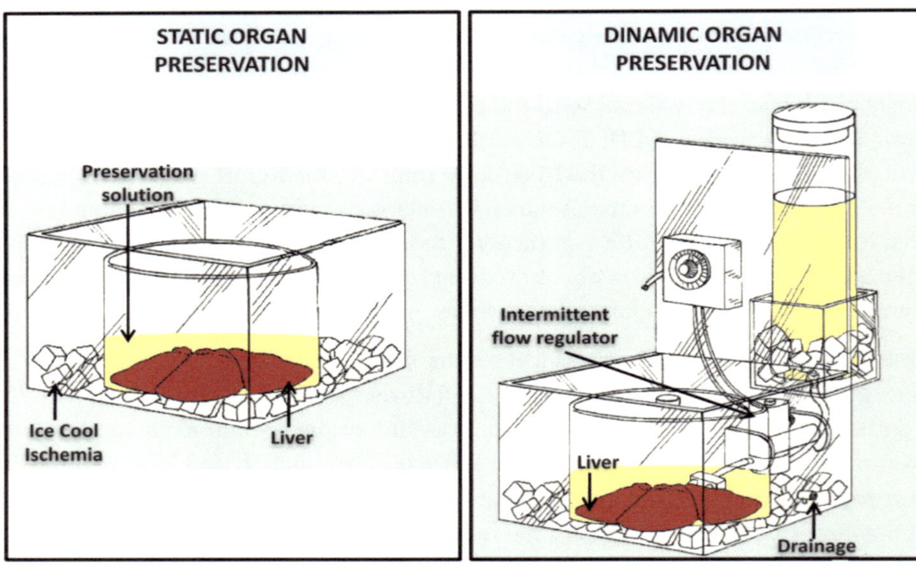

Figure 4. Illustrative modes of organ preservation. Static or dynamic organ preservation.

7.1. Static organ preservation

Static cold storage (SCS) is the most commonly used preservation method used for all organs. The principles underlying cold preservation are the slowing of metabolism (by cooling) and the reduction of cell swelling due to the composition of preservation solutions. The introduction of the University of Wisconsin (UW) solution by Belzer and Southard for SCS was a breakthrough and remains the conventional method of preservation. Reduction of metabolic activity (by cooling) is the major principle of organ preservation [57,58]. At the moment the flow of oxygenated blood is terminated, the supply of oxygen, cofactors and nutrients stops and the accumulation of metabolic waste products begins. Although metabolism is slowed 1.5- to 2-fold for every 10ºC drop in temperature, anaerobic metabolism continues, which leads to depletion of energy stores and concomitant build up of an acidotic milieu. Depletion of ATP causes loss of transcellular electrolyte gradients, influx of free calcium and the subsequent activation of phospholipases, and therefore is the main contributor for cell swelling and lysis. Ischaemia creates the basis for the subsequent production of toxic molecules after reperfusion, particularly reactive oxygen intermediates, the basis of the cascade of events that characterize the I/R injury. Even with the most effective preservation solutions, cold storage aggravates graft injury at the time of transplantation. This situation is due to two processes, one proportional to the duration of ischemia and the other specifically related to cooling [57]. Using this preservation method, however, organs undergo injury at several consecutive stages: warm ischemia prior to preservation, cold preservation injury, ischemic rewarming during surgical implantation and reperfusion injury. With the extension of criteria to include expanded criteria donor and donation after cardiac death organs, static preservation is associated with increased delayed graft function and graft loss. In organs retrieved from non-heart-beating donors (NHBD) -with an inevitable period of oxygen deprivation between cardiac arrest and organ perfusion – the deleterious effects of cold ischaemia are superimposed on the injury sustained during warm ischaemia [57]. Only a few studies have demonstrated the optimization of graft function and survival with modification of static preservation. It is doubtful that considerable improvements in organ preservation and especially in the rescue of marginal organs will be possible as long as the strategy is based on static principles [58]. In 1990s, Minor et al., developed a new method, called venous systemic oxygen persufflation (VSOP) to supply gaseous oxygen to livers during SCS preservation [59]. The oxygen was introduced into hepatic vasculature via the suprahepatic vena cava. This technique was employed on steatotic rat livers for 24 h, and resulting in improved preservation of mitochondria and sinusoidal endothelial linings, less KC activation and reduced hepatocellular enzyme release compared to SCS preservation. Recently, by assessing the enzyme release, energy storage, bile production, and cell death during isolated reperfusion, it was demonstrated that application of VSOP for 90 minutes may rescue the steatotic livers after extended (18 h) SCS preservation [60].

7.2. Machine perfusion

Machine liver perfusion is an alternative preservation method to SCS which can be further categorized based on the temperature employed and has emerged with promising data over the past decade because it has significant potential in graft preservation and optimization when the use of marginal organs is the objective. Machine perfusion involves pulsatile perfusion of the liver using a machine as opposed to SCS. This can be performed by perfusing the liver with a hypothermic perfusate or with a normothermic perfusate. There is experimental evidence in animal models that machine perfusion protects against liver I/R injury [61]. The safety and efficacy of machine perfusion compared to SCS to decrease liver I/R injury is yet to be assessed in humans by randomized controlled trials [61,62].

Compared with simple cold storage, machine perfusion confers many anticipated advantages such as the following: 1) provision of continuous circulation and better preservation of the microcirculation; 2) continuous nutrient and oxygen delivery; 3) removal of metabolic waste products and toxins; 4) opportunity to assess organ viability; 5) improved clinical outcomes via improved immediate graft function rates; 6) prolonged preservation time without increased preservation damage; 7) administration of cytoprotective and immunomodulating substances; and 8) lower graft dysfunction incidence, shorter hospital stays, and better graft survival rates [62].

7.3. Normothermic machine perfusion

In the first half of the 20th century, Alexis Carrel perfused different organs with normothermic, oxygenated serum and demonstrated viability for several days [63]. Actually, the first successful human LT carried out by Starzl [64], were transplanted after liver graft pretreatment by machine perfusion with diluted, hyperbaric oxygenated blood. Most perfusion circuits were assembled from standard cardiopulmonary bypass components. Principle constituents are a centrifugal pump, a membrane oxygenator and a heat exchanger. Other critical components of the perfusate include nutrition (glucose, insulin, aminoacids), drugs to prevent thrombosis or microcirculatory failure (heparin, prostacyclin) and agents to reduce cellular oedema, cholestasis and free radical injury [57]. Normothermic machine perfusion (NMP) provides a physiologically-relevant environment to the isolated donor organ, the quality of liver grafts can be manipulated more efficiently than those simply stored in an ice-box during SCS, because NMP maintains and mimics normal *in vivo* liver conditions and function during the entire period of preservation, thus avoiding hypothermia and hypoxia and minimizing preservation injury [58,62]. In contrast to cold storage preservation the concept of normothermic preservation is to maintain cellular metabolism. The underlying principle is the combination of continuous circulation of metabolic substrates for ATP regeneration and removal of waste products. There is accumulating evidence for the superiority of the more physiological approach of normothermia in association with an oxygenated blood-based perfusion solution [57].

Schön et al., [65] studied NMP to preserve pig livers for transplantation and to rescue them from warm ischemia in a model of donor after cardiac death. Short (5 h) or prolonged (20 h) NMP preservation is superior to SCS for normal and ischemically damaged livers, respectively [62]. The longest preservation of steatotic livers was the NMP preservation for 48 hours in a pig model by Jamisson et al., who employed blood containing additional insulin and vasodilators as perfusate, and observed a mild reduction of steatosis from 28% to 15%. The NMP circuit dually perfuses 1.5 L of autologous heparinized blood at physiological pressures, which allows hepatic blood flow autoregulation. Prostacyclin, taurocholic acid, and essential amino acids are infused continuously. Apart from logistics, one potential drawback of NMP is the mandatory use of oxygen carriers if blood is not available [62]. Perhaps the only weakness is that SCS prior to NMP revokes its beneficial effect. Therefore, immediately after cardiac asystole, normothermic perfusion in the donor should be installed, as described by Fondevila et al., [66] for the preservation of livers from uncontrolled donation after cardiac death. The use of

NHBDs as a source of liver grafts for transplantation has long been debated. The concept of normothermic recirculation in the context of NHBDs was first developed by Garcia-Valdecasas et al., [67]. With 4 h of NMP, hepatic damage incurred during 90 minutes of cardiac arrest can be reverted, achieving 100% graft survival after 5 days of postransplant follow-up. These results offer the hope that NMP will be able to increase the clinical applicability of NHBD LT over that offered by traditional cold storage [67].

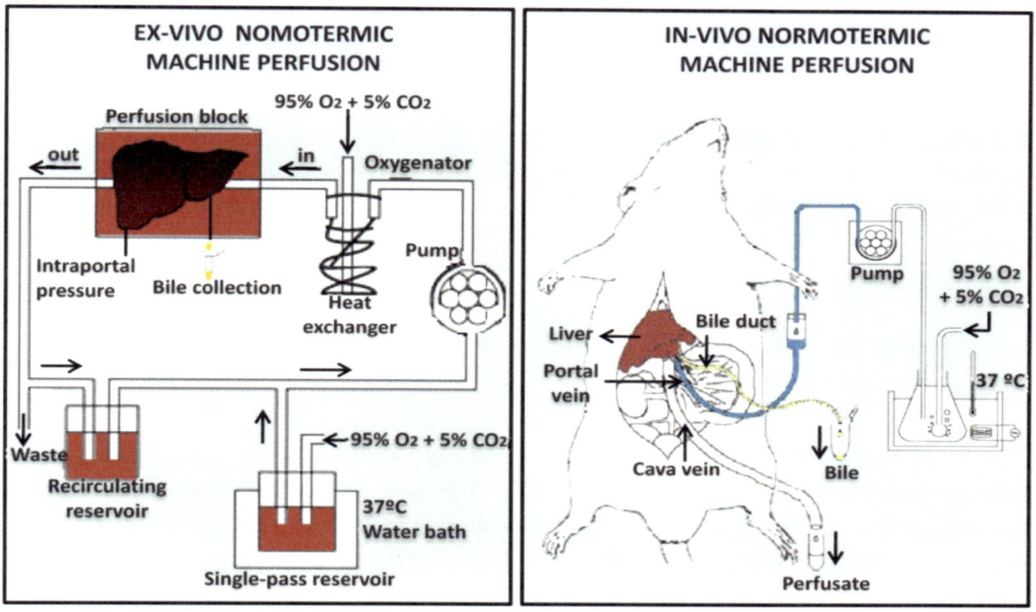

Figure 5. Esquematic illustration for *ex-vivo* and *in-vivo* normotermic machine perfusion

7.4. Hypothermic machine perfusion

For decades, cooling down organs to cold temperatures allowed successful organ transplantation within a limited period. The first and most prominent difference between SCS and (oxygenated) hypothermic machine perfusion (HMP) is the restoration of the tissue's energy charge and glycogen content while preventing ATP depletion [62]. In 1990, Pienaar et al., [68] reported that seven of eight dogs survived after LT with HMP preservation for 72 h and a similar outcome after 48 h of SCS. HMP is increasingly being used as an alternative method to SCS for the preservation of grafts obtained from nonoptimal donors. Indeed, several studies have reported a greater reduction in delayed graft function after HMP preservation than after SCS. Bessems et al., employed HMP preservation with UW-gluconate solution on steatotic rat livers for 24 h and alleviated I/R compared to SCS [69]. There is a substantial body of research, predominantly in rodents, demonstrating improved preservation by providing oxygen to livers [70]. Nevertheless, clear guidelines towards target values/ranges for oxygen levels regarding the optimal duration of oxygenation during HMP are lacking. HMP can also be applied at the end of the cold storage period, which is attractive for logistical reasons. The disadvantage here is the time-dependent increase in vascular resistance, bearing the risk of damage to the sinusoidal endothelium [58].

7.5. Subnormotermic machine perfusion

Subnormothermic machine perfusion (SNMP) preservation lies between HMP and NMP, but it remained relatively unexplored until recently despite holding promising applications [71]. In an isolated rat liver perfusion model, SNMP enhanced the functional integrity of steatotic livers compared with SCS findings. Organ protecting properties mediated by decreasing the temperature to a 20–28ºC have been observed previously. SNMP avoids some of the downsides of hypothermia while maintaining mitochondrial function and it may circumvent the logistical rest raints of NMP [62]. Vairetti et al., preserved steatotic rat livers by SNMP (20ºC) with Kreb-Henseleit solution for 6 hours and obtained reduced I/R damage compared to SCS [71].

8. Factors to be considered before the selection of an experimental model of hepatic I/R

Many investigators have used rodent models of warm (*in situ*) liver I/R to mimic some of the pathophysiological events that occur during LT. Although a great deal of useful information has been generated from these studies, an overriding question remains: Are the mechanisms responsible for transplant-mediated liver injury and dysfunction the same as those that have been reported for warm liver I/R injury? The answer is yes and no; that is, some of the mechanisms are similar, but many are dissimilar. It is important to make a distinction between the different types of ischemia, because there already is some controversy regarding the pathophysiological mechanisms depending on the type of ischemia (cold or normothermic), and it should be considered that the type of ischemia, the extent and time of ischemia, the type of liver submitted to I/R, and the presence of liver regeneration, all lead to differences in the pathophysiological mechanisms of hepatic I/R. These are discussed below to provide the reader with a guide to select the appropriate experimental model of hepatic I/R depending on the aims being pursued.

8.1. Relevance of the type of surgical procedure

The mechanisms responsible for hepatic I/R injury as well as the effects of pharmacological treatments are dependently of the liver surgical procedure. There is a range of potentially conflicting results with regard to the mechanisms responsible for ROS generation in liver I/R injury depending of the liver surgical procedure evaluated. XDH/XOD system is the main ROS generator in hepatocytes and LT-related lung damage [72]. However, results obtained in experimental models of the isolated perfused liver have underestimated the importance of the XDH/XOD system, and suggest that mitochondria could be the main source of ROS

http://dx.doi.org/10.5772/51829

[9]. In addition, studies by Metzger et al., in experimental models of normothermic hepatic ischemia showed that the increased vascular oxidant stress after 30 and 60 minutes of ischemia was attenuated by inactivation of KC but not by high dose of allopurinol in experimental models of normothermic hepatic ischemia [73].

It should be considered that the effectiveness of drugs on hepatic regeneration and damage could be different depending on the surgical conditions evaluated. Thus, gadolinium chloride treatment protected against hepatic damage in conditions of I/R without hepatectomy and improved liver regeneration after PH without I/R [74]. However, the same drug had injurious effects on hepatic damage and impaired liver regeneration in conditions of PH under I/R [75]. It should be also considered that the effectiveness of RAS blockers on hepatic regeneration and damage could be different depending on the surgical conditions evaluated. In conditions of PH under I/R, the AT1R antagonist for nonsteatotic livers and the AT1R and AT2R antagonists for steatotic ones improved regeneration in the remnant liver. The combination of AT1R and AT2R antagonists in steatotic livers showed stronger liver regeneration than either antagonist used separately and also provided the same protection against damage as that afforded by AT1R antagonist alone. However, the loss of protection of Ang II receptor antagonists against damage in conditions of PH under I/R (only AT1R antagonist protected steatotic liver against damage) compared with the study of I/R without hepatectomy (in which both Ang-II receptor antagonists reduced damage in both liver types) could be explained by the different surgical conditions. In the model of I/R without hepatectomy [33], the blood supply to the left and median liver lobes (70% hepatic mass) was interrupted, and the other hepatic lobes remained intact. However, in the conditions evaluated herein, only blood supply to the remnant liver (30% hepatic mass) was interrupted and the other hepatic lobes were excised. Compared with the study of I/R without hepatectomy [33], in PH under I/R, there are two main differences, the percentage of hepatic mass that is deprived of blood supply and hepatic resection. It is well known that the mechanisms of hepatic damage are different depending on the percentage of hepatic mass that is deprived of blood supply [76,77]. In addition, the inherent mechanisms of hepatic damage derived from the massive removal of hepatic mass should be considered. This may explain, at least partially, why the same drug, such as an Ang II receptor antagonist, may show differential effect on hepatic injury depending on surgical conditions [36]. In line with this, clinical and experimental studies revealed the injurious effects of NO on damage in the remnant liver in conditions of PH under I/R [36]. However NO protect against hepatic damage in an experimental model of I/R without PH [11]. In PH under I/R, Ang-II is an appropriate therapeutic target to protect steatotic livers against hepatic damage and regenerative failure. However, this target could be not appropriate in steatotic LT, since the results indicate a novel target for therapeutic interventions in LT within the RAS cascade, based on Ang 1-7, which could be specific for this type of liver. Indeed, Ang 1-7 receptor antagonist reduced necrotic cell death and increased survival in recipients transplanted with steatotic liver grafts [15].

The results, based on isolated perfused liver, indicated that the addition of epidermal growth factor (EGF) and isulin-like growth factor 1 (IGF-I) separately or in combination to UW reduced hepatic injury and improved function in both liver types. EGF increased IGF-I, and both additives up-regulated AKT in both liver types. This was associated with glycogen synthase kinase-3β (GSK3β) inhibition in non-steatotic livers and PPARγ over-expression in steatotic livers [78]. The benefits of EGF and IGF-I as additives in UW solution were also clearly seen in an experimental model of normothermic hepatic ischemia. However, the relationship between EGF and IGF-I was different dependently of the surgical procedure. Indeed, under these conditions, IGF-I increased EGF, thus protecting steatotic and non-steatotic livers against I/R damage. The beneficial role of EGF on hepatic I/R damage may be attributable to p38 inhibition in non-steatotic livers and to PPARγ overexpression in steatotic livers [79].

PPARα agonists as well as ischemic preconditioning (IP), through PPARα, inhibited mitogen-activated protein kinase expression following I/R in steatotic livers undergoing normothermic hepatic ischemia. This in turn inhibited the accumulation of adiponectin in steatotic livers and reduced its negative effects on oxidative stress and hepatic injury [13]. In line with this, adiponectin silent small interfering RNA (siRNA) treatment decreased oxidative stress and hepatic injury in steatotic livers. However, another study by Man et al., 2006 [80] in small fatty grafts, adiponectin treatment exerted anti-inflammatory effects that down-regulated TNFα mRNA and vasoregulatory effects that improved the microcirculation. Adiponectin anti-inflammatory effects also include the activation of cell survival signaling via the phosphorylation of Akt and the stimulation of NO production. Additionally, the studies by Man et al., [80] showed the anti-obesity and proliferative properties of adiponectin in small fatty transplants. Taken together, the aforementioned data indicate that the action mechanisms of adiponectin depend on the surgical conditions. Thus, on the basis of the different results reported to date in hepatic I/R, it is difficult to discern whether we should aim to inhibit adiponectin, or administer adiponectin to protect steatotic livers against cold ischemia associated with transplantation. Moreover, the adiponectin data reported for these experimental models of hepatic I/R [13,80] should not be extrapolated to cadaveric organ transplantation. For small liver grafts (which are relatively common) and under conditions of warm ischemia, the periods of ischemia range from 40 to 60 minutes; this range may not be accurate for cadaveric donor LT.

RBP4 is an adipokine synthesized by the liver, whose known function is to transport retinol in circulation. However, the role of RBP4 in hepatic I/R could depend on the liver surgical procedure. Steatotic liver grafts were found to be more vulnerable to the down-regulation of RBP4. RBP4 treatment-through AMP-activated protein kinase (AMPK) induction- reduced PPARγ over-expression, thus protecting steatotic liver grafts against I/R injury associated with transplantation. In terms of clinical application, therapies based on RBP4 treatment and PPARγ antagonists might open new avenues for steatotic LT and improve the initial conditions of donor livers with low steatosis that are available for transplantation [81]. On the other hand, the effects of RBP4 could depend on the surgical conditions. Indeed, RBP4 administration not only failed to protect both liver types from damage and regenerative failure, it exacerbated the negative consequences of liver surgery in PH under I/R [82]. Under these conditions, RBP4 affected the mobilization of retinol from steatotic livers, revealing actions of RBP4 independent of simple retinol transport. The injurious effects of RBP4 were

http://dx.doi.org/10.5772/51829

not due to changes in retinol levels. Thus, strategies based on modulating RBP4 could be ineffective and possibly even harmful in both liver types in PH under I/R or surgical conditions including small-for-size LT.

8.2. Relevance of the duration of hepatic ischemia

The severity of hepatocyte damage depends on duration of ischemia. Depending on the objectives of the research, it is important to consider a specific ischemia duration. In other words, if you want to study the mechanisms involved in hepatic I/R injury or the protective mechanisms of a drug, it is more appropriate to use a duration of ischemia associated with high survival. If the purpose is to study the relevance of a drug in hepatic I/R injury, then it is advisable to assess survival, and, therefore, it is more adequate to use experimental models in which the ischemic period is associated with low survival. These observations are based on the following data reported in the literature. It appears that short periods (60 minutes) of warm ischemia result in reversible cell injury, in which liver oxygen consumption returns to control levels when oxygen is resupplied after ischemia. Reperfusion after more prolonged periods of warm ischemia (120-180 minutes) results in irreversible cell damage. These observations agree with a previous report on rat liver subjected to I/R, indicating a cellular endpoint for hepatocytes after 90 minutes of ischemia [83]. In human LT, a long ischemic period is a predicting factor for posttransplantation graft dysfunction, and some transplantation groups hesitate to transplant liver grafts preserved for more than 10 h. Some studies in experimental models of LT indicate that cold ischemia for 24 h induces low survival. However, LT, following shorter ischemic periods, may also result in primary organ dysfunction [72].

It is important to distinguish between the types of Ischemia (warm and cold) because there is already some controversy about the pathophysiological mechanisms of cold ischemia, which may depend, for example, on the time. The mechanisms of hepatic I/R injury are also different depending on the duration of hepatic ischemia. Along these lines, in the same experimental model of LT, XDH/XOD plays a crucial role in hepatic I/R injury only in conditions under which significant conversion of XDH to XOD occurs (80–90% of XOD) such as 16 h of cold ischemia. However, this ROS generation system does not appear to be crucial for shorter ischemic periods such as 6 h of cold ischemia [72]. Similarly, it should also be noted that oxidative stress in hepatocytes and the stimulatory state of KCs after I/R depend on the duration of ischemia and may also differ between ischemia at 4ºC and that at 37ºC, which probably leads to different developmental mechanisms of liver damage.

Our previous results indicate that PPARα does not play a crucial role in I/R injury in nonsteatotic livers. This contrasts with a study published by Okaya and Lentsch [84], in which the authors reported the benefits of PPARα agonists on postischemic liver injury. Although the dose and pretreatment time of the PPARα agonist WY-14643 were similar in both studies, Okaya and Lentsch reported an ischemic period of 90 minutes; ours was 60 minutes, which is the ischemic period currently used in liver surgery [3]. Thus, 60 minutes of ischemia seems to be insufficient to induce changes in PPARα in nonsteatotic livers [13].

8.3. Relevance of the extent of hepatic ischemia

Another factor to consider before selecting the experimental model of hepatic I/R is the percentage of hepatic ischemia applied. The extent of hepatic injury as well as the hepatic I/R mechanisms, including the recovery of blood flow and energy charge during hepatic reperfusion is dependent on the extent of ischemia-whether total or partial (70%) hepatic ischemia is applied [36]. This fact could be explained by the stealing phenomenon. In contrast to 100% hepatic ischemia, during ischemia in the left and median lobes, the flow is shunted via the right lobes and following the release of the occlusion of the left and median lobes, a significant amount of shunting via the right lobes will continue during reperfusion until vascular resistance in the postischemic lobes decreases. This occurs because blood flows through the path of least resistance. The reasons for this may be cellular swelling endothelial, stasis, or other changes. Thus, the recovery of blood flow and hepatic perfusion of the preischemic lobe is later in the case of 70% hepatic ischemia than in 100% hepatic ischemia [76]. In line with these observations, the benefits of some drugs such as ATP-MgCl2 were dependent on the extent of hepatic ischemia used [32,77].

8.4. Relevance of the type of liver submitted to I/R

A variety of clinical factors including starvation, graft age, and steatosis have been studied in different experimental models of hepatic I/R because of the relevance of these factors in clinical practice. These factors enhance liver susceptibility to I/R injury, further increasing the patient risks related to reperfusion injury.

8.4.1. Starvation

The pre-existent nutritional status is a major determinant of the hepatocyte injury associated with I/R. In clinical LT, starvation of the donor, due to prolonged intensive care unit hospitalization or the lack of adequate nutritional support, increases the incidence of hepatocellular injury and primary nonfunction [85]. Based on the nutritional state status, several experimental and clinical studies support the hypothesis that the availability of glycolytic substrates is important for maintenance of hepatic ATP levels during I/R. Fasting exacerbates I/R injury because the low content of glycogen stores results in more rapid ATP depletion during ischemia. In addition, fasting causes alterations in tissue antioxidant defenses, accelerates the conversion of XDH to XOD during hypoxia and induces mitochondrial alterations [85]. Caraceni et al., [86] have shown that mitochondrial damage is greatly enhanced by fasting which decreases the hepatic content of antioxiants and therefore sensitizes the mitochondrial to the injurious effects of ROS. Considering these observations, an artificial nutritional support may represent a new approach for the prevention of reperfusion injury in fasted livers. On the contrary, fasting has been reported to improve organ viability and survival [87], as it reduces phagocytosis and the generation of TNF-α [87]. To understand these apparent contradictory results, it is important to consider the different experimental conditions in these investigations. A beneficial effect of high glycogen content can mainly be expected under conditions of long preservation times and long periods of warm ischemia. Under these conditions, high metabolic reserves of the liver may attenuate ischemic cell injury and preserve defense functions against cytotoxic mediators of KCs. Conversely, short ischemic periods require lower metabolic reserves, and the extent of KC activation can be the dominant factor in early graft injury.

8.4.2. Age

A number of distinct age-related alterations have been identified in the hepatic inflammatory response to hepatic I/R [88]. Under warm hepatic ischemia, mature adult mice had greatly increased neutrophil function, increased intracellular oxidant levels, and decreased mitochondrial function compared with the findings in young adult mice. These alterations contributed to the increased liver injury after I/R observed in mature adult mice compared with that in young adult mice. The results obtained in an experimental model of isolated perfused liver indicate that, during reperfusion, livers obtained from old rats generate a lower amount of oxyradicals than livers from young rats. This fact could be explained by the lower KC activity, the reduction of liver blood flow, and the impaired functions and structural alterations observed in the livers of old rats. In fact, in hepatocytes from mature adult mice, delayed activation of nuclear factor kappa B (NFκB) in response to TNF-α and virtually no production of macrophage inflammatory protein 2 have been detected, which may be due to an agerelated defect in hepatocytes [88].

8.4.3. Steatosis

The first step to minimize the adverse effects of I/R in steatotic livers is a full understanding of the mechanisms involved in I/R injury in these marginal organs. This can be achieved only with the selection of an appropriate method to induce steatosis in livers undergoing I/R. It is well known that the mechanisms involved in hepatic I/R injury are different depending on the type of liver (nonsteatotic versus steatotic livers). In addition to the impairment of microcirculation, mitochondrial ROS generation dramatically increases during reperfusion in steatotic livers [9,86]. Results obtained under warm hepatic ischemia indicate that apoptosis is the predominant form of hepatocyte death in the ischemic nonsteatotic liver, whereas the steatotic livers develop massive necrosis after an ischemic insult [9]. Steatotic livers differed from nonsteatotic livers in their response to the UPR and ER stress since IRE1 and PERK were weaker in the presence of steatosis [89]. Decreased ATP production and dysfunction of regulators of apoptosis, such that Bcl-2, Bcl-xL and Bax have been proposed to explain the failure of apoptosis in steatotic livers. Differences were also observed when we analyzed the role of the RAS, as the nonsteatotic grafts exhibited higher Ang-II levels than steatotic grafts whereas steatotic grafts exhibited higher Ang 1-7 levels [15]. In the context of I/R injury associated with LT, the axis ACE-Ang II-ATR and ACE2-Ang 1-7-Mas play a major role in nonsteatotic and steatotic grafts, respectively. From the point of view of clinical application, these findings may open up new possibilities for therapeutic interventions in LT within the RAS cascade, based on Ang 1-7 for steatotic livers and Ang II for non-steatotic ones [15]. Moreover, reduced RBP4 and increased PPARγ levels were observed in steatotic livers compared to non-steatotic livers [81]. The vulnerability of steatotic livers subjected to warm ischemia is also associated with increased adiponectin, oxidative stress, and IL-1 levels and a reduced ability to generate IL-10 and PPARα [13,90].

It should be considered that there are differences in the mechanisms involved in hepatic I/R injury depending on the method used to induce steatosis. In contrast with other experimental models of steatosis, both dietary high fat and alcohol exposure induced the production of SOD/catalase-insensitive ROS, which may be involved in the mechanism of steatotic liver failure after OLT [9]. Neutrophils have been involved in the increased vulnerability of steatotic livers to I/R injury, especially in alcoholic steatotic livers. However, neutrophils do not account for the differentially greater injury in non-alcoholic steatotic livers during the early or late hours of reperfusion. Similarly, the role of TNF in the vulnerability of steatotic livers to I/R injury may be dependent on the type of steatosis [1,9].

8.5. Relevance of regeneration in experimental models of hepatic I/R

It is known that different experimental models trigger different responses when a common mechanism or the same drug is investigated. This situation is witnessed when analyzing liver injury in models of I/R with or without hepatectomy. This situation is illustrated by Ramalho et al., [36] regarding the loss of protection of Ang-II receptor antagonists against liver damage in conditions of PH under I/R compared with the study of I/R without hepatectomy, in which Ang-II receptor antagonists reduced hepatic damage. These different results could not be explained by differences in the dose or frequency of drug administration but rather by differences in surgical conditions (percentage of hepatic ischemia and the presence or absence of hepatectomy). In the model of I/R without hepatectomy [33], the blood supply to the left and median liver lobes (70% hepatic mass) was interrupted, and the other hepatic lobes remained intact. However, in PH under I/R, only blood supply to the remnant liver (30% hepatic mass) was interrupted and the other hepatic lobes were excised [36].

According to the cell type and experimental or pathologic conditions, TNF-α may stimulate cell death or it may induce hepatoprotective effects mediated by antioxidant, antiapoptotic, and other anti-stress mediators coupled with a pro-proliferative biologic response. For example, although the deleterious effect of the TNF-α in local and systemic damage associated with hepatic I/R in experimental models of normothermic hepatic ischemia is well established [91], this mediator is also a key factor in hepatic regeneration [92], an important process in RSLT and PH associated with hepatic resections [93]. These differential effects observed for TNF-α can also be extrapolated to transcription factors. It is well known that NFκB can regulate various downstream pathways and thus has the potential to be both pro- and antiapoptotic [8]. Currently it is not clear whether the beneficial effects of NFκB activation in protection against apoptosis or its detrimental proinflammatory role predominate in liver I/R [8]. Hepatic neutrophil recruitment and hepatocellular injury are significantly NFκB activation is suppressed in mice following partial hepatic I/R. However, NFκB activation is essential for hepatic regeneration after rat LT, and reduces apoptosis and hepatic I/R injury [94].

http://dx.doi.org/10.5772/51829

9. Strategies applied in experimental models of hepatic I/R

9.1. Pharmacological treatment and additives in preservation solution

Numerous experimental studies have focused on the developing *in vivo* pharmacological strategies aimed at inhibiting the harmful effects of I/R [9,72,89,90,95-99]. Some of these studies are summarized in Table 1. However, none of these treatments has managed to prevent hepatic I/R injury. A large number of ingredients-which have been introduced into UW solution in experimental models of hepatic cold ischemia [9,95,100-102] (Table 1). However, none of these modifications to the UW solution composition have found their way into routine clinical practice. Further studies will be required to elucidate whether the use of perfluorochemicals (PFC) in preservation solutions might improve the viability of liver grafts undergoing transplantation. PFC are hydrocarbons with high capacity for dissolving respiratory and other nonpolar gases. A negligible O_2-binding constant of PFC allows them to release O_2 more effectively than hemoglobin into the surrounding tissue (acts as an oxygen-supplying agent). PFC differs from hemoglobin preparations in that it is a totally synthetic compound formed on a liquid hydrocarbon base. Unlike hemoglobin, acidosis, alkalosis, and temperature seem to have no or little effect on the oxygen delivery of PFC, allowing this compound to be used effectively during cold storage of organs [103]. A recently study, used Oxycyte, a PFC added to UW solution can be beneficial after cardiac death liver graft preservation in a rat model [103]. However, their effects on reperfusion injury were not evaluated in that study. In fact, the possibility that preoxygenated PFC exacerbates the ROS during reperfusion should not be discarded since the use of gaseous oxygen applied to the livers during the storage period was only effective in improving hepatic viability upon reperfusion when antioxidants were added to the UW rinse solution [104].

It should be also considered that the inclusion of some components in the UW solution has been both advocated and criticized. Indeed, simplified variants of the UW solution in which some additive were omitted were demonstrated to have similar or even higher protective potential during cold liver storage. Another limitation of the UW solution is that some of its constituent compounds, including allopurinol do not offer very good protection because they are not present at a suitable concentration and encounter problems in reaching their site of action [9]. The possible side effects of some drugs may frequently limit their use in human LT. For example, idiosyncratic liver injury in humans is documented for chlorpromazine, pernicious systemic effects have been described for NO donors, allopurinol therapy can cause hematological changes and gadolinium can induce coagulation disorders. Some case reports of acute hepatotoxicity attributed to rosiglitazone have been published [105]. The development of therapeutic strategies that utilize the protective effect of heme oxygenase-1 induction is hampered by the fact that most pharmacological inducers of this enzyme perturb organ function by themselves [106].

Pharmacological treatment-derived difficulties must also be considered. In this regard, SOD and GSH exhibit inadequate delivery to intracellular sites of ROS action [9]. The administration of anti-TNF antibodies does not effectively protect against hepatic I/R injury, and this finding has been related to the failure of complete TNF-α neutralization locally [11]. Although this also occurs in non-steatotic livers, modulating I/R injury in steatotic livers poses a greater problem. Differences in the action mechanisms between steatotic and non-steatotic livers mean that therapies that are effective in non-steatotic livers may prove useless in the presence of steatosis, and the effective drug dose may differ between the two liver types. Findings such as these must be considered when applying pharmacological strategies in the same manner to steatotic and non-steatotic livers because the effects may be very different. For example, caspase inhibition, a highly protective strategy in non-steatotic livers, had no effect on hepatocyte injury in steatotic livers [9]. Moreover, whereas in an LT experimental model, an NO donor reduced oxidative stress in non-steatotic livers, the same dose increased the vulnerability of steatotic grafts to I/R injury. Furthermore, there may be drugs that would only be effective in steatotic livers. This was the case of compounds such as cerulenin, which reduce UCP-2 expression in steatotic livers and carnitine [9].

Pharmacological Therapy – Warm Ischemia			
Species	**Drug**	**Ischemic Time**	**Effect**
Mice	Cerulenin *(Fatty acid synthase inhibitor)*	15 min	↓ UPC2, ↑ ATP
	Catalase and derivatives	30 min	↓ Oxidative stress
	Apocynin *(NAPH oxidase inhibitor)*		↓ Oxidative stress
	TBC-1269 *(Pan-selectin antagonist)*	90 min	↓ Inflammatory response, ERK ½
Rat	Lisinopril *(ACE inhibitor)*	30 min	↓ Oxidative stress
Rat	Ascorbate *(ROS scavenger)*		↓ Apoptosis
	Allopurinol *(XOD inhibitor)*	30 60 min	↓Oxidative stress
	Melatonin *(Hormone)*	40 min	↓ IKK, JNK pathways
	SOD *(antioxidant)*	45 min	↓ Microcirculatory disturbances, leukocyte acumulation
	L-arginine *(NO precursor)*		↑ NO, ATP ↓ Neutrophil accumulation
	Tocopherol *(Antioxidante)*	45 90 min	↓ Microcirculatory disturbances, Lipid peroxidation, SEC damage
	IL-10	60 min	↓ IL-1, Oxidative stress
	Anti-ICAM-1		↓ Adherence of leukocytes in postsinusoidal venules
	Gabexate mesilate *(Protease inhibitor)*		↓ TNF-α, Leukocyte activation
	OP-2507 *(Analogue of prostacyclin)*		↓ Microcirculatory disturbance
	WY-14643 *(PPARα agonist)*		↓ Oxidative stress, Inflammatory cytokines

http://dx.doi.org/10.5772/51829

	n-3 PUFA		↓ Liver injury, Oxidative stress
	Glutathione *(Antioxidant)*	60 90 min	↓ Microcirculatory disturbances ↑ Detoxification of ROS
	Spermine NONOate *(NO donor)*		↓ IL-1α, Oxidative stress
	FK506 *(Immunosupressant)*		↓ TNF
	Rosiglitazone *(PPARα agonist)*		↑ Autophagy ↓ Cytokines
	AMPK activators	90 min	↑ NO, ATP
	Adenosine		↑ NO
	Anti-TNF antiserum		↓ TNF, Leukocyte accumulation
	α-Lipoic acid *(Antioxidant)*		↑ Liver regeneration, ↓ Apoptosis
Pharmacological Therapy – Warm Ischemia with Hepatectomy			
Species	**Drug**	**Ischemic Time**	**Effect**
Rat	Tauroursodeoxycholate *(Bile acid)*	60 min	↓ Endoplasmic reticulum stress
	Sirolimus *(Immunossupressant)*		↓ Linfocytes
	IL-1ra *(IL-1 receptor antagonist)*	90 min	↓ TNF, Oxidative stress
Dog	FK 3311 *(Cox-2 inhibitor)*	60 min	↓ Neutrophil infiltration, Cox-2
Pharmacological Therapy – Liver Trasplantation			
Species	**Drug**	**Ischemic Time**	**Effect**
Mice	Cerulenin *(fatty acid synthase inhibitor)*	80 min	↓ UPC2, ↑ ATP
Rat	FK 409 *(NO donor)*	80 min	↑ HSP, IL-10, ↓ SEC damage, IL-1
	CS1 peptides *(FN-α4β1 interac blocker)*	4 h	↓ Neutrophil and lymphocyte T infiltration, TNF-α, iNOS
	Tocopherol *(antioxidante)*	5 h	↓ Lipid peroxidation, SEC damage, Microcirculatory disturbance
	Hemin *(HO-1 inducer)*	6 h	↑ Bcl-2
	Cobalt-protoporphyrin IX *(HO-1 inducer)*		↓ Macrophages infiltration and T cells
	PSGL-1 *(P-selectin blocker)*		↓ Neutrophil infiltration, TNF-α, INFγ, iNOS
	Anti-TNF antiserum	6, 24 h	↓ TNF, Leukocyte accumulation
	SOD *(antioxidant)*	8 h	↓ Microcirculatory disturbance, Leukocyte acumulation
	Tauroursodeoxycholate *(Bile acid)*		↓ Endoplasmic reticulum stress
	Allopurinol *(XOD inhibitor)*	8, 16 h	↓Oxidative stress

	Z-DEVD-FMK *(caspase 3 and 7 inhibitor)*	16 h	↑ Microvascular perfusión, Bcl-2 ↓ Apoptosis
	L-arginine *(NO precursor)*	18 h	↑ NO, ATP, ↓ Neutrophil accumulation
	Treprostinil *(Prostacyclin analogue)*		↓ Liver injury, Platelet deposition, microcirculatory disturbance
	ANP *(vasodilating peptide)*	24 h	↑ PI3K/Akt, ↓ Apoptosis
	Bucillamine *(antioxidant)*		↓Oxidative stress
	Chlorpromazine *(Ca^2 + channel antagonist)*		↑ ATP ↓ Mitocondrial dysfunction, Alterations in lipid metabolism
	sCR1 *(complement inhibitor)*		↓ Microcirculatory disturbance, Leukocyte adhesion
	Glutathione *(antioxidant)*		↓ Microcirculatory disturbance ↑ Detoxification of ROS
	N-acetylcysteine *(glutathione precursor)*		↓ Microcirculatory disturbance
	Anti-ICAM-1		↓ Adherence of leukocytes in postsinusoidal venules
	Glycine *(Kupfer cell modulator)*		↓ Neutrophil accumulation, TNF-α
	GdCl3 *(Kupffer cell blocker)*		↓ Neutrophil accumulation, TNF-α
	Cbz-Val-Phe methyl ester *(calpain inhibitor)*	24, 40h	↓ Calpain activation, SEC apoptotic
	EHNA *(adenosine deaminase inhibitor)*	24, 44 H	↑ Interstitial adenosine ↓ Microcirculatory disturbance, Leukocytes rolling
	CGS-21680 *(adenosine A2 receptor agonist)*	30 h	↑ cAMP, ↓ SEC Killing
	Sotrastaurin *(PKC Inhibitor)*		↓ Apoptosis, macrophage/neutrophil accumulation
	FR167653 *(IL-1β and TNF-α supressor)*	48 h	↓ TNF-α, IL-1α, Kupffer cell activation
	Doxorubicin *(Heat shock proteins inducer)*		↓ TNF-α, MIP-2, NKκB
Pig	Sodium ozagrel *(Thromboxane synthase inhibitor)*	8 h	↓ ET-1
Additives to UW solution – Liver Trasplantation			
Species	**Drug**	**Ischemic Time**	**Effect**
Mouse	Erythropoietin *(EPO)*	24 h	↓ Liver injury
Rat	Meloxicam *(COX-2 Inhibitor)*	1 h	↓ Apoptosis, Liver injury, Oxidative stress
	Simvastatin *(KLF2-inducer)*	1, 6, 16 h	↓ Inflammation, Liver injury, Oxidative stress,
	Tauroursodeoxycholate *(Bile acid)*	2 h	↓ Endoplasmic reticulum stress
	S-nitroso-N-acetylcysteine	2, 4, 6 h	↓ Liver injury

	LY294002 *(PI3K inhibitor)*	7, 9, 24 h	↓ Apoptosis
	8br-cAMP, 8br-cGMP *(nucleotide analogs)*	24 h	↓ TNF-α and neutrophil accumulation
	Ruthenium red *(mitochondrial Ca2+ uniporter inhibitor)*		↓ Mitocondrial dysfunction
	Melatonin *(Hormone)*		↓ Oxidative stress, Liver injury
	OP-4183 *(PGI2 analogue)*		↓ Oxidative stress
	SAM *(ATP precursor)*		↓ Oxidative stress
	IDN-1965 *(caspase inhibitor)*	24, 30 h	↓ Apoptosis
	Pifithrin-alpha *(p53 inhibitor)*	24, 48 h	↓ Apoptosis
	Sodium nitroprusside *(NO donor)*		↓ Microcirculatory dysturbances
	FR167653 *(p38 inhibitor)*	30 h	↓ Microcirculatory dysturbances
	GSNO *(NO donor)*	48 h	↓ SEC damage
Dog	Trifluoperazine *(calmodulin inhibitor)*	24 h	↓ Microcirculatory dysturbances
Pig	E5880 *(PAF antagonist)*	8 h	↓ Microcirculatory dysturbances
	EGF, IGF-1, NGF-α	18 h	↑ ATP

Table 1. In *vivo* pharmacological therapy and additives in preservation solution in experimental models of warm hepatic ischemia (with or whithout hepatectomy) and liver transplantation

9.2. Gene therapy

Advances in molecular biology provide new opportunities to reduce liver I/R injury by using gene therapy. Genome manipulation can be achieved by: A) germ line manipulation (oocyte injections); B) stem cell transformation and reintroduction into embryos, and C) targeting specific cells or organs with vectors or viruses (gene transfer). The first 2 approaches include germ-line alterations and are neither feasible nor accepted by society. The third approach would lend to the treatment of individual patients with either acquired or congenital diseases [12]. In the last years, significant advances in gene therapy vectors have occurred. Gene transfer can be accomplished by direct injection of DNA into a target organ or tissue, transduction by recombinant viral vectors carrying a specific gene of interest, e.g., adenovirus (Ad) or retrovirus, transfection of cells by chemical methods (e.g., cationic liposomes), or stem cell transduction and reintroduction of genetically-altered cells back into embryos [107] (Table 2). Currently, researchers in gene transfer have focused efforts toward targeting vectors to specific cells or organs without loss of transduction ability [108,109], allowing high level gene transduction of the liver without affecting other organs [12,107].

		Genetic material	Packaging capacity	Duration of experiment	Integration into genome	Transduction of postmitotic cells
Recombinant viruses	Oncoretrovirus	RNA	9 kb	Long	Yes	Low
	Lentivirus	RNA	10 kb	Long	Yes	Low
	Foamy	RNA	12 kb	Long	No	High
	Herpes virus	DNA	"/>30 kb	Transient	No	High
	Adenovirus	DNA	30 kb	Transient	Rarely	Moderate
	AAV	DNA	4.6 kb	Long postmitotic tissues	Rarely	Moderate
	Oncoretrovirus	RNA	9 kb	Long	Yes	Low
	Lentivirus	RNA	10 kb	Long	Yes	Low
Non-viral methods	siRNA	RNA	No limitation	Transient	No	Zero
	DNA injection	DNA	No limitation	Transient	No	Zero
	Cationic liposomes	DNA	No limitation	Transient	No	Zero
	Stem cell transduction	DNA	No limitation	Transient	No	Zero

Table 2. Summary of gene therapy vectors commonly used.

Antiapoptotic Strategies (Bcl-2/Bcl-Xl, Bag-1 and caspases): Bcl-2 blocks apoptosis and necrosis and has been implicated in the prolongation of cell survival [110]. Given its functional importance in the cell death cascade, it constitutes one of the key targets for cytoprotective therapeutic manipulation for the regulation of apoptosis [110,111]. As demostrated by Bilbao et al., [111] in a mouse hepatic I/R model, overexpression of Ad-mediated Bcl-2 gene significantly decreased hepatocyte apoptosis and necrosis, improved hepatic function, and prolonged survival as compared with controls. In addition, Bag-1 is a Bcl-2 binding protein resulting in a prolonged and stabilized antiapoptotic activity [112]. In addition, Bag-1 appears to exert an indirect silencing effect on TNF receptor R1 and hence suppresses the death receptor signal. A recent study by Sawitzki et al., [113] has demonstrated the cytoprotective effect of Ad-mediated Bag-1 gene transfer in rat liver I/R. Using a model of cold ischemia and OLT, Ad-Bag-1 transfer improved portal venous blood flow, increased bile production, and improved hepatic function with decreased neutrophil accumulation in the graft. Furthermore, Ad-mediated Bag-1 expression preserved hepatic architecture and reduced inflammation. The activation of T cells infiltrating the graft was inhibited, since decreased expression of TNF-α, CD25, IL-2, and IFNγ [107]. Caspase-8 is presumed to be the apex of the death-mediated apoptosis pathway, whereas caspase-3 belongs to the "effector" proteases in the apoptosis cascade. Contreras et al., demonstrated that inhibition of caspase-8 and caspase-3 by siRNA provided significant protection against warm hepatic I/R injury and decreased animal mortality. In addition, animals given siRNA caspase-8, or more significantly siRNA caspase-3, presented lower neutrophil infiltration and better histologic profiles [114].

Antioxidant therapy (SOD, HO-1, Ferritin): Oxidative stress can activate NF-κB and the AP-1 pathway and induce expression of proinflammatory genes including cytokines, adhesion molecules, and chemokines leading to neutrophil-mediated inflammation [115-117]. To inhibit the burst of ROS or its effect on hepatocytes, several oxygen stress inhibitory proteins have been studied, e.g., SOD and catalase have been transfected by either adenovirus, liposomes or polyethylene-glycol [8,12,118]. Using partial hepatic I/R models, Ad-mediated MnSOD administration reduced liver tissue damage and activation of both NF-κB and AP1 [119,120] when compared with lacZ-transduced controls. In another study, He et al., [121] demonstrated that SOD or catalase gene delivery by polylipid nanoparticles injected via the portal vein 1 day prior to the warm I/R procedure resulted in high levels of the transgene enzyme activity in the liver, and markedly attenuated hepatic I/R injury [121]. However, results with NFκB activation have been conflicting. Takahashi et al. reported that overexpression of IκB, an NFκB inhibitor (mediated by Ad-IκB) resulted in partial protection in hepatic I/R injury [122]. Heme oxygenase 1 (HO-1) is a stress responsive protein and can be induced by various conditions such as hypoxia [12,107]. Several studies have shown that HO-1 exhibits potent cytoprotective effects after hepatic I/R [123,124]. In a cold ex-vivo rat liver perfusion model and a syngeneic liver transplant OLT model, treatment of genetically obese Zucker rats with Ad-HO-1 improved portal venous blood flow, increased bile production, and decreased hepatocyte injury [123]. Unlike in untreated rats, upregulation of HO-1 correlated with preserved hepatic architecture, improved liver function, and depressed infiltration by T cells and macrophages. Ad-mediated HO-1 gene overexpression increased survival of recipients from 40% to 80% [12,107]. Ad-HO-1 gene transfer decreased macrophage infiltration in the portal areas and inducible nitric oxide synthetase (iNOs) expression; it also increased the expression of antiapoptotic genes Bcl-2/Bcl-xl and Bag-1, as compared with controls [107]. Iron chelation is another approach to ameliorate the I/R injury cascade. Free iron has been shown to play a role in the formation of the free radicals through the Fenton reaction; these contribute to endothelial cell damage. Ferritin induction is a result of the action of HO-1 on the heme porphyrin causing the release of Fe2+. Ferritin can reduce the availability of intracellular free Fe2+, which can participate in free radical generation [125]. Studies by Ke et al., [107] demostrated that overexpression of Ad vector carrying the ferritin heavy chain (H-ferritin) gene protects rat livers from I/R injury [126]. In these studies, the protective effect of H-ferritin was associated with the inhibition of endothelial cell and hepatocyte apoptosis. Evidence suggested that H-ferritin exerts an antiapoptotic role and may be used as a therapeutic measure to prevent I/R [107].

Immunoregulatory cytokines (IL-10 and IL-13) and IL-1 receptor antagonist (IL-1R): IL-13 regulates liver inflammatory I/R injury via the signal transducer and activator of transcription 6 (STAT6) pathway [127]. IL-10 induces antioxidant HO-1 gene expression in murine macrophages and exerts anti-inflammatory effects [128]. In recent studies, Ad-IL-13 gene transfer in cold ischemia models has shown powerful cytoprotective effects [129]. Gene transfer of IL-13 improved hepatic function, upregulated HO-1, and prevented hepatic apoptosis through the upregulation of Bcl-2/Bcl-xl [107]. The beneficial effects of IL-13 correlated with *in vivo* cross talk between innate TLR4 and adaptive Stat6 immunity [130]. In fact, using an experimental model of warm hepatic ischemia, Stat6-deficient mice with Ad-IL-13 failed to improve hepatic function and hepatic histological features. Transfer of Ad-IL-13 increased anti-oxidant HO-1 expression and inhibited TLR4 activation in WT mice, whereas low HO-1 and enhanced TLR4 expression was shown in Stat6-deficient mice [107]. It has been demonstrated that the pro-inflammatory cytokine IL-1 plays a critical role in the pathophysiological response to I/R. Experimental results have shown that blockade of the IL-1R reduced TNF production and liver damage [131]. In a partial hepatic I/R model, gene transfer of Ad-mediated IL-1R antagonist prolonged animal survival and improved hepatic function while preserving the histological architecture. In addition, a marked decrease in production of proinflammatory cytokines such as IL-1, TNF-α, and IL-6 was present [107].

T-cell co-stimulation blockade: CD40-CD154. A number of studies have shown that CD4+ T lymphocytes play an important role as key cellular mediators in I/R injury mediated inflammatory responses. The CD40–CD154 co-stimulation pathway provides the essential second signal in the initiation and maintenance of T-cell-dependent immune esponses [132]. Recent studies have demonstrated that CD40-CD154 is required for the mechanism of hepatic warm I/R injury [133]. In OLT, prolonged *in vivo* blockade of the CD40-CD154 interaction following pretreatment of liver isografts with Ad-CD40Ig exerted potent cytoprotection against I/R injury. Apoptosis was prevented and neutrophil accumulation was reduced. Evidence also demonstrated prevention of Th1-type cytokine (interferon γ (IFN-γ) and IL-2) upregulation and the local expression of antioxidant HO-1 and antiapoptotic Bcl-2/Bcl-xl genes were triggered [107].

Adipocytokine, sphyngolipid and TLR4 regulation: Massip-Salcedo et al., [13] demostrated though the systemic delivery of adiponectin in livers treated with adiponectin siRNA that steatotic livers by themselves can generate adiponectin as a consequence of I/R. This study reports evidence of the injurious effects of adiponectin in stetatotic livers under warm ischemic conditions, and results suggest the clinical potential of gene therapy for I/R damage in steatotic livers by siRNA-mediated adiponectin gene silencing [13]. Products of sphingolipid metabolism are important second messengers that regulate a variety of cell processes including cell death, proliferation, and inflammation. Using a mice warm hepatic I/R model, Shi et al., demonstrated that SK2 knockdown by siRNA effectively prevented hepatocyte death [134]. Jiang et al., [135] reported a hepatocyte-specific delivery system for the treatment of liver I/R, using galactose-conjugated liposome nanoparticles (Gal-LipoNP). Heptocyte-specific targeting was validated by selective *in vivo* delivery as observed by increased Gal-LipoNP accumulation and gene silencing in the liver. Gal-LipoNP TLR4 siRNA treatment reduced hepatic damage, neutrophil accumulation and the inflammatory cytokines IL-1 and TNF-α [135].

Advances in molecular biology have provided new opportunities to reduce liver I/R injury using gene therapy [9,12,13,96,114] (Table 3). However, the experimental data indicate that there are a number of problems inherent in gene therapy, such as vector toxicity, difficulties in increasing transfection efficiencies and protein expression at the appropriate time and site, and the problem of obtaining adequate mutants (in the case of NFκB) due to the controversy regarding NFκB activation [136]. Although non-viral vectors (such as naked DNA and liposomes) are likely to present fewer toxic or immunological problems, they suffer from in-

http://dx.doi.org/10.5772/51829

efficient gene transfer [136]. In addition, LT is an emergency procedure in most cases, which leaves very little time to pre-treat the donor with genetic approaches. Efforts to reduce the time between gene therapy and LT might open new venues for preventative gene therapy [12]. Currently, viral vectors hydrodynamic injection and cationic liposomes are the main methods for delivering siRNA *in vivo*. While viral vectors are associated with severe side effects, other methods require large volume and high injection speed, which are not clinically applicable [135]. Systemic administration of small interfering RNA (siRNA) may cause globally nonspecific targeting of all tissues, which impedes clinical use.

9.3. Cell therapy – Hepatocyte transplantation

The liver was among the first organs considered for strategies based on the transplantation of isolated cells. The first hepatocyte transplant was performed to treat the Gunn rat, the animal model for Crigler-Najjar syndrome, which is congenitally unable to conjugate bilirubin and consequently exhibits life long hyperbilirubinemia. The transplant resulted in a decreased plasma bilirubin concentration. Later, isolated hepatocytes were transplanted into rats with liver failure induced by dimethylnitrosamine. These experiments demonstrated that hepatocyte transplantation could potentially be used for the treatment of liver failure and innate defects of liver-based metabolism. More than 30 years later, these models are still used in work to improve hepatocyte engraftment and/or function [137].

Many studies have shown that hepatocytes transplanted into rodents via the spleen or the portal vasculature enter through portal vein branches and are entrapped in proximal hepatic sinusoids; consequently, the hepatocytes are distributed predominantly in periportal regions of the hepatic lobules. Transplanted hepatocytes cause both portal hypertension and transient I/R injury. The portal hypertension, in experimental animals at least, usually resolves within 2 to 3 hours with no obvious long-term detrimental effects, and microcirculatory abnormalities disappear within 12 hours. Numerous hepatocytes (up to 70% of transplanted cells) remain trapped in the portal spaces, and most of them are destroyed by the phagocytic responses of KC, which are activated shortly after deposition of hepatocytes in liver sinusoids [138]. The remaining cells translocate from sinusoids into the liver plates through a process involving disruption of the sinusoidal endothelium and release of vascular endothelial growth factor by both host and transplanted cells. In rodents, hepatic remodeling is complete within 3 to 7 days, and the engrafted cells become histologically indistinguishable from host cells. Transplantation of 2×10^7 hepatocytes in rats has led to the engraftment of about 0.5% of the transplanted cells in the recipient livers [139]. Only hepatocytes harboring a selective advantage for survival/proliferation can efficiently repopulate a recipient liver, and as a result, many repopulation strategies have been developed using approaches involving the induction of acute or chronic liver injury [137]. Despite decades of research, the processes and factors underlying cell engraftment and *in situ* proliferation are only partially understood, and a good understanding of these mechanisms is essential for the development of new and efficient treatments of human liver diseases. The prevention of early loss of transplanted cells would undoubtedly improve hepatocyte transplantation. First, it has been recently shown that cell-cell interactions between transplanted hepatocytes and hepatic stellate cells modulate hepatocyte engraftment in rat livers. After cell transplantation, soluble signals activating hepatic stellate cells are rapidly induced along with early up-regulated expression of matrix metalloproteinases and their inhibitors [140]. Second, the interaction between integrin receptors and the extracellular matrix plays a role in cell engraftment. Third, hepatocytes express soluble and membrane-bound forms of tissue factor–dependent activation of coagulation and exert tissue factor–dependent hepatocyte-related procoagulant activity [137].

Gene	Specie	Ischemia	Vector	Effect
Bcl-2	Mouse	Warm ischemia	Adenovirus	↓ Apoptosis and Necrosis ↑ Survival
eNOS	Mouse	Warm ischemia	Adenovirus	↓ Liver injury
SOD	Mouse/Rat	Warm ischemia	Adenovirus	↓ Liver injury
IL-13	Mouse/Rat	Cold ischemia	Adenovirus	↓ Liver injury, Neutrophil infiltration, TLR4 activation, Apoptosis ↑ HO-1 expression, Survival
Bag-1	Rat	Cold ischemia	Adenovirus	↓ Liver injury, Neutrophil infiltration
CD40Ig	Rat	Cold ischemia	Adenovirus	↓ Liver injury, Neutrophil accumulation, Apoptosis and Necrosis
IkB	Rat	Cold ischemia	Adenovirus	↓ Liver injury
HO-1	Rat	Cold ischemia	Adenovirus	↓ Liver injury, Macrophage infiltration, iNOS ↑ Survival
Ferritin	Rat	Cold ischemia	Adenovirus	↓ Liver injury, Apoptosis
IL-1R antagonist	Rat	Warm ischemia	Cationic liposomes	↓ Liver injury ↑ Survival
SOD	Mouse	Warm ischemia	Polyplexes	↓ Liver injury ↑ Antioxidative enzyme activity
Catalase	Mouse	Warm ischemia	Polyplexes	↓ Liver injury ↑ Antioxidative enzyme activity
SK2	Mouse	Warm ischemia	siRNA	↓ Liver injury, Apoptosis ↑ survival
Caspase-3	Mouse	Warm ischemia	siRNA	↓ Liver injury, Neutrophil infiltration
Caspase-8	Mouse	Warm ischemia	siRNA	↓ Liver injury, Neutrophil infiltration
TLR4	Mouse	Warm ischemia	siRNA	↓ Liver injury, Neutrophil infiltration, ROS, Inflammation
Adiponectin	Rat	Warm ischemia	siRNA	↓ Liver injury

Table 3. Summary of gene therapy using specific target genes in hepatic ischemia-reperfusion

In recent years, the development of different animal models has allowed significant progress in hepatocyte transplantation. In rats, the occlusion of portal branches of the two anterior liver lobes results in a regeneration response in the remaining nonoccluded lobes leading to their hypertrophy. This procedure, portal branch ligation, favors efficient retroviral transduction of hepatocytes *in vivo*. Furthermore, hepatic tissue engineering using primary hepatocytes is an emerging therapeutic approach to liver diseases. Two recent studies reported engraftment of functional hepatocytes in a neovascularized subcutaneous cavity in mice. A method to manipulate uniform sheets of hepatic tissue allowing the formation, *in vivo*, of a 3-dimensional miniature liver system that maintained its biological function for several months has been also described [137,139]. In the view of clinical practice, treatment of fulminant hepatic failure patients by hepatocyte transplantation has been attempted by a number of investigators [141]. In one report, patients who received a hepatocyte transplant, one patient fully recovered and three were successfully bridged to OLT [141]. In a prospective study of five patients who were transplanted with cryopreserved human hepatocytes, three patients were successfully bridged to OLT [142]. Other reports have described clinical improvement and relatively longer survival in hepatocyte- transplanted patients [143] but poor final outcome has also been reported, possibly related to immunosuppression, inadequate number of transplanted cells, and limited engraftment time [137].

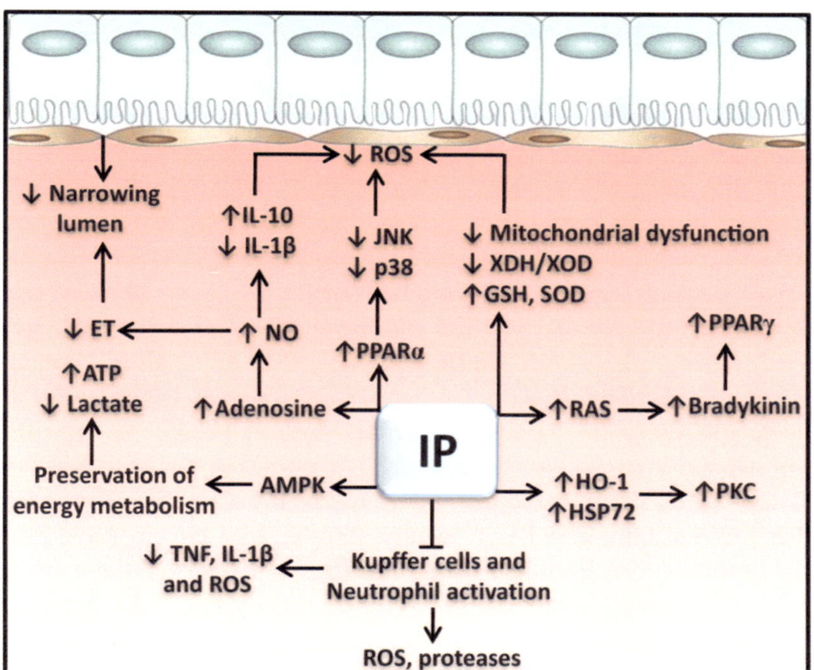

Figure 6. *Mechanisms of Ischemic preconditioning in hepatic ischemia-reperfusion injury.* AMPK, AMP-activated protein kinase; ATP, adenosine triphosphate; ET, endothelin; GSH, glutathione; HO-1, heme oxygenase 1; HSP72, heat shock protein 72; IL, interleukin; JNK, c-Jun N-terminal kinase; NO, nitric oxide; PKC, protein kinase C; PPAR, peroxisome proliferator-activated receptor; RAS, renin-angiotensin system; ROS, reactive oxygen species; SOD, superoxide dismutase; TNF, tumor necrosis factor; XDH/XOD, xanthine/xanthine oxidase

9.4. Surgical strategies

The response of hepatocyte to ischemia never ceases to surprise. In fact, contrary to what might be expected, the induction of consecutive periods of ischemia in the liver does not induce an additive effect in terms of hepatocyte lesions. Ischemic preconditioning (IP) based on brief periods of ischemia followed by a short interval of reperfusion prior to a prolonged ischemic stress protects the liver against I/R injury by regulating different cell types and multiple mechanisms such as energy metabolism, microcirculatory disturbances, leukocyte adhesion, KC activation, proinflammatory cytokine release, oxidative stress, apoptosis and necrosis [96] (Figure 6). This is an advantage in relation with the use of drugs that exerts its action on a specific mechanism. The benefits of IP observed in experimental models of hepatic warm and cold ischemia [96] prompted human trials of IP. To date, IP has been successfully applied in human liver resections in both steatotic and non-steatotic livers but unfortunately, it proved ineffective in elderly patients [144]. Preliminary clinical studies have reported the benefits of IP in LT [145,146]. IP may also have a role in the transplantation of small grafts whose pathophysiology overlaps with I/R injury. Additional randomized clinical studies are necessary to confirm whether this surgical strategy can be commonly used in clinical liver surgery.

10. Conclusion and perspectives

From the data obtained in experimental models of hepatic I/R, we can state that I/R injury is a multifaceted and intriguing phenomenon. The increasing use of marginal donors in major liver surgery and the fact that these organs are more susceptible to ischemia highlight the need for further research directed at the mechanisms of I/R injury. Machine perfusion has been criticized for its complicated logistics and for possibly damaging the organ and vital structures such as the endothelium. On the contrary, NMP fulfils all ideal organ preservation criteria by avoiding hypoxia and hypothermia. Responses to the strategies aimed at reducing hepatic I/R injury might depend on the surgical procedure, type of liver and percentage of hepatic ischemia. Further research is required to elucidate whether the pharmacological approaches presented in this review can be translated into liver surgery associated with hepatic resections and LT. Advances in molecular biology have provided new opportunities to reduce liver I/R injury using gene therapy. However, there are a number of problems inherent in gene therapy, such as vector toxicity and difficulties in increasing transfection. Liver-cell transplantation is at an early stage. Numerous approaches to isolating stem cells of hepatic or extrahepatic origin, including embryonic stem cells, are being developed. However, extensive work is still required to assess the number of cells that need to be expanded and differentiated, and the functionality of the different cell types needs to be carefully addressed in animal models. Surgical strategies such as IP affect multiple aspects of I/R injury, whereas pharmacological approaches often affect only a few mediators and might have systemic side effects.

http://dx.doi.org/10.5772/51829

Acknowledgments

Jiménez-Castro M.B. and Elias-Miró M., contributed equally to this work. Jiménez-Castro M.B., is in receipt of a fellowship from SETH Foundation (Sociedad Española de Transplante Hepatico) Spain.

Author details

M.B. Jiménez-Castro[1], M. Elias-Miró[1], A. Casillas-Ramírez[1] and C. Peralta[1,2*]

*Address all correspondence to: cperalta@clinic.ub.es

1 August Pi i Sunyer Biomedical Research Institute, Barcelona, Spain

2 Networked Biomedical Research Center of Hepatic and Digestive Diseases, Barcelona, Spain

References

[1] Serafin A., Rosello-Catafau J., Prats N., Xaus C., Gelpi E., Peralta C. Ischemic preconditioning increases the tolerance of fatty liver to hepatic ischemia-reperfusion injury in the rat. *American Journal of Pathology* 2002;161(2) 587–601.

[2] Clavien P., Harvey P., Strasberg S. Preservation and reperfusion injuries in liver allografts. An overview and synthesis of current studies. *Transplantation* 1992;53(5) 957-978.

[3] Huguet C., Gavelli A., Chieco P., Bona S., Harb J., Joseph J., et al. Liver ischemia for hepatic resection: where is the limit? *Surgery* 1992;111(3) 251-259.

[4] Busuttil R., Tanaka K. The utility of marginal donors in liver transplantation. *Liver Transplantation* 2003;9(7) 651–663.

[5] Ploeg R., D'Alessandro A., Knechtle S., Stegall M., Pirsch J., Hoffmann R., et al. Risk factors for primary dysfunction after liver transplantation-a multivariate analysis. *Transplantation* 1993;55(4) 807-813.

[6] Behrns K., Tsiotos G., DeSouza N., Krishna M., Ludwig J., Nagorney D. Hepatic steatosis as a potential risk factor for major hepatic resection. *Journal of Gastrointestinal Surgery* 1998;2(3) 292-298.

[7] Jaeschke H. Molecular mechanisms of hepatic ischemia-reperfusion injury and preconditioning. *American Journal of Physiology Gastrointestinal and Liver Physiology* 2003;284(1) G15–G26.

[8] Fan C., Zwacka R., Engelhardt J. Therapeutic approaches for ischemia/reperfusion injury in the liver. *Journal of Molecular Medicine* 1999;77(8) 577-592.

[9] Elias-Miro M., Massip-Salcedo M., Jiménez-Castro MB., Peralta C. Does adiponectin benefit steatotic liver transplantation?. *Liver Transplantation* 2011;17(1) 993-1004.

[10] Jaeschke H. Mechanisms of reperfusion injury after warm ischemia of the liver. *Journal ofHepatobiliary and Pancreatic Surgery* 1998;5(4) 402–408.

[11] Peralta C., Fernandez L., Panes J., Prats N., Sans M., Pique J., et al. Preconditioning protects against systemic disorders associated with hepatic ischemia-reperfusion through blockade of tumor necrosis factor-induced P-selectin up-regulation in the rat. *Hepatology* 2001;33(1) 100–113.

[12] Selzner N., Rudiger H., Graf R., ClavienP. Protective strategies against ischemic injury of the liver. Gastroenterology 2003;125(3) 917–936.

[13] Massip-Salcedo M., Zaouali M., Padrissa-Altés S., Casillas-Ramírez A., Rodés J., Roselló-Catafau J., Peralta C. Activation of peroxisome proliferator-activated receptor-alpha inhibits the injurious effects of adiponectin in rat steatotic liver undergoing ischemia-reperfusion *Hepatology* 2008;47(2) 461-472.

[14] Bader M., Peters J., Baltatu O., Müller D., Luft FC., Ganten D. Tissue rennin-angiotensin systems: New insights from experimental animal models in hypertension research. *Journal of Molecular Medicine* 2001;79 76-102.

[15] Alfany-Fernández I., Casillas-Ramírez A., Bintanel-Morcillo M., Brosnihan K., Ferrario C., Serafin A., et al. Therapeutic targets in liver transplantation: angiotensin II in nonsteatotic grafts and angiotensin-(1-7) in steatotic grafts. *American Journal of Transplantation* 2009;9(3) 439-451.

[16] Quijano-Collazo Y. Trasplante hepatico experimental. Brasil:Atheneu Hispánica; 2006.

[17] Abdo E., Cunha J., Deluca P., Coelho A., Bacchella T., Machado M. Protective effect of N2-mercaptopropionylglycine on rats and dogs liver during ischemia/reperfusion process. *Arquivos de Gastroenterologia* 2003;40(3) 177–180.

[18] Malarkey D., Johnson K., Ryan L., Boorman G., Maronpot R. New insights into functional aspects of liver morphology. *Toxicologic Pathology* 2005;33 27-34.

[19] Saxena R., Theise N., Crawford J. Microanatomy of the human liver – exploring the hidden interfaces. Hepatology 1999; 30(6) 1339-1346.

[20] Lin Y., Nosaka S., Amakata Y., Maeda T. Comparative study of the mammalian liver innervations: an immunohistochemical study of protein gene product 9.5, dopamine β-hydroxylase and tyrosine hydroxylase. *Comparative Biochemistry and Physiology* 1995;110A(4) 289-298

[21] Bentley P., Calder I., Elcombe C., Grasso P., Stringer D., Wiegand H. Hepatic peroxisome proliferator in rodents and its significance for humans. *Food and Chemical Toxicology* 1993:31(11) 857-907.

[22] Hasmall S., James N., Macdonald N., Soames A., Roberts R. Species differences in response to diethylhexylphthalate:suppression of apoptosis, induction of DNA synthesis and peroxisome proliferator activated receptor alpha-mediated gene expression. *Archives of Toxicology* 2000;74 85-91.

[23] Yahanda A., Paidas C., Clemens M. Susceptibility of hepatic microcirculation to reperfusion injury: A comparison of adult and suckling rats. *Journal of Pediatric Surgery* 1990;25(2) 208–213.

[24] Vidal M. Traitement chirurgical des ascites. *La Presse Médicale* 1903;11 747–749.

[25] Blakemore A., Lord J. The technic of using vitallium tubes in establishing portacaval shunts for portal hypertension. *Annals of Surgery* 1945;122(4) 449–475.

[26] Burnett W., Rosemond G., Weston J., Tyson R. Studies of hepatic response to changes in blood supply. *Surgical Forum* 1951;94 147–153.

[27] Bernstein D. Cheiker S. Simple technique for porto-caval shunt in the rat. *Journal of Applied Physiology* 1959;14(3) 467–470.

[28] Spiegel H., Bremer C., Boin C., Langer M. Reduction of hepatic injury by indomethacin-mediated vasoconstriction: a rat model with temporary splenocaval shunt. *Journal of Investigative Surgery* 1995;8(5) 363-369.

[29] Bengmark S., Börjesson B., Olin T., Sakuma S., Vosmic J. Subcutaneous transposition of the spleen: An experimental study in the rat. *Scandinavian Journal of Gastroenterology* 1970;7 175–179.

[30] Meredith C., Wade D. A model of portal-systemic shunting in the rat. *Clinical and Experimental Pharmacology and Physiology* 1981;8 651–652.

[31] Suzuki S., Nakamura S., Sakaguchi T., Mitsuoka H., Tsuchiya Y., Kojima Y., et al. Pathophysiological appraisal of a rat model of total hepatic ischemia with an extracorporeal portosystemic shunt. *Journal of Surgical Research* 1998;80(1) 22–27.

[32] Hasselgren P., Jennische E., Fornander J., Hellman A. No beneficial affect of ATP-MgCl2 on impaired transmembrane potential and protein synthesis in liver ischemia. *Acta Chirurgica Scandinavica* 1982;148(7) 601–607.

[33] Casillas-Ramírez A., Amine-Zaouali M., Massip-Salcedo M., Padrissa-Altés S., Bintanel-Morcillo M., Ramalho F., et al. Inhibition of angiotensin II action protects rat steatotic livers against ischemia-reperfusion injury. *Critical Care Medicine* 2008;36(4) 1256-1266.

[34] Peralta C., Bartrons R., Riera L., Manzano A., Xaus C., Gelpí E., Roselló-Catafau J. Hepatic preconditioning preserves energy metabolism during sustained ischemia.

American Journal of Physiology -Gastrointestinal and Liver Physiology 2000(279)1 G163–G171.

[35] Palmes D., Spiegel H. Animal models of liver regeneration. *Biomaterials* 2004;25 1601-1611.

[36] Ramalho F., Alfany-Fernandez I., Casillas-Ramírez A., Massip-Salcedo M., Serafín A., Rimola A., et al. Are angiotensin II receptor antagonists useful strategies in steatotic and nonsteatotic livers in conditions of partial hepatectomy under ischemia-reperfusion?. *Journal of Pharmacology and Experimental Therapeutics* 2009;329(1) 130-140.

[37] Czaja MJ. Liver regeneration following hepatic injury. London: Chapman and Hall; 1998.

[38] Spiegel H. Palmes D. Surgical techniques of orthotopic rat liver transplantation. *Journal of Investigative Surgery* 1998;11(2) 83-96.

[39] Cannon J. Organs. *Transplantation Bulletin* 1956;3 7. En: Cordier G., Garnier H., Clot J., Camplez P., Gorin J., Clot P. Orthotopic liver graft in pigs. 1st results. *Mémories de l'Académie Nationale de Chirurgie* 1966;92(27) 799-807.

[40] Garnier H., Clot J., Bertrand M., Camplez P., Kunlin A., Gorin J., et al. Liver transplantation in the pig: surgical approach. *CR Hebd Seances Academic Science* 1965;260(21) 5621-5623.

[41] Hori T., Nguyen J., Zhao X., Ogura T., Hata T., Yagi S., et al. Comprehensive and innovative techniques for liver transplantation in rats: A surgical guide. *World Journal of Gastroenterology* 2010;16 (25) 3120-3132.

[42] Aller M., Mendez M., Nava M., Lopez L., Arias J., Arias J. The value of microsurgery in liver research. *Liver International* 2009;29(8) 1132-1140.

[43] Lee S., Charters A., Chandler J., Orloff M. A technique for orthotopic liver transplantation in the rat. *Transplantation* 1973;16(6) 664-669.

[44] Lee S., Charters A., Orloff M. Simplified technic for orthotopic liver transplantation in the rat. *American Journal of Surgery* 1975;130(1) 38-40.

[45] Zimmermann F., Butcher G., Davies H., Brons G., Kamada N., Turel 0. Techniques for orthotopic liver transplantation in the rat and some studies of the immunologic responses to fully allogeneic liver grafts. *Transplantation Proceedings* 1979;11 571-577.

[46] Kamada N.. Calne R. Orthotopic liver transplantation in the rat. Technique using cuff for portal vein anastomosis and biliary drainage. *Transplantation* 1979;28(1) 47-50.

[47] Miyata M., Fischer J., Fuhs M., lsselhard W., Kasai Y. A simple method for orthotopic liver trasplantation in the rat. Cuff technique for three vascular anastomoses. *Transplantation* 1980;30 335-338.

[48] Engemann R., Ulrichs K., Thiede A., Muller-Ruchholtz W., Hamelmann H. Value of a physiological liver transplant model in rats. Induction of specific graft tolerance in a fully allogeneic strain combination. *Transplantation* 1982;33 566-568.

[49] Kitakado Y., Tanaka K., Asonuma K., Uemoto S., Matsuoka S. A new bioabsorbable material for rat vascular cuff anastomosis: Establishment for the long-term orthotopic liver transplantation model. *Archives Ipn Chirurgie* 1992;61 445-453.

[50] Ma Y., Wang G., Guo Z., Guo Z., He X., Chen C. Surgical techniques of arterialized orthotopic liver transplantation in rats. *Chinese Medical Journal* 2007;120(21) 1914-1917.

[51] Urakami H., Abe Y., Grisham M. Role of reactive metabolites of oxygen and nitrogen in partial liver transplantation: lessons learned from reduced-size liver ischemia and reperfusion injury. *Clinical and Experimental Pharmacology and Physiology* 2007;34(9) 912-919.

[52] Bismuth H., Houssin D. Reduced-sized orthotopic liver graft in hepatic transplantation in children. *Surgery* 1984;95(3) 367–370.

[53] Couinaud L. Le foie; études Anatomiques et Chirurgicales. France:Masson; 1957

[54] Gong N., Chen X. Partial liver transplantation. *Frontier Medical* 2011;5(1) 1-7.

[55] Broelsch C., Emond J., Whitington P., Thistlethwaite J., Baker A., Lichtor J. Application of reduced-size liver transplants as split grafts, auxiliary orthotopic grafts, and living related segmental transplants. *Annals of Surgery* 1990;212(3) 368-375.

[56] Lo C., Fan S., Liu C., Lo R., Lau G., Wei W., et al. Extending the limit on the size of adult recipient in living donor liver transplantation using extended right lobe graft. *Transplantation* 1997;63(10) 1524-1528.

[57] Vogel T., Brockmann J., Friend P. Ex-vivo normothermic liver perfusion: an update. *Current Opinion in Organ Transplantation* 2010;15(2) 167-172.

[58] Rougemont O., Lehmann K., Clavien P. Preconditioning, organ preservation, and postconditioning to prevent ischemia-reperfusion injury to the liver. *Liver Transplantation* 2009;15(10) 1172-1182.

[59] Minor T., Saad S., Nagelschmidt M., Kotting M., Fu Z., Paul A., et al. Successful transplantation of porcine livers after warm ischemic insult in situ and cold preservation including postconditioning with gaseous oxygen. *Transplantation* 1998;65(9): 1262-1264.

[60] Minor T., Stegemann J., Hirner A., Koetting M. Impaired autophagic clearance after cold preservation of fatty livers correlates with tissue necrosis upon reperfusion and is reversed by hypothermic reconditioning. *Liver Transplantation* 2009;15(7) 798-805.

[61] Gurusamy K., Gonzalez H., Davidson B. Current protective strategies in liver surgery. *World Journal of Gastroenterology* 2010;16(48) 6098-6103.

[62] Monbaliu D., Brassil J. Machine perfusion of the liver: past, present and future. *Current Opinion in Organ Transplantation* 2010;15 160-166.

[63] Carrel A. The culture of whole organs. *Science* 1935;14 621–623.

[64] Starzl T., Groth C., Brettschneider L., Moon J., Fulginiti V., Cotton E., Porter K. Extended survival in 3 cases of orthotopic homotransplantation of the human liver. *Surgery* 1968;63 549–563.

[65] Schön M., Kollmar O., Wolf S., Schrem H., Matthes M., Akkoc N., et al. Liver transplantation after organ preservation with normothermic extracorporal perfusion. *Annals of Surgery* 2001;2338(1) 114–123.

[66] Fondevila C., Hessheimer A., Ruiz A., Calatayud D., Ferrer J., Charco R., et al. Liver transplant using donors after unexpected cardiac death: novel preservation protocol and acceptance criteria. *American Journal of Transplantion* 2007;7(7) 1849-1855.

[67] García-Valdecasas J., Fondevila C. In-vivo normothermic recirculation: an update. *Current Opinion in Organ Transplantation* 2010;15(2) 173-176.

[68] Pienaar B., Lindell S., Van Gulik T., Southard J., Belzer F. Seventy-two-hour preservation of the canine liver by machine perfusion. *Transplantation* 1990;49(2) 258–260.

[69] Bessems M., Doorschodt B., van Marle J., Vreeling H., Meijer A., van Gulik T. Improved machine perfusion preservation of the non-heart-beating donor rat liver using Polysol: a new machine perfusion preservation solution. *Liver Transplantation* 2005;11 1379–1388.

[70] Vekemans K., Liu Q., Brassil J., Komuta M., Pirenne J., Monbaliu D. Influence of flow and addition of oxygen during porcine liver hypothermic machine perfusion. *Transplantation Proceedings* 2007;39(8) 2647-2651.

[71] Vairetti M., Ferrigno A., Carlucci F., Tabucchi A., Rizzo V., Boncompagni E., et al. Subnormothermic machine perfusion protects steatotic livers against preservation injury: a potential for donor pool increase?. *Liver Transplantation* 2009;15(1) 20–29.

[72] Fernández L., Heredia N., Grande L., Gómez G., Rimola A., Marco A., et al. Preconditioning protects liver and lung damage in rat liver transplantation: role of xanthine/xanthine oxidase. *Hepatology* 2002;36(3) 562–572.

[73] Metzger J., Dore S. Lauterburg B. Oxidant stress during reperfusion of ischemic liver: no evidence for a role of xanthine oxidase. *Hepatology* 1998;8(3) 580–584.

[74] Rai R., Yang S., McClain C., Karp C., Klein A., Diehl A. Kupffer cell depletion by gadolinium chloride enhances liver regeneration after partial hepatectomy in rats. *American Journal of Physiology* 1996;270 G909–G918.

[75] Watanabe M., Chijiiwa K., Kameoka N., Yamaguchi K., Kuroki S., Tanaka M. Gadolinium pretreatment decreases survival and impairs liver regeneration after partial hepatectomy under ischemia/reperfusion in rats. *Surgery* 2000;127 456–463.

[76] Hayashi H., Chaudry I., Clemens M., Baue A. Hepatic ischemia models for determining the effects of ATP-$MgCl_2$ treatment. *Journal of Surgical Research* 1986;40(2) 167–175.

[77] Chaudry I., Clemens M., Ohkawa M., Schleck S., Baue A. Restoration of hepatocellular function and blood flow following hepatic ischemia with ATP–$MgCl_2$. *Advances in Shock Research* 1982;8 177–186.

[78] Zaouali M., Padrissa-Altés S., Ben Mosbah I., Alfany-Fernandez I., Massip-Salcedo M., Casillas Ramirez A., et al. Improved rat steatotic and nonsteatotic liver preservation by the addition of epidermal growth factor and insulin-like growth factor-I to University of Wisconsin solution. *Liver Transplantation* 2010;16(9) 1098-111.

[79] Casillas-Ramírez A., Zaouali A., Padrissa-Altés S., Ben Mosbah I., Pertosa A., Alfany-Fernández I., et al. Insulin-like growth factor and epidermal growth factor treatment: new approaches to protecting steatotic livers against ischemia-reperfusion injury. *Endocrinology* 2009;150(7):3153-3161.

[80] Man K., Zhao Y., Xu A., Lo C., Lam K., Ng K., et al. Fat-derived hormone adiponectin combined with FTY720 significantly improves small-for-size fatty liver graft survival. *American Journal of Transplantation* 2006;6(3) 467-476.

[81] Casillas-Ramírez A., Alfany-Fernández I., Massip-Salcedo M., Juan M., Planas J., Serafin A., et al. Retinol-Binding protein 4 and peroxisome proliferator-activated receptor-γ in steatotic liver transplantation. *Journal of Pharmacology and Experimental Therapeutics* 2011;338(1) 143-153.

[82] Elias-Miró M., Massip-Salcedo M., Raila J., Schweigert F., Mendes-Braz M., Ramalho F, et al. Retinol binding protein 4 and retinol in rat steatotic and non-steatotic livers in partial hepatectomy under ischemia-reperfusion. *Liver Transplantation* 2012; doi: 10.1002/lt.23489.

[83] Gonzalez-Flecha B., Cutrin J., Boveris A. Time course and mechanism of oxidative stress and tissue damage in rat liver subjected to in vivo ischemia-reperfusion. *Journal of Clinical Investigation* 1993;91(2) 456-464.

[84] Okaya T., Lentsh A. Peroxisome proliferator-activated receptor-alpha regulates postischemic liver injury. *American Journal of Physiology - Gastrointestinal and Liver Physiology* 1994;286 G606-G612.

[85] Stadler M., Nuyens V., Seidel L., Albert A., Boogaerts J. Effect of nutritional status on oxidative stress in an ex vivo perfused rat liver. *Anesthesiology* 2005;103(5) 978–986.

[86] Caraceni P., Domenicali M., Vendemiale G., Grattagliano I., Pertosa A., Nardo B., et al. The reduced tolerance of rat fatty liver to ischemia reperfusion is associated with mitochondrial oxidative injury. *Journal of Surgical Research* 2005;124(2) 160–168.

[87] Sankary H., Chong A., Foster P., Brown E., Shen J., Kimura R. et al. Inactivation of Kupffer cells after prolonged donor fasting improves viability of transplanted hepatic allografts. *Hepatology* 1995;22(4) 1236–1242.

[88] Okaya T., Blanchard J., Schuster R., Kuboki S., Husted T., Caldwell C., et al. Age-dependent responses to hepatic ischemia/reperfusion injury. *Shock* 2005;24(5) 421–427.

[89] Ben Mosbah I., Alfany-Fernández I., Martel C., Zaouali M., Bintanel-Morcillo M., Rimola A., et al. Endoplasmic reticulum stress inhibition protects steatotic and non-steatotic livers in partial hepatectomy under ischemia-reperfusion. *Cell Death and Disease* 2010;1 e52(1-12).

[90] Serafin A., Rosello-Catafau J., Prats N., Gelpi E., Rodes J., Peralta C. Ischemic preconditioning affects interleukin release in fatty livers of rats undergoing ischemia/reperfusion. *Hepatology* 2004;39(3) 688–698.

[91] Peralta C., Leon O., Xaus C., Prats N., Jalil E., Planell E., et al. Protective effect of ozone treatment on the injury associated with hepatic ischemia-reperfusion: antioxidant-prooxidant balance. *Free Radical Research* 1999;31(3) 191–196.

[92] Teoh N., Leclercq I., Pena A., Farell G. Low-dose TNF-alpha protects against hepatic ischemia-reperfusion injury in mice: implications for preconditioning. *Hepatology* 2003;37(1) 118–128.

[93] Tian Y., Jochum W., Georgiev P., Moritz W., Graf R., Clavien P. Kupffer cell-dependent TNF-alpha signaling mediates injury in the arterialized small-for-size liver transplantation in the mouse. *Proceedings of the National Academy of Sciences* 2006;103 4598-4603.

[94] Bradham C., Schemmer P., Stachlewitz R., Thurman R., Brenner D. Activation of nuclear factor-kappaB during orthotopic liver transplantation in rats is protective and does not require Kupffer cells. Liver *Transplantation and Surgery* 1999;5(4) 282–293.

[95] Casillas-Ramírez A., Ben Mosbah I., Ramalho F., Rosello-Catafau J., Peralta C. Past and future approaches to ischemia-reperfusion lesion associated with liver transplantation. *Life Science* 2006;79 1881–1894.

[96] Bahde R., Spiegel H. Hepatic ischaemia-reperfusion injury from bench to bedside. *British Journal of Surgery* 2010;97(10) 1461-1475.

[97] Zúñiga J., Cancino M., Medina F., Varela P., Vargas R., Tapia G., et al. N-3 PUFA supplementation triggers PPAR-α activation and PPAR-α/NF-κB interaction: anti-inflammatory implications in liver ischemia-reperfusion injury. *PLoS One* 2011;6(12) e28502.

[98] Ghonem N., Yoshida J., Stolz D., Humar A., Starzl T., Murase N., Venkataramanan R. Treprostinil, a prostacyclin analog, ameliorates ischemia-reperfusion injury in rat orthotopic liver transplantation. *American Journal of Transplantation* 2011;11(11) 2508-2516.

[99] Kamo N., Shen X., Ke B., Busuttil R., Kupiec-Weglinski J. Sotrastaurin, a protein kinase C inhibitor, ameliorates ischemia and reperfusion injury in rat orthotopic liver transplantation. *American Journal of Transplantation* 2011;11(11) 2499-2507.

[100] Stoffels B., Yonezawa K., Yamamoto Y., Schäfer N., Overhaus M., Klinge U., et al. Meloxicam a COX-2 inhibitor, ameliorates ischemia/reperfusión injury in non-heart-beating donor livers. *European Surgical Research* 2011;47(3) 109-117.

[101] Li W., Meng Z., Liu Y., Patel R., Lang J. The hepatoprotective effect of sodium nitrite on cold ischemia-reperfusion injury. *Journal of Transplantation* 2012; 635179.

[102] Eipel C., Hübschmann U., Abshagen K., Wagner K., Menger M., Vollmar B. Erythropoietin as additive of HTK preservation solution in cold ischemia/reperfusion injury of steatotic livers. *Journal of Surgical Research* 2012;173(1) 171-179.

[103] Bezinover D., Ramamoorthy S., Uemura T., Kadry Z., McQuillan P., Mets B., et al. Use of a third-generation perfluorocarbon for preservation of rat DCD liver grafts. *Journal of Surgical Research* 2011; 1-7.

[104] Minor T., Kötting M. Gaseous oxygen for hypothermic preservation of predamaged liver grafts: fuel to cellular homeostasis or radical tissue alteration?. *Cryobiology* 2000;40 182-186.

[105] Reynaert H., Geerts A., Henrion J. Review article: the treatment of non-alcoholic steatohepatitis with thiazolidinediones. *Alimentary Pharmacology and Therapeutics* 2005;22(10) 897-905.

[106] Schmidt R. Hepatic organ protection: from basic science to clinical practice. *World Journal of Gastroenterology* 2010;16(48) 6044-6045.

[107] Ke B., Lipshutz G., Kupiec-Weglinski J. Gene therapy in liver ischemia and reperfusion injury. *Current Pharmacology* 2006;12 2969-2975.

[108] Mizuguchi H., Hayakawa T. Targeted adenovirus vectors. *Human Gene Therapy* 2004;15(11) 1034-1044.

[109] Drazan K., Csete M., Da Shen X., Bullington D., Cottle G., Busuttil R., Shaked A. Hepatic function is preserved following liver-directed, adenovirus-mediated gene transfer. *Journal of Surgical Research* 1995;59(2) 299-304.

[110] Kroemer G. The proto-oncogene Bcl-2 and its role in regulating apoptosis. *Nature Medicine* 1997;3: 614-20.

[111] Bilbao G., Contreras J., Eckhoff D., Mikheeva G., Krasnykh V., Douglas J., et al. Reduction of ischemia-reperfusion injury of the liver by in vivo adenovirus-mediated gene transfer of the antiapoptotic Bcl-2 gene. *Annals of Surgery* 1999;230 185-93.

[112] Takayama S., Sato T., Krajewski S., Kochel K., Irie S., Millan J., et al. Cloning and functional analysis of BAG-1: a novel Bcl-2-bonding protein with anti-cell death activity. *Cell* 1995;80 279-84.

[113] Sawitzki B., Amersi F., Ritter T., Fisser M., Shen X., Ke B., et al. Upregulation of Bag-1 by ex vivo gene transfer protects rat livers from ischemia/reperfusion injury. *Human Gene Therapy* 2002:13 1495-504.

[114] Contreras J., Vilatoba M., Eckstein C., Bilbao G., Anthony J., Eckhoff D. Caspase-8 and caspase-3 small interfering RNA decreases ischemia/reperfusion injury to the liver in mice. *Surgery* 2004;136(2) 390-400.

[115] Palmer H., Paulson K. Reactive oxygen species and antioxidants in signal transduction and gene expression. *Nutrition Reviews* 1997;55 353-361.

[116] Zwacka R., Zhang Y., Zhou W., Halldorson J., Engelhardt J. Ischemia/reperfusion injury in the liver of BALB/c mice activates AP-1 and nuclear factor kappaB independently of IkappaB degradation. *Hepatology* 1998;28 1022-30.

[117] Baeuerle P., Henkel T. Function and activation of NF-kappa B in the immune system. *Annual Review of Immunology* 1994;12 141-79.

[118] Okaya T., Lentsch A. Hepatic expression of S32A/S36A Ikappa B alpha does not reduce postischemic liver injury. *Journal of Surgical Research* 2005;124(2) 244-249.

[119] Zwacka R., Zhou W., Zhang Y., Darby C., Dudus L., Halldorson J., et al. Redox gene therapy for ischemia/reperfusion injury of the liver redices AP1 and NF-κB activation. *Nature Medicine* 1998;4 698-704.

[120] Wheeler M., Katuna M., Smutney O., Froh M., Dikalova A., Mason R., et al. Comparison of the effect of adenoviral delivery of three superoxide dismutase genes against hepatic ischemia-reperfusion injury. *Human Gene Therapy* 2001;12 2167-2177.

[121] He S., Zhang Y., Venugopal S., Dicus C., Perez R., Ramsamooi R., et al. Delivery of antioxidative enzyme genes protects against ischemia7reperfusion-induced liver injury in mice. *Liver Transplantation* 2006;12(21) 1869-1879.

[122] Takahashi Y., Ganster R., Ishikawa T., Okuda T., Gambotto A., Shao L., et al. Protective role of NF-kappaB in liver cold ischemia/reperfusion injury: effects of IkappaB gene therapy. *Transplantation Proccedings* 2001;33(1) 602.

[123] Amersi F., Buelow R., Kato H., Ke B., Coito A., Shen X., et al. Upregulation of heme oxygenase-1 protects genetically fat Zucker rat livers from ischemia/reperfusion injury. *Journal of Clininical Investigation* 1999;104(11) 1631-1639.

[124] Tsuchihashi S., Fondevila C., Kupiec-Weglinski J. Heme oxygenase system in ischemia and reperfusion injury. *Ann Transplant* 2004;9(1) 84-87.

[125] Halliwell B., Gutteridge J. Biologically relevant metal ion-dependent hydroxyl radical generation. An update. *FEBS Letter* 1992;307(1) 108-112.

[126] Berberat P., Katori M., Kaczmarek E., Anselmo D., Lassman C., Ke B., et al. Heavy chain ferritin acts as an antiapoptotic gene that protects livers from ischemia reperfusion injury. *FASEB Journal* 2003;17 1724-1726.

[127] Kato A., Yoshidome H., Edwards M., Lentsch A. Regulation of liver inflammatory injury by signal transducer and activator of transcription-6. *American Journal of Pathology* 2000;157 297-302.

[128] Lee T., Chau L. Heme oxygenase-1 mediates the anti-inflammatory effect of interleukin-10 in mice. *Nature Medicine* 2002;8 240-246.

[129] Ke B., Shen X., Lassman C., Gao F., Busuttil R., Kupiec-Weglinski J. Cytoprotective and antiapoptotic effects of IL-13 in hepatic cold ischemia/reperfusion injury are heme oxygenase-1 dependent. *American Journal of Transplantation* 2003;3 1076-1082.

[130] Ke B., Shen X., Gao F., Busuttil R., Kupiec-Weglinski J. Interleukin 13 gene transfer in liver ischemia and reperfusion injury: role of Stat6 and TLR4 pathways in cytoprotection. *Human Gene Therapy* 2004;15 691-698.

[131] Harada H., Wakabayashi G., Takayanagi A., Shimazu M., Matsumoto K., Obara H., et al. Transfer of the interleukin-1 receptor antagonist gene into rat liver abrogates hepatic ischemia-reperfusion injury. *Transplantation* 2002;74 1434-1441.

[132] Ke B., Shen X., Gao F., Busuttil R., Lowenstein P., Castro M., et al. Gene therapy for liver transplantation using adenoviral vectors: CD40-CD154 blockade by gene transfer of CD40Ig protects rat livers from cold ischemia and reperfusion injury. *Molecular Therapy* 2004;9 38-45.

[133] Shen X., Ke B., Zhai Y., Amersi F., Gao F., Anselmo D., et al. CD154-CD40 T cell costimulation pathway is required in themechanism of hepatic ischemia/reperfusion injury, and its blockade facilitates and dependents on heme oxgenase-1 mediated cytoprotection. *Transplantation* 2002;74 315-319.

[134] Shi Y., Rehman H., Ramshesh V., Schwartz J., Liu Q., Krishnasamy Y., et al. Sphingosine kinase-2 inhibition improves mitochondrial function and survival after hepatic ischemia-reperfusion. *Journal of Hepatology* 2012;56(1) 137-145.

[135] Jiang N., Zhang X., Zheng X., Chen D., Zhang Y., Siu L., et al. Targeted gene silencing of TLR4 using liposomal nanoparticles for preventing liver ischemia reperfusion injury. *American Journal of Transplantation* 2011;11(9) 1835-1844.

[136] Somia N., Verma I. Gene therapy: trials and tribulations. *Nature Reviews: Genetics* 2000;1(2) 91–99.

[137] Weber A., Groyer-Picard M., Franco D., Dagher I. Hepatocyte transplantation in animal models. *Liver Transplantation* 2009;15 7-14.

[138] Joseph B., Malhi H., Bhargava K., Palestro C., McCuskey R., Gupta S. Kupffer cells participate in early clearance of syngeneic hepatocytes transplanted in the rat liver. *Gastroenterology* 2002;123 1677-1685.

[139] Allen K., Soriano H. Liver cell transplantation: the road to clinical application. *Journal of Laboratory and Clinical Medicine* 2001;138 298-312.

[140] Benten D., Kumaran V., Joseph B., Schattenberg J., Popov Y., Schuppan D., et al. Hepatocyte transplantation activates hepatic stellate cells with beneficial modulation of cell engraftment in the rat. *Hepatology* 2005;42 1072-1081.

[141] Soriano H. Liver cell transplantation: human applications in adults and children. London: Kluwer Academic Publishers; 2002.

[142] Strom S., Fisher R., Thompson M., Sanyal A., Cole P., Ham J., et al. Hepatocyte transplantation as a bridge to orthotopic liver transplantation in terminal liver failure. *Transplantation* 1997;63(4) 559–569.

[143] Bilir B., Guinette D., Karrer F., Kumpe D., Krysl J., Stephens J., et al. Hepatocyte transplantation in acute liver failure. *Liver Transplantation* 2000;6(1) 32–40.

[144] Clavien P., Selzner M., Rudiger H., Graft R., Kadry Z., Rousson V., et al. A prospective randomized study in 100 consecutive patients undergoing major liver resection with versus without ischemic preconditioning. *Annals of surgery* 2003;238(6) 843–850.

[145] Azoulay D., Del Gaudio M., Andreani P., Ichai P., Sebag M., Adam R., et al. Effects of 10 minutes of ischemic preconditioning of the cadaveric liver on the graft's preservation and function: the ying and the yang. *Annals of Surgery* 2005;242(1) 133–139.

[146] Amador A., Grande L., Martí J., Deulofeu R., Miquel R., Solá A., et al. Ischemic preconditioning in deceased donor liver transplantation: a prospective randomized clinical trial. *American Journal of Transplantation* 2007;7(9) 2180-2189.

Chapter 7

The Aim of Technology During Liver Resection — A Strategy to Minimize Blood Loss During Liver Surgery

Fabrizio Romano, Mattia Garancini, Fabio Uggeri, Luca Gianotti, Luca Nespoli, Angelo Nespoli and Franco Uggeri

Additional information is available at the end of the chapter

http://dx.doi.org/10.5772/54301

1. Introduction

Liver resection is considered the treatment of choice for liver tumours. Despite standardized techniques and technological advancing for liver resections, an intra-operative haemorrhage rate ranging from 700 and 1200 ml is reported with a post-operative morbidity rate ranging from 23 and 46% and a surgical death rate ranging from 4 and 5% [l],[2],[3],[4],[5],[6].

The parameter "**Blood loss**" has a central role in liver surgery and different strategies to minimize it are a key to improve these results. Bleeding has to be considered a major concern for the hepatic surgeon because of several reasons. At first it is certainly the major intra-operative surgical complication and cause of death and historically one of the major postoperative complication together with bile leaks and hepatic failure [5],[6],[7],[8],[9].

Besides a high intra-operative blood loss is associated with higher rate of post-operative complication and shorter long-term survival [10],[ll],[l2],[l3]. Furthermore it is associated with an extensive use of vessel occlusion techniques, directly correlated with higher risk of post-operative hepatic failure. Last, a higher value of intra-operative blood loss is associated with a higher rate of peri-operative transfusions; host immunosuppression associated with transfusions with a dose-related relationship is correlated with a higher rate of complication (in particular infections) and recurrence of malignancies in neoplastic patients [11],[l2],[l4],[l5],[l6],[17],[18],[19],[20],[21]. In order to reduce transfusions hepatic surgeon has also not to misinterpret post-operative fluctuations of blood parameter: Torzilli at al. demonstrated that haemoglobin rate and haematocrit after liver resection show a steady and significant decrease until the third post-operative day and then an increase; so this situation has to be explained as physiological and does not justifies blood administration [22].Although the mechanism of bleeding in surgical interventions is multifactorial, technical factors may be responsible for a significant amount of intraoperative and early postoperative bleeding. The main progress in reducing perioperative blood loss has been made through improved surgical and anesthetic techniques and through better understanding of hemostatic disorders in patients who have liver disease. developments in surgical, anesthesiologic, and pharmacologic strategies that have contributed to a reduction of blood loss during liver surgery in cirrhotic and noncirrhotic patients. The clinical relevance of different types of strategies may vary, depending on the stage of the operation. For example, topical hemostatic agents have a role in reducing blood loss from the hepatic resection surface after partial liver resection, whereas surgical techniques play a more important role during transection of the liver parenchyma (Fig. 1).

2. How can we reduce bleeding in liver surgery?

Figure 1 shows the amount of blood loss during the different phases of liver surgery. It is clear that the higher risk for bleeding and the greater amount of blood loss occur during the parenchymal transection phase of the procedure.

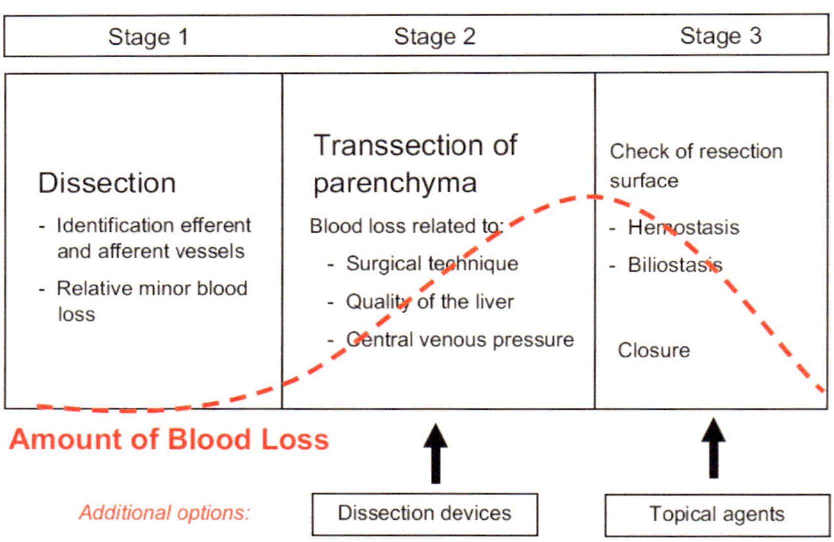

Figure 1. The mechanisms of bleeding and the relative amount of blood loss (dotted line) during the three surgical stages of partial liver resections. In general, most bleeding can be encountered during transsection of the liver parenchyma. In this stage of the operation, blood loss is mainly caused by bleeding from the resection surface of the liver.

The aim of the study is to investigate the principal solutions to the problem of high blood loss in hepatic resection, considering the role of surgeons and anestesiologists. Table 1 resume all the methods to prevent or reduce bleeding during liver surgery. Moreover we focused our attention on the technological aspects of liver parenchima transection. We will describe each technology and instrument discussing the principle of functioning, the technical characteristics and analysed the advantages (**A**) and the disadvantages (**D**) correlated to their employment during liver transection. We divided the instruments taking into account the energy employed for their functioning.

Surgical
Vascular clamping techniques
Inflow occlusion
Continuous Pringle maneuver
Continuous Pringle maneuver after ischemic preconditioning
Intermittent Pringle maneuver
Total vascular occlusion
Dissection devices for transsection of liver parenchyma
Classic methods
Scalpel
"Finger-fracture" method
Clamp crushing
Ultrasonic dissection
Hydro-jet dissection
Electro coagulation (monopolar, bipolar,Argon coagulation)
Radiofrequency ablation-based devices
Staplers
Topic hemostatic agents
Anesthesiologic
Maintaining low central venous pressure by using
Volume contraction
Phlebotomy
Vasodilatation
If needed, forced diuresis
Blood products
Use of pharmacologic agents
Antifibrinolytics
Recombinant factor VIIa

Table 1. Surgical and anesthesiologic methods used to reduce blood loss in liver surgery

Moreover we tried to compare the different instruments and technologies basing on literature data to identify the best instruments for each type of liver resection (open surgery, laparoscopic surgery, resective surgery, oncologic surgery, liver transplantation).

3. The role of the surgeon

Most blood loss during liver resection occurs during parenchymal transection. Hepatic surgeon has different ways to control bleeding:

Vessel occlusion techniques: Those technique are based on the idea that to limit the blood flow through the liver during parenchymal transection can reduce the haemorrhage. Although various forms and modified techniques of vascular control have been practiced, there are basically two main strategies; inflow vascular occlusion and total vascular exclusion23-24 Inflow vascular occlusions are techniques that limit anterograde blood flow with the clamping of all the triad of the hepato-duodenal ligament (*Pringle 's manoeuvre, PM*), only of the vascular pedicles (selective clamping of the portal vein and the hepatic artery or *Bismuth technique*) or *intravascularportal clamping*. During Pringle's manouvre the hepatoduodenal ligament is encircled with a tape, and then a vascular clamp or tourniquet is applied until the pulse in the hepatic artery disappears distally. The PM has relatively little general haemodynamic effect and no specific anaesthetic management is required. However, bleeding can still occur from the backflow from the hepatic veins and from the liver transection plane during unclamping. The other concern is the ischaemic-reperfusion injury to the liver parenchyma, especially in patients with underlying liver diseases25. The continuous Pringle manoeuvre (CPM) can be safely applied to the normal liver under normothermic conditions for up to 60 minutes and up to 30 minutes in pathological (fatty or cirrhotic) livers, although much longer durations of continuous clamping 127 minutes in normal livers and 100 minutes in pathological livers have been reported to be safe26-27. One way to extend the duration of clamping and to reduce ischaemia to the remnant liver is by the intermittent Pringle manoeuvre (IPM). It involves periods of inflow clamping that last for 15-20 minutes followed by periods of unclamping for five minutes (mode 15/5 or 20/5), or five minutes clamping followed by one minute unclamping (mode 5/1)28-29 IPM permits a doubling of the ischaemia time, when compared with CPM and the total clamping time can be extended to 120 minutes in normal livers and 60 minutes in pathological livers. The disadvantage of IPM is that bleeding occurs from the liver transaction surface during the unclamping period and, thus, the overall transection time is prolonged as more time is spent in achieving haemostasis. Belghiti et al (1999) revealed that there was no significant difference in total blood loss or volume of blood transfusion between CPM and IPM (mode 15/5). However, they noticed that pathological livers tolerated CPM poorly.

A newer perspective on inflow occlusion comes from the concept of ischaemic preconditioning (IP). It refers to an endogenous self-protective mechanism by which a short period of ischaemia followed by a brief period of reperfusion produces a state of protection against subsequent sustained ischaemia-reperfusion injury [30]-[31]. The IP is performed with ten minutes of ischaemia followed by ten minutes of reperfusion before liver transaction with CPM [32].

Hemihepatic clamping (half-Pringle manoeuvre) interrupts the arterial and portal inflow selectively to the right or left liver lobe that is to be resected [33]-[34]. It can be performed with or without prior hilar dissection. It can also be combined with simultaneous occlusion of the ipsilateral major hepatic vein. The advantage of this technique is that it avoids ischaemia in the remnant liver, avoids visceral congestion and allows clear demarcation of the resection margin. The disadvantage is that bleeding from the parenchymal cut surface can occur from the nonoccluded liver lobe.

Segmental vascular clamping entails the occlusion of the ipsilateral hepatic artery branch and balloon occlusion of the portal branch of a particular segment. The portal branch is identified by intra-operative ultrasound and puncture with a cholangiography needle through which a guide wire and balloon catheter is passed [35],[36].

Total vascular exclusion (TVE) combines total inflow and outflow vascular occlusion of the liver, isolating it completely from the systemic circulation. It is done with complete mobilisation of the liver, encircling of the suprahepatic and infrahepatic IVC, application of the Pringle manoeuvre, and then clamping the infrahepatic IVC followed by clamping of the suprahepatic IVC. TVE is associated with significant haemodynamic changes and warrants close invasive and anaesthetic monitoring. Occlusion of the IVC leads to marked reduction of venous return and cardiac output, with a compensatory 80% increase in systemic vascular resistance and 50% increase in heart rate and, thus, not every patient can tolerate it. TVE can be applied to a normal liver for up to 60 minutes and for 30 minutes in a diseased liver. The ischaemic time can be extended when combined with hypothermic perfusion of the liver [37]-[38]. Apart from the unpredictable haemodynamic intolerance, post-operative abdominal collections or abscesses and pulmonary complications are more common in TVE, when compared with CPM.

Inflow occlusion with extraparenchymal control of hepatic veins is a modified way of performing TVE. The main and any accessory right hepatic vein, the common trunk of the middle and left hepatic veins, or the separate trunks of the middle and left hepatic veins (15% of cases) are first dissected free and looped. It has been reported that the trunks of the major hepatic veins can be safely looped in 90% of patients [39]-[40]. The loops can then be tightened or the vessels clamped after inflow occlusion is applied, so that the liver lobe is isolated from the systemic circulation without interrupting the caval flow. It can be applied in a continuous or intermittent manner. The maximal ischaemia time is up to 58 minutes under continuous occlusion. This technique is more demanding than TVE, but it can avoid the haemodynamic drawbacks of TVE while at the same time provide almost a bloodless field for liver transection.

Instruments and technique for resections: Although a large part of improvements of these last decades in liver surgery can be correlated to a better knowledge of the surgical hepatic anatomy (Couinaud's segmentation of liver [41]), better monitoring during anaesthesia and introduction of intra-operative ultrasonography and of other imaging techniques, the choice of surgical technique for sectioning the liver has surely important repercussions on the intervention's outcome. Furthermore in the last two decades improvements in technology allowed the development of a large number of instruments with the aim to reduce blood loss during surgical procedure. The main part of these tools have been developed or applied to liver surgery. The rationale in liver transection is to employ an instrument that can selectively eliminate parenchyma leaving vital structures intact. In other words, a resistance modulated device, able to fragment low-resistance tissue (hepatic parenchyma) preserving fibrous (high-resistance) components such as vessels and biliary ducts, successively ligated by the surgeon. To date, no single instrument has been designed to adequately satisfy both of these tasks.

There are two techniques we could define traditional: the *finger fracture method* and the *clamp crushing method*. These are the oldest techniques for hepatic transection and are still employed especially by long experienced surgeons. Techniques of liver transection gained marked attention since the introduction of the clamp-crushing technique in the 1970s.10,11 As a refinement of the finger fracture method, it has served as the reference technique for liver transection ever since.

The use of traditional techniques to isolate bile ducts and vascular pedicles from the surrounding parenchyma provides for employment of clips or sutures for sealing bile ducts and vascular vessels and for other haemostasis techniques to stop haemorrhage from the resection's surface. There are several studies those sustain that traditional methods are still competitive with new technique based on utilization of special devices [1],[42],[96] In a recent Metanalysis Rahbari and coll concluded that the clamp-crushing technique could be still reccomended as the reference method for the transection of the parenchyma during liver surgery [12], [4].

Introduction of new devices for liver dissection surely have an important role, in particular for reduction of intra-operative blood loss. Actually the most important devices useful for liver resection are the followings, presented as they are from a technical point of view and analysed to find the advantages (A) and the disadvantages (D) correlated to their employment and divede according to the source of energy employed. There are two types of transection devices: those mainly used for dissection (e.g. the haemostatic clamps or ultrasonic dissector) and mainly used for haemostasis and coagulation (e.g. sutures, endo-staplers, sealers, etc.) (table 2). Moreover the water-jet, the ultrasonic aspirator (CUSA®) and the blunt dissection can be categorised under selective dissection techniques. Non-selective techniques cannot discriminate between duct structures and parenchyma. To mention are finger fracture and mechanical instruments as the scalpel, the scissors and with reservation the linear stapler as well as thermal instruments as the high-frequency electrocoagulator, the laser, the bipolar forceps or the scissors of the UltraCision®

Preparation	**Transection**
Finger fracture	ligation
crush/clamp	clips
suction knife	electrocoagulation (mono/bipolar)
CUSA	Microwave tissue coagulation
Water Jet	Ultracision
Jet-Cutter	Ligasure
Tissuelink	Gyrus
Aquamantys	

Table 2. Surgical techniques for preparation and tissue transection of the liver

Furthermore most attempts have involved use of radiofrequency ablation-based instruments in a "precoagulation strategy" in which the energy device is used to burn and seal the parenchyma before sharp dissection. In the second strategy, ultrasonic-activated instruments cut through the liver while sealing the vessels. Both method suffer from the fact that large vessels are poorly visualized and can bleed on transection. In addition, blood or biliary vessels from adiacent parts of the liver meant to be salvage can be inadvertently injured by this "blind" coagulation.

3.1. Tools based on ultrasound technology

Harmonic Scalpel, HS (Johnson and Johnson Medical, Ethicon, Cincinnati, USA): Also known as "Ultrasonically Activated Scalpel" or "Ultrasonic Coagulation Shears", this instrument was introduced in the early 1990s. The ultrasound scissors System includes a generator with a foot switch, the reusable handle for the scalpel and the cutting device with scissors. The scissors are composed by a moveable blade and by a fixed longitudinal blade that vibrates with a ultrasonic frequency of 55,5 kHz (55.500 vibrations per second). HS can simultaneously cut and coagulate causing protein denaturation by destroying the hydrogen bonds in proteins and by generation of heat in vibrating tissue. This generated heat denatures proteins and forms a sticky coagulum that covers the edges of dissection. Although the heat produces no smoke and thermal injury is limited, the depth of marginal necrosis is greater than incurred by either the water jet or CUSA The lateral spread of the energy is 500 micrometers.

A: HS is the only instrument that can simultaneously cut and coagulate (it can coagulate vessel until 2-3 mm of diameter [43]); it's useful on cirrhotic liver [44]; no electricity passes through the patient and there's no smoke production (especially useful in laparoscopic surgery); it can be used in laparoscopic and laparotomic surgery. **D**: The instrument results in a continuous bleeding risk related to the blind tissue penetration to coagulate vessels hidden into the hepatic parenchyma. Studies demonstrate that HS is not capable to reduce blood loss and operating time compared to traditional techniques [45]-[46], cannot coagulate vessel over 2-3 mm of diameter which have to be clipped, legated or sealed with other instruments; HS is not easy to use as a blunt dissector and have substantially demonstrated its usefulness only during the resection of the superficial part of liver (2, 3 cm) free from large vessels and bile ducts; besides some studies have demonstrated that HS increases the rate of post-operative bile leaks [47]-[48] raising concern that HS may not be effective in sealing bile ducts. this postoperative bile leakage occurred because Glisson's sheath was not completely sealed when the HA is used blindly in the deep liver parenchymal layer. It was difficult to seal the sheath precisely in the deep liver parenchymal layer.

The use of HS in liver cirrhosis is controversial. The greatest concern with the use of the harmonic scalpel is the risk of shearing [49]. Slight errors of movement can shear parenchyma without completely coagulating vessels and/or ducts. Moreover it's expensive (the generator costs US$ 20.000 and the handle US$ 250). An evolution fo the harmonic Scalpel is the Harmonic FOCUS. Using this device the liver parenchyma is crushed by the nonactivated HF, which blades are similar to Kelly forceps, and the tiny areas of residual tissue are checked and completely sealed with the activated HF without changing to forceps. This device allow, after accurate exposure, a sealing "under view" of tiny vasculatures and biliary structures and this seems to reduce bleeding and postoperative bile leakages. [125-126] This new technique has been called "fusion technique".The attempt to accomplish both the task of division and of hemostasis is provided by a recently introduced device, which intends to crush liver parenchyma simul taneously sealing the vessels without the need to change the instrument, the so called focus-clysis or 'fusion technique'

Functionally, the instrument should be compared to a Kelly, in which the surgeon can adjust the precision and depth of cutting by modulating blade pressure; parenchyma crushing exposes the tiny vessels that can be coagulated employing the harmonic technology provided in high power (1–2 mm vessels) and low power (up to 5 mm). Vessels larger than 5 mm in diameter should be divided and ligated in a traditional fashion. It seems that the 'fusion technique' could reduce blood loss and the incidence of biliary fistula, with a cost comparable to other technologies.

Cavitron Ultrasonic Surgical Aspirator, CUSA (Valleylab) (Fig 2): The use in liver surgery of this instrument, also known as Ultrasonic Dissector, was described for the first time in literature in 1979 by Hodgson [50]. CUSA is a surgical system in which a pencil-grip surgical hand piece contains a transducer that oscillates longitudinally at 23 kHz and to which a hollow conical titanium tip is attached. The vibrating tip of the instrument causes explosion of cells with a high water content (just like hepatocytes) and fragmentation of parenchyma sparing blood and bile vessel because of their walls prevalently composed by connective cells poor of water but rich of intracellular bonds. This device (together with hydrojet dissector) should be considered among that tools able to selectively divide parenchyma from vessels according to their different mechanical resistance (in which hepatocytes contain less fibrous tissue than the vessel, thus offering less resistance to crushing during parenchymal division), the so called selective dissection technique.

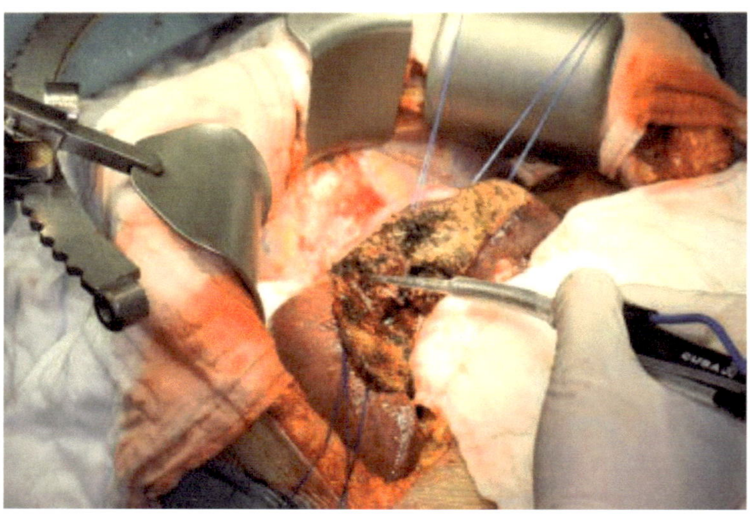

Figure 2. Parenchima transection using CUSA

The device is equipped by a saline solution irrigation system that cools the hand piece and wash the transection plane and by a constant suction system that removes fragmented bits of tissue and permits excellent visualization. **A**: CUSA is capable to dissect offering excellent visualization resulting useful in particular during non-anatomical resections and approaching the deeper portion of the transaction plane [51]-[52]. The instrument allows surgeons to see clearly blood and biliary vessels as they dissect through the liver [53], (2) use of the instrument allows them to avoid prolonged extrahepatic vascular control, and (3) the operation actually takes less time because the vessels are continuously controlled during the dissection and there is little need for a prolonged search for bleeding or biliary vessels after the specimen has been removed.

A previous retrospective study from Fan showed that the ultrasonic dissector resulted in lower blood loss, lower morbidity, and lower mortality compared with the clamp crushing technique [54] Furthermore, ultrasonic dissection resulted in a wider tumor-free margin because of a more precise transection plane.

D: CUSA can't coagulate or realize haemostasis so it need to be used in couple with an other instruments to achieve hemostasis and biliostasis. Even if some studies sustain it to be capable to reduce intra-operative blood loss, operating time and duration of vessel occlusion [55], important studies demonstrate that CUSA can't offer these advantages if compared with traditional techniques; a prospective trial by Rau et al. showed no statistical difference in reduction of blood loss with the use of CUSA as compared to conventional methods [56]; and another trial by Takayama et al. [52], in fact, noted a greater median blood loss. CUSA causes more frequent tumour exposure at the surgical margin than traditional techhiques[1] and it's less useful for cirrhotic livers because the associated fibrosis prevents easy removal of hepatocytes [57]; besides some authors found using CUSA method (compared to clamp crushing method) an increase of venous air embolism without evidence of hemodynamic compromise but with increased risk of paradoxical embolism in cirrhotic patients [58]. Moreover CUSA should be used in association with other devices which are able to perform hemostasis. The instrument seems cumbersome and complicated to inexperienced operating room personnel. Therefore, it is easy for the instrument to malfunction. The fact that the instrument works by removing a margin of liver tissue makes it, by nature, less attractive for harvesting liver for living-donor transplantation.

3.2. Tools based on radiofrequency technology

Tissuelink Monopolar Floating Ball, TMFB (Floating Ball, TissueLink medical, Dover, NH, USA) (Fig 3): This new instrument put on the market in 2002 is a linear device that employs Radiofrequency energy focused at the tip to coagulate target tissue. The tip is provided with a low volume (4-6 ml/min) saline solution irrigation that makes easier the conduction of RF in surrounding tissue and cools the tip itself avoiding formation of chars. TMFB can seal vascular and bile structures up to 3 mm in diameter by collagen fusion. These qualities makes this device an excellent instrument for achieving haemostasis and in particular for pre- coagulating (with a painting movement) parenchyma and vessels prior to transection, preventing blood loss.

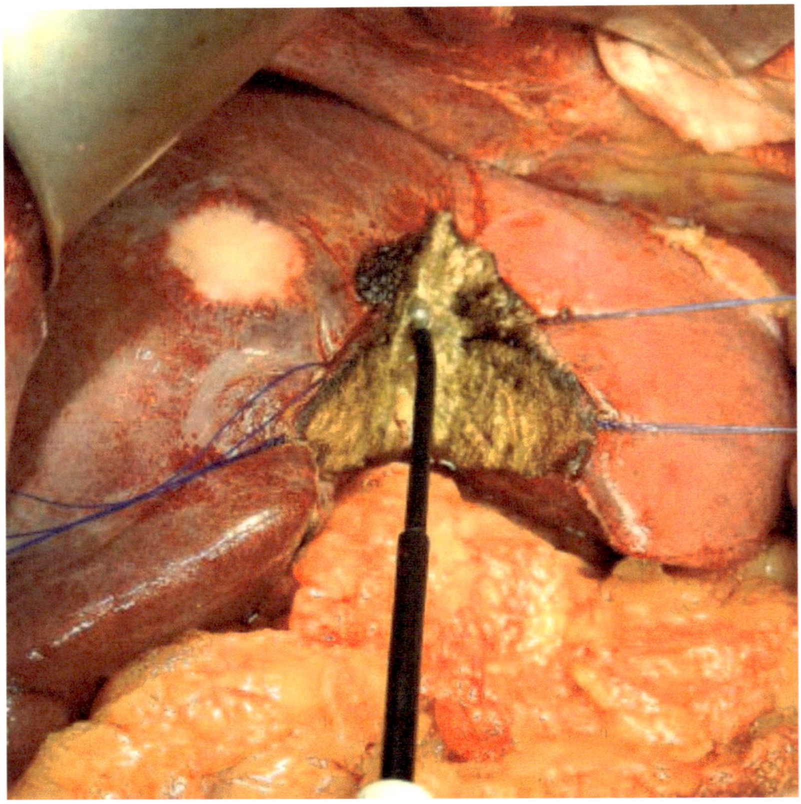

Figure 3. The Tissue Link working performing a liver resection

Otherwise continuously heating tissue underneath a cool layer, however, causes a build up of steam that can result in tissue destruction. The latter phenomenon is known as steam popping [59].

There are two models on the market, the DS3.0 with blunt tip that simply coagulates and the DS3.5-C Dissecting Sealer that is provided with sharp tip that can also dissect. **A**: The instrument is, in a sense, "friendlier" to most surgeons. In other words, surgeons, who are usually adept at using cautery, can easily understand this mechanism of action and use it accordingly. TMFB can coagulate (and the Dissecting Sealer can also cut) tissues and seals blood and bile ducts up to 3 mm in diameter, is able to reduce blood loss and the recourse to vessel occlusion techniques if compared to traditional technique s [60],[61],[62], offers good results also in cirrhotic livers and cystopericystectomy [63] and has a saline irrigation that avoids production of smoke, chars and sticky coagulum to which the device could stick causing new bleeding when it's moved away. TMFB, used on the cut liver surface after dissection, destroys eventual additional cancer cells at the margin of resection; in order to assure sterile margins, extra tissue destruction at the margins of resection may be desirable for tumor excisions. Otherwise this could be a disadvantage in case of living donor liver transplantation. It's available for both laparotomic and laparoscopic surgery and it's quite cheap and compatible with most electrosurgical generator currently available.

D: TMFB is not able to coagulate vessel over 2-3 mm of diameter which have to be clipped, legated or sealed with other instruments [64]. So the instrument should be used in combination with other instruments or clips or ties. Moreover studies do not demonstrate it's efficacy to reduce operating time if compared with traditional techniques [65].

Bipolar Vessel Sealing Device, BVSD (LigaSure, Valleylab Inc. Boulder, Colorado, USA) (fig 4): The use in liver surgery of this instrument was described for the first time in literature in 2001 by Horgan [67]. The LigaSure System includes a generator with a foot switch and a clamp-form hand piece that can be used for parenchymal fragmentation and isolation of blood and bile structures just like in clamp crushing technique before application of energy; it employs RF to realize permanent occlusion of vessels or tissue bundle. The LigaSure generator has a Valleylab's Instant Response technology, a feedback-controlled response system that diagnoses the tissue type in the instrument jaws and delivers the appropriate amount of energy to effectively seal the vessel: when the seal cycle is complete, a generator tone sound, and output to the handset is automatically discontinued. BVSD is capable to obliterate the lumen of veins and arteries up to 7 mm in diameter by the fusion of elastin and collagen proteins of the vessel walls; that makes BVSB the only safe and real alternative to sutures and clips for sealing vessel [68],[69],[70].

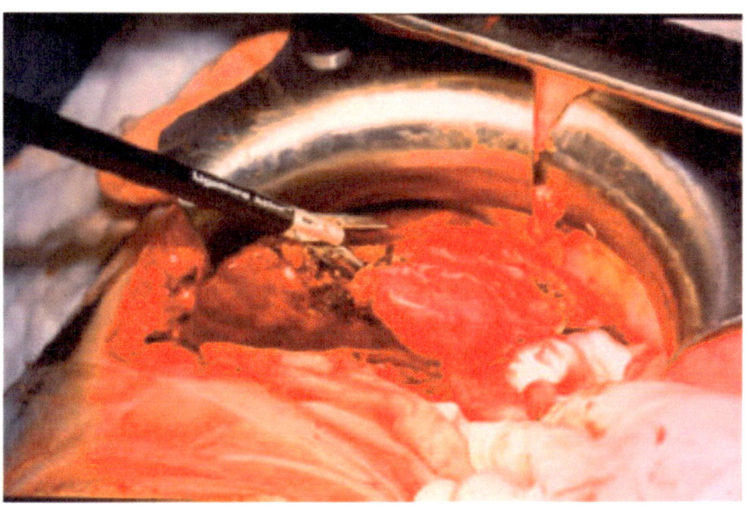

Figure 4. The Ligasure Atlas during parenchyma transection

A: BVSD coagulates sealing vessels up to 7 mm in diameter with minimal charring, thermal spread or smoke, it's capable to reduce blood loss and the need for vessel occlusion techniques if compared to traditional techniques [8],[71],[72], A recently published randomized controlled trial demonstrated that the use of Ligasure in combination with a clamp crushing technique resulted in lower blood loss and faster transaction speed in minor liver resections compared with the conventional technique of electric cautery or ligature for controlling vessels in the transection plane [73]. Otherwise a more recent randomized trial from the same team was not able to show a real difference between the traditional techniques and the Ligasure vessel sealing system [74]. The instrument is available for both laparotomic and laparoscopic surgery [75]. Furthermore the use of Ligasure System is not correlated with an increase of the rate of post-operative bile leaks and in some study bile leakage was nihill [76]-[127] and that proves his effectiveness in obliterate also bile vessel. **D**: after the application the coagulated tissue often sticks to the instrument's jaws causing new bleeding when the device is moved away; BVSD seems to be less effective in presence of cirrhosis for two reasons: first the portal hypertension correlated with cirrhosis causes thinning of the dilate portal vein's walls and makes their obliteration less effective; second cirrhosis makes crushing technique difficult and the hepatic tissue between the blades may disperse the power applied causing vessel to bleed [128]; moreover it seems to be ineffective in cystopericystectomy [77] (even if some surgeons sustain his effectiveness in this surgery [78]). Ligasure vessels sealing system has been widely use during liver transection in a "blind" way [70]-[71], achieving parenchymal fracture and vessel sealing in the same time without identification of tiny vasculatures and bile ducts. This could be considered a limits of this tools which do not allow the surgeon to clearly check the structures which are going to be sealed. To overcome this limit a technique similar to the "fusion technique" used with Harmonic FOCUS has been developed for the Ligasure vessel sealing system [130]., using the Ligasure precise. With this technique using LigaSure itself, the hepatic parenchyma was widely and gently crushed and confirmed that the remnant vessels and tiny vessels (2mm in diameter) were divided by the LigaSure under direct vision. This allow to coagulate only vessels appropriate for sealing with this instrument and imprtant vascular pedicles to adjacent segments can be visualized and protected. Larger vessels (3mm in diameter) were tied by absorbable braid. This approach seems to reduce transection time and is the so called "postcoagulation technique" [138].

Habib's technique: This technique, invented by Habib in 2002, is also known as Bloodless Hepatectomy Technique [10],[88]. Resection is conducted using cooled tip RadioFrequency probe those contain a 3 cm exposed tip to coagulate liver resection margins. Once a 2 cm-wide coagulative necrosis zone is created by multiple applications of the probes in adjacent zones and at different depths, the division of the parenchyma with a surgical scalpel is possible without any bleeding. Both the remnant liver and the removed specimen have on the margin of resection a portion of necrotic coagulated liver l cm thick.

A: The primary problem with each of the previous devices is that whilst small vessels can be coagulated during transection, larger vessels are often left patent and injured, which can result in considerable blood loss requiring tedious clipping and suturing in order to achieve haemostasis.

Habib's Technique allows hepatic resections with marginal blood loss, without any vessel occlusion technique or intra or post-operative transfusions, coagulating each vessel encountered in the field of energy application; In a preliminary study of 15 cases of mainly segmental or wedge resection reported by Weber et al., the mean blood loss was only 30±10 ml, and no complications such as bile leakage were observed [88]. Another group also reported low blood loss using this technique in liver resection [89]. Haemostasis is obtained only by RF thermal energy: no additional devices like stitches, knots, clips or fibrin glue are needed [10],[88],[90],[91]; it's effective also in the cirrhotic liver and the l-cm-thick of burned coagulated surface assures margins free from tumour. The technique has the advantage of simplicity compared with the aforementioned transection techniques. As the RF assisted technique allows parenchymal sparing during the first resection, this in turn results in more repeat liver resections being possible for recurrences. It also enables nonanatomical resections during these repeat resections.

D: Habib's technique cannot be applied near the hilum or the cava vein for fear of damaging this structures and because the blood flow of large vessels subtracts RF energy and involves an incomplete coaugulative necrosis [92],[93] (up to now the technique has been experienced only for segmental resection); the l-cm-thick of burned coagulated layer in the surface involves the loss of part of healthy parenchyma and a higher rate of post-operative abdominal abscesses [91],[94]. Moreover one potential disadvantage of this technique is the sacrifice of parenchymal tissue in the liver remnant, with a 1 cm wide necrotic tissue at the transection margin, which may be critical in cirrhotic patients who require major liver resection or in case of liver resection for living donor liver transplantation. An evolution of the Habib probe is the Habib 4X [92]which adress the problem of time consuming and the risk of skin burns from the grounding pad related to previous device.The device was introduced perpendicularly into the liver, abutting the transection line (Figure 5). The generator was programmed to produce an alert signal when energy delivery had been automatically stopped, thus avoiding over coagulation and carbonation. The probe was gently moved to and fro in its vertical axis for 3e5 mm throughout the coagulation process to avoid adherence of the probe to the liver parenchyma. The probe was then reintroduced adjacent to the last coagulated area in a serial fashion, until the area to be transected was fully ablated. The number of applications required to create a complete zone of desiccation was related to the size of the cut surface of the resection margin.

1. A second line of ablation, parallel to the first line and closer to the tumour edge, was then done to ensure complete tissue coagulation and perfect haemostasis prior to transection

2. The Habib 4X was then applied perpendicularly to the previous two lines of ablation, so as to ensure complete coagulation of any residual normal liver parenchyma. This allowed a margin of coagulated liver parenchyma to remain; ensuring vessels and bile ducts remained sealed. For deeper tumours the device was applied at an angle of 45 degrees to the surface. This technique allow to achieve a very low rate of blood transfusion in a very large series [88]

Gyrus plasmakinetic pulsed bipolar coagulation device: Gyrus /Gyrus medical inc., Maple Groves, Mn, USA) is a bipolar cautery device which seals the hepatic parenchima using a combination of pressure and energy that results in the fusion of collagen and elastin in the walls of the hepatic vasculature and bile ducts [98]. The device can reliably seals vessels up to 7 mm in diameter minimizing the amount of blood loss during the transection of the liver. Thermal spread and sticking to tissues is reduced by a cooling period after each pulse as the impedance of the coagulated tissue increased. This instrument has been previously widely used in gynaecological procedures and it's use in liver surgery is relatively new.

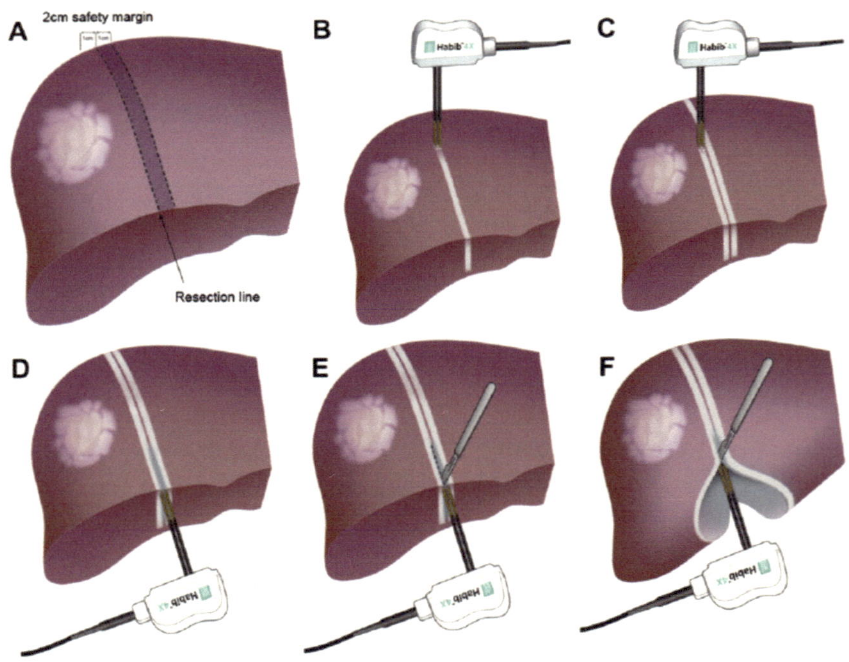

Figure 5. Habib technique for liver resection

A: It could be used in a similar manner to the clamp-crush technique to transect hepatic parenchyma. After incising the hepatic capsule with bovie the instrument is inserted into the liver in an open manner and bipolar energy is applied as the forceps are slowly closed over the parenchyma. The cauterized liver is subsequently transected with Metzenbaum scissors. The device was used for the entire hepatic parenchymal transection; only named vascular and biliary structures required additional attention and were stapled or suture ligated. The device exhibits a minimal thermal spread of 2–3 mm and was frequently used for parenchymal transection abutting the hepatic hilum. With the exception of large, named vascular and biliary structures which were routinely stapled or ligated, excellent haemostasis and biliary duct fusion were achieved uniformly.

In a recent series median blood loss rate compare favourably with those in several large series using the traditional clamp-crush technique [99]. Moreover blood loss and transfusion rates were comparable with those cited in recent report of alternative parenchymal transection, as showed by results of Tan et Al [100]. In this study Gyrus compared favourably with Harmonic scalpel in term of Bile leakage and the author underlined the concorrential cost of the device. Moreover it seems to be useful even in case of cirrhotic patients. Corvera et al. [98] have also reported the use of the Gyrus device in cirrhotic livers comparing it to the clamp and crush

http://dx.doi.org/10.5772/54301

technique. They evaluated five patients in each group showing similar results between the two groups in terms of operating time, blood loss and major post-operative complications.

D: as the ligasure vessel sealing device one of the limit of this device is the "blind" use without clear identification of vascular and biliary structures before sealing

The Aquamantis System: The Aquamantys System employs Transcollation ® technology (fig 6) to simultaneously deliver RF (radiofrequency) energy and saline for haemostatic sealing and coagulation of soft tissue and bone at the surgical site. Transcollation technology is used in a wide variety of surgical procedures, including orthopaedic joint replacement, spinal surgery, orthopaedic trauma and surgical oncology.Transcollation technology simultaneously integrates RF (radiofrequency) energy and saline to deliver controlled thermal energy to the tissue. This allows the tissue temperature to stay at or below 100°C, the boiling point of water. Unlike conventional electrosurgical devices which operate at high temperatures, Transcollation technology does not result in smoke or char formation when put in contact with tissue. Blood vessels contain Type I and Type III collagen within their walls. Heating these collagen fibers causes radial compression, resulting in a decrease in vessel lumen diameter. Using the Aquamantys generator with patented bipolar and monopolar sealers, surgeons can achieve broad tissue-surface haemostasis by applying Transcollation technology in a painting motion, or it can be used to spot-treat bleeding vessels. This is capable of sealing structures 3–6 mm in diameter without producing high temperature or excessive charring and eschar. Structures more than 6 mm in diameter should be divided in conventional manner with clips or ties. Constant suction is required to clear the saline used for irrigation.

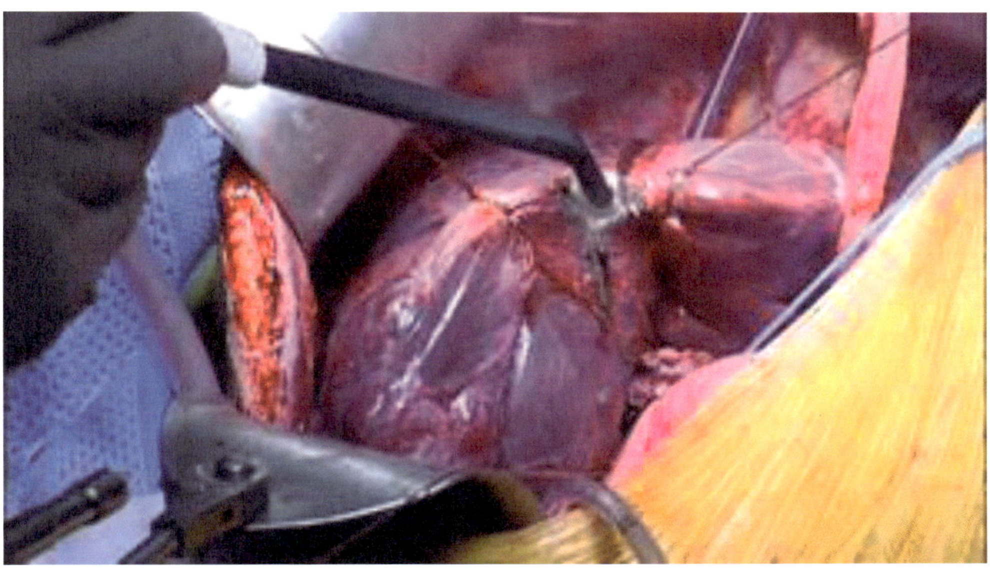

Figure 6. Aquamantys transcollation technology performing liver resection

A: it's use is "friendlier" to most surgeons, easy to learn most surgeons are comfortable after 5–6 procedures. It seals blood and bile ducts up to 6 mm in diameter, is able to reduce blood loss and the recourse to vessel occlusion techniques. Moreover it offers good results also in cirrhotic livers [66] and destroys eventual additional cancer cells at the margin of resection.

D: it is expensive and pace of liver transection could be low. Moreover there is a lack of data reported in literature due to the relative novelty of this device.

Coolinside: The new Coolinside® device (Apeiron Medical, Valencia, Spain) is a hand-held device which simultaneously coagulates (using RF) and cuts (by means of a cold scalpel) the liver. This device and its manipulation is built for both laparotomic and laparoscopic procedures.Coagulation is performed by a blunttip metallic electrode positioned at the distal edge, which is electrically connected to a Cosman CC-1 coagulator system (Radionics, Burlington, MA, USA) operating at a maximum power of 90W. The liver tissue is cut using a thin blade at the distal edge. Inside it the active electrode has a closed hydraulic circuit containing saline solution at a temperature of 0 ºC, which is propelled to the distal edge by a Radionics continuous perfusion pump (Burlington, MA, USA) at a speed of approximately 130 mL/min. The cold liquid keeps the surface of the tissue below 100 ºC by refrigerating the active electrode. The feedback system for the warm saline solution means that it can never come into contact with the patient (as in the case of the Tissuelink® device).

A: The key to the performance of the device is in the fact that the depth of hepatic parenchymal transection is adapted to the coagulation effect achieved by the proximal edge of the active electrode, that part which first comes into contact with the tissue. In this way, every time the surgeon moves the device over the surface of the liver, the parenchyma is cut and coagulated simultaneously [132]. In this study 11 hepatic resection were performed entirely with coolinside without the need for ligature or clips or pringle manouver, with no bile leak complication and high transection speed. This device combines coagulation and transection capacity and it does not need to be combined with other devices (not even stitches or clips). Moreover, it is not necessary to perform vascular occlusion, parenchymal coagulation is homogeneous and, lastly, there is the possibility of using it in laparoscopic surgery.

D:As with other RF devices, tissue pre-coagulation can change structures so that it can be difficult to identify the main hepatic vessels or conduits. Moreover, the amount of hepatic tissue that is sacrificed may be greater than in the case of other techniques, given that with this device the coagulated area may be up to 5 mm, which might limit but not contraindicate this technique in cirrhotic patients. Moreover this could be considered a disadvantages in case of liver resection during living donor liver transplantation

3.3. Others source of energy

Water Jet Scalpel, WJS: The WJS was introduced in 1982 by Papachristou [79]. This tools could achieve, as well as CUSA, a selective dissection.

The dissection modalities which take advantage of the anatomic conditions are called selective. The water-jet effects hereby like an intelligent knife and separates the more resistant duct- and

http://dx.doi.org/10.5772/54301

vessel structures automatically from the parenchyma which thus become visible. When visible they can be closed easily under controlled conditions.

The device consists of a pressure generating pump and a flexible hose connected to the hand piece. The liquid (saline solution) flows at a steady stream and is projected through the nozzle at the tip of the hand piece. The jet hits the liver at the desired line of transection and washes away the parenchyma, leaving the intra-hepatic ducts and vessel undamaged; then the vascular and bile structures can be legated and the transection plane coagulated. The tip is reinforced by a suction tube which removes excess fluid; besides splashing is avoided by covering the area of dissection with a transparent sheet or a Petri dish. Compared to the CUSA, the water jet leaves a smoother cut surface and little hepatic degeneration or necrosis at the borders.

A: WJS can dissect offering excellent visualization and is effective also in the cirrhotic liver. In the only available prospective randomized trial of water jet in the literature, in which 31 patients underwent liver resection using water jet and another 30 patients underwent liver resection using CUSA, water jet transection reduced blood loss, blood transfusion, and transection time compared with CUSA [80]. water jet techniques is quite good for dissecting out major hepatic veins when tumors are in proximity. This allows for delineation of hepatic veins, particularly at the junction with the inferior vena cava, and prevents positive margin. It allow the so called selective dissection technique.

D: WJS can't coagulate or realize haemostasis and some study demonstrate that it cannot achieve a reduction of intra-operative blood loss and operating time if compared with traditional techniques [81],[82]; using this technique is possible cancerous seeding of the healthy abdominal organs and infection of the operators by hepatic viruses. Moreover in literature some cases of gas embolism are described using this device [83]. Furthermore the instrument may be more effective than the CUSA with respect to operating in the presence of cirrhosis. Papachristou and Barters [79] initially reported that the water jet was likely to be ineffective when there is increased fibrotic tissue. Later papers, however, describe successful resections with cirrhosis by using higher jet pressures. Une et al. [80] report that one does not need to use higher water jet pressures to dissect cirrhotic tissue effectively; instead, the same pressures as for normal parenchyma just need to be applied longer. The major concern of surgeons using the water jet is the associated splash. The latter effect is caused by solution bouncing off tissues. Besides the obvious infectious concerns of the possibility of contaminating operating room personnel, the splash brings up the notion of the possibility of cancerous seeding. This possibility must be considered in operations for malignancy and one needs to take additional care not to expose the gross tumor during the dissection.

Staplers (fig 7): Since the nineties vascular staplers to divide hepatic veins and portal branches during hemihepatectomy are considered an achievement that aids in minimizing blood loss and thereby reduces the need for inflow occlusion. Further, staplers seem to be advantageous in the unroofing of hepatic cysts since any inadvertently injured bile duct or blood vessel is sealed [84].

Staplers can be used in liver surgery for control of inflow and outflow vessels, or to divide liver parenchyma [84],[85]. The stapler is rarely used as the principal instrument in hepatic resection. The device can add speed to the operation in open or laparoscopic surgery. Its primary use is for achieving control of hepatic vasculature, particularly the hepatic veins.The use of vascular staplers to divide hepatic veins and portal branches is considered an achievement that has aided in minimizing blood loss and thereby reduced the need for inflow occlusion. Recent publications reporting a number of techniques using stapling devices in liver surgery showed them to be extraordinarily useful in the safe ligation of inflow and outflow vessels.

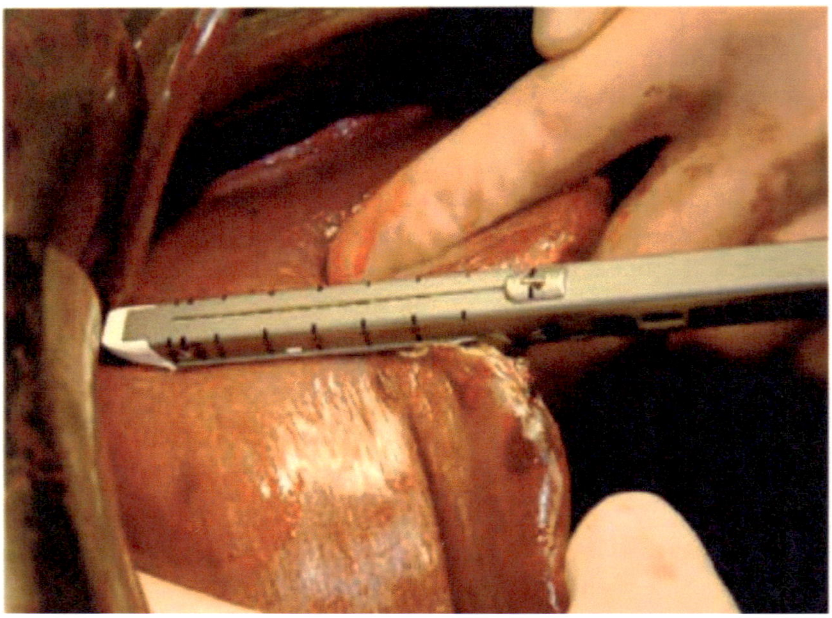

Figure 7. Parenchima transection performed using a Stapler

Biliary radicals can be incorporated efficiently into the staple line. Division of the hepatic veins with a stapler as opposed to direct ligation proffers several advantages. First, it eliminates the risk of dissecting the hepatic veins and minimize the risk of slipped ligature. Furthermore the stapler simultaneously divides multiple venous branches, especially on the right side, that are too short to allow for a safe and rapid more traditional ligation.

A: It is particularly useful in dividing the major trunk of hepatic veins or the middle hepatic vein deep in the transaction. Vascular staplers also can be used to divide the hepatic duct pedicle in right or left hepatectomy [7]. The procedure starts by dividing the liver capsule by diathermy the use of a stapler for transection of the liver parenchyma following by fracturing the liver tissue with a vascular clamp in a stepwise manner and subsequently divided with an EndoGIA vascular stapler. In a large series of 300 stapler hepatectomies, including 193 major hepatectomies, mortality of 4% and morbidity of 33% were reported which is comparable with conventional liver resection techniques. Vascular control was necessary in only 10% of the series, with an overall median blood loss of 700 mL [86]. The rate of biliary leakage seems to be very low, with a 8% reported in the largest series [86]. Moreover the trasection speed is the highest among all the techniques employed. Most recently, an ultrasound-directed transparenchymal application of vascular staplers to selectively divide major intrahepatic blood vessels before the parenchymal phase of liver resection has been shown to minimize blood loss, warm ischemia time, and operative time [131].

More to the point, in cases of difficult parenchymal transection with ongoing bleeding, the stapler device offers faster specimen removal giving the surgeon the opportunity to control the loss of blood from the raw liver surface

D:Although the technique appears attractive, the financial cost is a serious drawback. One problem associated with the use of a stapler for liver transection is increased risk of bile leak, since the stapler is not very effective in sealing small bile ducts [87]. Otherwise other studies report a very low rate of biliary injury and leakage. Moreover the surgeon must also be selective in the use of a stapler for the treatment of tumors particularly near the hilum in order to obtain sufficient margin. In case of stapler malfunction the surgeon should be ready with a back up technique to achieve vein control in case of sudden hemorrage. Serious blood loss can theoretically occur when the stapler has sealed only half the diameter of the vessel or after misfire of the device.

Chang's needle technique: This technique presented by Chang in 2001 [95] is based on the utilization of a special instrument equipped with a 18 cm straight inner needle with an hook near its top; Chang needle can be applied repeatedly to make overlapping interlocking mattress sutures with N° l silks along the inner side of the division line. After this phase liver parenchyma can be divided directly by scissors, electrocautery or traditional resection methods applying new suture only for tubular structures of significant size.

A: Chang's needle technique can be performed without application of any vessel occlusion techniques, without any other haemostatic technique and reducing blood transfusions; this method seems to be capable to reduce both intra-operative blood loss and resection time; besides it's surely cheap and is reported to be simple too [96].

D: It can't be applied if the lesion is too close to inferior cava vein [97]

3.4. Combined techniques

In the last decades a combined use of the devices previously analyzed has been reported in literature to increase the efficacy of each device, based on consideration that we have 2 different kind of instruments (as shown in table 3): those that allow a preparation of vascular structures achieving a selective dissection and those that allow a non-selective dissection (with a blind coagulation of the vasculature and biliary structures). Efficient and safe liver parenchymal transection is dependent on the ability to simultaneously address 2 tasks: parenchymal division and hemostasis. Because no single instrument has been developed that is adequate for both of these tasks, most hepatic parenchymal transections are performed using a combination of instruments and techniques.

Aloia e coll developed a 2-surgeons technique which combine saline-linked cautery and ultrasonic dissection [133]. This techniques allowed a reduction in the operative time when compared to ultrasonic dissection alone. Moreover blood loss and lenght of operation seems to be reduced.

Reference	Patients	Technique	Blood loss/ transfused patients	Operative time, min	Transection speed, cm^2/s
Takayama et al. [8]	132	Clamp-crush technique	452^a/NA	54^b	1.0
	(66 vs. 66)	Cavitron ultrasonic surgical aspirator	515^a/NA	61^b	1.1
Rau et al. [9]	61	Hydrojet dissector	NA/1.5	28^b	NA
		Cavitron ultrasonic surgical aspirator	NA/2.5	46^b	
Koo et al. [22]	50	Clamp-crush technique	792^a/NA	119	NA
	(25 vs. 25)	Cavitron ultrasonic surgical aspirator	875^a/NA	139	
Lesurtel et al. [16]	100	Clamp-crush technique	1.5^cNA	NA	3.9
	(4 groups,	Cavitron ultrasonic surgical aspirator	4^c/NA		2.3
	25 each)	Hydrojet dissector	3.5^c/NA		2.4
		Radiofrequency dissecting sealer	3.4^c/NA		2.5
Arita et al. [21]	80	Clamp-crush technique	733^a/0	80	0.89
	(40 vs. 40)	Radiofrequency dissecting sealer	665^a/2	79	0.99
Smyrniotis et al. [20]	82	Clamp-crush technique	460^a/15	211	NA
	(41 vs. 41)	Sharp transection	500^a/13	205	
Lupo et al. [23]	50	Clamp-crush technique	NA/8	292	NA
	(26 vs. 24)	Radiofrequency dissecting sealer	NA/13	278	

Only randomized trials are reported. NA = Not available in the study.
[a] Blood loss is expressed in ml.
[b] Value refers only to transection time.
[c] Blood loss is expressed in ml/cm^2. The number of patients transfused is expressed as a mean only in the trial by Rau et al. [9].

[a] Blood loss is expressed in ml.

[b] Value refers only to transection time.

[c] Blood loss is expressed in ml/cm^2. The number of patients transfused is expressed as a mean only in the trial Rau et al. [9].

Table 3. Only randomized trials are reported. NA= Not available in the study.

In January 2004, Sakamoto et al retrospectively compared their experience with 16 liver resections in which SLC was used in combination with a bipolar vessel-sealing device and a matched set of 16 patients undergoing liver resections in which a crush-clamp technique was used.[134] They found that fewer patients in the SLC group required inflow occlusion and that blood loss was reduced. Differences in total operative time were not reported, but liver transection time was prolonged in the SLC group. Aldrighetti et al. [135] published a relatively larger series comparing clamp-crushing with ultrasonic plus harmonic scalpel dissection. The latter resulted in longer operative time, but with a reduced blood loss (and consequently a lower transfusion rate) and with a lower rate of biliary fistula. However, the retrospective method of the study, and the relatively long period of inclusion may have biased these results against the clamp-crush technique. Lesurtel and Tanai combined ultrasonic dissection with bipolar coagulation [136-137]. They concluded that UD associated with efficient bipolar forceps cautery is probably one of the safest and the most efficient device for liver transection, even if its superiority over the clamp crushing technique has not been well established. In a recent paper Yokoo et coll [139] combined the use of ultrasonically activated scalpel with a saline linked radiofrequency dissecting sealer versus bipolar cautery with a saline-irrigation system and ultrasonically activated. Scalpel. The first technique resulted in shorter operative time and lower postoperative complication rate. Moreover Gruttadauria and coll developed a combination of utrasonic surgical aspirator in association with a monopolar floating ball in elderly patients. This new technique reduced length of stay, procedure length, and use of perioperative blood in a cohort of patients [140]. Nagano and coll evaluated the efficacy of combination of CUSA plus argon beam colagulator in comparison with CUSA plus bipolar coagulation, and showed that the first approach allowed to a shorter transection time and lower blood loss [141]

Haemostasis techniques: Coagulation of vessels over 1 mm of diameter can be achieved positioning clips or sutures before division, or using devices like LigaSure, TMFB or HS for their target vessels or staplers for the largest veins. Clips and sutures are used especially during transection through traditional techniques.

During and after liver's transaction haemostasis of the vascular structures under 1 mm of diameter is another important concern of the surgeon: first because the continuous bleeding from the little vessels in the parenchyma represents a considerable part of intra-operative blood loss, and second because it makes hard for the surgeon the visualization of the surgical field. The stop of tearing small vessels that causes oozing from the cut surface can be achieved with normal monopolar or bipolar electrocoagulator, better if equipped with saline irrigation that makes them less traumatic and avoids formation of sticky coagulum An alternative is represented by employment of Argon Beam Coagulator or TMFB that probably is the best device for stopping tearing of small vessels on the cut surface of the liver.

After the resection other two precautions can be taken: application of mattress sutures for providing to a mechanical compression of the bare surface and application of biological glue for realizing complete haemostasis through a chemical/biological action.

Choice of surgical strategy: The choice of surgical strategy is based on the pre-operative evaluation and on the now indispensable Intra-Operative Ultrasonography (IOUS); in fact several studies have demonstrated that the IOUS is capable to change surgical strategy in over 40% of cases finding new lesions or diagnosing as inoperable lesions those were thought operable at the previous evaluation [101-104].The kind of surgical strategy chosen for the intervention on the base of affects strongly influences the operative outcome and the amount of operative blood loss. The most considerable aspect is the amplitude of the resection: a large resection like a right hemi-hepatectomy (or another typical resection) involves a higher bleeding and risk of complications. From this point of view the choice of segmental or wedge limited resections, when they are possible in respect of radical oncology standards, has to be consedered the best option [105,106]. Usual surgical margins for removal of liver tumours are 1 cm of healthy parenchyma surrounding the lesion. Kokudo et al. in 2002 demonstrated that for colorectal metastases the surgical margin can be, in particular situations, lowered to 2 mm with increase of the pathology recurrence rate from O% for 5 mm margin to 6% for 2 mm margin [107].

This finding, combined with a contrast-enhanced IOUS during the resection, could be a rationale incentive for practising limited resections [108-110], and the possibility of an accurate investigation of the remnant liver through the IOUS

Drug administration for reducing intra-operative blood loss: Liver resection may cause a variable degree of hyperfibrinolytic states; this phenomenon occurs in the days immediately after hepatectomy and is more pronounced in patients with a diseased liver or in patients who have undergone to a wider hepatectomy extent [111-116]So some authors propose the utilization of drugs with antifibrinolytic effect like Aprotinin that is reported to be capable to reduce intra-operative blood loss (especially during liver resection time) and transfusions [117-119]. Other authors propose utilization of the cheaper Tranexamic acid reporting similar results [120]. Although a theoretical risk of thromboembolic complications is present, no adverse drug effects like deep venous thrombosis, pulmonary embolism or other circulatory disturbances were detected in both these studies.

3.5. Comparison of different liver transection techniques

The choice of transection techniques is currently a matter of preference of surgeons, as there are few data from prospective randomized trials that compared different techniques. It has been shown in small prospective randomized trials that clamp crushing or water jet may be preferable to CUSA in terms of quality of transection or speed of transection [1],[122]. Moreover Water-jet dissection.

Seems to be considerably faster than CUSA® or blunt dissection and Pringle-time and blood loss can be reduced by using this device [83]. However, the results of these trials remain to be validated by larger-scale trials. CUSA dissection is still a widely used technique worldwide.

Several studies have been addressed to clarify these critical points, underlining the advantages and the drawbacks of each device. One of the first randomized studies [52] comparing the ultrasonic dissector versus the clamp-crush technique showed that the ultrasonic dissector is more frequently associated with tumor exposure at the resection margin and with incomplete appearance of landmark hepatic veins on the cut surface. The authors did not find any difference in postoperative morbidity and blood loss, concluding that clamp-crushing technique resulted in a higher quality of hepatectomy, thus being the option of choice.

Aldrighetti et al. [135] published a relatively larger series comparing clamp-crushing with ultrasonic plus harmonic scalpel dissection. The latter resulted in longer operative time, but with a reduced blood loss (and consequently a lower transfusion rate) and with a lower rate of biliary fistula. However, the retrospective method of the study, and the relatively long period of inclusion may have biased these results against the clamp-crush technique.The study performed by Takayama and colleagues found no difference in transection speed between the crush/clamp technique and ultrasonic dissection. This same study also demonstrated that the crush/clamp technique resulted in increased precision and improved quality of hepatectomy according to a grading system considering such factors as positive surgical margins, appearance of landmark hepatic veins on the cut hepatic surface, and postoperative morbidity. Koo and colleagues also demonstrated that no difference existed with blood loss, transfusion requirements, speed of resection, or total operative time between crush/clamp and the ultrasonic dissector

A randomized study [73] comparing LigaSure with the conventional method, demonstrated no statistical difference ($p = 0.185$) in blood loss and mortality rate between the two groups. But, LigaSure was slightly superior in terms of transection speed, number of ties per cm 2 and hemostasis time. The resulting total operating time decreased by 27 min, and hospital stay was shortened by 2 days in the LigaSure group. The authors performed also a cost analysis which found a highly cost-effective ratio in favor of LigaSure due to shorter operative time, hospital stay and low capital cost of the disposable device. They considered 3 mm as the range of maximal effectiveness in sealing portal triads (without increasing the rate of biliary fistula). A more recent randomized study [74] did not demonstrate this difference in blood loss, operating time and hospital stay, failing to find a superiority of one technique over the other. In this particular situation, the cost-effectiveness of LigaSure in the clamp-crush method was not confirmed, favoring once again the latter. Radiofrequency-assisted hepatic transection has also been studied in a randomized, controlled fashion. The results of this study indicated that postoperative morbidity, including abscesses and biliary complications, was significantly higher with the use of radiofrequency-assisted resection compared to crush/clamp.

As recently described in non-randomized settings [85]-[86], liver transection could be also performed with the stapling technique. As reported, the technique appears to be safe and quicker. Commonly, staplers are considered to be expensive tools, but they increase only the total material cost. However, owing to decreased blood loss, transfusion rate, shorter operative time and in-hospital stay, the global cost for a hepatectomy (especially for the major ones) has considerably decreased especially in high-volume centers. It should also be noticed that the stapling technique [142] can reduce the time of vascular control (i.e. Pringle). This fact turns out to be relevant when the resection is conducted in injured parenchyma due to prolonged chemotherapy (hepatic steatosis, sinusoidal obstruction syndrome, steatohepatitis, etc.). Cataldo et al [143] comparing stapler, crush/clamp and dissecting sealer demostrate that liver trasnection with stapler was quicker, but mean blood loss and oncological margin were similar for the three techniques. A recent study of clearly demonstrate that there is no benefit of any alternative method that has so far been compared with the clamp-crushing technique within a RCT regarding morbidity, mortality, and transfusion rates. Moreover, available RCTs failed to show an advantage of these novel devices to reduce blood loss, parenchymal injury, operation time, and hospital stay.Recently, a randomized trial compared four methods of liver transection, namely clamp crushing, CUSA, Hydrojet, and dissecting sealer, with 25 patients in each group [121]. In that study, clamp crushing was associated with the fastest transection speed, lowest blood loss, and lowest blood transfusion requirement. Furthermore, clamp crushing was the most cost-effective technique. However, in that study, clamp crushing was performed with the Pringle maneuver, whereas the other techniques were performed without the Pringle maneuver. This might have resulted in bias in favor of clamp crushing. An other recent comparative study between clamp crushing technique (CRUSH), ultrasonic dissection

(CUSA) or bipolar device (LigaSure), failed to show any difference between the three techniques in terms of intraoperative blood loss, blood transfusion, postoperative complications and mortality [72]. Further prospective randomized studies are needed to determine which transection technique is the best. Moreover a recent review of the Cochrane conclude that Clamp-crush technique is advocated as the method of choice in liver parenchymal transection because it avoids special equipment, whereas the newer methods do not seem to offer any benefit in decreasing the morbidity or transfusion requirement. Otherwise in the comparison of different techniques, apart from the efficacy in transaction with low blood loss, the relative speed of transection and the potential complications are other parameters to be considered. [122] Furthermore, the use of special instruments for transection is costly, especially when two instruments are used in combination for transection and hemostasis. It is difficult to compare the relative cost of different transection instruments because some are reusable whereas others are designed for single use, and the cost of the same instrument varies substantially in different countries. The clamp–crush and sharp dissection techniques do not involve any additional instruments. A cost comparison between the clamp–crush technique and other techniques revealed that clamp–crush is two to six times cheaper than other methods, depending on the number of surgeries performed each year. Nonetheless, the cost of these various techniques should play a part in the surgeon's decision as to whether to use them or not.

Besides reduction of blood loss and perioperative complications, radical resection with tumor-free margins is a major goal in surgery for malignant hepatic lesions. Disease-positive resection margins are a strong prognostic factor for local tumor recurrence and overall survival. Unfortunately, pathohistological data on resection margins were only available for two trials.Takayama et al. demonstrated comparable resection margins in their comparison of the clamp-crushing to the ultrasonic dissector technique.[52] However, Smyrniotis et al. reported far greater length of the narrowest tumor-free margin in their sharp transection group. [144] The question of whether any alternative transection technique provides a benefit in longterm survival of cancer patients needs further evaluation within clinical trials.

4. The role of the anaesthesiologist

Patients those are subjected to liver surgery are usually pre and intra-operatorially treated with infusion of liquids, plasma expanders and blood products: normally hepatic resections are in fact conduced in condition of euvolaemia or hypervolaemia to protect patients from the risk of consistent haemorrhage and haemodynamic's instability.

Despite this idea several studies have demonstrated that a condition of Low Central Venous Pressure (LCVP) can reduce bleeding, recourse to vessel occlusion techniques and transfusions during resection [111,112,113]. It has been scientifically demonstrated that intra-operative blood loss is correlated with inferior retro-hepatic vena cava pressure [114].

Mendelez obtained very low blood loss results in major hepatic resections managed keeping theCVP under 5 mmHg: this is possible with abstention from practising any infusion but intra-operative liquid infusion at the low speed of 75 ml/h and without any drug administration but employing hypotensive effects of normal anaesthetics (like Isoflurane, morphine and Fentalyn). It's obvious that LCVP technique needs a strict monitoring of several parameters: in particular systolic arterial pressure has constantly to be kept over 90 mmHg and diuresis over 25 ml/h. After the specimen is removed and after the realization of complete haemostasis starts the infusion of liquids, and if necessary of plasma expanders and blood products until euvolaemia is obtained and haemoglobin value is over 8-10 g/dl [115].

LCVP has to be abandoned in case of uncontrollable haemorrhage (over 25% of total blood volume) or application of total vascular exclusion technique. Mendelez using LCVP reports a 0,4% rate of gas embolism [116]. This illustrates the importance of collaboration between surgeons and anaesthetists for a successful hepatectomy.

5. Conclusions

Improvement in the techniques of liver transection is one of the most important factors for improved safety of hepatectomy in recent years. The use of intraoperative ultrasound aids delineation of the proper transection plane and allow to transect tumor close to main vessels without bleeding. Clamp crushing and ultrasonic dissection are currently the two most popular techniques of liver transection. The role of new instruments such as ultrasonic shear and RFA devices in liver transection remains unclear, with few data available in the literature.

The role of vascular exclusion including Pringle's manouver seems to be decreasing with improved transection technique. However, it remains a useful technique in reducing bleeding from inflow vessels, especially for surgeons with less experience in liver resection, and recent results show safety of this technique even for prolonged total time of ischemia. Maintenance of low central venous pressure remains an important adjunctive measure to reduce blood loss in liver transection.

As clear data for comparison of various liver transection techniques are lacking, currently the choice of technique is often based on the individual surgeon's preference. However, certain general recommendations can be made based on existing data and the author's experience. Clamp crushing is a lowcost technique but it requires substantial experience to be used effectively for liver transection, especially in the cirrhotic liver. CUSA can be used in both cirrhotic and non-cirrhotic liver, is associated with low blood loss and it has a well established safety record, with low risk of bile leak. It is particularly useful in major hepatic resections when dissection of the major branches of the hepatic veins is required, or in cases where the tumor is in close proximity to a major hepatic vein, as it allows clear dissection of the hepatic vein from the tumor. This could be the preferred

5.1. Technique in oncological resection

5.1.1. The main disadvantage of the CUSA technique is slow transection

Newer instruments such as the Harmonic Scalpel, Ligasure and TissueLink Dissector enhance the capability of hemostasis and allow faster transection. However, they lack the preciseness of CUSA in dissection of major hepatic veins, and, HS more than others may be associated with increased risk of bile leak. Moreover they are particularly useful in laparoscopic liver resection. They can also be used in combination with CUSA for sealing of vessels, but this increases the cost substantially. RFA-assisted transection is probably the most speedy liver transaction technique. However, the risk of thermal injury to major bile duct is a serious concern and its use is probably restricted to minor resection Gyrus and Aquamantis are relatively new instrument and literature do not allow to draw any conclusion about their efficacy and safety.

The experience of the surgeon in practising hepatic surgery, whatever is the method to perform it, is still a factor of primary importance. In spite of that, the advent of new diagnostic instruments, new devices for resection and coagulation, a better knowledge of the liver's anatomy and pathology and a closer collaboration with the anaesthetist make the hepatic surgery a kind of surgery more defined and rational. From this point of view new studies based on the use of different surgical strategies, association of different devices and employment of different diagnostic and anaesthetic techniques is desirable.

5.2. Summary of advantages and disadvantages of the parenchymal-division instruments (table 4)

Table.4lists the primary advantages and disadvantages of five instruments used for parenchymal division during liver resection. The CUSA has the principal advantage of precise identification of both vascular and biliary vessels so that they may be controlled by ligature or other methods. In addition, the CUSA provides some haptic feedback to the surgeon so that dissection planes may remain clear. The principal disadvantages of the CUSA are threefold: (1) While the instrument permits removal of a large margin around tumors, the proof of adequate margins ends up in the suction container; (2) due to its mechanism of action, the CUSA is not very good for dissection through the fibrotic tissues found in cirrhotic livers; (3) without considerable education of the operating room personnel, the complexity of the mechanism may be cause for delays or malfunctions during procedures. The water jet affords many of the same advantages as the CUSA. Additionally, it produces minimal marginal necrosis, making it an ideal instrument in certain scenarios. The most important concern with this instrument, however, is the splash, for reasons described above. The harmonic scalpel's primary advantage is its ability to simultaneously cut and coagulate. The associated coagulum, however, may cause delayed complications. Originally devised for laparoscopic use, the harmonic scalpel's design is not particularly advantageous for open cases. Used as an adjunctive instrument, the stapler provides the possibility for speedier dissections. On the other hand, the stapler is a relatively imprecise instrument that also has the potential to malfunction during procedures. The floating ball is a surgeon-friendly instrument, particularly for the novice liver resectionist. Its mode of action may be particularly helpful in cirrhosis. The instrument acts by "controlled" burning and therefore is, by nature, an imprecise instrument; plus, there are concerns both for delayed complications related to the coagulum and for steam popping.

http://dx.doi.org/10.5772/54301

5.3. Ranking the clinical usefulness of the five instruments (table 5)

Table 2 subjectively ranks the five instruments according to perceived usefulness in various clinical scenarios. For resection of malignancies, we rank the CUSA number one because of its ability to stay within tissue planes during resections while preserving vessels for ligature. The water jet was second due to concerns about the splash. Third on the list is the floating ball because of its user friendliness. The harmonic scalpel lands fourth on our list because we expect laparoscopic liver resections to increase. We find the water jet to be the most useful instrument for living-donor resections because of the minimal necrotic margin. After the water jet, we advocate the more traditional, fine instrument (e.g., mosquito clamp) dissections. We rank the CUSA third because with experience, the surgeon may minimize the disadvantage of tissue removal.

Instrument	Advantages	Disadvantages
CUSA	permits identification of vessels; tactile feedback	pathologic confusion, use difficult in cirrhosis mechanically complicated do not coagulate, need a combined technique
Water Jet	selective dissection minimal marginal necrosis	splash; possible electolyte imbalances
Harmonic scalpel	cut and coagulate simultaneosly	coagulum precoagulation technique; blind dissection
Ligasure	cut and coagulate simultaneosly	coagulum precoagulation technique; blind dissection
Gyrus	ut and coagulate simultaneosly	coagulum precoagulation technique; blind dissection
TissueLink	friendliness to novices	imprecision, steam popping precoagulation technique
Aquamantys	Friendliness	precoagulation technique
Stapler	speed	imprecision, malfunction
Habib technique	coagulate large vessels	speed

Table 4. Advantages and disadvantages of most common devices

The harmonic scalpel tops the instruments for laparoscopic surgery, primarily because the scalpel is designed for laparoscopic surgery. Another reason the scalpel is particularly useful here is that the principal tumors being removed now via the laparoscope are small benign ones.

Therefore, the imprecision of this instrument is not so much of a disadvantage. The CUSA comes in second primarily because its suction competes with insufflation. Staplers are number three because of their ability to gain quick control over vessels during laparoscopic dissections. Finally, because laparoscopic hepatic surgery is rapidly evolving, we believe there will soon be new uses for old instruments or development of new instruments that will be particularly useful for this approach. For cirrhotic livers, we rank the floating ball number one due to its effective burning of fibrotic tissue. The harmonic scalpel may also be effective. Because of their relative precision, we rank the water jet and CUSA lower than the other two. Staplers do also have a role here.

Scenario	Instrument ranking
resection of malignancies	Cusa
	Water Jet
	Habib
	Tissuelink
	HS and Ligasure
Living donor resections	Tissuelink and Aquamantis
	Water jet
	CUSA
	HS and Ligasure and Gyrus
	Habib
Laparoscopic procedures	HS and Ligasure
	CUSA
	Stapler
Cirrhosis	Tissuelink and Aquamantis
	Habib
	HS and Gyrus
	Water Jet
	CUSA

Table 5. Instrument ranking in various clinical scenarios based on perceived usefulness

Author details

Fabrizio Romano, Mattia Garancini, Fabio Uggeri, Luca Gianotti, Luca Nespoli, Angelo Nespoli and Franco Uggeri

Department of Surgery, University of Milan Bicocca, San Gerardo Hospital Monza, Milan, Italy

References

[1] Poon RT, Fan ST, Lo CM, et al. Improving perioperative outcome expands the role of hepatectomy in management of benign and malignant hepatobiliary diseases: analysis of 1222 consecutive patients from a prospective database. Ann Surg. 2004;240:698 –708

[2] Rees M, Plant G, Wells J et al; One hundred and fifty hepatic resections: evolution of tecnique towards bloodless surgery. British Joumal of Surgery 1996; 83:1526-1529

[3] Doci R, Gennari L, Bignami P et al. Morbidity and Mortality after Hepatic Resection of Metastases from Colorectal Cancer. Br L Surg l995;377-381

[4] Belghiti J, Hiramatsu K, Benoist S, et al. Seven Hundered Hepatectomies in tehe 1990s: an update to evaluate the actual risk of Liver Resection. Journal of American Surgeon 2000,19138-46

[5] Gozzetti G, Mazziotti A, Grazi L et al: Liver Resection without Blood Transfusion. Br J Surg 1995;82:1105-1110

[6] Cunningham JD, Fong Y, Shriver C et al: One Hundred consecutive Hepatic Resections: Blood Loss, Transfusion and Operative Technique. Archives of Surgery 1994;129:1050-1056

[7] Descottes B, Lachachi F, Durand-Fontanier S et al: Right hepatectomies without vascular clamping: report of 87 cases. Journal of Hepatobiliary Pancreatic Surgery 2003; 10:90-94

[8] Romano F, Franciosi C, Caprotti R, Uggeri F, Uggeri F. Hepatic surgery using the Ligasure Vessel System. World Journal of Surgery 2005; 29:110-112

[9] Jarnagin WR, Gonen M, Fong Y, et al: Improvement in Perioperative Outcome after Hepatic Resection: Analysis of 1803 consecutive cases over the past decade. Annals of Surgery 2002;236:397-406

[10] Navarra G, Spalding D, Zacharoulis D, Nicholls JP, Kirby S, Costa 1, Habib NA. Bloodlcss Hcpatectomy Technique. HPB Surg 2002;4:95-97

[11] Rosen CB, Nagomey DM, 1`aswell HF, I-Iegelson S, Ilstrup D, Van Heerden JA. Perioperative blood trasfusion and determinants of survival after liver resection for metastatic colorectal carcinama. Annals of Surgery 1992: 216:493-505

[12] Stephenson KR, Steinberg SM, Hughes KS, Vetto JT, Sugarbaker PH, Chang AE. Perioperative blood trasfusions are associated with decreased time to recurrence and decreased survival after resection for colorectal liver metastases. Annals of Surgery 1988; 208: 679-687

[13] Torzilli G, Makuuchi M, Midorikawa Y et al: Liver Resection Without Total Vascular Exclusion: Hazardous or Bencfuical? An analysis of our Experience. Annals of Surgery 2001; 233:167-175

[14] Kooby DA, Stockman J, Ben-Porat L, Gonen M, Jamagin WR, Dematteo RP, Tuorto S, Wuest D, Blumgart LH, Fong Y. Influence fo Trasfusions on Perioperative and Long-Term Outcome in Patients Following Hepatic Resection for Colorectal Metastases. Annals of Surgery 2003; 237:860-870

[15] Fujimoto J, Okamoto E, Yamanaka N et al: Adverse Effect of Perioperative Blood Transfusions on Survival after hepatic Resection for Hepatocellular Carcinoma. Hepato- Gastroenterlogy 1997; 44:1390-1396

[16] Ohio M, Contini P, Mazzei C et al; Soluble HLA class I, HLA class II and FAS Ligand in Blood Components. A possible key to explain the lmmunomodulatory Effects of Allogenic Blood Transfusionsl Blood 1999; 93:1770-1777

[17] Tait BD, d'Apice AJF, Morrow L, Kennedy L. Changes in suppressor cell activity in renal dialysis patients after blood transfusion. Transplant Proc 1984; 16:995-997

[18] Kaplan J, Samaik S, Levy J. Transfusion-induced immunologic abnormalities not related to the AIDS virus. N Engl J Med 1985; 313:1227

[19] Donnelly PK, Shenton BK, Alomran AM, Francis DM, Proud G, Taylor RM. A new mechanism of humoral immuno-depression in chronic renal failure and its importance to dialysis and transplantation. Proceedings of the European Dialysis and transplant Association 1983; 20:297-304

[20] Lenliard V, Gemsa D, Opelz G. Transfusion-induced release of prostaglandin E2 and its role in the activation ofT suppressor cells. Transplant Proc 1985; 17:2380-2382

[21] Lawrence RJ, Cooper AJ, Lozidou M, Alexander P, Taylor 1. Blood transfusion and recurrence of colorectal cancer: the role of platelet-derived growth factors. British Journal of Surgery 1990; 77:1106-1 109

[22] Torzilli G, Gambetti A, Del Fabbro D, Leoni P, Olivari N, Donadon M, Montorsi M, Makuuch M. _Techniques for Hepatectomies Without Blood Transfusion, Focusing on lnterpretation of Postoperative Anemia. Archives of Surgery 2004; 139:1061-1065

[23] Abdalla EK, Noun R, Belghiti J. Hepatic vascular occlusion: which technique? Surg Clin North Am 2004; 84; 563-85.

[24] Smyrniotis V, Farantos C, Kostopanagiotou G, Arkadopoulos N. Vascular control during hepatectomy: Review of methods and results. World J Surg 2005; 29: 1384-96.

[25] Kim YI. Ischemia-reperfusion injury of the human liver during hepatic resection. J Hepatobiliary Pancreat Surg 2003; 10: 195-9.

[26] Smyrniotis VE, Kostopanagiotou GG, Contis JC, Farantos CI, Voros DC, Kannas DC, Koskinas JS. Selective hepatic vascular exclusion (SHVE) versus Pringle manoeuvre in major liver resections: A prospective study. World J Surg 2003; 27: 765-9.

[27] torzilli

[28] Belghiti J, Noun R, Malafosse R, Jagot P, Sauvanet A, Pierangeli F, et al. Continuous versus intermittent portal triad clamping for liver resection: a controlled study. Ann Surg 1999; 229: 369-75.

[29] Capussotti L, Muratore A, Ferrero A, Massucco P, Ribero D, Polastri R. Randomized clinical trial of liver resection with and without hepatic pedicle clamping. Br J Surg 2006; 93:685-689

[30] Clavien PA, Yadav S, Sindram D, Bentley RC. Protective effects of ischaemic preconditioning for liver resection performed under inflow occlusion in humans. Ann Surg 2000; 232: 155-62

[31] Nuzzo G, Giuliante F, Vellone M, De Cosmo G, Ardito F, Murazio M, et al. Pedicle clamping with ischemic preconditioning in liver resection. Liver transpl 2004; 10: S53-S57.

[32] Clavien PA, Selzner M, Rudiger HA, Graf R, Kadry Z, Rousson V, Jochum W. A prospective randomized study in 100 consecutive patients undergoing major liver resection with versus without ischemic preconditioning. Ann Surg 2003; 238: 843-52.

[33] Makuuchi M, Mori T, Gunven P, Yamazaki S, Hasegawa H. Safety of hemihepatic vascular occlusion during resection of the liver. Surg Gynecol Obstet 1987; 164: 155-8.

[34] Horgan PG, Leen E. A simple technique for vascular control during hepatectomy: The half-Pringle. Am J Surg 2001; 182: 265-7.

[35] Castaing D, Garden OJ, Bismuth H. Segmental liver resection using ultrasound-guided selective portal venous occlusion. Ann Surg 1989; 210: 20-23.

[36] Goseki N, Kato S, Takamatsu S, Dobashi Y, Hara Y, Teramoto K, et al. Hepatic resection under the intermittent selective portal branch occlusion by balloon catheter. J Am Coll Surg 1994; 179: 673-8.

[37] Huguet C, Addario-Chieco P, Gavelli A, Arrigo E, Harb J, Clement RR. Technique of hepatic vascular exclusion for extensive liver resection. Am J Surg 1992; 163: 602-05.

[38] Eyraud D, Richard O, Borie DC, Schaup B, Carayon A, Vezinet C, et al. Hemodynamic and hormonal responses to the sudden interruption of caval flow: Insights from a prospective study of hepatic vascular exclusion during major liver resections. Anesth Analg 2002; 95: 1173-8.

[39] Torzilli G, Makuuchi M, Midorikawa Y, Sano K, Inoue K, Takayama T, Kubota K. Liver resection without total vascular exclusion: hazardous or beneficial? An analysis of our experience. Ann Surg 2001; 233: 161-75.

[40] Elias D, Dube P, Bonvalot S, Debanne B, Plaud B, Lasser P. Intermittent complete vascular exclusion of the liver during hepatectomy: Technique and indications. Hepatogastroenterology 1998; 45: 389-95.

[41] Couinaud C; Le foie: etudes anatomique et chirurgicales. Paris: Masson, 1957

[42] Meyers WC, Shekherdimian S, Owen SM, Ringe BH, Brooks AD. Sorting through methods of dividing the liver. European Surgery 2004; 36:289-295

[43] Schmidbauer S, Hallfeldt KK et al: Experience with Ultrasound Scissors and Blades (UltraCision) in open and laparoscopic liver resection. Annals of Surgery 2002; 235(1): 27-30

[44] H Sugo,Y Mikami, F Matsumoto et al: Hepatic resection using Harmonic Scalpel. Surgery Today 2000; 30:959-962

[45] Kim J, Ahamad SA, Lowy AM et al: Increased biliary fistulas after liver resection with the Harmonic Scalpel. The American Surgeon 2003; 69(9):815-819

[46] Okamoto T, Nakasato Y, Yanagisawa S et al: Hepatectomy using the Coaugulating Shears type of Ultrasonically Activated Scalpel. Digestive Surgery 2001; l8(6):427- 430

[47] Fun ST, Lai ECS, Lo CM et al. Hepatectomy with an Ultrasonic Dissector for hepatocellular carcinoma. British Journal of Surgery 1996; 83:117-120

[48] Nakayama H, Masuda H, Shibata M, Amano S, Fukuzawa M. Incidence of bile leakage after three types of hepatic parenchymal transection. Hepatogastroenterology 2003; 50:15l7-1520

[49] W. Schweiger, A. El-Shabrawi, G. Werkgartner, H. Bacher, H. Cerwenka, M. Thalhammer and H. J. Mischinger Impact of parenchymal transection by Ultracision® harmonic scalpel in elective liver surgery. Eur Surg 2004;36:285-288

[50] Hodgson WJB, Aufses A Jr. Surgical ultrasonic dissection of liver. Surgical Rounds 1979; 2:68

[51] Fusulo F, Giori A, Fissi S et al:-Cavitron Ultrasonic Surgical Aspirator'(CUSA) in liver resection. International Surgery 1992; 77:64-66

[52] Takayama T, Makuuchi M, Kubota K, Harihara Y, Hui AM, Sano K, et al. Randomized comparison of ultrasonic vs clamp transection of the liver. Arch Surg 2001; 136: 922-8.

[53] E Felekouras, E Prassas, M Kontos, I Papaconstantinou, E Pikoulis, A Giannopoulos, C Tsigris, M Tzivras, C Bakogiannis, M Safioleas, E Papalambros, E Bastounis.Liver Tissue Dissection: Ultrasonic or RFA Energy? World J Surg 2006;30:2210-2216

[54] Fan ST, Lai EC, Lo CM, Chu KM, Liu CL, Wong J.Hepatectomy with an ultrasonic dissector for hepatocellular carcinoma Br J Surg. 1996:117-20.

[55] Yamamoto Y, Ikai I, Kume M et al: New simple technique for hepatic parenchymal resection using a Cavitron Ultrasonic Surgical Aspirator and Bipolar Cautery Equipped with a Chamnel for Water Dripping. World Journal of Surgery 1999; 23:1032-1037

[56] Rau HG, Wichmann MW, Schinkel S, Buttler E, PickelmannS, Schauer R, et al. Surgical techniques in hepatic resections: Ultrasonic aspirator versus Jet-Cutter. A prospective randomized clinical trial. Zentralbl Chir 2001;/126:/586_90.

[57] Wrightson WR, Edwards MJ, McMasters KM. The role of the ultrasonically activated shears and vascular cutting stapler in hepatic resection. Am Surg 2000;66:1037–1040.

[58] Koo BN, Kil HC, Choi JS, Kim JY, Chun DH, Hong YW. Hepatic resection by the Cavitron Ultrasonic Surgical Aspirator increases the incidence and severity of venous air embolism. Anesth Analg 2005; 101.966-970

[59] Topp SA, McClurken M, Lipson D, Upadhya GA, Ritter JH, Linehan D, Strasberg SM (2004) Saline-linked surface radiofrequency ablation: factors affecting steam popping and depth of injury in the pig liver. Ann Surg 239: 518–527

[60] Sakamoto Y, Yamamoto J et al: Bloodless liver resection using the Monopolar Floating Ball plus Ligasure Diathermy: preliminary results of 16 liver resections. World Joumal of Surgery

[61] Di Carlo I, Barbagallo F, Toro A et al. Hepatic resection using a water-cooled, high-density, Monopolar Device: a new technology for safer surgery. Joumal of gastrointestinal surgery 2004; 5 596-600

[62] Aloia TA, Zorzi D, Abdalla EK, Vauthey JN. Two surgeon technique for hepatic parenchymal transection of the non-cirrhotic liver using a salin-linked cautery and ultrasonic dissection. Ann Surg 2005;242;172-177

[63] Torzilli G, Donadon M, Marconi M, Procopio F, Palmisano A, Del Fabbro D, Botea F, Spinelli A, Montorsi M. Monopolar floating ball versus bipolar forceps for hepatic resection: a prospective trial. J Gastrointest Surg. 2008 Nov;12(11):1961-6

[64] Arita J, Hasegawa K, Kokudo N. Randomized clinical trial of the effect of a saline-linked radiofrequency coagulator on blood loss during hepatic resection. Br J Surg. 2005;92:954–959.

[65] Sandonato L, Soresi M, Cipolla C, Bartolotta TV, Giannitrapani L, Antonucci M, Galia M, Latteri MA. Minor hepatic resectio for hepatocellular carcinoma in cirrhotic patients: kelly clamp crushing resection versus heat coagulative necrosis with bipolar radiofrequency devices Am Surg. 2011;1490-5

[66] Geller DA, Tsung A, Maheshwari V, et al. Hepatic resection in 170 patients using saline-cooled radiofrequency coagulation. HPB 2005;7:208.

[67] Horgan PG: A novel technique for parenchymal division during hepatectomy. The American Journal of Surgery 2001; 181: 236-237

[68] Strasberg SM, Drebin JA, Linehan D. Use of Bipolar Vessel-Sealing Device for Parenchymal Transecticn During Liver Surgery. Journal of Gastrointestinal Surgery 2002,6:569-574

[69] Nanashima A, Tobinaga S, Abo T, Nonaka T, Sawai T, Nagayasu T. Usefulness of the combination procedure of crash clumping and vessel sealing for hepatic resection. J Surg Oncol. 2010 Aug 1;102:179-83

[70] Tepetes K, Christodoulidis G, Spryridakis EM. Tissue Preserving Hepatectomy by a Vessel Sealing Device Journal of Surgical Oncology 2008;97:165–168

[71] Patrlj L, Tuorto S, Fong Y. Combined blunt-clump dissection and Ligasure ligation for hepatic parenchyma dissection: postcoagulation technique. J Am Coll Surg. 2010;210:39-44

[72] Doklestić K, Karamarković A, Stefanović B, Stefanović B, Milić N, Gregorić P, Djukić V, Bajec D. The Efficacy of Three Transection Techniques of the Liver Resection: A Randomized Clinical Trial. Hepatogastroenterology. 2011 ;59:117-121.

[73] Saiura A, Yamamoto J, Koga R, Sakamoto Y, Kokudo N, Seki M, et al. Usefulness of LigaSure for liver resection: analysis by randomized clinical trial. Am J Surg 2006;/192:/41-45.

[74] M Ikeda, K Hasegawa, K Sano, H Imamura, Y Beck, Y Sugawara,, N Kokudo, M Makuuchi. The Vessel Sealing System (LigaSure) in Hepatic Resection. A Randomized Controlled Trial Ann Surg 2009;250:199-203

[75] Slakey DP. Laparoscopic liver resection using a bipolar sealing device: Ligasure. HPB 2008;10:253-5.

[76] S Evrard, Y Bécouarn, R Brunet, M Fonck, C Larrue, S Mathoulin-Pélissier. Could bipolar vessel sealers prevent bile leaks after hepatectomy? Langenbecks Arch Surg; 392: 41–44

[77] Andoh H, Sato Y, Yasui O et al: Laparoscopic right hemihepatectomy for a case of polycystic disease with right predominance. Joumal of Hepatobiliary Pancreatic Surgery 2004; 11:1l6-118

[78] Garancini M, Gianotti L, Mattavelli I, Romano F, Degrate L, Caprotti R, Nespoli A, Uggeri F. Bipolar vessel sealing system vs. clamp crushing technique for liver parenchyma transection. Hepatogastroenterology. 2011 Jan-Feb;58:127-32

[79] Papachristou DN, Barters R: Resection of the liver with a waterjet. British journal of Surgery 1982; 69:93-94

[80] Une Y, Uchino J, Shimamura T et al: Water Jet Scalpel for liver resection in Hepatocellular Carcinoma with or without Cirrhosis. Intemational Surgery 1996; 81:45-48

[81] Izumi R, Yabushita K, Yagi M et al: Hepatic resection using a water jet dissector. Surgery today 1993; 23:31-35

[82] Rau HG, Wichmann MW, Schinkel S, Buttler E, Pickelmann S, Schauer R, Schildberg FW. Surgical techniques in hepatic resections: Ultrasonic aspirator versus Jet-Cutter. A prospective randomized clinical trial]. Zentralbl Chir. 2001 Aug;126:586-90..

[83] Rau HG, Duessel AP, Wurzbacher S. The use of water-jet dissection in open and laparoscopic liver resection. HPB 2008;10:275-80

[84] Fong Y, Blumgart LH. Useful stapling techniques in liver surgery. J Am Coll Surg 1997;/185:/93 -100.

[85] Kaneko H, Otsuka Y, Takagi S, Tsuchiya M, Tamura A, Shiba T. Hepatic resection using stapling devices. Am J Surg 2004;/ 187:/280 4.

[86] P Schemmer, H Friess, U Hinz, A Mehrabi, T W. Kraus, K Z'graggen, J Schmidt, W Uhl, MW. Bu chler. Stapler hepatectomy is a safe dissection technique. Analysis of 300 patients. World J Surg 2006;30;419-430

[87] Wang WX, Fan ST. Use of the Endo-GIA vascular stapler for hepatic resection. Asian J Surg 2003;/26:/193 6.

[88] Weber JC, Navarra G, Jiao NR, Nicholls JP, Jensen SL, Habib NA. New technique for liver resection using heat coagulative necrosis. Annals of Surgery 2002,236: 1-4

[89] Stella M, Percivale A et al: Radiofrequency-assisted liver resection. Journal of Gastrointestinal Surgery 2003; 7:797-801

[90] Haghighi KS, Wang F, King J, Daniel S, Morris DL. In-line radiofrequency ablation to minimize blood loss in hepatic parenchymal transection. Am J Surg 2005;/190:/43 7.

[91] Pai M, Frampton AE, Mikhail S, Resende V, Kornasiewicz O, Spalding DR, Jiao LR, Habib NA. Radiofrequency assisted liver resection: analysis of 604 consecutive cases.. Eur J Surg Oncol. 2012;38:274-80

[92] Pai M, Jiao LR, Khorsandi S, et al. Liver resection with bipolar radiofrequency device: Habibtrade mark 4X. HPB 2008;10: 256–60.

[93] A Ayav, L Jiao, R Dickinson, J Nicholls, M Milicevic, R Pellicci, P Bachellier,N Habib. Liver Resection With a New Multiprobe Bipolar Radiofrequency Device. Arch Surg 2008;143:396-401

[94] Ayav A, Bachellier P, Habib NA, et al. Impact of radiofrequency assisted hepatectomy for reduction of transfusion requirements. Am J Surg. 2007;193:143-148.

[95] Chang YC, Nagasue N, Lin XZ et al: Easier hepatic resection with a straight needle. American Journal of Surgery 2001; 182:260-264

[96] Chang YC, Nagasue N, Chen CS, Lin XZ. Simplified hepatic resection with the use on Chang's Needle. Annals of Surgery 2006; 243:169-172

[97] Y. C. Chang, N. Nagasue. Blocking intrahepatic inflow and backflow using Chang's needle during hepatic resection: Chang's maneuver. HPB 2008;10:244-248

[98] CU Corvera, SA Dada, JG Kirkland, BS Ryan, D Garrett, BA Lawrence, W Way, L Stewart. Bipolar Pulse Coagulation for Resection of the Cirrhotic Liver. Journal of Surgical Research 2006;136, 182-186

[99] MR Porembka, MB Majella Doyle, NA Hamilton, PO Simon, SM Strasberg, DC Linehan, WG Hawkins. Utility of the Gyrus open forceps in hepatic parenchymal transection. Hpb 2009;11:258-263

[100] J Tan, A Hunt, R Wijesuriya, L Delriviere, A Mitchell. Gyrus PlasmaKinetic bipolar coagulation device for liver resection ANZ J Surg 2010;80:182-185

[101] Shukla PJ, Pandey D, Rao PP, Shrinkhande SV, Thakur MH, Arya S, Ramani S, Mehta S, Mohandas KM. Impact of intra-operative ultrasonography in liver surgery. Indian J oumal of Gastroenterology 2005; 24(2):62-65

[102] Bismuth H, Castaing D, Garden OJ. The use of operative ultrasound in surgery of primary liver tumors. World Journal of Surgery 1987;11:6l0-614

[103] Staren ED, Gambla M, Deziel DJ et al: Intraoperative ultrasound in the management of liver neoplasm. American Surgeon 1997;63:591-596

[104] Parker GA, Lawrence W Jr, Florsley JS et al. Intraoperative ultrasound of the liver affects operative decision making. Annals of Surgery l989;209:569-577

[105] DeMatteo RP. Anatomic segmental hepatic resection is superior to wedge resection as an oncologic operation for colorectal liver metastases. Journal of Gastrointestinal Surgery 2000; 4:178-184

[106] Kokudo N. Anatomical Major resection versus nonanatomical limited resection for liver metastases from colorectal carcinoma. American Journal of Surgery; 181:153-159

[107] Kokudo N, Miki Y, Sugai S, Yanagisawa A, Kato Y, Sakamoto Y, Yamamoto J, Yamaguchi T, Muto T, Makuuchi M. Genetic and histological assessment of surgical margins in resected liver metastases from colorectal carcinoma: minimum surgical margins for successful resection. Archives of Surgery 2002; 137:833-840

[108] Torzilli G, Del Fabbro D, Olivari N, Calliada F, Montorsi M, Makuuchi M. Contrast-enhanced ultrasonography during liver surgery. British Journal of Surgery 2004; 91:1165-1167

[109] Torzilli G, Olivari N, Del Fabbro D, Gambetti A, Leoni P, Montorsi M, Makuuchi M. Contrast-enhanced intraoperative ultrasonography in surgery for hepatocellular carcinoma in cirrhosis, Liver Transplantation 2004; 10:534-38

[110] Torzilli G, Del Fabbro D, Palmisano A, Donadon M, Bianchi P, Roncalli M, Balzarini L, Montorsi M. Contrast-enhanced intraoperative ultrasonography during hepatectomies for colorectal cancer liver metastases. Journal of Gastrointestinal Surgery 2005; 9:1148-1153

[111] Melendez JA, Arslan V, Fischer ME, Wuest D, Jarnagin WR, Fong Y, Blumgart LH. Perioperative Outcomes of Major Hepatic Resection under Low Central Venous Pressure Anesthesia: Blood Loss, Blood Trasfusion, and the Risk of Postoperative Renal Dysfunction. Journal of American College of Surgeons 1998; 187:620-625

[112] Terai C, Anada H, Matsushima S et al: Effect of mild Trendelemberg on Central Hemodynamics and Intemal Jugular velocity, cross sectional area, and Flow. American Journal of Emergency Medicine 1995; 13:255-258

[113] Hughson RL, Maillet A, Gauquelin G, et al: Investigation of hormonal effects during 10-h head-down tilt on heart rate and blood pressure variability. Journal of Applicated Physiology 1995; 78:583-596

[114] Smymiotis V, Kostopanagiotou G, Theodoraki K, Tsantoulas D, Contis JC. The role of central venous pressure and type of vascular control in blood loss during major liver resections. American Journal of Surgery 2004; 187:398-402

[115] Chen H, Merchant NB, Didolkar MS. Hepatic resection using intermittent vascular inflow occlusion and low central venous pressure anesthesia improves morbidity and mortality. Journal of Gastrointestinal Surgery 2000; 4:162-167

[116] Johnson M, Mannar R, Wu AVO. Correlation between Blood Loss and Interior Vena Cava Pressure during Liver Resection. British Journal of Surgery 1998; 85:188-190

[117] Paputheodoridis GV, Burroughs AK. Hemostasis in hepatic and biliary disorders. In: Blumgart LH, Fong Y, eds. Surgery of the liver and biliary tract, 3rd ed. London: Saunders, 2000:199-213

[118] Oguro A, Taniguchi H, Daidoh T et al. FActcrs relating to coagulation, fibrinolysis and hepatic damage after liver resection. Hepatobiliary Pancreatic Surgery 1993; 7:43-49

[119] Lentschener C, Benhamou D, Mercier FJ Boyer-Neumann C, Naveau S, Smadja C, Wolf M, Franco D. Aprotinin reduces blood loss in patients undergoing elective liver resection. Anesth Analg 1997; 84:875-881

[120] Wu CC, Ho WM, Cheng SB, Yeh DC, Wen MC, Liu TJ, P'eng FK. Perioperative parenteral Tranexamic Acid in liver tumour resection: a prospective randomized trial toward a "blood transfusion"-free hepatectomy. Annals of Surgery 2006; 243:173- 180

[121] Lersutel M, Selzner M, Petrowsky S, McCormack L, Clavien PA. How should transection of the liver be performed?: a prospective randomized study in 100 consecutive patients: comparing four different transection strategies. Ann Surg 2005;/242:/814_22.

[122] KS Gurusamy, V Pamecha, D Sharma, BR Davidson. Techniques for liver parenchymal transection in liver resection. Cochrane Library Copyright © 2009 The Cochrane Collaboration. Published by JohnWiley & Sons, Ltd.

[123] Torzilli G, Procopio F, Donadon M, Del Fabbro D, Cimino M, Montorsi M. Safety of intermittent Pringle maneuver cumulative time exceeding 120 minutes in liver resection: a further step in favor of the "radical but conservative" policy.Ann Surg. 2012 Feb;255:270-80

[124] Rahbari NN, Koch M, Schmidt T, Motschall E, Bruckner T, Weidmann K, Mehrabi A, Büchler MW, Weitz J. Meta-analysis of the clamp-crushing technique for transection of the parenchyma in elective hepatic resection: back to where we started? Ann Surg Oncol 2009;16:630-639

[125] Jagannath P,ChhabraDG, Sutariya KR et al. (2010)Fusion technique for liver transection with Kelly-clysis and harmonic technology. World J Surg 34:101–105.

[126] N Gotohda, M Konishi, S Takahashi, T Kinoshita, Y Kato, T Kinoshita. Surgical Outcome of Liver Transection by the Crush-Clamping Technique Combined with Harmonic FOCUS. World J Surg (2012) 36:2156–2160

[127] Romano F, Garancini M, Caprotti R, Bovo G, Conti M, Perego E, Uggeri F. Hepatic resection using a bipolar vessel sealing device: technical and histological analysis.HPB 2007;9:339-44

[128] Romano F, Franciosi C, Caprotti R, Uggeri F, Uggeri F. Hepatic surgery using the Ligasure vessel sealing system. World J Surg. 2005 Jan;29:110-2

[129] Pai M, Jiao LR, Khorsandi S, et al. Liver resection with bipolar radiofrequency device: Habibtrade mark 4X. HPB 2008;10: 256–60.

[130] A Nanashima,S Tobinaga, T Abo, T Nonaka, T Sawai, T Nagayasu. Usefulness of the Combination Procedure of Crash Clamping and Vessel Sealing for Hepatic Resection. Journal of Surgical Oncology 2010;102:179–183

[131] Smith DL, Arens JF, Barnett CC, et al. A prospective evaluation of ultrasound directed transparenchymal vascular control with linear cutting staplers in major hepatic resections. Am J Surg 2005;190:23–29.

[132] MÁ Martínez-Serrano, L Grande, F Burdío, E Berjano, I Poves, R Quesada. Sutureless hepatic transection using a new radiofrequency assisted device. Theoretical model, experimental study and clinic trial. CIR ESP. 2011;89:145–151

[133] Aloia TA, Zorzi D, Abdalla EK, Vauthey JN. Two-surgeon technique for hepatic transection of the noncirrhotic liver using salinelinked cautery and ultrasonic dissection. Ann Surg 2005; 242: 172–177.

[134] Sakamoto Y, Yamamoto J, Kokudo N, et al. Bloodless liver resection using the monopolar floating ball plus ligasure diathermy: preliminary results of 16 liver resections. World J Surg. 2004;28:166–172.

[135] Aldrighetti L, Pulitano C, Arru M, Catena M, Finazzi R, Ferla G. ''Technological'' approach versus clamp crushing technique for hepatic parenchymal transection: a comparative study. J Gastrointest Surg. 2006;10:974–9.

[136] Lesurtel M, Belghiti J. Open hepatic parenchymal transection using ultrasonic dissection and bipolar coagulation. HPB, 2008; 10: 265- 270

[137] Taniai N, Onda M, Tajiri T, Akimaru K, Yoshida H, Mamada Y. Hepatic parenchymal resection using an ultrasonic surgical aspirator with electrosurgical coagulation. Hepatogastroenterology 2002;/49:/1649 -1651

[138] Patrlj L, Tuorto S, Fong Y. Combined blunt clamp dissection and ligasure ligation for hepatic parenchyma dissection: postcoagulation technique. J Am Coll Surg 2010;210:39-44

[139] Yokoo H, Kamiyama T, Nakanishi K, Tahara M, Fukumori D, Kamachi H, Matsushita M, Todo S. Effectiveness of using ultrasonically activated scalpel in combination with radiofrequency dissecting sealer or irrigation bipolar for hepatic resection. Hepatogastroenterology. 2012 ;59:831-5

http://dx.doi.org/10.5772/54301

[140] Gruttadauria S, Doria C, Vitale CH, Cintorino D, Foglieni CS, Fung JJ, Marino IR. Preliminary report on surgical technique in hepatic parenchymal transection for liver tumors in the elderly: a lesson learned from living-related liver transplantation. J Surg Oncol. 2004 Dec 15;88:229-33

[141] Nagano Y, Matsuo K, Kunisaki C, Ike H, Imada T, Tanaka K, Togo S, Shimada H. Practical usefulness of ultrasonic surgical aspirator with argon beam coagulation for hepatic parenchymal transection. World J Surg. 2005 Jul;29:899-902

[142] Schemmer P, Bruns H, Weitz J, Schmidt J, Büchler MW. Liver transection using vascular stapler: a review. HPB (Oxford) 2008; 10:249-252

[143] Cataldo ET, Earl TM, Chari RS, Gorden DL, Merchant NB, Wright JK, Feurer ID, Wright Pinson C. A clinica comparative analisys of crush/clamp, stapler and dissections sealer hepatic transection method. HPB 2008;10:321-326

[144] Smyrniotis V, Arkadopoulos N, Kostopanagiotou G, Farantos C, Vassiliou J, Contis J, et al. Sharp liver transection versus clamp rushing technique in liver resections: a prospective study. Surgery. 2005;137:306–11

Chapter 8

The Role of Ultrasound in Hepatic Surgery

Mattia Garancini, Luca Gianotti, Fabrizio Romano,
Vittorio Giardini, Franco Uggeri and Guido Torzilli

Additional information is available at the end of the chapter

http://dx.doi.org/10.5772/54420

1. Introduction

The first experiences of ultrasonography (US) during surgical operations dated at the first years of the sixties, when some surgeons employed ultrasound in order to identify urinary or biliary stones [1,2]. These experiences gave birth to 2 important areas of application of ultrasound in the surgical field: intra-operative ultrasonography (IOUS) and interventional ultrasonography.

The first reports concerning the usage of IOUS in liver surgery dated at 1980-81 [3,4].

Hepatic surgery became the most important field of development of IOUS and nowadays the ultrasounds are employed for several goals: the precise localization of lesions and their relationship with surrounding biliary and vascular structures, the examination of the liver anatomy in order to plan the surgical strategy in respect of the oncologic principles, the intra-operative re-staging with identification of new nodules.

In 1968 Gramiak and Shah firstly introduced the ultrasound contrast agents (USCA); later, the introduction of ultrasound contrast agents for the study of the liver in 1999 [5], and then the intra-operative contrast enhanced ultrasound (CEIOUS) [6] offered further development to this important technique.

Nowadays the IOUS is considered an invaluable tool for hepatic surgery and its usage should be considered mandatory. CEIOUS demonstrates great potentialities but its role has not been established yet, even considering recent developments of multi-slice computerized tomography and magnetic resonance with liver-specific contrast agents.

2. IOUS and CEIOUS: Technical aspects

If compared to the trans-abdominal conventional US, IOUS offers several advantages. First, the higher resolution of the ultrasonographyc images, because the probe is in direct contact with the liver avoiding the absorption of acoustic waves by the abdominal wall. Second, during conventional US the liver has to be "spied" within the acoustic windows (es: transcostal), meanwhile during IOUS the proper intra-operative probes [Fig 1] can be placed in contact with the anterior, superior, inferior or posterior liver surface and a lesion can be studied from different point of view; consequently, IOUS performed after liver mobilization offers much more information. Third, during IOUS, information obtained with the ultrasound study and information gained by inspection and palpation can complement each other.

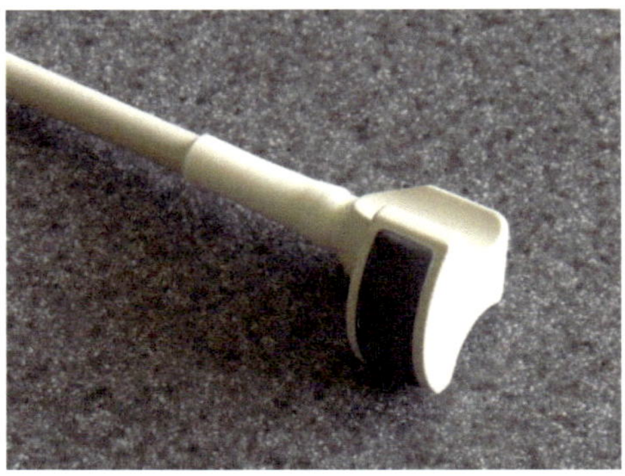

Figure 1. Intra-operative ultrasound probe

The non-panoramic nature of the study represents the main limitation of every US examination, included the IOUS. A great attention should be paid to examine the whole liver parenchyma, avoiding to leave some portion of the liver unexplored. For this reason, information gained by IOUS should always be integrated with the ones obtained from the pre-operative and panoramic study like computerized tomography (CT) and magnetic resonance (MR).

Before IOUS of the liver, partial hepatic mobilization with section of the round and falciform ligaments is always suggested.

Firstly, the liver should be explored using a standard convex (frequencies: 3.75-10 MHz) or micro-convex probe (frequencies: 3.75-10 MHz), in order to obtain a wide ultrasonographyc imaging. The probe should be initially placed between segment 4a and 4b to visualize the hepatic hilum, and then moved on the liver surface evaluating presence of eventual anatomical abnormalities of portal, arterial or biliary pedicles and of sub-hepatic venous system. Then the liver should be explored and mapped searching for focal lesions; precise localization of the lesions detected at pre-operative staging must be confirmed and new lesions must be mapped. A standardized sequential study of each segment is suggested for that, avoiding to leave unexplored portion of liver.

http://dx.doi.org/10.5772/54420

Afterwards, when indicated, the CEIOUS can be performed; main goals of the CEIOUS are characterization of lesions of uncertain nature and detection of new lesions not previously visualized.

The contrast agent (example: 4.8 ml of Sulfur Hexafluoride) has to be injected in a peripheral vein (cannula of 21 gauge or larger) and the arterial, portal and late phases are monitored (CEIOUS phases are reported in Table 1 and Figure 2); if necessary the USCA can be repeated twice.

Phase	Time (seconds)
Injection	0
Arterial phase	10-45
Portal phase	45-90
Late phase	90-240

Table 1. CEUS and CEIOUS vascular phases

The main advantage of the trans-abdominal contrast enhanced ultrasound (CEUS) and of the CEIUOS is that they allow a continuous real-time imaging; consequently they offer much more information for characterization of nodules than contrast-enhanced CT and MR, whose main limitation is that they are non-continuous techniques.

3. CEIOUS: The contrast agents

The acoustic difference between the intra-vascular gas microbubbles and the surrounding blood and tissues represents the basis for use of ultrasound contrast agents (USCA). The gas content of first-generation USCA (eg: Levovist, Schering AG, Berlin, Germany) is air, and the outward diffusion of air results in a relatively rapid decrease in the acoustic reflection and hence limited clinical utility. The stability of newer USCA like Optison (GE Healthcare, Amersham, Buckinghamshire, England), SonoVue (Bracco, Milan, Italy), and Definity (Bristol-Myers Squibb, Billerica, MA) is achieved by use of highmolecular-weight gases, and the slower outward diffusion of these gases makes such second generation USCAs more effective and long lived in the vascular system.

In recent years microbubbles taken up by Kupffer cells, thus possessing a "post-vascular" phase, were registered as a new second-generation USCA in Japan (Sonazoid, GE Healthcare). During the post-vascular Kupffer-phase, the tumour appears as a contrast defect image due to the lack of Kupffer cells and can consequently be characterized.

The usage of some USCAs is not approved in Italy, and authors' experience hare reported is limited to the Sulfur Hexafluoride (SonoVue, Bracco, Milan, Italy).

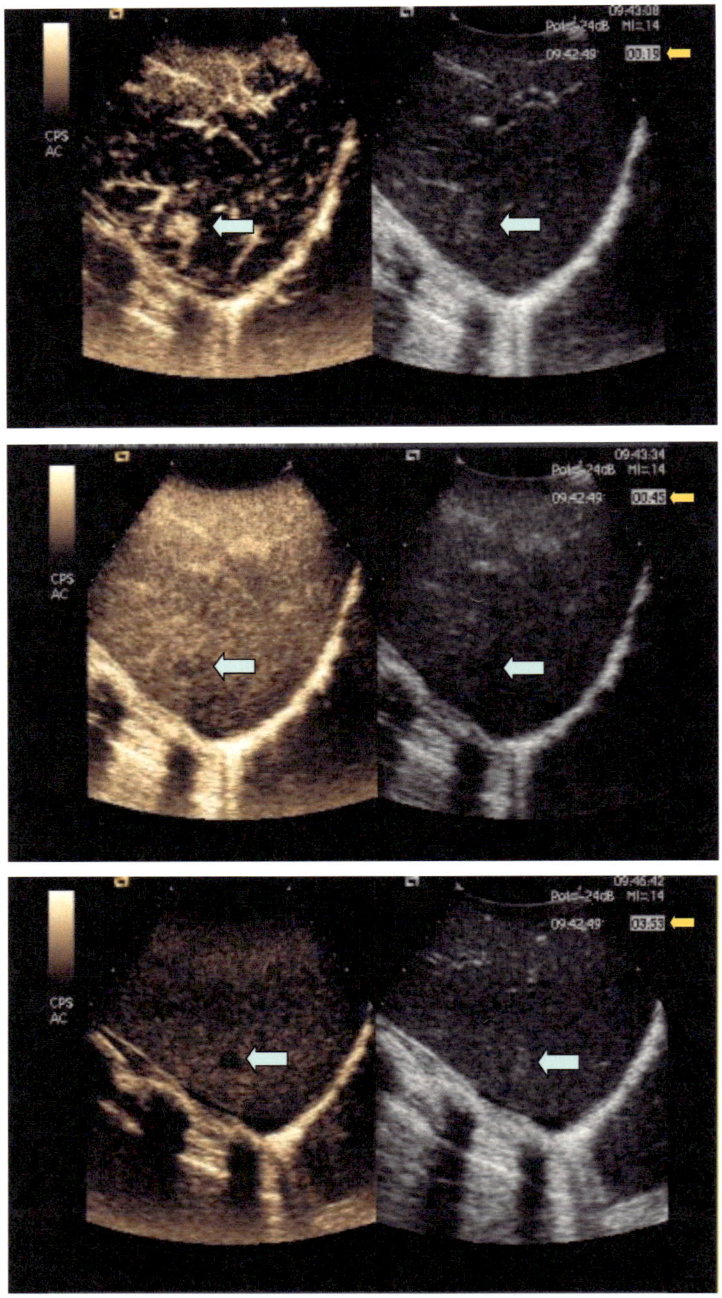

Figure 2. This picture shows a colorectal liver metastases (indicated by azure-blu arrows) in the arterial, portal and tardive phases (time passes form the injection of contrast agents is indicated by yellow arrows) during an contrast-enhanced intra-operative ultrasound study.

4. IOUS and CEIOUS: The intra-operative re-staging

Nowadays, IOUS is still considered the most accurate diagnostic technique for detecting focal liver lesions [7,8]. Nevertheless, it's remarkable that recent technical ameliorations in radiology allowed better outcomes in terms of sensitivity and specificity regarding the detection of primitive and metastatic liver lesions. In particular, the recent availability of multidetector-row Computerized Tomography (CT) with more than 64 channels and of liver specific contrast agents in Magnetic Resonance (MR) represent a great improvement in the diagnostic accuracy of liver tumours.

Hepatocellular carcinoma (HCC) and colo-rectal liver metastases (CRLM) represent the most common malignant liver lesions and the most common indication to liver resection worldwide, and consequently in this chapter the attention will be focused to the staging of these tumours.

4.1. Colorectal liver metastases

Concerning the detection of synchronous liver metastases, the contrast enhanced CT is reported to have a sensitivity and the specificity of respectively 64-72% and 64-72% [9,10], although some recent studies conducted on smaller populations showed values of sensibility of 71.7–92% [11-14]. On the other hand, concerning the detection of metachronous liver metastases, the efficacy of contrast enhanced CT revealed to be unimpressive in term of sensibility [15].

MR showed sensibility ranging from 42 and 100%; the sensibility of MR with liver-specific non-superparamagnetic contrast agents ranges between 64 and 98%, resulting generally superior when compared to the sensibility of CT scan, and a specificity of 75-79% [16-20].

In literature the data regarding the sensibility of the Positron Emission Tomography (PET) – CT appear contrasting, meanwhile the specificity is considered higher than the ones obtained by contrast enhanced CT and MR [21-23].

The trans abdominal CEUS showed high values of sensibility (80-98%) and specificity (66%-98%) for the detection of CRLM; for lesions larger than 20 mm, when sulphur-hexafluoride microbubbles (SonoVue®, Bracco, Milan, Italy) SonoVue is employed as contrast agent, the sensibility is 100% and consequently superior to conventional ultrasound and comparable to contrast enhanced CT [24-29]. It's remarkable that the studies included in these reviews regard mostly comparisons between different radiologic techniques without the anatomo-pathologic or follow up data.

Several studies demonstrated that IOUS of the liver is useful for the intra-operative re-staging of patients undergoing to liver resection for CRLM [7,8] and of patients undergoing to colorectal resection of the primitive neoplasm even in absence of liver lesions detected during pre-operative work-up [30-31]. The superiority of the IOUS compared to pre-operative studies in terms of sensibility leads to a modification of the surgical strategy [32]. The main limitation of the IOUS is the difficult characterization of the nodules; it has been ridden out after the introduction of the USCAs.

Several studies demonstrated that the CEIOUS is the most accurate diagnostic technique for detection and characterization of liver nodules; both the sensibility and specificity of CEIOUS in studies based on the comparison with other diagnostic techniques like CT and MR rises up to 100% and downsize the diagnostic accuracy of the pre-operative staging and even of the IOUS [33-37].

Preliminary results of a prospective study [59] based on the comparison among CEIOUS, CEUS, CT and RM with liver-specific contrast agent for the detection of liver metastases in patients submitted to colorectal resection for cancer, showed that CEIOUS has higher sensibility and specificity when singularly compared to any other pre-operative technique [Table 2]. These results are consistent with the ones previously published in similar setting of patients. In this survey, when the pre-operative work up is analysed on the whole (CT + RM + CEUS), CEIOUS did not offer an amelioration in terms of sensibility but showed an increased value of specificity for better characterization of liver lesions. Moreover, the CEIOUS modified the surgical strategy in 44.4% of patients even when the pre-operative work up is analysed on the whole (CT + RM + CEUS).

	TC	RM	CEUS	CEIOUS
Sensibility	80%	90%	80%	100%
Specificity	93%	79%	100%	100%

Table 2. Sensibility and specificity of CT, RM, CEUS and CEIOUS

Consequently, all patients undergoing liver resection for CRLM and all patients undergoing colorectal resection for cancer should be submitted to IOUS of the liver; moreover, among these patients, all the ones studied during the pre-operative staging with only one radiologic technique, all the ones studied with more than one technique reporting contrasting results and all the ones with new hepatic nodules during IOUS should be submitted to CEIOUS.

4.2. Hepatocellular carcinoma

Studies regarding the accuracy of pre-operative radiologic examinations for HCC assessed values of sensitivity and specificity of 60-93% and 50-95% for CT and of 52-100% and 42-97% for MR respectively; regarding the RM the best results have been obtained employing liver-specific contrast agents [39-40]. On the other side, it's remarkable that the studies included in these reviews regard mostly comparisons between different radiologic techniques without the anatomo-pathologic or follow up data.

Several studies reported that IOUS detects additional nodules in 33-41% of patients undergoing liver resection for HCC [41-43]. In cirrhotic patients with HCC, IOUS is a useful tool to detect new nodules but cannot differentiate malignant lesions from other liver nodules which account for 70–80% [44]. In fact, the risk nowadays is to overestimate the tumour stage with IOUS or laparoscopic ultrasonography considering that, except for those nodules with mosaic ultrasonographic pattern which are malignant in 84% of cases, only 24–30% of hypoechoic nodules, and 0–18% of those hyperechoic are malignant [45]. To overcome this problem even biopsy seems not to be adequate. When sulphur-hexafluoride microbubbles (SonoVue®, Bracco, Milan, Italy), the CEIOUS analysis of nodules vascularization may provide crucial information for their differentiation.

In this sense, Torzilli et al proposed in 2007 [41] a classification for the patterns of enhancement during CEIOUS in 4 categories: A1 (full enhancement in the arterial phase and washout in the delayed phases), A2 (intralesional signs of neovascularization during all phases), A3 (no nodular enhancement but detectability during the liver enhancement), and B (undetectability during the liver enhancement). Following this classification, resection is recommended for A1-3 nodules for high risk of malignancy and no treatment is recommended for B nodules.

With its intra-operative re-staging, CEIOUS shows sensibility of 100%, specificity of 69-100% and can modify the surgical strategy up to 79% of patients [41-43]. All patients undergoing liver resection for HCC should be submitted to IOUS; moreover, all the patients carriers of liver tumours of uncertain differentiation at pre-operative work up and all patients with new nodules at IOUS should be submitted to CEIOUS.

5. Echo-guided liver resection

The modern liver surgery is based on two concepts: a liver resection has to be radical following the oncologic principles and has to be conservative in a parenchyma sparing policy [46]. Consequently the exact resection plane should be carefully planned before the resection using the invaluable ultrasound guidance.

An ultrasound probe is placed on the liver surface and the target lesion to be removed has to be visualized. The surgeon draws on the liver surface the resection plane that includes the tumour; this procedure is simplified by the usage of a linear probe, because if the acoustic waves are parallel, to define the projection of the lesion or of the resection's area on the liver surface is easier (Fig). After that, the parenchymal transection can start, but during the resection the echo-guidance should be used to check if the resection plane is correct or has to be modified.

It's remarkable that the oncologic principles those have to be respected can vary depending on the type of liver tumour.

In presence of CRLM, the most important aspect regards the tumour margin. Positive hepatectomy margin has been indicated as an independent negative prognostic factor for carriers of CRLM [47], but the minimum safe width of free margin has to be established yet. Data regarding the presence of micro-metastases around CRLM are contrasting, reporting rates of micro-metastases ranging from 2% to 58% of patients; consequently, these authors suggested different widths of free margin ranging from 2 to 10 mm [48,49]. If the presence of micrometastases around a CRLM could be related to the cytoreduction after some type chemotherapy has to be clarified yet. The rate of cut edge recurrence is reported to be up to

13.3% for a margin inferior to 2 mm, but if the surgical margin could represents a prognostic factor for patients survival is still debated [48,49]. Anyway, all the authors agree that micro-metastases are confined to a short distance from the tumour (mostly less than 5-10 mm) and that a tumour margin of 10 mm is safe without risk of cut-edge recurrence. The more reasonable approach for carriers of CRLM should be to guarantee a 10 mm margin when possible, so the surgeon during the echo-guided definition of the resection plane should consider this margin. Anyway, because liver resection plus chemotheraphy provides the best chance of cure for carriers of CRLM, complete removal of the tumour with a minimum margin (even less than 2 mm) is justified when technically unavoidable for tumours size, location or number. This aspect is of paramount importance in presence of tumours next to or in contact with major vessels; in these cases, in absence of clear signs of vascular invasion at the IOUS, the vessel resection and consequent major liver resection should be avoided, offering with a parenchyma sparing policy lower post-operative morbidity and mortality. Moreover the avoidance of major hepatectomy allows the possibility of further repeated hepatectomies in patients with disease recurrence, those have shown similar morbidity and mortality compared to first hepatectomy [50].

In presence of HCC, the most important aspect regards the type of surgical resection to be performed, anatomic or non-anatomic. Anatomic resection should be considered the gold standard approach for liver resection in patients with HCC, meanwhile non-anatomic resection should be indicated only in selected patients with HCC set on cirrhosis with poor liver function. Indeed, tumour dissemination from the main lesion through the portal branches demands an anatomic approach with removal of at least the portal area which includes the lesion. The surgical margin per se does not represent a main aspect, because an anatomic resection (segmentectomy or sub-segmentectomy) can be considered adequate even in presence of a narrow margin, while a non-anatomic resection of a nodule with a 10 or even 20 mm margin could be inadequate if the portal branch feeding the nodule has not be removed. HCCs are usually associated with liver cirrhosis, and several series reported that liver resection in cirrhotic patients is related to not negligible postoperative mortality and morbidity [51,52]. The main problem to overcome when planning a surgical approach is to find a balance between the liver volume to be resected, which should be drastically reduced, and the need to perform, if possible, an anatomic resection. The use of IOUS as guidance is indispensable in this sense, but there are several methods up to now available for this procedure. The most diffused technique is the puncture technique proposed by Makuuchi et al in 1981 [53,54]. With this technique, the portal branch feeding the tumour to be resected is punctured under IOUS-guidance, through a free-hand technique or with a proper device, and then dye (usually indigo-carmine) is injected into the vessel while the hepatic artery at the hepatic hilum is clamped. The stained area becomes evident on the liver surface, it is marked with the electrocautery, and hepatic artery clamping is released. The main disadvantage of this technique, other than the quite high skill in puncturing millimetric vessels, is the fact that if the ink regurgitates or is injected into the wrong portal branch, it could be difficult to identify the proper area to be removed. Furthermore, clamping of the hepatic artery is recommended but not always feasible without the need for a hilar dissection to tape the vessel to be clamped. Other methods have been proposed such as a balloon catheter inserted transhepatically to occlude the feeding portal branch [55], or, more recently, through the mesenteric vein [56]. Mazziotti et al. proposed for segment 8 resection the division of the liver along the main portal fissure, and subsequently to approach the segment 8 glissonian pedicle intraparenchymally [57]. Santambrogio et al. have even recently suggested ablation of the feeding portal and arterial branches [58].

More recently Torzilli et al. proposed the ultrasound-guided finger compression technique, consisting in the demarcation of the resection area (segmental either subsegmental) by IOUS-guided finger compression of the vascular pedicle feeding the tumor at the level closest to the tumour but oncologically suitable. This maneuver is constantly monitored in real-time by simply using the same IOUS probe and it is maintained until the surface of the targeted liver area begins to discolor and can be easily marked with the electrocautery [59]. Torzilli's technique offers several advantages, including the non-invasiveness (no intravascular catheter) and rapid reversibility, and consequently can be repeated if necessary.

In general, any other type of primitive or metastatic liver tumours, when a surgical treatment is indicated, can be managed by means of a surgical resection with adequate margins, but in literature data concerning other specific tumours are still lacking.

One more and recent application of IOUS in hepatic surgery concerns the management of liver tumours involving an hepatic vein (HV) next to the caval confluence. These lesions traditionally require a major hepatectomy, with resection of the involved vein and the portion of parenchyma drained by that vein. Nevertheless, as previously reported, morbidity and mortality after major hepatic resections are not negligible, especially in cirrhotic patients [51,52]. A careful intra-operative study of the liver anatomy can offer alternatives to major hepatectomy. In 1987 Makuuchi M et al. introduced a new hepatectomy procedure for resection of the right hepatic vein (when invaded by a tumour) and preservation of the inferior right hepatic vein, an accessory hepatic vein draining segment VI present in 20-25% of patients [60]. Then, in 2010 Torzilli et al. suggested a set of criteria to be met for a parenchyma-sparing liver resection in presence of liver tumours invading any HV at its caval confluence [61]. The criteria are based on the direct or indirect signs of presence of venous anastomoses connecting adjacent HV, those had been previously highlighted in 1958 by Couinaud C et al. during studies performed on liver specimens [62] and can now be detected intra-operatively during IOUS [63].

A segment of a HV can be resected while avoiding the removal of the complete portion of the liver drained by that vein when, during HV finger compression at the hepatocaval confluence, at least one of these criteria is satisfied:

1. Reversal flow direction in the peripheral portion of the hepatic vein to be removed, which suggests drainage through collateral circulation in adjacent HV or inferior cava vein (IVC)

2. Hepatopetal flow in the portal branch feeding the areas to be spared

3. Detectable connecting veins with adjacent HV or IVC

It is remarkable how every surgical procedure performed on the liver is strictly dependent from the knowledge of the liver anatomy and from the ultrasounds; definitely in liver surgery the ultrasounds represent the link between the surgical anatomy and the surgical intervention.

6. Laparoscopic ultrasound

Due to improvements in technologies and increasing surgeon's experiences, the number of hepatectomy performed laparoscopically increased exponentially around the world in the recent years, and consequently the usage of laparoscopic ultrasound (LUS) of the liver [64]. Main goals of LUS are the same of ones presented in open liver surgery; anyway LUS has a few theoretical drawbacks if compared to traditional IOUS, including the difficulty in the ultrasound study of the superior and posterior segments and the limited diffusion of laparoscopic probe equipped for the contrast enhanced study.

Other indications to LUS include the re-staging before laparotomic liver surgery or before laparoscopic resection of gastrointestinal cancer (more frequently of colorectal cancer). Diagnostic laparoscopy combined with LUS is considered an adequate staging modality for primary liver malignancies and permits to avoid unnecessary laparotomies [65]. Nevertheless, the LUS seems to play a limited role in staging patients with potentially resectable CRLM candidates for open liver resection; this is owing mainly to the low sensitivity rate of 59% [66]. Consequently there may be a role for laparoscopy for diagnosing suspected peritoneal disease, but LUS should not be used routinely in patients with CRLM candidates for open liver resection.

The LUS of the liver at the time of primary resection of colorectal cancer is reported to yield more lesions than preoperative contrast-enhanced computerized tomography and could be considered for routine use during laparoscopic oncologic colorectal surgery [67].

One further indication for LUS is laparoscopic radiofrequency in patients carriers of HCC and not amenable to liver resection or percutaneous ablation; in these patients, LUS is an invaluable tool, either in the pre-treatment imaging to re-stage the patient, evaluate the relationship of the tumour with the surrounding structures and to guide the insertion of the electrode into the tumour, either for the post-treatment imaging evaluation [68].

7. Conclusions

Ultrasonography is an invaluable tool in hepatic surgery, either for the intra-operative re-staging, either for the guidance during the surgical procedure. The only major drawback of this IOUS-guided liver surgery is the need for hepatic surgeons to be trained in the use of ultrasound. Indeed, to be fully profitable, IOUS and CEIOUS should be carried out by the surgeon himself who can then use the information obtained by the ultrasound exploration

http://dx.doi.org/10.5772/54420

in a surgical perspective. Organization of a training program for liver surgeons is far from being carried out worldwide, but it should be considered a main goal for hepato-biliary surgeons, because the liver surgeons must be equipped with ultrasound skills as like as with surgical technical skills.

Author details

Mattia Garancini[1], Luca Gianotti[1], Fabrizio Romano[1], Vittorio Giardini[1], Franco Uggeri[1] and Guido Torzilli[2]

*Address all correspondence to: mattia_garancini@yahoo.it

1 Department of General Surgery, Ospedale San Gerardo, Monza, Italy

2 Third Department of Surgery, University of Milan School of Medicine, IRCCS Istituto Clinico Humanitas, Rozzano, Milan, Italy

References

[1] Eiseman B, Greenlaw RH, Gallagher JQ. Localization of common duct stones by ultrasound. Arch Surg 1965;91:195

[2] Schliegel TU, Diggdon P, Cuellar J. The use of ultrasound for localizing renal calculi. J Urol 1961;86:367

[3] Sigel B, Coelho JCU, Spigos DG, et al. Real-time ultrasonography during biliary surgery. Radiology 1980;137:531

[4] Makuuchi M, Hasegawa H, Yamazaki S. Intraoperative ultrasonic examination for hepatectomy. Jap J Clin Oncol 1981;11:367

[5] Blomley MJK, Albrecht T, Cosgrove DO, et al. Improved detection of liver metastases with stimulated acoustic emission in the late phase of enhancement with the US contrast agent SH U 508A: early experience. Radiology 1999;210:409-416

[6] Torzilli G, Olivari N, Moroni E, Del Fabbro D, Gambetti A, Leoni P, Montorsi M, Makuuchi M. Contrast-enhanced intraoperative ultrasonography in surgery for hepatocellular carcinoma in cirrhosis. Liver Transpl 2004;10(2 Suppl 1):S34-38

[7] Sahani DV, Kalva SP, Tanabe KK, et al. Intraoperative US in patients undergoing surgery for liver neoplasms: comparison with MR imaging. Radiology 2004; 232:810–814.

[8] Torzilli G, Makuuchi M. Intraoperative ultrasonography in liver cancer. Surg Oncol Clin N Am 2003;12:91–103.

[9] Bipat S, van Leeuwen MS, Comans EFI, et al. Colorectal liver metastases: CT, MR imaging, and PET for diagnosis--meta-analysis. Radiology 2005;237(1):123-131

[10] Kinkel K, Lu Y, Both M, Warren RS, Thoeni RF. Detection of hepatic metastases from cancers of the gastrointestinal tract by using noninvasive imaging methods (US, CT, MR imaging, PET): a meta-analysis. Radiology 2002;224(3):748-756

[11] Ashraf K, Ashraf O, Haider Z, Rafique Z. Colorectal carcinoma, preoperative evaluation by spiral computed tomography. J Pak Med Assoc 2006;56(4):149-153

[12] Scott DJ, Guthrie JA, Arnold P, et al. Dual phase helical CT versus portal venous phase CT for the detection of colorectal liver metastases: correlation with intra-operative sonography, surgical and pathological findings. Clin Radiol 2001;56(3):235-242

[13] Soyer P, Poccard M, Boudiaf M, et al. Detection of hypovascular hepatic metastases at triple-phase helical CT: sensitivity of phases and comparison with surgical and histopathologic findings. Radiology 2004;231(2):413-420.

[14] Wicherts DA, de Haas RJ, van Kessel CS, et al. Incremental value of arterial and equilibrium phase compared to hepatic venous phase CT in the preoperative staging of colorectal liver metastases: An evaluation with different reference standards. Eur J Radiol 2011;77(2):305-311

[15] Glover C, Douse P, Kane P, et al. Accuracy of investigations for asymptomatic colorectal liver metastases. Dis Colon Rectum 2002;45(4):476-484

[16] Bartolozzi C, Donati F, Cioni D, et al. Detection of colorectal liver metastases: a prospective multicenter trial comparing unenhanced MRI, MnDPDP-enhanced MRI, and spiral CT. Eur Radiol 2004;14(1):14-20

[17] Balci NC, Befeler AS, Leiva P, Pilgram TK, Havlioglu N. Imaging of liver disease: comparison between quadruple-phase multidetector computed tomography and magnetic resonance imaging. J Gastroenterol Hepatol 2008;23(10):1520-1527

[18] Regge D, Campanella D, Anselmetti GC, et al. Diagnostic accuracy of portal-phase CT and MRI with mangafodipir trisodium in detecting liver metastases from colorectal carcinoma. Clin Radiol 2006;61:338-347

[19] Rappeport ED, Loft A, Berthelsen AK, et al. Contrast-enhanced FDG-PET/CT vs. SPIO-enhanced MRI vs. FDG-PET vs. CT in patients with liver metastases from colorectal cancer: a prospective study with intraoperative confirmation. Acta Radiol 2007;48(4):369-378

[20] Koh DM, Brown G, Riddell AM, et al. Detection of colorectal hepatic metastases using MnDPDP MR imaging and diffusion-weighted imaging (DWI) alone and in combination. Eur Radiol 2008;18(5):903-910

[21] Selzner M, Hany TF, Wildbrett P, et al. Does the novel PET/CT imaging modality impact on the treatment of patients with metastatic colorectal cancer of the liver? Ann Surg 2004;240(6):1027-1034; discussion 1035-1036

[22] D'souza MM, Sharma R, Mondal A, et al. Prospective evaluation of CECT and 18F-FDG-PET/CT in detection of hepatic metastases. Nucl Med Commun 2009;30(2): 117-125

[23] Kong G, Jackson C, Koh DM, et al. The use of 18F-FDG PET/CT in colorectal liver metastases-comparison with CT and liver MRI. Eur J Nucl Med Mol Imaging 2008;35(7):1323-1329

[24] Albrecht T, Blomley MJK, Burns PN, et al. Improved detection of hepatic metastases with pulse-inversion US during the liver-specific phase of SHU 508A: multicenter study. Radiology 2003;227(2):361-370

[25] Larsen LPS, Rosenkilde M, Christensen H, et al. The value of contrast enhanced ultrasonography in detection of liver metastases from colorectal cancer: a prospective double-blinded study. Eur J Radiol 2007;62(2):302-307

[26] Konopke R, Kersting S, Bergert H, et al. Contrast-enhanced ultrasonography to detect liver metastases : a prospective trial to compare transcutaneous unenhanced and contrast-enhanced ultrasonography in patients undergoing laparotomy. Int J Colorectal Dis 2007;22(2):201-207

[27] Gültekin S, Yücel C, Ozdemir H, et al. The role of late-phase pulse inversion harmonic imaging in the detection of occult hepatic metastases. J Ultrasound Med 2006;25(9): 1139-1145

[28] Oldenburg A, Hohmann J, Foert E, et al. Detection of hepatic metastases with low MI real time contrast enhanced sonography and SonoVue. Ultraschall Med 2005;26(4): 277-284

[29] Rappeport ED, Loft A, Berthelsen AK, et al. Contrast-enhanced FDG-PET/CT vs. SPIO-enhanced MRI vs. FDG-PET vs. CT in patients with liver metastases from colorectal cancer: a prospective study with intraoperative confirmation. Acta Radiol 2007;48(4):369-378

[30] Milsom JW, Jerby BL, Kessler H, et al. Prospective, blinded comparison of laparoscopic ultrasonography vs. contrast-enhanced computerized tomography for liver assessment in patients undergoing colorectal carcinoma surgery. Dis Colon Rectum 2000;43(1):44-49

[31] Stone MD, Kane R, Bothe A, et al. Intraoperative ultrasound imaging of the liver at the time of colorectal cancer resection. Arch Surg 1994;129(4):431-435; discussion 435-436

[32] Agrawal N, Fowler AL, Thomas MG. The routine use of intra-operative ultrasound in patients with colorectal cancer improves the detection of hepatic metastases. Colorectal Dis 2006;8(3):192-194

[33] Torzilli G, Del Fabbro D, Palmisano A, et al. Contrast-enhanced intraoperative ultrasonography during hepatectomies for colorectal cancer liver metastases. J Gastrointest Surg 2005;9(8):1148-1153; discussion 1153-1154

[34] Leen E, Ceccotti P, Moug SJ, et al. Potential value of contrast-enhanced intraoperative ultrasonography during partial hepatectomy for metastases: an essential investigation before resection? Ann Surg 2006;243(2):236-240

[35] Fioole B, de Haas RJ, Wicherts DA, et al. Additional value of contrast enhanced intraoperative ultrasound for colorectal liver metastases. Eur J Radiol 2008;67(1):169-176

[36] Conlon R, Jacobs M, Dasgupta D, Lodge JPA. The value of intraoperative ultrasound during hepatic resection compared with improved preoperative magnetic resonance imaging. Eur J Ultrasound 2003;16(3):211-216

[37] Torzilli G. Contrast-enhanced intraoperative ultrasonography in surgery for liver tumors. Eur J Radiol 2004;51 Suppl:S25-29

[38] Garancini M. Contrast-enhanced intra-operative ultrasound vs pre-operative imaging for the detection of liver metastases in patients with colo-rectal cancer: a prospective study. Specialization thesis. University of Milano-Bicocca; 2011. (available at: http://www.slc.livermeta.net/index.php/congressi) [accessed 21/09/2012]

[39] Bolog N, Andreisek G, Oancea I, Mangrau A. CT and MR imaging of hepatocellular carcinoma. J Gastrointestin Liver Dis 2011;20:181-189.

[40] Willatt JM, Hussain HK, Adusumilli S, Marrero JA. MR Imaging of hepatocellular carcinoma in the cirrhotic liver: challenges and controversies. Radiology 2008;247(2): 311-330

[41] Torzilli G, Palmisano A, Del Fabbro D, Marconi M, Donadon M, Spinelli A, Bianchi PP, Montorsi M. Contrast-Enhanced Intraoperative Ultrasonography Durino Surgery for Hepatocellular Carcinoma in Liver Cirrhosis: Is It Useful or Useless? A Prospective Cohort Study of Our experience. Ann Surg Oncol 2007;14:1347–1355

[42] Lu Q, Luo Y, Yuan CX, Zeng Y, Wu H, Lei Z, Zhong Y, Fan YT, Wang HH, Luo Y. Value of contrast-enhanced intraoperative ultrasound for cirrhotic patients with hepatocellular carcinoma: A report of 20 cases. World J Gastroenterol 2008;14:4005–4010.

[43] Wu H, Lu Q, Luo, He XL, Zeng Y. Application of contrast-enhanced intraoperative ultrasonography in the decision-making about hepatocellular carcinoma operation. World J Gastroenterol 2010;16:508–512.

[44] Takigawa Y, Sugawara Y, Yamamoto J et al. New lesions detected by intraoperative ultrasound during liver resection for hepatocellular carcinoma. Ultrasound Med Biol 2001;27:151–156

[45] Kokudo N, Bandai Y, Imanishi H, et al. Management of new hepatic nodules detected by intraoperative ultrasonography during hepatic resection for hepatocellular carcinoma. Surgery 1996;119:634–640

[46] Torzilli G, Montorsi M, Donadon M, Palmisano A, Del Fabbro D, Gambetti A, Olivari N, Makuuchi M. "Radical but conservative" is the main goal for ultrasonography-

guided liver resection: prospective validation of this approach. J Am Coll Surg 2005;201(4):517-528.

[47] Hughes KS, Rosenstein RB, Songhorabodi S, Adson MA, Ilstrup DM, Fortner JG, Maclean BJ, Foster JH, Daly JM, Fitzherbert D, et al. Resection of the liver for colorectal carcinoma metastases. A multi-institutional study of long-term survivors. Dis Colon Rectum 1988;31:1-4.

[48] Kokudo N, Miki Y, Sugai S, Yanagisawa A, Kato Y, Sakamoto Y, Yamamoto J, Yamaguchi T, Muto T, Makuuchi M. Genetic and histological assessment of surgical margins in resected liver metastases from colorectal carcinoma: minimum surgical margins for successful resection. Arch Surg 2002;137(7):833-40.

[49] Wakai T, Shirai Y, Sakata J, Valera VA, Korita PV, Akazawa K, Ajioka Y, Hatakeyama K. Appraisal of 1 cm hepatectomy margins for intrahepatic micrometastases in patients with colorectal carcinoma liver metastasis. Ann Surg Oncol 2008;15(9): 2472-2481.

[50] Lopez P, Marzano E, Piardi T, Pessaux P. Repeat hepatectomy for liver metastases from colorectal primary cancer: a review of the literature. J Visc Surg 2012;149:97-103

[51] Poon RT, Fan ST, Lo CM, et al (2002) Extended hepatic resection for hepatocellular carcinoma in patients with cirrhosis: is it justified? Ann Surg 236:602–611

[52] Schroeder RA, Marroquin CE, Bute BP, et al. Predictive indices of morbidity and mortality after liver resection. Ann Surg 2006;243:373–379.

[53] Makuuchi M, Hasegawa H, Yamazaki S. Intraoperative ultrasonic examination for hepatectomy. Jpn J Oncol 1981;11:367–390.

[54] Makuuchi M, Hasegawa H, YamazakiS, et al. Ultrasonically guided systematic subsegmentectomy. Surg Gynecol Obstet 1985;161:346-350

[55] Shimamura Y, Gunve´n P, Takenaka Y, et al. Selective portal branch occlusion by balloon catheter during liver resection. Surgery 1986;100:938–941.

[56] Ou JR, Chen W, Lau WY. A new technique of hepatic segmentectomy by selective portal venous occlusion using a balloon catheter through a branch of the superior mesenteric vein. World J Surg 2007;31:1240 –1242.

[57] Mazziotti A, Maeda A, Ercolani G, et al. Isolated resection of segment 8 for liver tumors: a new approach for anatomical segmentectomy. Arch Surg 2000;135:1224 – 1229.

[58] Santambrogio R, Costa M, Barabino M, et al. Laparoscopic radiofrequency of hepatocellular carcinoma using ultrasound-guided selective intrahepatic vascular occlusion. Surg Endosc 2008;22:2051–2055.

[59] Torzilli G, Procopio F, Cimino M, Del Fabbro D, Palmisano A, Donadon M, Montorsi M. Anatomical segmental and subsegmental resection of the liver for hepatocellular

carcinoma: a new approach by means of ultrasound-guided vessel compression. Ann Surg 2010;251(2):229-235

[60] Makuuchi M, Hasegawa H, Yamazaki S, et al. Four new hepatectomy procedures for resection of the right hepatic vein and preservation of the inferior right hepatic vein. Surg Gynecol Obstet 1987;164:68–72.

[61] Torzilli G, Palmisano A, Procopio F, Cimino M, Botea F, Donadon M, Del Fabbro D, Montorsi M. A new systematic small for size resection for liver tumors invading the middle hepatic vein at its caval confluence: mini-mesohepatectomy. Ann Surg 2010;251(1):33-39

[62] Couinaud C, Nogueira C. Les veines sus-hepatique chez l'homme. Acta Anat (Basel) 1958;34:84-110

[63] Torzilli G, Garancini M, Donadon M, Cimino M, Procopio F, Montorsi M. Intraoperative ultrasonographic detection of communicating veins between adjacent hepatic veins during hepatectomy for tumours at the hepatocaval confluence. Br J Surg 2010;97(12):1867-1873

[64] Nguyen KT, Nguyen KT, Gamblin TC, Geller DA (2009) World review of laparoscopic liver resection: 2804 patients. Ann Surg 250:831–841

[65] de Castro SM, Tilleman EH, Busch OR, van Delden OM, Laméris JS, van Gulik TM, Obertop H, Gouma DJ. Diagnostic laparoscopy for primary and secondary liver malignancies: impact of improved imaging and changed criteria for resection. Ann Surg Oncol 2004;11:522-529.

[66] Hariharan D, Constantinides V, Kocher HM, Tekkis PP. The role of laparoscopy and laparoscopic ultrasound in the preoperative staging of patients with resectable colorectal liver metastases: a meta-analysis. Am J Surg 2012;204:84-92.

[67] Milsom JW, Jerby BL, Kessler H, Hale JC, Herts BR, O'Malley CM. Prospective, blinded comparison of laparoscopic ultrasonography vs. contrast-enhanced computerized tomography for liver assessment in patients undergoing colorectal carcinoma surgery. Dis Colon Rectum 2000;43(1):44-49.

[68] Santambrogio R, Opocher E, Costa M, Cappellani A, Montorsi M. Survival and intrahepatic recurrences after laparoscopic radiofrequency of hepatocellular carcinoma in patients with liver cirrhosis. J Surg Oncol 2005;89:218-225; discussion 225-226.

Chapter 9

Segmental Oriented Liver Surgery

O. Al-Jiffry Bilal and Khayat H. Samah

Additional information is available at the end of the chapter

http://dx.doi.org/10.5772/51775

1. Introduction

Understanding the vascular and biliary anatomy of the liver is mandatory for a successful anatomical liver resection. It is also extremely important in complex liver operations, althaugh it might not be in cases of simple wedge resection for benign disease. As the presence of HCC is usually in the background of liver cirrhosis, the importance of anatomical resection to be able to clear the tumour and have sufficient amount of liver to avoid post-operative liver failure. In this chapter we will try to illustrate the importance of anatomical liver resection and give an idea of the latest liver anatomy with a demonstration on how to identify and resect each part of the liver.

2. Why anatomical liver resection

As many general surgeons might like to do wedge non anatomical liver resections because it is less complicated and gets the tumour out. There are several reasons to perform anatomical resection:

1. In Hepato-Cellular carcinoma (HCC) which is the most common reason to perform liver resections, were it is the first line of treatment nowadays [1,2]. As the HCC are able to invade the portal veins and disseminate through its inter segmental branches [3] (cough reflux), segmentectomy is preferable. Intrahepatic metastasis [4,5] and invasion to the portal and hepatic venous system will affect the post operative prognosis. To improve the post surgical outcome the segmental liver resection is indicated. It involves the removal of the whole segment containing the tumor with its vasculature which might be affected by the tumor invasion [1,4 - 6]. Satellite micro metastasis will also be removed as their feeding vessel for that segment [3].

Anatomic liver resection is superior to non anatomic from the oncologic and anatomic aspects [7]. Anatomically based hepatectomy is the best means of achieving a negative margin[8].The recurrence rate within 2 years associated with aggressive tumor biology such as high tumor grade, satellite lesions and microvascular invasion [7], is higher in non anatomical resection.

In small HCC <4cm anatomic resection achieves better disease-free survival than limited resection without increasing the postoperative risk [9-10].

The overall survival and the disease-free survival rates were significantly better in the anatomic resection compared to the non anatomic resection group [1,11-12],as well as the recurrence disease free survival [10].

A meta-regression analysis was done and published in June 2012 that was conducted on 9036 patients from 1990-2011 and demonstrated that the 5 years disease free survival and the 5 year survival was significantly better in the anatomic resection group than the non anatomic resection group with no effect on the post operative mortality and morbidity[13].

2. Less bleeding with almost no need for transfusion in the intra-operative period as there is no transaction of the vessels. Also there is few vessels present in the inter segmental planes. Relatively the inter segmental area is a non-vascular plane, so segmental identification, control of the feeding vessels and the vascular pedicle will decrease the blood loss. This is one of the direct causes of decreased post operative morbidities and mortalities [3,14 - 16].

3. Segmental resection will preserve as much of the liver parenchyma [3] and will enable sufficient liver volume especially in cirrhotic patients [16] and in patients with multiple liver lesions [17] or in patients who will need another resection in the future. Also it will decrease the post operative liver insufficiency from small liver remnant in cirrhotic patients [3,14,15,16].

4. In colorectal metastasis segmental resection is superior to non anatomical resection as it results in better tumour clearance and free margins. Multiple studies demonstrated that it did affect the disease free survival, and the control of micro-metastasis through segmental portal branches. Segmentectomy offered disease-free and overall survival rates similar to those after major resection. [3,14]

For metastasis it has been found that with wedge resection the recurrence rate and positive margins were higher compared to the segmental resection. This resulted in inadequate tumour resection especially in deep lesions where the incidence of inadvertently cutting into the tumour is higher. Also the bleeding rate is high due to the difficult control of the venous branches that will obscure the resection plane.

Wedge resections are usually inadequate and potentially dangerous, especially for large tumours, and are often associated with greater blood loss and a greater incidence of positive histological margins.[8,11]. Liver failure due to parynchymal necrosis or small liver remnant are observed in non anatomical (wedge) liver resection. It also results in higher incidence of biliary fistula and infection because of the remnant devitalized liver tissue [18].

http://dx.doi.org/10.5772/51775

Non-anatomical liver resection (Wedge) can be done in certain circumstances; in resections where the tumour is small (<3cm) and located peripherally at the edge of a cirrhotic liver or when the tumour is situated at the border of several segments and its resection requires the removal of large volume which is not possible due to the liver status.

Also, in cases of benign liver resection were no safety margin is required and the surgeon would like to preserve as much liver volume as possible, so the lesion can be enucleated. However, care should be taken not to injure nearby vessels or bile ducts.

3. Segmental liver anatomy

3.1. The history

The understanding of liver segments was first established in 1953 by Healy [19] and was further reinforced by Couinaud in 1957 [20]. When trying to understand their description it might be somewhat confusing, however we will try to make it as simple as possible.

They both used the new division by Cantlie who disapproved the old terminology of the right and left liver which was divided by the falciform ligament and used his description of the right and left liver divided by the midline which is oblique and extended from the gallbladder bed to the right side of the inferior vena cava. Healy then divided the liver using the arteriobiliary segmentation. This lead to the division of the right liver into the two segments, the right anterior and the right posterior segments (called now sections). The left side was divided by the falciform into the left medial and left lateral segments (called now sections). However, Couinaud used the hepatic veins and divided the right liver into right anterior and right posterior sectors. The left side was divided by the left hepatic vein into the left medial and left lateral sectors, and the middle hepatic vein was running in the midplane of the liver (Cantile line). Then recently the terminology of segments that was described by Healy was changed to sections leading the way to the word section and sector that you see in all papers involving the liver anatomy. They both divided these sectors or sections to segments according to the portal vein anatomy and we reached to our 8 segments that we know today. **Figure.1**

When looking at these two description you will find that both agreed on the anatomy of the right liver cause there was no difference between the right anterior (segment 5&8) and the right posterior (segments 6&7) section or sector. However, on the left side there was a difference, because of the anatomical variations and we believe this is what led to this misunderstanding. The left medial section (segment 4) is not the same as the left medial sector (segment 3&4), and the left lateral section (segment 2&3) is not the same as the left lateral sector (segment 2). They also both agreed on the separation of segment 1 (caudate Lobe) as it has its own blood supply and drains directly to the inferior vena cava.

Another thing when looking to the terminology is the word "Lobe". Some authors use the term left lobectomy to describe the resection of segments 2&3, which is the functional left lateral section. Also the right lobe as segments 4 to 8 were it is an extended right trisectionectomy.

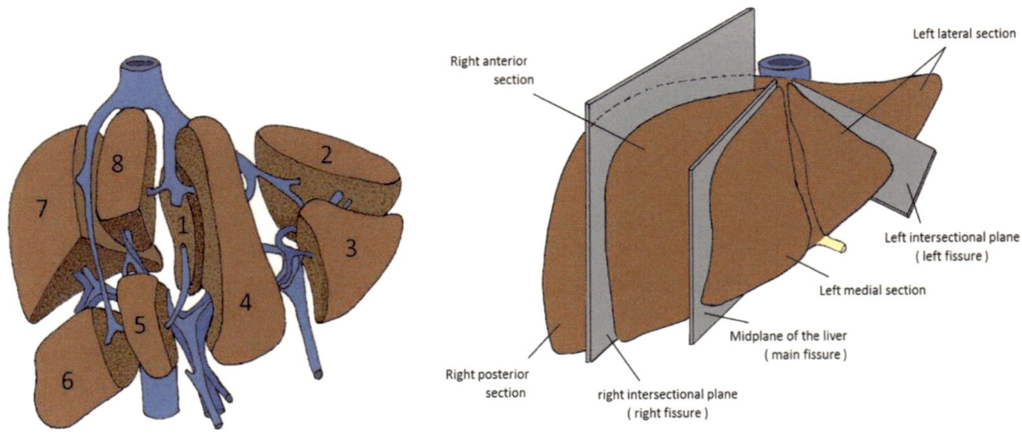

Figure 1. Liver sections, plane and segments

This description was based on the anatomical land mark of the liver using the falciform ligament and not the functioning liver segments as described above.

3.2. The new terminology

The use of many different terminologies and difficulty in understanding the description described above, were the European societies adopted Couinaud's description and the American societies used the Healy's description. So the scientific committee of the International Hepato-Pancreato-Biliary Association with experts around the world came up with the Brisbane 2000 Terminoloy of Liver Anatomy and resection which we have been using and will use for our description in this chapter [21].

To understand this terminology, first the liver is divided into two parts, the main liver and the caudate lobe (called the dorsal sector by Cauinaud). Then the main liver is divided into the right and left liver.

This part is called the first order division, where the liver is divided into the right liver or right hemiliver, and the left liver or the left hemiliver. Notice the word lobe has been removed completely for the confusion we mentioned above, so the resection of the right side is called right hepatectomy or right hemihepatectomy (segments 5 to 8). The left side is called; left hepatectomy or left hemihepatectomy (segments 2 to 4). **Figure.2**

The second order division, where the right liver is divided into two parts. The right anterior section giving the right anterior sectionectomy (segment 5&8), the right posterior section leading to the resection of the right posterior sectionectomy (segments 6&7). On the left side there will be the left medial section giving the left medial sectionectomy (segment 4), and the left lateral section leading to the resection of the left lateral sectionectomy (segment 2&3). **Figure.3**

http://dx.doi.org/10.5772/51775

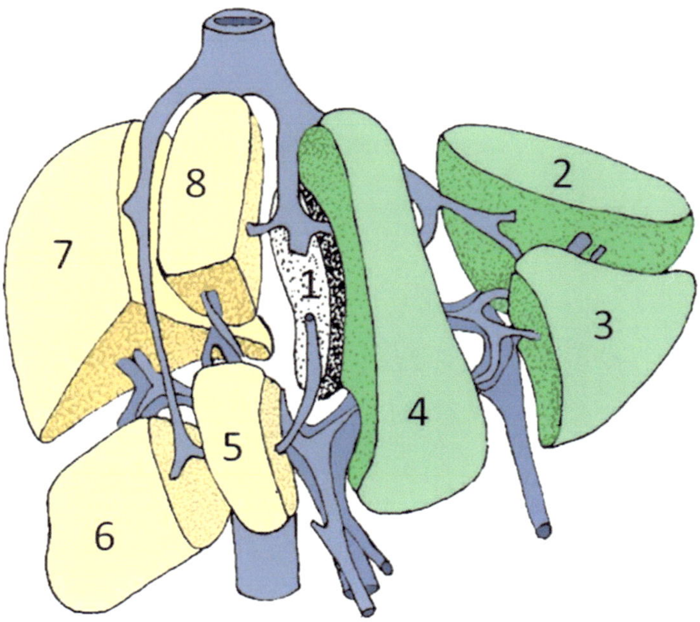

Figure 2. Right (yellow) and left liver (green)

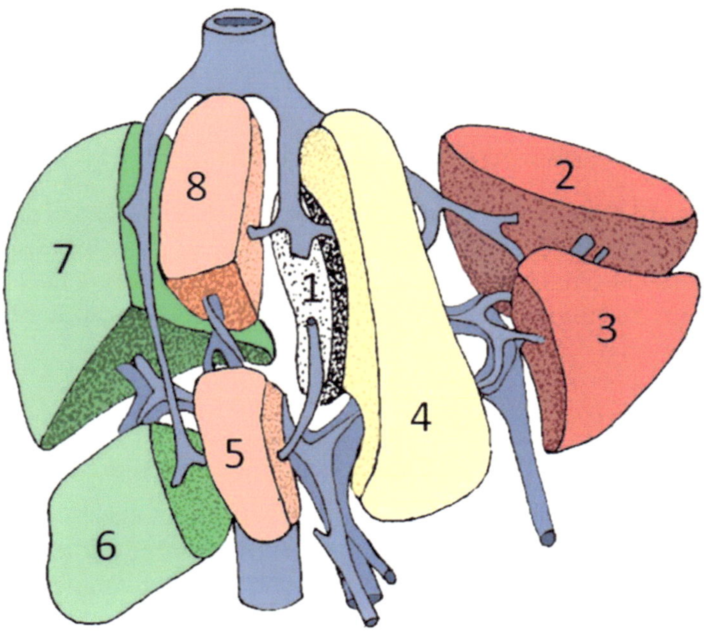

Figure 3. Sections Green: right posterior, orange: right anterior Yellow: left medial, red: left lateral

The third order division, is the division of each of these sections into segments as we mentioned above. The resection of any of these segments is called a segmentectomy and if two or more segments were resected that are not related as described in the second order division it is called bisegmentectomy or trisegmentectomy. This should not be coinfused with the trisectionectomy of the right or left side were we resect three sections and not segments. **Figure.4**

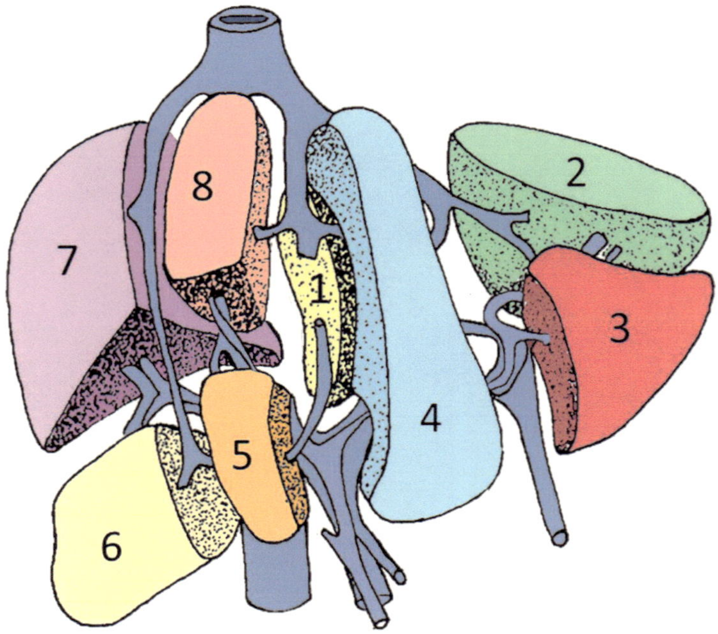

Figure 4. Segments, each with a different color

An addition was added also if the word sector were to be used instead of section. This is the same on the right side and on the left we had a left medial sector with a left medial secterectomy (segment 3&4), and the left lateral sector giving rise to the resection of the left lateral secterectomy (segment 2). So the term section or sector has to be used very cautiously on the left side to describe exactly what you mean.

3.3. Clinical applications

1. As each liver segment can be resected separately, liver resection can be segment based
2. Segement 4, is divided into 4A and 4B. This was made because of multiple indications were segment 4A is rsected without the resection of segment 4B like in cases of gallbladder cancer. Also the resection of segment 4A is counted as the most difficult liver resection as it lies between the middle and the left hepatic vein.
3. This terminology has gained wide acceptance and has removed most of the confusion that use to exist in the past.

http://dx.doi.org/10.5772/51775

3.4. Intrahepatic glissonian triads

The extra hepatic portal triad is consisted of the portal vein, the hepatic artery and the common hepatic duct. These structures are enclosed in a connective tissue and peritoneum up to the hepatic hilum. The term Glissonian sheath is reserved for the part that extendeds into the intrahepatic portion of the liver beyond the hilum. This sheath surrounds the portal triad structure before they enter into each section, giving rise to the resection of each segment (liver unit) separately without affecting the other segments [22]. This gives rise to the aberrance of the central segments 4, 5 and 8 ramifications like a bush and fan shaped. Consequently, a single segment resection will require several Glissonian sheath at various depth and is much more difficult. Were the priphral segments 6, 7, 2 and 3 have long branches that travels a distance reaching to these segments giving the appearance of tree like making their resection less complicated and usually requiring a single Glissonian sheath ligation [23].

3.5. Portal vein and liver resection

On the right side the portal vein is similar to the arteriobiliary segmentation. On the left side they differ from each other. The left portal vein consists of a transverse and an umbilical portion. The transverse portion only sends small branches to segment 4 and one or two branches to segment 1. All the larger branches arise beyond the attachment of the ligamentum venosum (umbilical portion of the left portal vein). **Figure.5**. This part of the vein gives right branches to segment 4 and on the left side it gives one branch to segment 2 and more than one to segment 3. The portal vein terminates where it joins the ligamentum teres at the edge of the liver. This unique structure explains the duael function of the left portal vein during in-utero and then in-adult life.

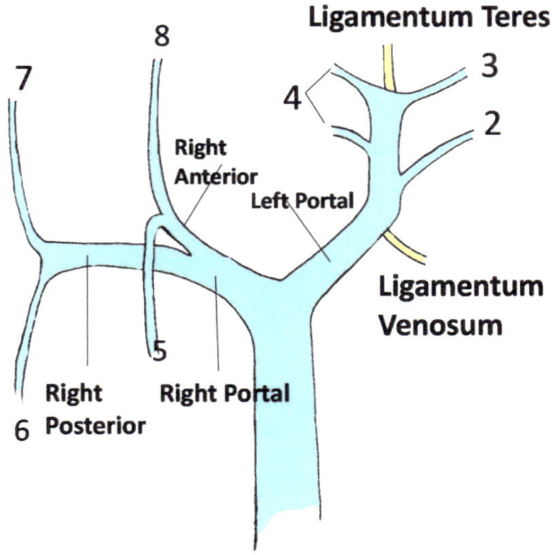

Figure 5. Portal vein with its divisions

On the right side the portal vein is usually very short and gives rise to the right anterior and right posterior branches. Each of these branches gives rise to two main segmental divisions. The right anterior gives both segment 5 and 8, where the right posterior gives segment 6 and 7. **Figure.6.**

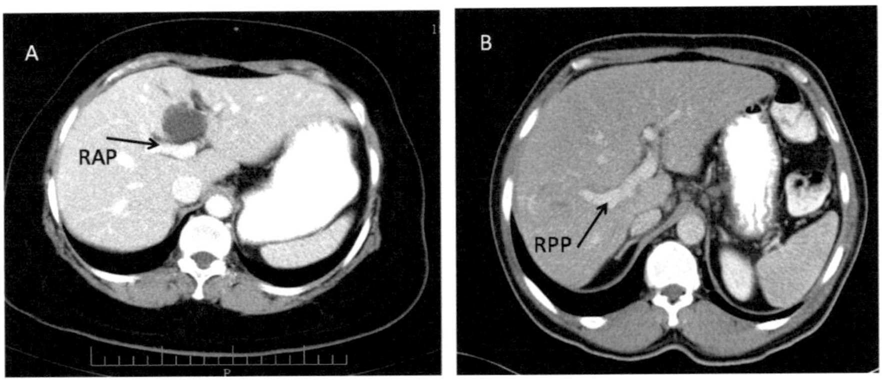

Figure 6. A) right anterior portal branch (RAP) B) right posterior portal branch (RPP)

Usually there are very little variations in the portal vein. The commonest one is where the right anterior branch joins the left portal vein. This is very important to recognise especially when doing a left hepatectomy causes injury could happen to the right anterior section leading to the loss of segments 5 and 8. Another common anomaly is the absence of the main right portal vein giving rise to a trifurcation at the hilum of the portal vein to the left main, right anterior and the right posterior branches. This is important when doing a right hepatectomy to transect each branch separately not to injure the left portal vein [24-25].

4. Clinical identification of the liver segments

For the clinical description of this part we will try to simulate what happens in clinical practice by dividing it to pre-operative radiology and intra-operative by intra-operative ultrasound.

4.1. Pre–operative

To try and make this part as simple as possible for the reader we will try to identify land marks that you should look for in the ultrasound, CT or MRI. The ultrasound is the usual screening tool used to see the whole liver and identify cystic from solid lesions. Then most centres will request a Triphasic CT scan of the liver in the hope to identify the nature of the lesion and the location. A physician should not comment on any lesion seen until full examination of all three phases (arterial, venous and delayed) are examined and the lesion is seen on all three phases to give the best chance of reaching the right diagnosis.

http://dx.doi.org/10.5772/51775

As we described the anatomy of the liver by the first order division and its landmark the middle hepatic vein, it is the same here. The middle hepatic vein can be seen on any of the above mentioned x-ray investigation. This will lead to the division of the liver to the right and left liver and identifying the lesion in which liver it lies. **Figure.7**.

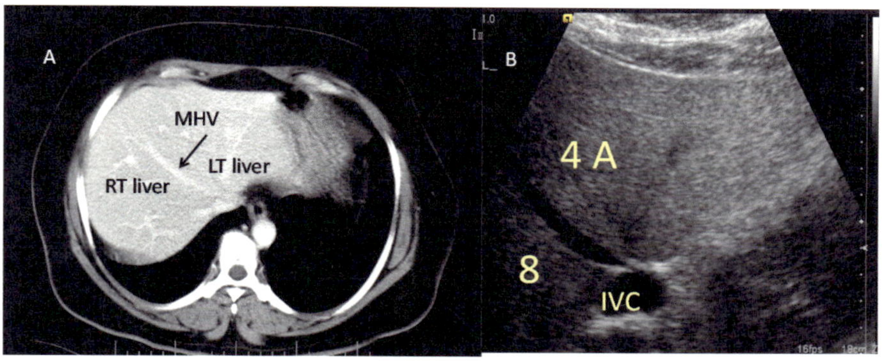

Figure 7. Middle hepatic vein (MHV) A) CT B) Ultrasound

The next step is to identify the falciform ligament and the right hepatic vein. This will divide the left liver to the medial and lateral sections and the right liver to the anterior and posterior sections alternatively. By this any lesion will be clearly seen in each section of the hemi-liver. **Figure.8**.

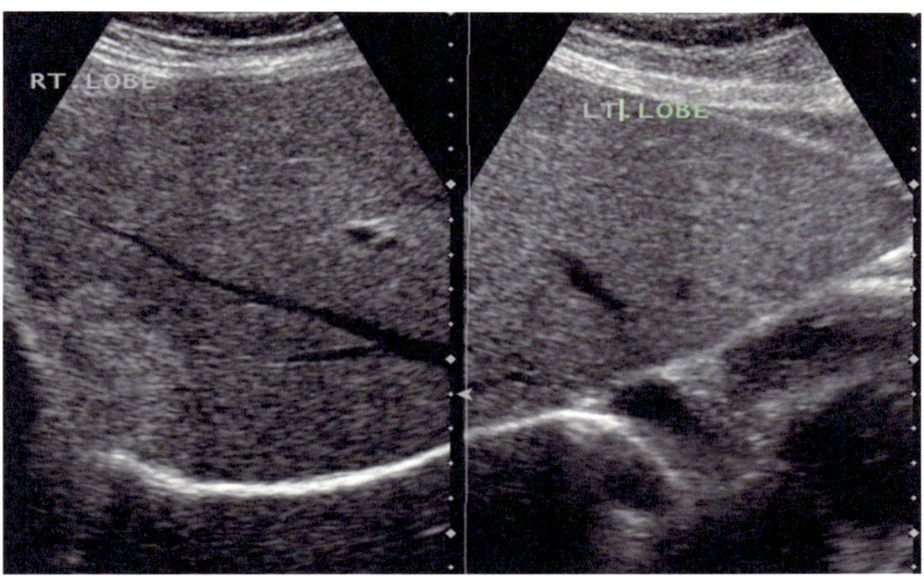

Figure 8. A) right hepatic vein (RHV) – with a lesion in seg 7 B) falciform (FL)

The last step is to identify the main portal vein and follow it till you reach to the bifurcation of the right and left branches which corresponds to the line that divides the liver into the upper and lower segments. This will give rise to the division of each section to its corresponded segments as described before in the anatomy part **Figure.9**.

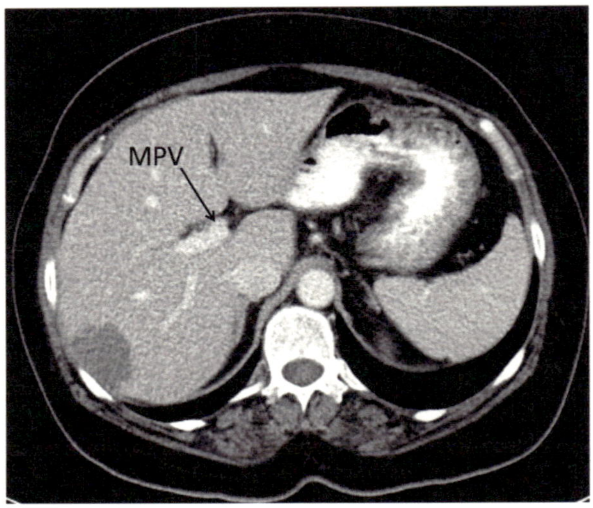

Figure 9. Main portal vein (MPV), with a lesion seen in the right posterior lower segment (segment6)

If this simple technique is adopted a full idea of the lesions identity and location could be achieved with a high degree of certainty making the surgical planning much more feasible. **Figure.10**.

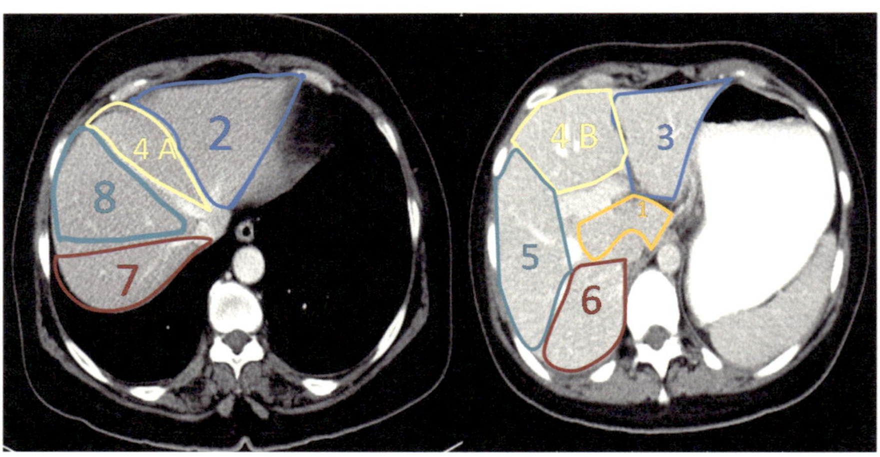

Figure 10. All segments identified on CT pre-opretive

http://dx.doi.org/10.5772/51775

4.2. Intra–operative

This is usually carried out by the intra-operative ultrasound [26-30], which we believe no liver resection should be done without mastering its use especially in malignant liver lesions. There are six simple steps that should be followed to get the best results of the ultrasound. 1) General inspection the whole liver as CT is not the ideal tool to identify superficial liver lesions. 2) A systemic recognition of all three hepatic veins and the main portal veins with its branches to identify all the liver segments. 3) Localize the tumour and determine which segments are involved. 4) Determine which segments needs to be resected to achieve good margins and balance it with the state of the liver trying at all times to go thru the anatomical lines to get an anatomical liver resection when possible to achieve the advantages mentioned before. 5) Mark the liver resection line on the liver surface. 6) Redetermine the distance from the tumour and the resection lines to be certain not to be close or even worse go thru the lesion.

To identify the segments the same method that was done pre-operative on CT is adopted by the localisation of the middle hepatic vein and drawing a line on it to get the right and left livers. **Figure.11**.

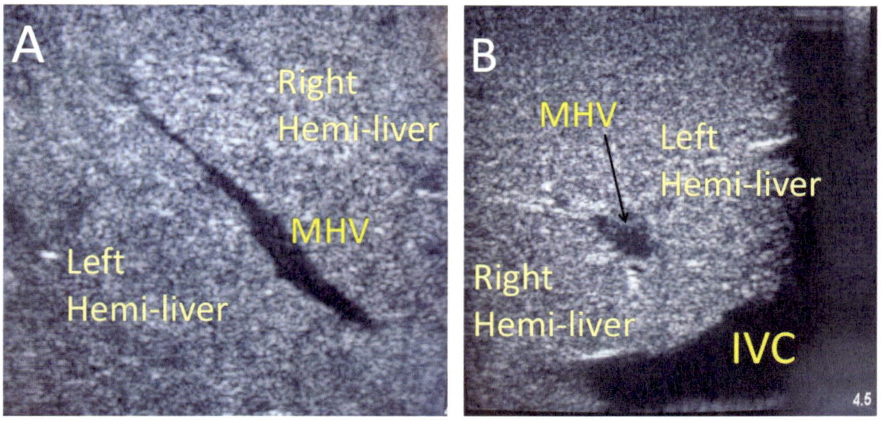

Figure 11. Intra operative ultrasound middle hepatic vein. A) longitudinal B) sagetal

The falciform ligament which divides the left liver to the medial and lateral sections can be seen on the surface. The left hepatic vein that divides segment 2 and 3 can be identified. On the right side the right hepatic vein is seen and a line is made to divide the right liver to the anterior and posterior sections. **Figure.12**.

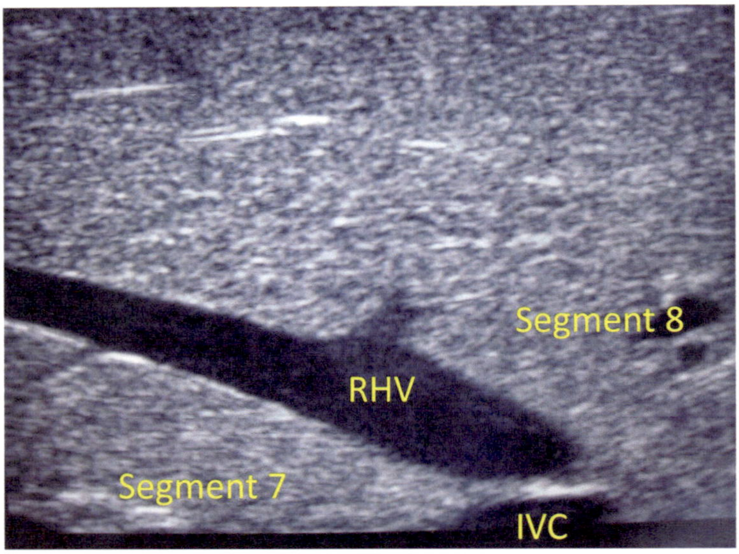

Figure 12. Intra operative ultrasound right hepatic vein.

The portal vein is then identified and followed to get all its branches and a line is made horizontally to get the upper and lower segments of the liver. **Figure.13**. After connecting all these lines the liver segments will be seen on the surface with the exception of segment 1 which is separate as we indicated before and can be seen over the IVC as the caudate lobe [31]. **Figure.14**

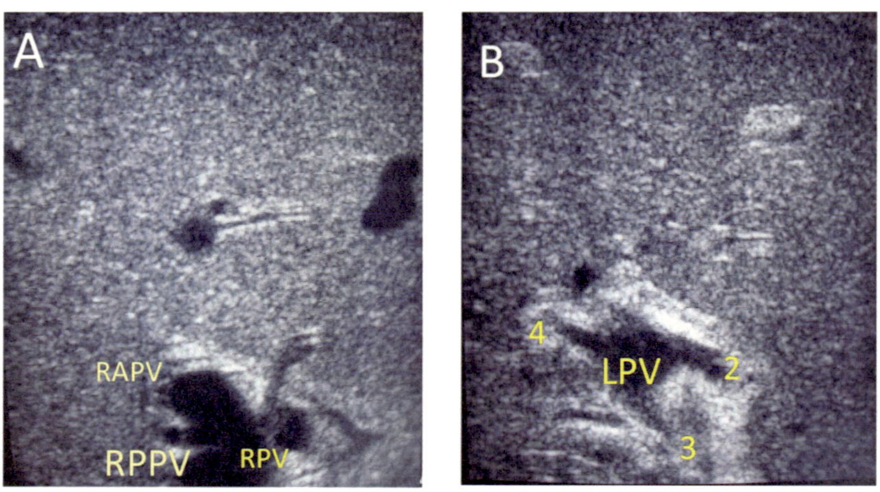

Figure 13. A) Right Portal veins (RPV) and its bifurcation to right anterior (RAPV) and right posterior (RPPV). B) Left portal vein (LPV) with its segmental branches

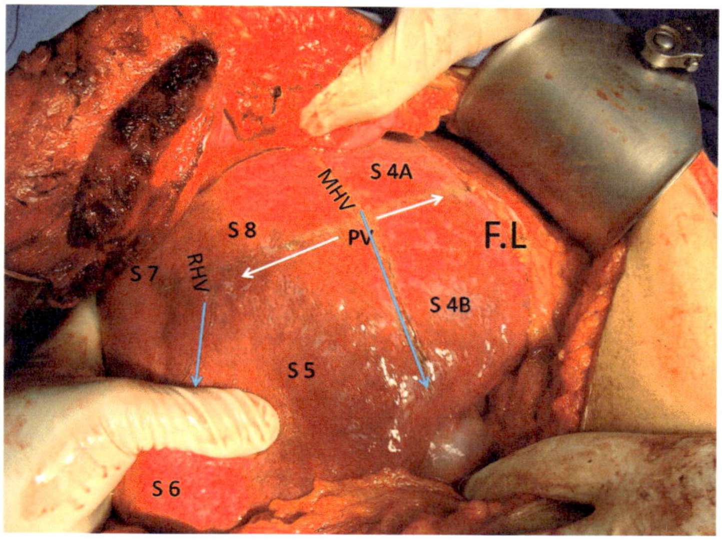

Figure 14. Liver segments on the liver intra operatively Portal vein (PV) in weight, middle hepatic vein (MHV), falciform ligament (FL), right hepatic vein (RHV)

5. Liver resection

A full pre-operative evaluation is necessary before embarking on a liver resection especially that most of the patients with HCC are also cirrhotic. There are multiple models to evaluate these patients and the most widely used one is the Child-Pugh score. This model stratifies patients into stage A, B, and C. Also the size of the tumour and the patient's physiological function are very important. Therefor most recent staging systems for HCC has included three important factors to evaluate the patient before any liver resection, the tumour, the liver status and the patient factor. Although chronic liver disease is not an absolute contraindication to liver resection, the morbidity and mortality increases prohibitively with increasing hepatic dysfunction. Childs class C or late B patients are generally excluded from major resections whereas Childs A or early B patients may be candidates [8,31].

As we mentioned above radiological studies are important in determining the presence of portal hypertension, ascitis, tumour localization, feasibility of the resection, tumour extension, distance from the pedicles and segments necessary to be resected as well as extra-hepatic metastasis [8].

5.1. Position and skin incision

The patient is usually in supine position, with the arms extended 90° when possible [8]. To minimize risk of air embolism from disrupted hepatic veins[8] and to minimize blood loss from the resected raw liver surface[3]. The resection is performed with the patient in the

Trendelenburg position and as recommended by all liver surgeon with a low central venous pressure of 0-5 mmHg(15°).**Figure.15**.

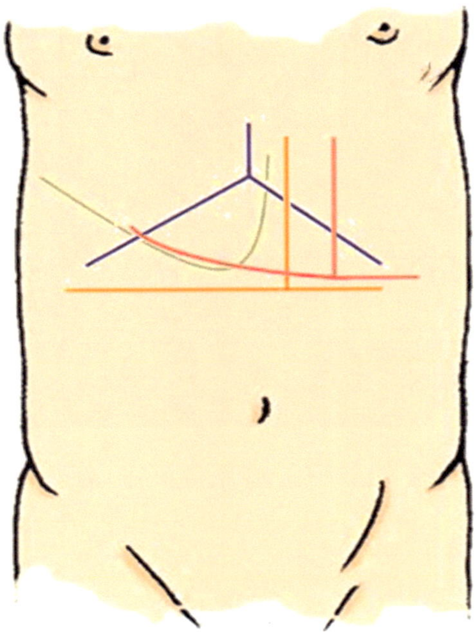

Figure 15. Skin incisions for liver surgery

Preparation of the operative field includes the area from the lower abdomen up to and including the chest, extending from axillary line to axillary line [8]. The majority of liver resections are performed with either a right subcostal incision with upper midline extension (inverted hockey stick) or a chevron (Mercedes) incision [8]. Intra-operative ultrasound is done as described above and the necessary ligaments are released according to the segments of the liver that needs to bee resected. Usually the falciform ligament is released to allow free mobilization of the liver and a better access for the ultrasound.

5.2. Approaches to liver resection

A liver surgeon should be familiar with all the techniques of liver resection because each has advantages and disadvantages making different resections more feasible.

5.2.1 Anterior approach

This technique is started by dissection of the portal triad and the hilar plate, where the right and left portal veins are identified.Figure.16. This makes the ligation of each portal branch more feasible. Then the vascular line of demarcation is seen and with the aid of intra-operative ultrasound to identify the rest of the vascular structures and the tumour. The liver is then

http://dx.doi.org/10.5772/51775

mobilized according to the part being resected. Parynchymal transaction is then carried out followed by ligation of the hepatic veins. This type is usually applied in patients with less liver fibrosis and a right or left liver resection is needed.

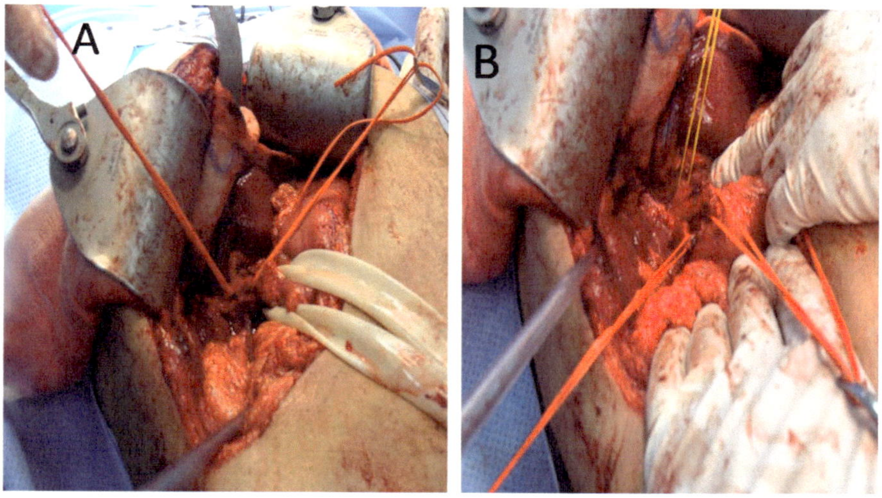

Figure 16. Anterior Approach. A) the tape is around the main and right hepatic artery. B) The yellow tape is around the left portal vein

5.2.2 Posterior approach

The liver is mobilized according to the part being resected. This will give access to the right or left hepatic vein which is usually circled and controlled. Then two ways can be done, were some surgeons transect the vein followed by Pringle and transect the liver parenchyma by the fast technique in about 10-15 min. This is usually fast and has less bleeding and can be done in patients with right, left and both left lateral and right posterior (peripheral sections) liver resections specially if the patient has liver fibrosis because of the time and bleeding. However, this technique requires the excellent use of ultrasound to avoid injury to the main vascular structures, and prevent a long Pringle time for the unresected part of the liver.

The other way is to start with the liver transaction. This will not require the routine use of Pringle, however it can be associated with more blood lose, and longer transection time to control the bleeding. This is usually done in non cirrhotic patients specially in living related liver transplant.

By using also the posterior approach the portal pedicle will be transacted at the end in the liver. This will decrease the injury or the narrowing of the unresected pedicle.

5.2.3 Hanging technique

This approach was adopted recently and was mainly applied in the right liver donors for living related liver transplant. This technique usually relies on the principle of keeping the liver well vascularised till the last minute to keep the liver viable.

The approach is done by using the avascular plane on the anterior part of the inferior vena cava and the window between the right and middle hepatic vein. This makes the passage of a tape from the inferior part of the liver to the superior part over the inferior vena cava. **Figure. 17**. The live is then transacted over the tape slowly while maintaining good haemostasis. Then the right hepatic vein and the right pedicle are transacted.

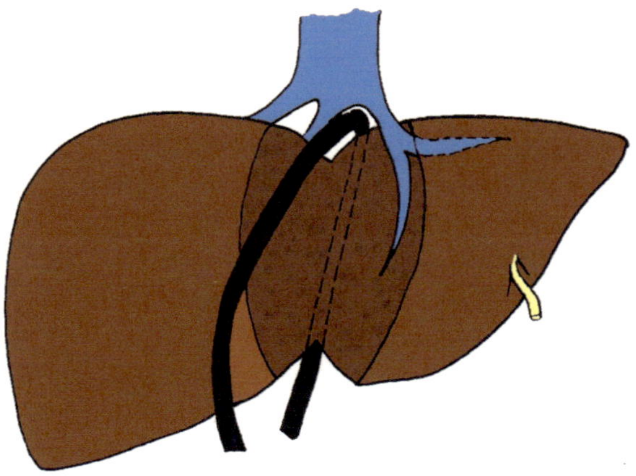

Figure 17. Hanging technique

This method is used mainly in right liver resection, and the tape can be moved in any plane wanted with the aid of the ultrasound. It also has a non touch like technique, were the liver is not mobilized till the vascular inflow and outflow are transacted. However, it requires time and very experienced surgeon not to injure the inferior vena cava during insertion of the tape. It's also time consuming and not applied in cirrhotic liver because bleeding will be more.

5.2.4. Hilar plate dissection

This technique is started by hilar plate dissection and reaching to each sectional branch or even to each segmental branch. Control of the inflow is done first followed by mobilization of the part intended to be resected. The liver resection is then carried out and the outflow is then transacted. **Figure.18**

This method is best for central liver resection, however the hilar dissection requires experience and cannot be carried out in cirrhotic livers as bleeding will be difficult to control. Intra-operative ultrasound is very important to locate the portal branches and the outflow veins to decrease its injury, also the tumor localization is important not to cut through it.

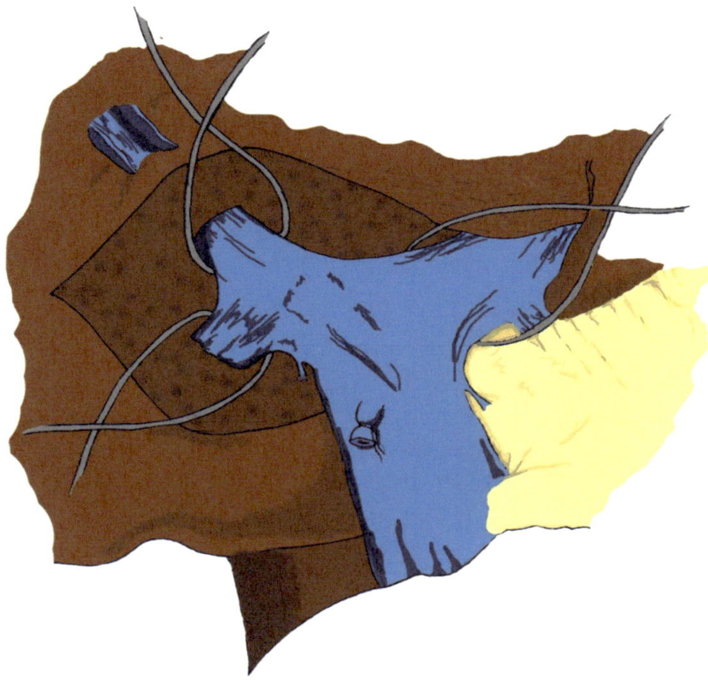

Figure 18. Hillar dissection. Tapes around the sectional portal branches on the right and the main left portal vein on the left

5.2.5. Intra–hepatic ligation

Peripheral and non anatomical liver resections are usually done by this approach. Intra-operative ultrasound is done to see the tumour and its blood supply. Mobilization followed by parenchymal transaction, were the inflow and outflow vessels are transacted in the liver.

5.2.6. Radio–frequency assisted liver resection

The first description of RFA-assisted liver resection was published by Habib's group [32]. This technique showed a major improvement of liver surgery with low/no morbidity and mortality observed [33]. It also showed decrease in the anesthetic time, operative time, hospital stay, and blood loss. Liver resection became a comparatively safer procedure [34].

Liver resection utilizing radiofrequency-induced resection plane coagulation as a safe alternative to the established resection techniques. The residual zone of coagulation necrosis remains basically unchanged during a follow up of three years, with a safety margins of 0.5-3.5 cm and Histopathological proof [35].

The RadioFrequency Assisted liver resection has 5 steps [32, 36]:

Step 1: First or inner line is made on the liver capsule with argon diathermy to mark the periphery of the tumor. This is done by bimanual palpation and intraoperative ultrasound.

Step 2: Second or outer line, again using argon diathermy, is made on the liver capsule 2 cm outside (away from) the inner line to mark the site where the probe is positioned to achieve coagulative necrosis.

Step 3: Coagulative necrosis is produced along a line that follows the second or outer line. The cooled-tip RF probe and a 500-kHz RF Generator, which produces 100 W of power and allows measurements of the generator output, tissue impedance, and electrode tip temperature. The probe contains a 3-cm exposed electrode, a thermocouple on the tip to monitor temperature and impedance. Two coaxial cannulae through which chilled saline is circulated during RF energy application to prevent tissue boiling and cavitation immediately adjacent to the needle.

Step 4: Further probe applications are deployed to obtain a zone of necrosis according to the depth of the liver parenchyma to be resected. Application of the RF energy should begin with the area deepest and farthest from the upper surface of the liver. Once the deepest 3 cm of tissue is coagulated, the probe is withdrawn by 3 cm to coagulate the next cylinder of tissue, and so on until the upper surface of the liver is reached. Each application requires about 60 seconds of RF energy.

Before each probe removal, the saline infusion is stopped to increase the temperature close to the electrode. This results in coagulation of the needle tract during withdrawal and reduces the possibility of bleeding from the probe tract and the liver capsule.

Step 5: The liver parenchyma is divided using the scalpel. The plane of division should be situated midway between the first and second line so as to leave a 1-cm resection margin away from the tumor and leave in situ 1 cm of burned coagulated surface.

5.2.7. Total hepatic vascular exclusion

This method combines total inflow and outflow vascular occlusion of the liver, isolating it completely from the systemic circulation. It is achieved after complete liver mobilization, application of inflow occlusion by Pringle manoeuvre, and then placing a clamp across the infra-hepatic IVC above the renal veins and the right adrenal vein followed by a supra-hepatic IVC clamp above the opening of the major hepatic veins. After the parenchymal transection and hemostasis, the clamps are removed in the reverse order[37]. **Figure 19**.

This results in a significant haemodynamic instability, with a substantial reduction in cardiac output, though blood pressure is usually maintained [38]. Around 10% of patients cannot tolerate it haemodynamically[39].

The ischaemic limit is 60-90 mins for patients with normal liver function [40]. In patients with cirrhosis, the maximal ischaemic time is halved and, in addition, the liver function before surgery must be at the better end of the spectrum[41]

However this technique is not done nowadays with the advanced surgical techniques except in rare conditions like tumour thrombus reaching the IVC or the atrium **Figure 20**. It also prevents intra-operative thrombus migration, and allows major hepatic veins or IVC reconstruction [37].

http://dx.doi.org/10.5772/51775

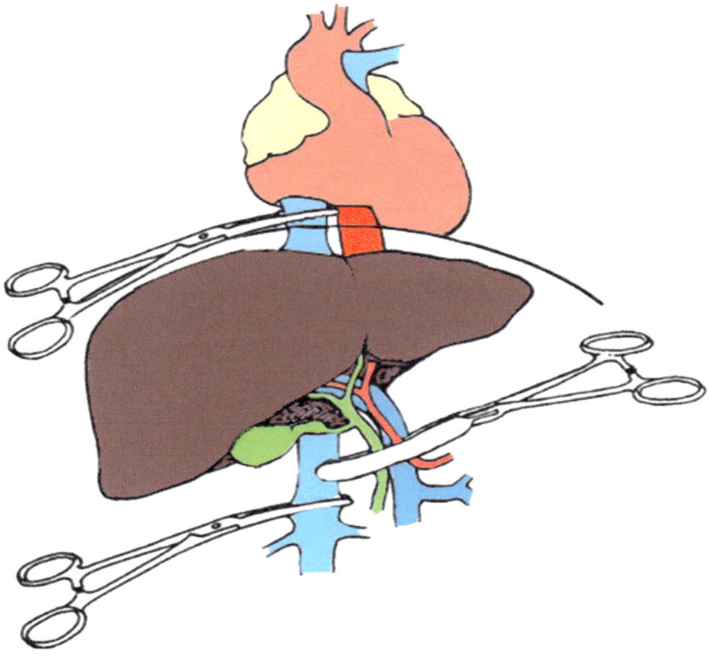

Figure 19. Total hepatic vascular occlusion

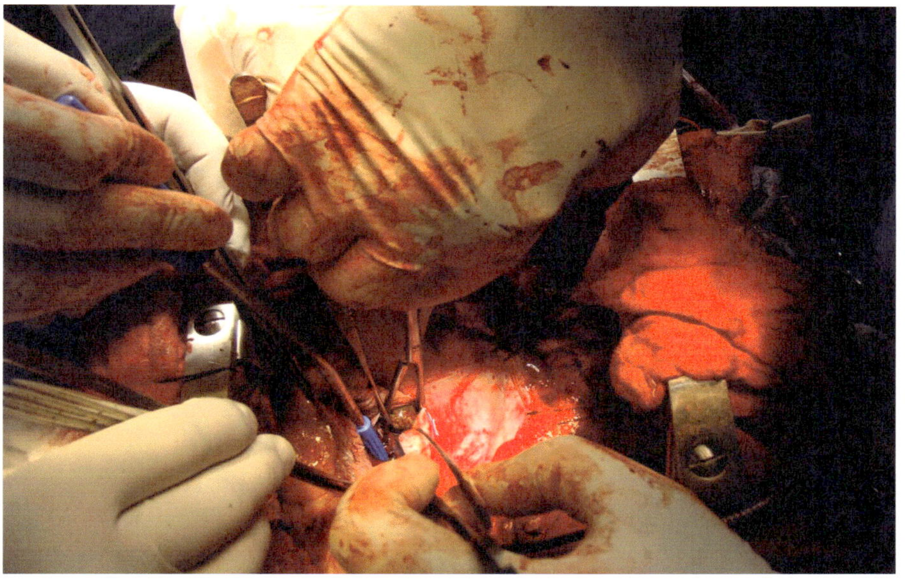

Figure 20. A case of HCC with atrial thrombus with total vascular occlusion. The thrombus is being removed from the right atrium.

However, with the development of liver surgery there has been use of some part of vascular occlusion done selectively or in compinations:

1. In-flow control:

2. Pringle manoeuvre; This is done by occluding the total inflow to the liver. This is usually in cases of central liver resection or majour resections where a large volume of blood is suspected to be lost. **Figure 21**

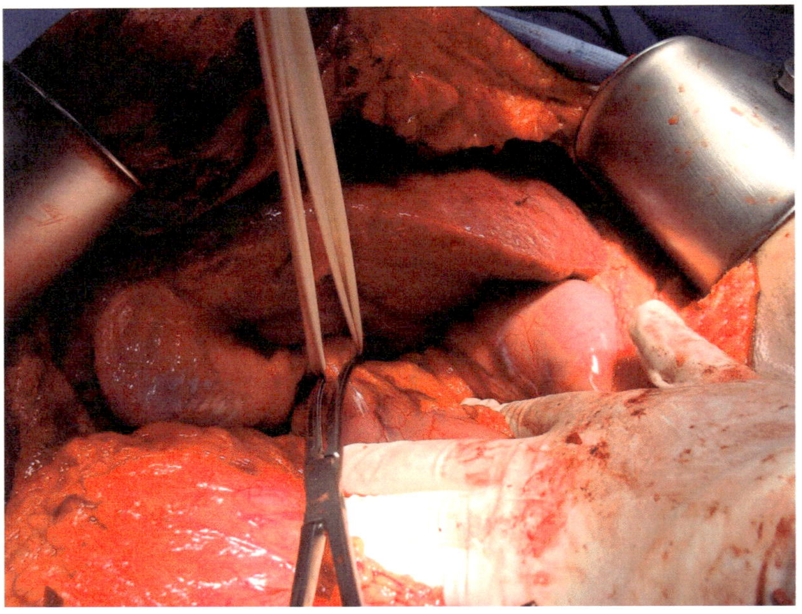

Figure 21. Pringles manoeuvre

1. Hemi-Hepatic control; This is done as described before in the right or left hemi-hepatectomy by controlling the right or left pedicle at the glissonian sheath. **Figure 16**

2. Sectional control; This is done by isolating and controlling the sectional branches as described in the (Hilar Plate Disection) as described above to be able to isolate each section without affecting other parts of the liver. **Figure 17**

3. Out-Flow Control:

4. Total hepatic control; this is achieved by either clamping of the IVC above and below or clamping the hepatic veins without affecting the flow of the IVC as nowadays done in piggy-back liver transplant.

5. Isolated hepatic vein control; this is done as described in the posterior approach where full mobilization of the liver is done and the right or left hepatic vein is isolated and clamped with-out affecting the IVC or the other hepatic veins

http://dx.doi.org/10.5772/51775

These all can be done separately or combined to achieve a bloodless liver resection and maintain patient stability.

5.3. Parynchymal transaction

Meyer-May described the use of Kocher-like clamps to crush liver parenchyma in 1939 [12,42] and haemostatic clamps such as Kelly clamps [43] are still used to crush small areas of the parenchyma, leaving the vessels intact.

Lortat-Jacob used the handle of a scalpel[9] and Lin described the use of finger fracture to remove parenchyma under inflow occlusion to isolate vessels and bile ducts for ligation[44,45].

Ultrasonic dissection has been developed using the CUSA (Cavitron Ultrasonic Surgical Aspirator)[42], this allows for delineation of the hepatic veins, particularly at the junction with the inferior vena cava, and prevents positive margin [45]. It has been shown to be very effective for division of the parenchyma with low blood losse [46,47].

Water-jet dissection [48-49] reduced blood loss, blood transfusion, and transaction time compared with CUSA, but there is increased risk of venous air embolism [45].

Harmonic Scalpel allows sealing of small vessels during the transaction of liver parenchyma. It can be used alone or in combination with clamp crushing or CUSA. It also have been adopted for laparoscopic resections [50,51] with limitation in the dissection around the main trunk of the hepatic veins [52]. **Figure.22**

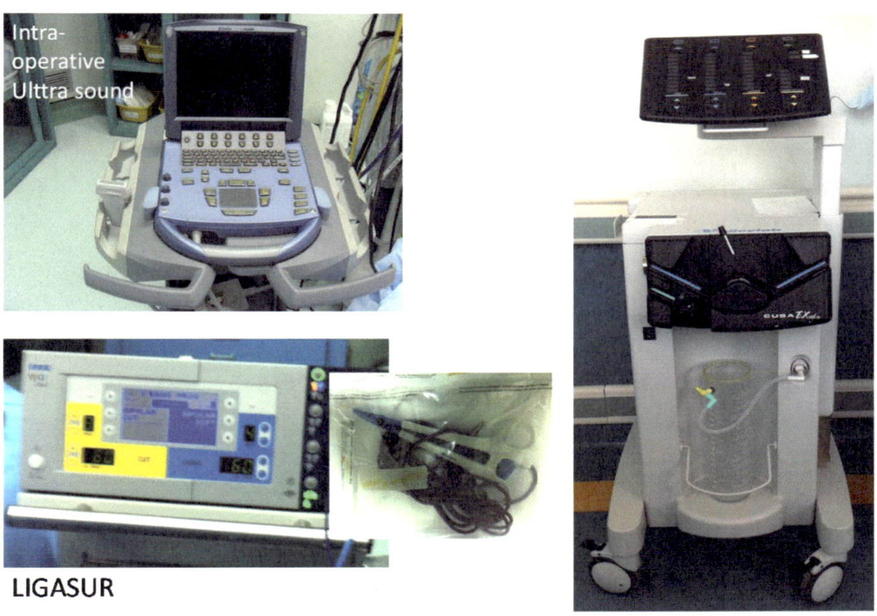

Figure 22. Instruments used for liver resection

Ligasure designed to seal small vessels by a combination of Ultrasonic dissection of liver parenchyma using compression pressure and bipolar radiofrequency (RF) energy [45], it was found to be more useful in laparoscopic resection than open.

Tissue Link dissecting sealer, where saline runs to the tip of the electrode to couple RF energy to the liver surface and achieve coagulation [45].

All these instruments have been used and according to many authors each has been claimed to be better than the other. Our believe is that a surgeon should be familiar with all techniques and instruments as each hospital has its own and when instrument malfunction occurs he will have the ability to adopt and rise up to the situation.

5.4. Specific liver resections

5.4.1. Right hepatectomy

Resection of the right hemiliver (segments 5, 6, 7 & 8) is one of the most common types of liver resection. It involves removing all hepatic parenchyma to the right of the middle hepatic vein [8]. This can be done by the Anterior, Posterior or the hanging techniques described above. However, it is important to see which approach will be better for each patient taking into consideration the tumour and the status of the liver.

This starts with mobilization of the right liver by division of the falciform, coronary and right triangular ligaments. Then vascular inflow and outflow control should take place. Three general approaches have been described for achieving vascular inflow control: 1) extrahepatic dissection within the porta hepatis, with division of the right hepatic artery and right portal vein prior to division of the parenchyma (anterior approach) 2) intrahepatic control of the main right pedicle within the substance of the liver prior to parenchymal transection (Intra-Hepatic ligation); and 3) intrahepatic control of the pedicle after parenchymal transaction (hanging technique or posterior approach) [8].

Then the right hepatic artery, right portal vein and the right hepatic duct are lighted and divided extrahepatic. The right liver is then dissected from the inferior vena cava either before or after according to which approach is being adopted. The short hepatic veins that drain from the right hemi liver to the inferior vena cava should be ligated and divided as well as the Hepato-caval ligament. The right hepatic vein is then dissected extrahepatic and ligated. After this step a clear line of demarcation will appear as the right hemi liver will became darker and ischemic. Liver parenchyma transaction will be done on the right border of the middle hepatic vein. Some vascular anomalies can cause the demarcation line of a right hepatectomy to be along the left border of the middle hepatic vein so care must tacked to preserve segment 4 branches or it will become congested. Blood loss control can be achieved by pringle's maneuver, using of low central pressure or extrahepatic clamping of the middle and left hepatic veins.**Figure.23**

http://dx.doi.org/10.5772/51775

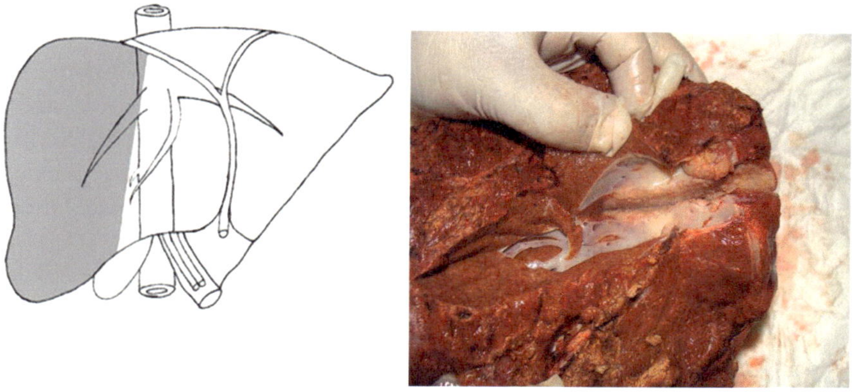

Figure 23. Right Hepatectomy; a right liver specimen with tumor invasion in the right hepatic vein

5.4.2. Extended right hepatectomy (Right trisectionectomy)

Right hepatectomy + extrahepatic ligation and division of the branches of the hepatic artery, portal vein and bile ducts to segment 4 with the division of the right and middle hepatic veins leaving the left hepatic vein and portal triad supplying the left lateral section intact [18].

The left triangular ligament may be preserved to prevent liver rotation and venous outflow occlusion post resection [42].**Figure.24**

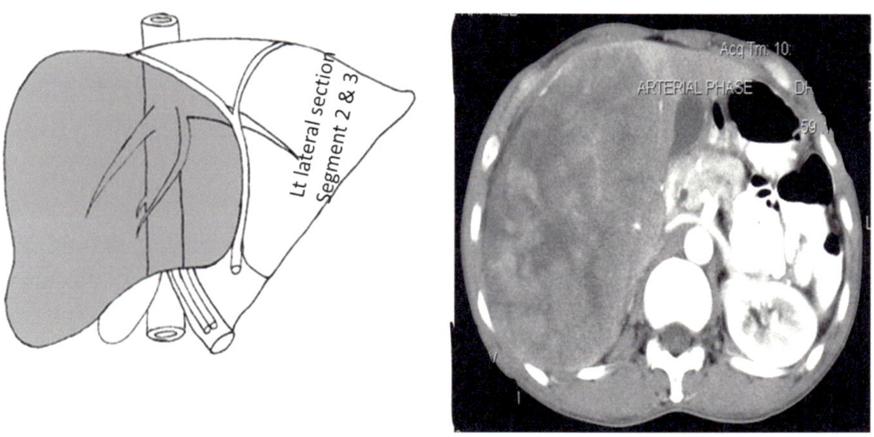

Figure 24. Right extended tri-sectionectomy; a CT scan of a liver tumor that was resected as shown in the drawing

5.4.3. Left hepatectomy

This can be done in the same manner as the right liver resection, however it will require the identification of the left portal triad. Starting with mobilization of the left liver by division of the falciform and the left triangular ligaments. Extrahepatic division of the extrahepatic branches of the left hepatic artery, left portal vein and left hepatic duct. Isolation of the trunk of the middle and left hepatic vein. Parynchymal transaction done along the plane demarcated by the ischemic left liver along a plan on the left side of the middle hepatic vein. The same should be considered as the line of demarcation can be on the right of the middle hepatic vein. The left hepatic vein is ligated intrahepaticly. Blood Loss can be reduced by using Pringle's maneuver plus either low central venous pressure or selective hepatic vascular occlusion by clamping the right hepatic vein. **Figure 25**

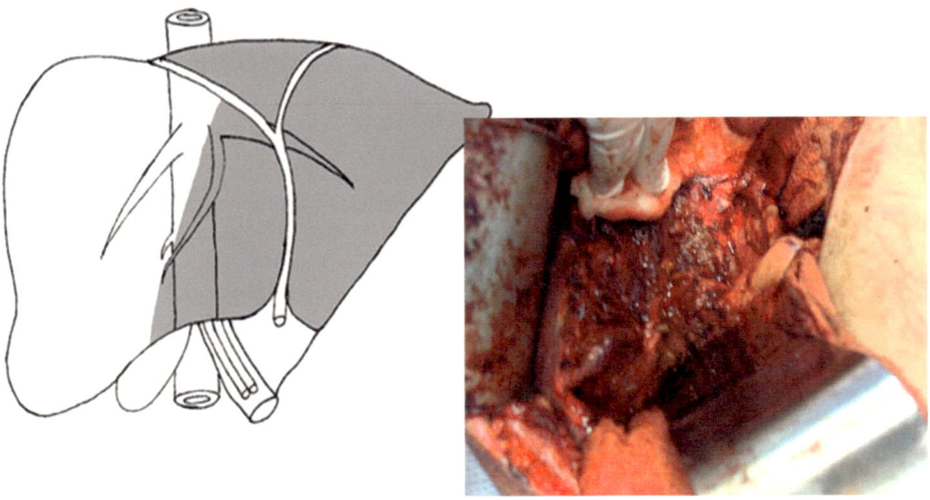

Figure 25. A case of Left Liver resection; the middle hepatic vein seen in the remnant liver with a schematic demonstration

5.4.4. Extended left hepatectomy (Left trisectionectomy)

Similar to left hepatectomy in addition of the right anterior section. Care should be done to preserve the hepatic arterial, portal venous and bile duct branches to the right posterior section and the right hepatic vein. If the right inferior hepatic vein is large it should be preserved so the venous drainage to segment 6 will not be affected [18].

5.4.5. Left lateral sectionectomy

Isolated segment II or III resection is uncommonly performed because of the ease of combined segment II and III (left lateral section) and the small volume of each segment. In the presence of cirrhosis or when multiple segmental resections are performed, isolated resection may be necessary. The left hepatic vein is identified extrahepaticaly and the left lateral sectional portal triad is ligated at the umbilical vein and the falciform ligament.**Figure.26**. Then the hepatic transaction is carried out with very minimal blood lose.

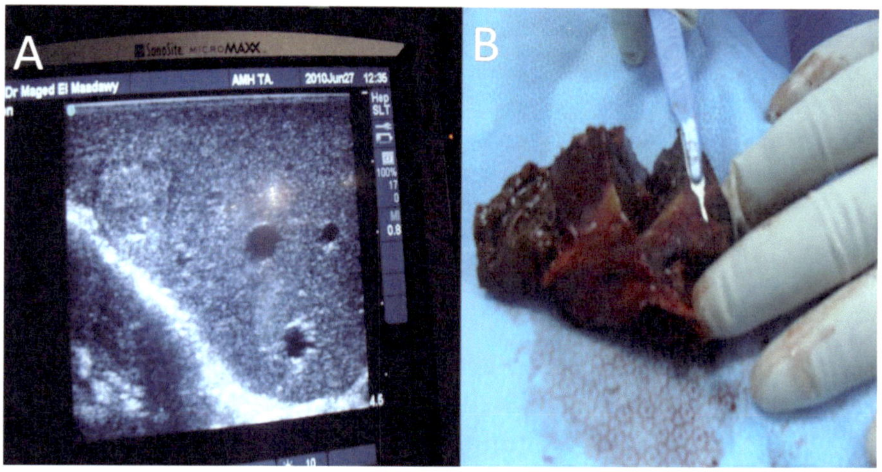

Figure 26. A) left lateral section as seen on intra-operaive ultrasound. B) the specimen with tumour to check for margins

5.4.6. Right posterior sectionectomy (Segment VI and VII)

This can be achieved by most techniques described above depending on the tumour size and the status of the Liver. Full mobilization of the right liver with division of the posterior draining veins. The right portal pedicle is exposed, and the anterior and posterior branches are identified (Hilar plate approach). The posterior pedicle is clamped, and the line of demarcation is evident. The pedicle may be divided, and parenchymal dissection may be performed in standard fashion. The line of transection is horizontal and posterior to the right hepatic vein. However, the right vein may be sacrificed during this procedure since the anterior section will be adequately drained by the middle hepatic vein[8]. If the liver is cirrhotic we would advise the use of an extrahepatic approach like the posterior approach to minimize the blood lose and injury to the right anterior portal triad.

5.4.7. Right anterior sectionectomy (Segment V and VIII)

This is extreamly rare and very difficult because of its location between both the right and middle hepatic veins with the importance of not injuring any of them. This is why if it is done it is combined with segment IV (Central liver resection) to remove the middle hepatic vein and have a safe distance from the right hepatic vein. The approach is similar to the right posterior sectionectomy were the right anterior portal triad is seen and ligated to stop the inflow and get the line of demarcation.

5.4.8. Isolated segment II or III resection

For removal of either segment II or III, the inflow pedicle is ligated, but the main left hepatic vein is preserved because it provides the only venous drainage to the remaining segment. The inflow pedicles to segments II and III branches directly from the umbilical portion of the left main portal vein. To isolate these pedicles, the left lateral section is shifted cephalad using traction on the divided falciform ligament. If present, the parenchymal bridge between segment III and IV is divided with electrocautery. Dissection of the umbilical fissure to the left of the portal vein is performed. Ligation of either segment II or III pedicles demarcates the boundary between them. The left hepatic vein may be clamped to reduce blood loss, but clamping is generally unnecessary if the central venous pressure is low. Liver transection then proceeds in an oblique antero-cranial plane with attention to preserve the left hepatic vein [3].

5.4.9. Isolated segment VII

To expose this segment dissection of the right triangular ligament is necessary. The vascular pedicle of segment VII originate from the right lateral glissoian pedicle and enters the parenchyma in a common trunk at segment VI, this will run deep and divide to two branches anterior to segment VI and posterior to segment VII.

After mobilizing the infindibulum of the gall bladder and dividing the lateral peritoneum of the hepato-duodenal ligament the lateral pedicle can be easily freed as well as the artery. Once this is identified with the bile duct, the right branch of the portal vein is freed. The bile ducts will never be dissected outside the parenchyma but only transparenchymaly at the end of the resection to prevent damage to the adjacent hepatic ducts. Clamping of the arterial branch will lead to blanching of the entire right anterior section. The fissure of the right hepatic vein will indicate the upper resection margin. The vein could be left in place or removed in case of neoplasm infiltration, also isolated resection of segment VII with ligation of the right hepatic vein can be safely performed, venous out flow of segment VI should be insured by preserving the accessory hepatic veins and the right inferior hepatic vein(present in 25%) to prevent the transitory venous congestion of segment VI with hemorrhage from the resection margins after isolated removal of segment VII. After clamping of the lateral glissonian pedicle the trunk of the right hepatic vein will be clamped and divided. Parenchymal dissection will follow the appearing ischemic demarcation line and the dissection plane will start from the top downward between segment VII and VIII. The pedicle will be exposed with the dissection once it have been divided the arterial and portal branches at the hilum can be unclamped, segment VI returns to its normal color and the inferior demarcation line will become evident.

5.4.10. Isolated segment VI

Similar to segment VII, after mobilization of the right liver, ligation of the inferior or accessory suprahepatic vein if present and clamping of the arterial and portal brances which will produce the ischemic demarcation line.

The parenchyma is divided starting from the lower margin of the liver proceeding along an oblique plane from the right to the left and from the front to back. Deep in the parenchyma the lateral pedicle is ligated. The glissonian pedicle is then unclamped at the hilum and segment VII will return to the normal colour, the upper dissection margin will follow the ischemic line between the two segments VI and VII.

http://dx.doi.org/10.5772/51775

5.4.11. Isolated segment IV

Segment IV is divided into two subsegments, IVA and IVB, based on the inflow pedicles. Isolated resection of IVB is usually done in a intra-hepatic ligation method and most often with segment V in cases of gallbladder carcinoma. Were outflow control for segment IV resection is usually not obtained until the liver is divided. After dissection of the hepatoduodenal ligament the left branches of the hepatic artery are identified and then the middle branch is ligated and divided. Dissection will be carried out along the gall bladder-inferior vena cava plane. Glissonian capsule divided above the hilar plate. The portal branch is usually seen with the hilar plate and dissection with control by Bull-dog clamps to see the line of demarcation. At this point segment IV will only be attached to the Middle Hepatic vein which will be transfixed.

5.4.12. Isolated segment I ''Caudate lobe''

This is the least popular liver resection as all the other segments can be done in an intra-hepatic ligation method or in a non-anatomical approach. However, the Caudate liver resection has its own unique location above the inferior vena cava and its own blood supply giving it the excellent challenge for any liver surgeon. There are 5 approaches:

1. Bilateral approach: For isolated caudate lobectomy, the caudate lobe is approached from both right and left side after complete mobilization of the liver with controll of the suprahepatic and intrahepatic inferior vena cava as well as the right hepatic vein and the common trunk of the middle and left hepatic veins. Then the caudate lobe is detached from the inferior vena cava along the anterior surface of the retro-haptic IVC and the short hepatic veins are identified and divided. The hepatogastric ligament is detached from the undersurface of the liver and the fibrous hepatocaval ligament need to be divided to free the spieglian lobe from the IVC and the diaphragm. All short hepatic veins are ligated and divided. So the caudate lobe is free from the inferior vera cava. The branches of the to the para caval portion of the caudate lobe from the right portal vein, right hepatic artery and duct, branches to the spiegelian lobe from the left portal vein, left hepatic artery and duct are ligated and divided. By carefull dissection the liver is detached from the surroundings and the right, middle and left hepatic veins. In this step; 2 important land marks for this dissection : A) the angle between the right hepatic vein and the inferior vans cava i.e the top of the caudate lobe. B) the meeting point between the caudate process and the right liver. An imaginary line joining these two points is considered as the caudate boundary for the liver transection. Meticulous care should be applied not to injure the major vessels or induce bleeding which will be difficult to control.

2. Left sided approach: Similar to the bilateral approach whit the exception that the dissection is mainly from the left side of the liver. In small tumours <3cm, if an isolated partial caudate lobecetomy or left hepatectomy combined with complete caudate lobecetomy is carried out. **Figure 27**

3. Right sided approach: Similar to the bilateral approach whit the exception that the dissection is mainly from the right side of the liver. In thin patients with right hepatectomy combined with caudate lobecetomy.

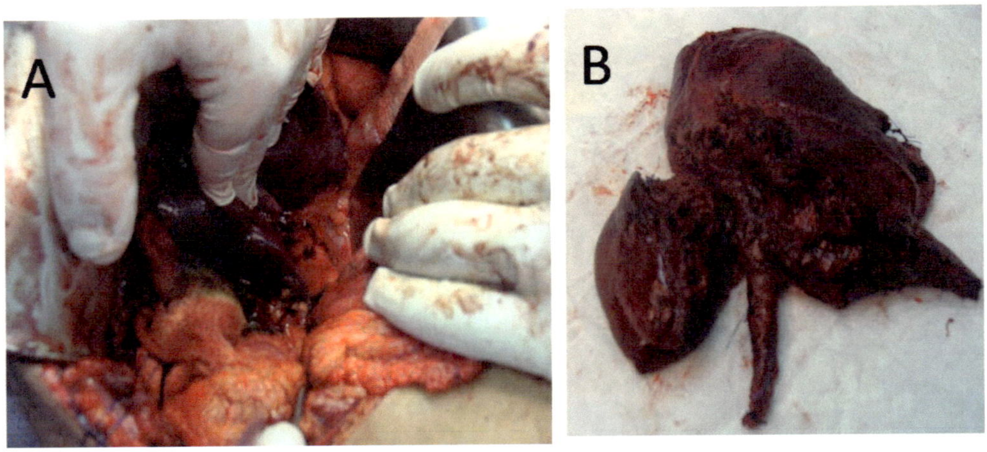

Figure 27. Caudate liver resection, A) the lobe is removed from the IVC and lifted up (left approach). B) The specimen of the caudate with the left liver and the CBD for cholangiocarcinoma

4. Anterior approach: This approach provides a better operative field by opening the mid plane of the liver widely so the major hepatic veins and the Hilar plate will be exposed to direct vision thus will facilitate tumour resection from the main vessels. For tumours >4cm especially when the tumour is located in the paracaval portion or in close contact with the major hepatic veins. With tha same technique of the bilateral approach. After freeing the caudate lobe from the reto-hepatic inferior vena cava, pringle's meneuver is then applied. The liver is transacted through the mid plane starting from the point between the root of the right and middle hepatic veins to the fossa of the gall bladder. This is better done using the hanging technique. When the transection reaches the Hilar plate at the hilum, the portal triade of the caudate lobe is isolated and divided. The caudate lobes then separated from the major hepatic veins in one block with the tumour. After removal of the specimen all bleeding points and bile leak should be controlled individually.

5. Retrograde caudate lobectommy: Used if the tumour is closely adherent to or infiltrating the inferior vena cava, or if the tumour is too large in size to be turned from one side to the other. Mobilization of the liver by the division of all the ligaments, control of the hepatoduodenal ligament, suprahepatic and intrahepatic inferior vena cava for possible occlusion if necessary. The liver is transected along the mid plane 1cm from the tumour, the hepatic veins are exposed under direct vision and carefully dissected from the specimen, ligation and division of the caudate portal triad from the right/left hepatic arteries and veins. In combined Left/right hepatectomy with caudate lobecetomy the hepatic pedicel can be transected accordingly. The specimen will be attached only to the inferior vena cava. The last step here will be the division of the short hepatic veins, and if the tumour is attached to the IVC part of it could be resected with the tumour and then it'll be repaired or reconstructed.

http://dx.doi.org/10.5772/51775

5.4.13. Central liver resection

Segments IV, V, and VIII (also known as mesohepatectomy) is rarely performed. This resection involves ligation of inflow vessels from both the right and left portal pedicles. The resection is performed by combining the techniques of segment IV resection and right anterior sectionectomy. Dissection begins at the hilum and the umbilical fissure with the goal of inflow control. The right anterior sectional pedicle is isolated, as are the segment IV pedicles. The division of the liver parenchyma begins to the right of the umbilical fissure (or within it if the tumor is nearby). **Figure.28.**Care should be given to avoid ligating the left main portal umbilical branch. Dissection is continued upward to the main trunk of middle hepatic vein. The right anterior sectional pedicle is ligated to demarcate the boundary of the liver resection on the right side. Liver transection proceeds in the plane of the right hepatic vein until it meets the left resection plane. At this point, one should be cautious with handling the freely dangling central lobe. Excessive traction may tear the thin-walled middle hepatic vein, resulting in massive hemorrhage. Gently hold the lobe and divide the base of the middle hepatic vein. This procedure removes the gallbladder, central lobe, and middle hepatic vein en bloc, leaving the caudate, right posterior section, and left lateral section intact. The raw liver surface may be covered with a flap of omentum.

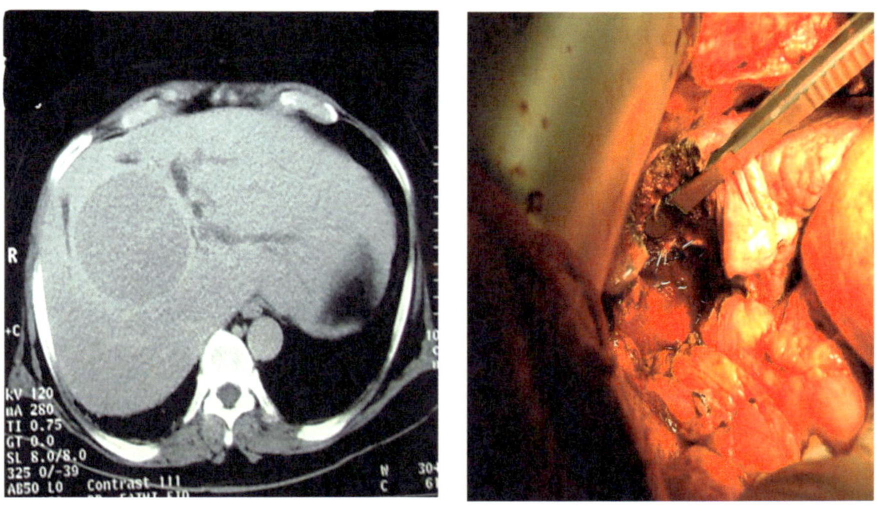

Figure 28. Central liver lesion as seen on CT scan and the same patient intra-operatively after resection

5.5. Control of bleeding

To minimize blood loss from the resected raw liver surface the patient is placed 15 degres in the Trendelenburg position [3]. Low venous pressure is maintained by minimizing fluid infusion and restricting intraoperative blood transfusion unless more than 25% of the blood volume is lost [53,54]. Systolic blood pressure is kept above 90 mm Hg, and intraoperative urine output is maintained at about 25 mL/hour [3].

Dissection and control of the hepatic veins performed prior to parenchymal transaction.[8].

Venous outflow draining is divided after dividing the inflow vessels[8], unless the posterior approach is adopted with a Pringles manoeuvre to prevent liver congestion.

Control of the suprahepatic and intrahepatic inferior vena cava [18], pringle's maneuver[3,18], and mobilization with parenchymal transection performed with a low central venous pressure < 5 mm Hg [3,11] can decrease the bleeding amount significantly.

Author details

O. Al-Jiffry Bilal[1,2] and Khayat H. Samah[2]

1 Surgery, Taif University, Taif, Saudi Arabia

2 Surgery, AlHada Military Hospital, Taif, Saudi Arabia

References

[1] Prognostic impact of anatomical resection for hepatocellular carcinomaKiyoshi Hasegawa, Norihiro Kokudo, Hiroshi Imamura, Yutaka Matsuyama, Masami Minagawa, Keiji Sano, Yasuhiko Sugawara, Tadatoshi Takayama, Masatoshi Makuuchi. Ann surg. (2005). , 242, 252-259.

[2] Eltawil et alDifferentiating the impact of anatomic and non-anatomic liver resection on early recurrence in patients with Hepatocellular Carcinoma. World journal of surgical oncology (2010).

[3] Segment-Oriented approach to liver resectionK.H. Liau, L.H. Blumgart, R.P. dematteo. Surg clin N Am (2004). , 84(2004), 543-561.

[4] Ultrasonically guided subsegmentectomyMakuuchi M, Hasegawa H, Yamaxaki S. Surg Gynecol Obstet. (1986). , 161, 346-359.

[5] Segmental liver resection using ultrasound-guided selective portal vein occlusion-Casting D, Garden J, Bismuth H. Ann Surg. (1989). , 210, 20-23.

[6] Segment-Oriented hepatic resection in the management of Malignant neoplasms Billigsley KGJarnagin WR, Fong Y, Blumgart LH. of the liver. J Am Coll Surg (1998). Nov; , 187(5), 471-81.

[7] Anatomic versus limited nonanatomic Resection for solitary hepatocellular carcinomaTanaka K, Shimada H, Matsumoto K, Nagano Y, Endo I, Togo SSurgery (2008).

[8] Techniques of Hepatic ResectionHoward m. Karpoff, William r. Jarnagin, José melendez, Yuman fong, Leslie h. Blumgart. Hepatobiliary Cancer.

[9] Ueno, S, et al. (2008). Efficacy of anatomic resection vs nonanatomic resection for small nodular hepatocellular carcinoma based on gross classification. J Hepatobiliary Pancreat Surg , 15(5), 493-500.

[10] Extent of liver resection influences the outcome in patients with cirrhosis and small hepatocellular carcinomaRegimbeau JM, Kianmanesh R, Farges O, Dondero F, Sauvanet A, Belghiti J. Surgery (2002). Mar;, 131(3), 311-7.

[11] Dematteo, R. P, Palese, C, Jarnagin, W. R, et al. Anatomic segmental hepatic resection is superior to wedge resection as an oncologic operation for colorectal liver metastases. J Gastrointest Surg (2000). , 4, 178-84.

[12] Imamura, H, Matsuyama, Y, Miyagawa, Y, et al. Prognostic significance of anatomical resection and des-_-carboxy prothrombin in patients with hepatocellular carcinoma. *Br J Surg*. (1999). , 86, 1032-1038.

[13] Cucchetti, A, et al. Acomprehensive meta-analysis on outcome of anatomic resection versus nonanatomic resection for hepatocellular carcinoma. Annal of Surgical oncology 27 June (2012).

[14] Segmental liver resection for Colorectal metastasis, Daniel V. Kosov, Georgi L. Kabakov. Gastrointestin Liver Dis.December (2009). , 18(4)

[15] Anatomic segmental resection compared to major hepatectomy in the treatment of liver neoplasmsThomas S. Helling, Benoit Blondeau. HPB,(2005). , 7, 222-225.

[16] Postoperative liver dysfunction and future remnant liver: where is the limit? Results of a prospective studyFerrero A, Vigano L, Polastri R, et al. World J Surg (2007). , 31, 1643-1651.

[17] Expanding criteria for resectability of colorectal liver metastasesPawlik TM, Schulick RD, Choti MA. Oncologist (2008). , 13, 51-64.

[18] Applied anatomy in liver resection and liver transplantW.Y. Lau 978-7-11712-875-9R-12876

[19] Healey JE JrSchriy PC. Anatomy of the biliary ducts within the human liver: analysis of the prevailing pattern of branching and the major variations of the biliary ducts. Arch Surg (1953). , 66, 599-616.

[20] Couinaud, C. Lefoie. Etudes Anatomiques et Chirugicales. Paris:Masson & Cie, (1957).

[21] The brisbane (2000). Terminology of Liver Anatomy and ResectionTerminology committee of the IHPBA, HPB 2000; , 333-9.

[22] The importance of Glisson's capsule and its sheaths in the intrahepatic approach to resection of the liverLaunois B, Jamieson G. Surg Gynecol Obstet (1992). , 174, 7-10.

[23] Kida, H, Uchimura, H, & Okamoto, K. Intrahepatic architecture of bile and portal vein. J Biliary tract and pancreas (1987). , 8, 1-7.

[24] Jamieson, G, & Launois, B. Liver resection and liver transplantation: the anatomy of the liver and associated structures. In :The anatomy of general surgical operations. Ed. Jamieson GG, Ilsevier Edinburgh, (2006). Chapter , 2, 8-23.

[25] Strsberg, S. M. liver terminology and Anatomy. In Hepatobiliary Carcinoma. Editor: W.Y. Lau World scintific Singapore (2007). chapter 2, , 25-50.

[26] The impact of intraoperative ultrasonography on surgery for liver neoplasmsKane R, Hughes L, Qcua E. J Ultrasound Med (1994).

[27] Laparoscopic staging and intraoperative ultrasonography for liver tumor managementRavikumar T. Surg Oncol Clin North Am (1996).

[28] Liver resection by ultrasonic dissection and intraoperative ultrasonographyHanna SS, Nam R, Leonhardt C. HPB Surg (1996). , 9, 121-8.

[29] Intraoperative ultrasonography and other techniques for segmental resectionsTakayama T, Makuuchi M. Surg Oncol Clin North Am (1996). , 5, 261-9.

[30] The use of operative ultrasound as an aid to liver resection in patients with hepatocellular-carcinomaMakuuchi M, Hasegawa H, Yamazaki S, Takayasu K, Moriyama N. World J Surg (1987). , 11, 615-21.

[31] Operative risks of major hepatic resectionsCapussotti L, Polastri R. Hepatogastroenterology (1998). , 45, 184-90.

[32] Weber, J. C, Navarra, G, Jiao, L. R, Nicholls, J. P, Jensen, S. L, & Habib, N. A. New technique for liver resection using heat coagulative necrosis. Ann Surg (2002).

[33] Navarra, G, Lorenzini, C, Curro, G, Basaglia, E, & Habib, N. H. Early results after radiofrequency-assisted liver resection. Tumori (2004).

[34] Tepel, J, Klomp, H. J, Habib, N, Fandrich, F, & Kremer, B. Modification of the liver resection technique with radiofrequency coagulation. Chirurg (2004).

[35] Radiomorphology of the Habib Sealer-Induced Resection Plane during Long-Time Followup: A Longitudinal Single Centere Experience after 64 Radiofrequency-Assisted Liver ResectionsRobert Kleinert, RogerWahba, Christoph Bangard, Klaus Prenzel,Arnulf H. H°olscher,1, 2 and Dirk Stippel.

[36] Radiofrequency ablation-assisted liver resection: review of the literature and our experiencePeng Yao & David L. Morris. HPB, (2006).

[37] Methods of vascular control technique during liver resection: a comprehensive review, Wan-Yee Lau, Eric C. H. Lai and Stephanie H. Y. Lau. Hepatobiliary Pancreat Dis Int,October 15,(2010). (5)

[38] Delva, E, Barberousse, J. P, Nordlinger, B, Ollivier, J. M, Vacher, B, Guilmet, C, et al. Hemodynamic and biochemical monitoring during major liver resection with use of hepatic vascular exclusion. Surgery (1984).

[39] Belghiti, J, Noun, R, Zante, E, Ballet, T, & Sauvanet, A. Portal triad clamping or hepatic vascular exclusion for major liver resection. A controlled study. Ann Surg (1996). , 224, 155-61.

[40] Huguet, C, Gavelli, A, Chieco, P. A, Bona, S, Harb, J, Joseph, J. M, et al. Liver ischemia for hepatic resection: where is the limit? Surgery (1992). , 111, 251-9.

[41] Emond, J, Wachs, M. E, Renz, J. F, Kelley, S, Harris, H, Roberts, J. P, et al. Total vascular exclusion for major hepatectomy in patients with abnormal liver parenchyma. Arch Surg (1995). discussion 830-1., 130, 824-30.

[42] A review of techniques for liver resection. AG Heriot, ND Karanjia. Ann R Coll Surg Engl 2002; 84: 371-380.

[43] One hundred consecutive hepatic resectionsBlood loss, transfusion, and operative technique. Cunningham JD, Fong Y, Shriver C, Melendez J, Marx WL, Blumgart LH. Arch Surg (1994). , 129, 1050-6.

[44] A simplified technique for hepatic resection. Lin T. Ann Surg 1974; 180: 225-9.

[45] Current techniques of liver transactionRONNIE T.P. POON. HPB, (2007).

[46] Cavitron ultrasonic surgical aspirator (CUSA) in liver resectionFasulo F, Giori A, Fissi S, Bozzetti F, Doci R, Gennari L. Int Surg (1992). , 77, 64-6.

[47] Resection of colorectal liver metastasesScheele J, Stang R, Altendorf-Hofmann A, Paul M. World J Surg (1995). , 19, 59-71.

[48] New water-jet dissector: initial experience in hepatic surgery Baer HUMaddern GJ, Blumgart LH. [published erratum appears in Br J Surg 1994; 81: 1103]. Br J Surg (1991). , 78, 502-3.

[49] A comparison of different techniques for liver resection: blunt dissection, ultrasonic aspirator and jet-cutter. Rau HG, Schardey FM, Buttler E, Reuter C, Cohnert TU, Schildberg FW.Eur J Surg Oncol 1995; 21: 183-7.

[50] Experience with ultrasound scissors and blades (UltraCision) in open and laparoscopic liver resectionSchmidbauer S, Hallfeldt KK, Sitzmann G, Kantelhardt T, Trupka A Ann Surg (2002).

[51] Cherqui, D, Husson, E, Hammoud, R, Malassagne, B, Stephan, F, Bensaid, S, et al. Laparoscopic liver resections: a feasibility study in 30 patients. Ann Surg (2000).

[52] Hepatic resection using the harmonic scalpelSugo H, Mikami Y, Matsumoto F, Tsumura H, Watanabe Y, Kojima K, et al. Surg Today (2000).

[53] Perioperative outcomes of major hepatic resections under low central venous pressure anesthesia: blood transfusionand the risk of postoperative renal dysfunction. Melendez JA, Arslan V, Fischer ME, Wuest D, Jarnagin W, Fong Y, et al. JAmColl Surg (1998). , 187, 620-5.

[54] Recent advances in hepatic resectionDeMatteo RP, Fong YM, Jarnagin WR, Blumgart LH. Semin Surg Oncol (2000). , 19, 200-7.

Chapter 10

Two-Step Hanging Maneuver for an Isolated Resection of the Dorsal Sector of the Liver

Hideaki Uchiyama, Shinji Itoh and Kenji Takenaka

Additional information is available at the end of the chapter

http://dx.doi.org/10.5772/51768

1. Introduction

Resection of malignant lesions arising in the dorsal sector of the liver is a challenging procedure because the sector is located deep in the abdominal cavity and surrounded by the inferior vena cava (IVC) and the major hepatic veins [1 – 9]. A hanging maneuver is an innovative procedure in hepatic surgeries, in which the liver parenchyma is hung by a tape, thereby making a straight cutting line [10 – 14]. This technique was applied in two patients who had a hepatocellular carcinoma (HCC) in the dorsal sector. Patient 1 was a 46-year-old female, who was found to have an HCC, approximately 3 cm in diameter, located just above the IVC. The patient had a large inferior right hepatic vein (IRHV). The superior right hepatic vein (SRHV) and the IRHV were individually controlled with a tape after dividing several short hepatic veins from the right side of the IVC. A cotton tape was introduced from the groove between the SRHV and the middle hepatic vein (MHV) to the right and left Glisson sheaths via the space just next to the left side of the IRHV. The liver was split into the right and left hemilivers by pulling the tape upwards. Next, the tape was introduced from the space behind the confluence of the MHV and the left hepatic vein (LHV) to the space behind the left Glisson sheath via the fissure of the ligamentum venosum after dividing a few small Glisson branches into the caudate lobe from the left Glisson sheath. The liver parenchyma was divided between the medial sector and the dorsal sector by pulling the tape medially, Finally, the dorsal sector including the tumor was resected by dividing the short hepatic veins from the left side of the IVC. Patient 2 was a 59-year-old male, who was found to have an HCC, approximately 3 cm in diameter, located in the Spiegel lobe (a part of the dorsal sector) during a follow-up for chronic hepatitis B. The tumor compressed the left side of the IVC and protruded inferomedially. Cotton tape was introduced from the groove between the MHV and the LHV to the groove between the right and left Glisson sheaths via the posterior surface of the liver after dividing all the short hepatic veins from the right side of the IVC. The liver was split into the right and left hemilivers by pulling the tape upwards. The liver parenchyma was divided between the medial sector and the dorsal sector as in Patient 1. The operation time was 623 and 435 minutes and the intraoperative blood loss was 834 and 1320 grams, respectively. No complications occurred in the two patients. The application of hanging maneuvers enables surgeons to safely resect tumors located deep in the dorsal sector of the liver.

This surgical technique requires a lot of indispensable procedures for hepatic surgeries. This chapter presents the step-by-step surgical procedures regarding hanging maneuvers for an isolated resection of the dorsal sector.

2. Patients

The patients' characteristics and preoperative laboratory data are summarized in Table 1. Patient 1 had a cirrhotic liver caused by hepatitis B and had undergone laparoscopic splenectomy approximately two months before hepatectomy to control intractable ascites caused by splenomegaly accompanied with cirrhosis. Patient 2 had a fibrotic liver caused by chronic hepatitis B. Both patients had a solitary HCC in the dorsal sector.

	Patient 1	**Patient 2**
age	46	59
gender	female	male
native liver disease	cirrhosis caused by hepatitis B	chronic hepatitis B
white blood cell (/μl)	4900	5400
hemoglobin (g/dl)	7.9	14.7
platelet (× 10^3 /μl)	235	171
total bilirubin (mg/dl)	0.49	0.42
albumin (g/dl)	3.2	4.6
prothrombin time – international normalized ratio	1.05	0.95
indocyanine green dye retention at 15 minutes (%)	27	13
tumor diameter (cm)	3	3

Table 1. Patient characteristics and preoperative laboratory data

http://dx.doi.org/10.5772/51768

3. Surgical procedures in patient 1

The HCC, approximately 3 cm in diameter, was located just above the IVC (Figure 1). A limited hepatectomy was selected because the patient had a relatively advanced cirrhotic liver and the preoperative evaluations predicted that an extended hepatectomy would have led to postoperative liver failure.

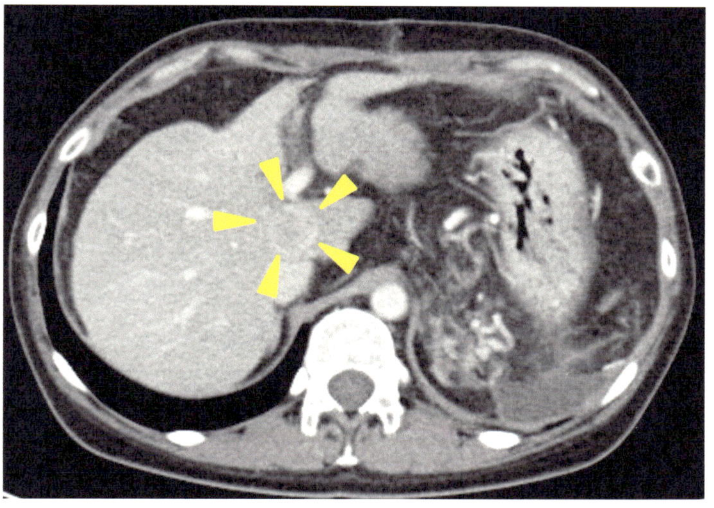

Figure 1. Hepatocellular carcinoma in Patient 1 located just above the inferior vena cava

Figure 2 shows a schematic diagram of the surgical procedure. Patient 1 had a relatively large IRHV. This vein was kept intact because its division could have caused congestion of the posterior sector. The liver was split into the right and left hemilivers by dividing the liver parenchyma along the right side of the middle hepatic vein using a hanging maneuver with a cotton tape introduced into the space between the posterior surface of the liver and the anterior surface of the IVC. The liver parenchyma was divided between the medial sector and the dorsal sector using a hanging maneuver with a cotton tape placed in the fissure of the ligamentum venosum.

The patient was placed in the supine position. The abdomen was opened by bilateral subcostal incisions with an upper midline extension. There was a small amount of ascites and the liver had a cirrhotic appearance. Cholecystectomy was performed and a tube was inserted into the cystic duct for cholangiography. The right lobe was mobilized clockwise by dividing the right triangular ligament. The IVC ligament was divided, and the SRHV and the IRHV were individually encircled with a tape. A thin cotton tape was introduced from the groove between the SRHV and the confluence of the MHV and the LHV to the left-side space of the IRHV (Figure 3).

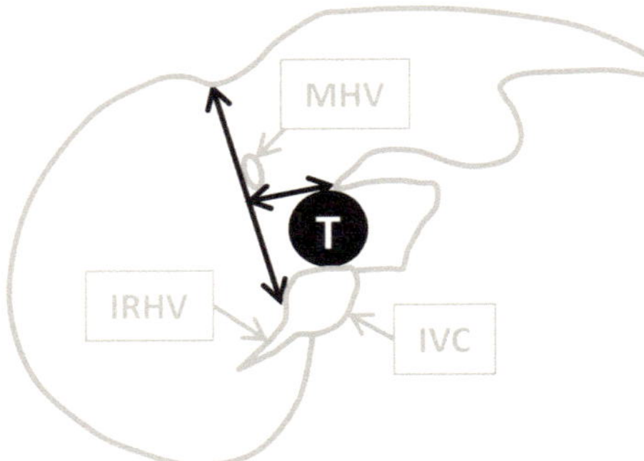

Figure 2. Schematic diagram of the hanging maneuvers for the isolated resection of the dorsal sector used in Patient 1 IRHV, the inferior right hepatic vein; IVC, the inferior vena cava; MHV, the middle hepatic vein; T, tumor

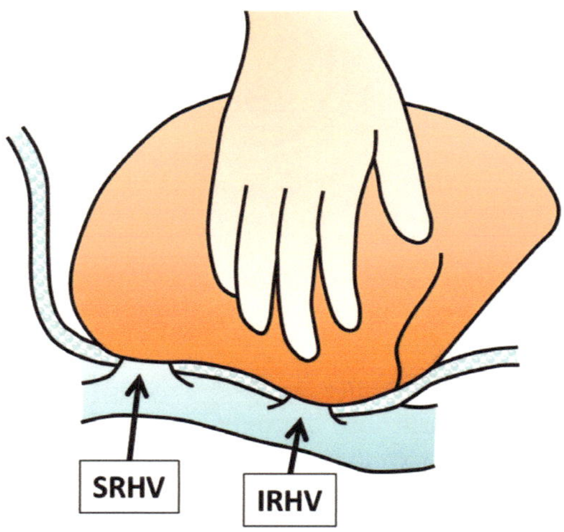

Figure 3. Introducing a cotton tape along the left-side spaces of the superior and the inferior hepatic veins SRHV, the superior right hepatic vein; IRHV, the inferior right hepatic vein

The procedure moved on to the hepatic hilum. The right Glisson sheath was encircled with a tape. A small notch was made on the lowest part of the dividing plane as a hook for the hanging tape (Figure 4).

The left lateral lobe was mobilized counterclockwise by dividing the left triangular ligament. The ligamentum venosum was divided near the LHV (Figure 5). Thereafter, the confluence of the MHV and the LHV was encircled with a tape.

http://dx.doi.org/10.5772/51768

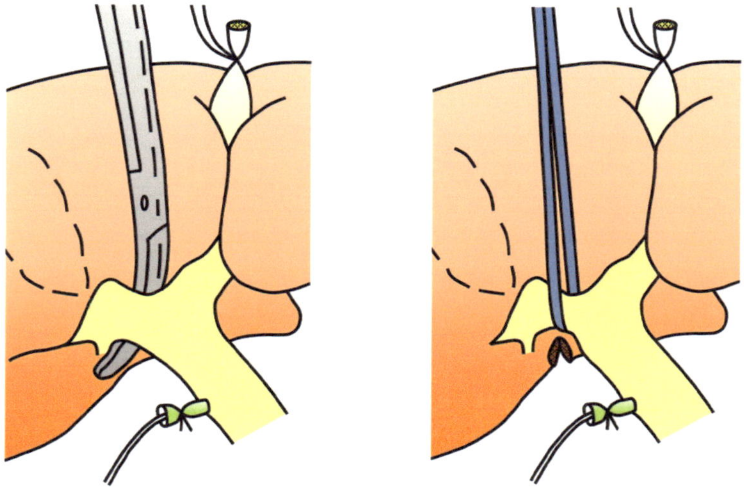

Figure 4. Taping of the right Glisson sheath

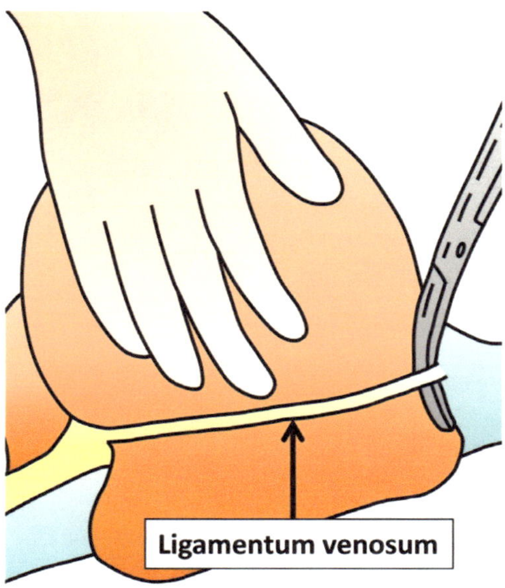

Figure 5. Division of the ligamentum venosum

The tail of the cotton tape was introduced into the groove between the right and the left Glisson sheath. The liver was split into the right and the left hemilivers by pulling up the cotton tape upwards (Figure 6, 7).

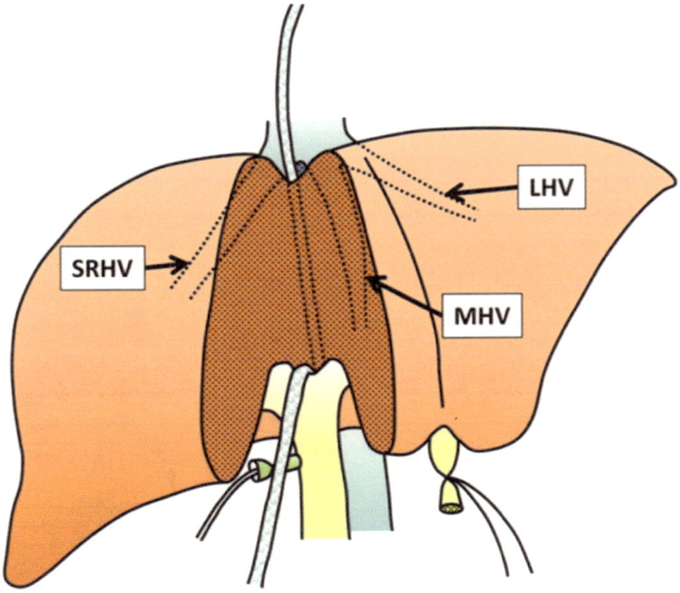

Figure 6. Splitting of the liver into the right and left hemilivers using a hanging maneuver (schematic diagram) LHV, the left hepatic vein; MHV, the middle hepatic vein; SRHV, the superior right hepatic vein

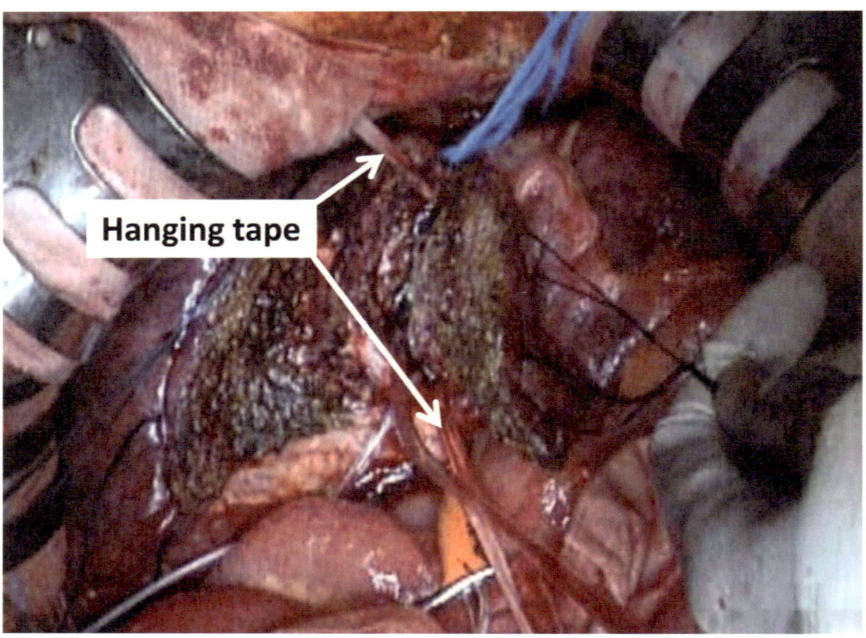

Figure 7. Splitting of the liver into the right and left hemilivers using a hanging maneuver (photograph)

http://dx.doi.org/10.5772/51768

Splitting the liver into the two hemilivers revealed a few caudate branches from the left Glisson sheath (Figure 8). These branches were divided to make a space behind the left Glisson sheath (Figure 9). A cotton tape was introduced from the space behind the confluence of the MHV and the LHV to the space behind the left Glisson sheath via the fissure of the ligamentum venosum. The liver parenchyma was transected between the medial sector and the dorsal sector by medially lifting the cotton tape (Figure 10).

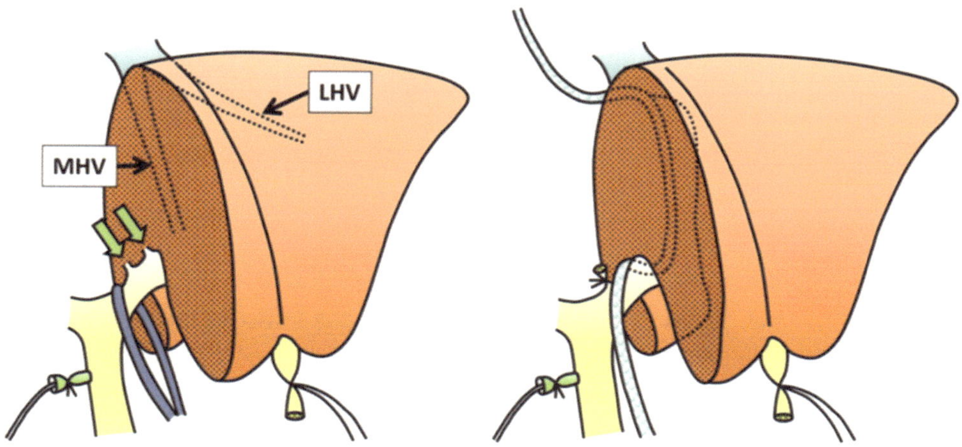

Figure 8. Division of the caudate branch from the left Glisson sheath (left) and a hanging maneuver for transecting the liver parenchyma between the medial sector and the dorsal sector (right) Green arrows indicate the caudate branch from the left Glisson sheath. LHV, the left hepatic vein; MHV, the middle hepatic vein

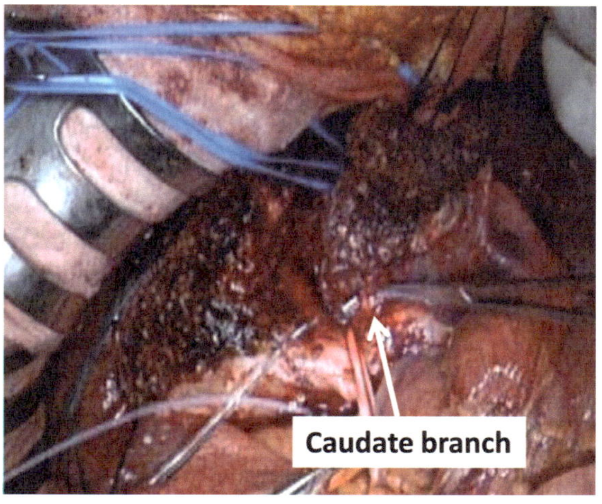

Figure 9. Division of the caudate branch from the left Glisson sheath

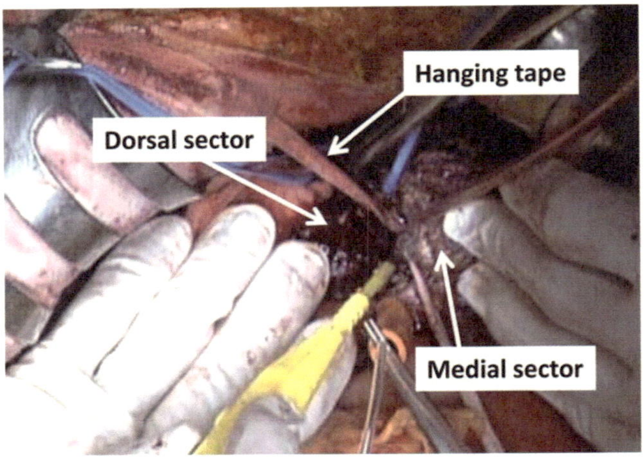

Figure 10. A hanging maneuver for transecting the liver parenchyma between the medial sector and the dorsal sector

All the short hepatic veins from the dorsal sector were divided from the left side of the IVC (Figure 11, 12). The IVC ligament was divided, and the dorsal sector including the tumor was retrieved from the surgical field (Figure 13).

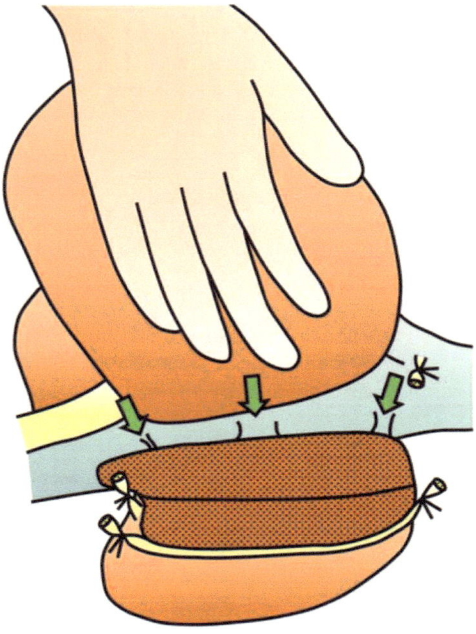

Figure 11. Division of the short hepatic veins from the left side of the inferior vena cava (schematic diagram) Green arrows indicate the short hepatic veins to be divided.

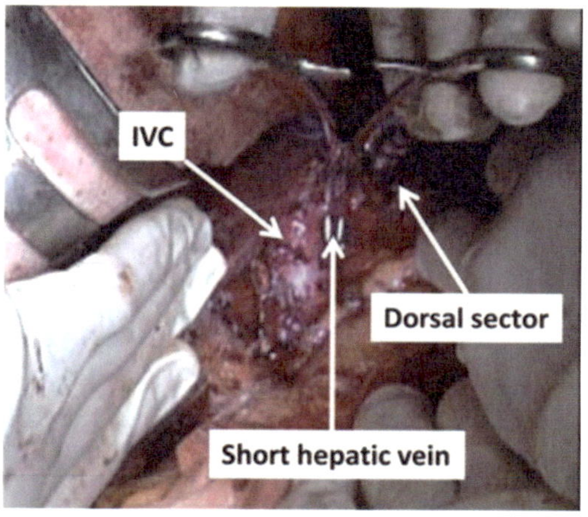

Figure 12. Division of the short hepatic veins from the left side of the inferior vena cava (photograph) IVC, the inferior vena cava

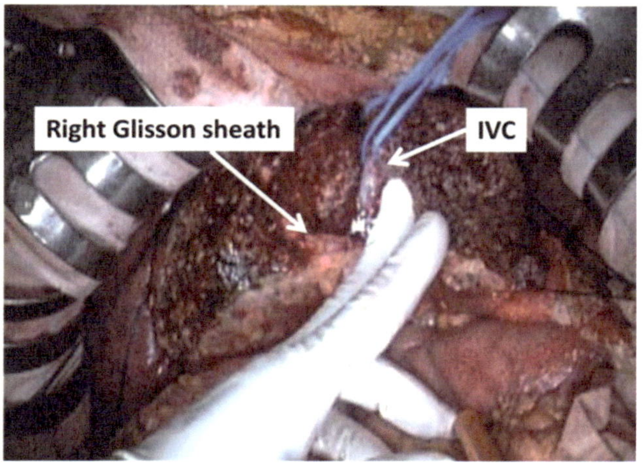

Figure 13. Completion of the isolated resection of the dorsal sector IVC, the inferior vena cava

4. Surgical procedures in patient 2

The surgical procedures in Patient 2 were reported previously [15]. The procedures differed in two points from the procedures used in Patient 1: All the short hepatic veins were divided from the right side of the IVC and the liver was split into hemilivers along the left side of the MHV by introducing cotton tape through the groove between the MHV and the LHV.

5. Surgical results

The surgical results are summarized in Table 2. Patient 1 required transfusion of two units of red blood cell because of pre-existing anemia. The resected specimens had an acceptable tumor-free surgical margin. Kinetics of the laboratory data are shown in Figure 14 and 15. Both patients exhibited rapid recovery of laboratory data. Follow-up CT after the surgeries demonstrated that there were no perfusion abnormalities in the livers (Figure 16).

	Patient 1	Patient 2
operation time (minutes)	623	435
intraoperative blood loss (grams)	834	1320
blood transfusion	two units of concentrated red blood cell	none
length of postoperative hospital stay (days)	13	15
complications	none	none

Table 2. Surgical results

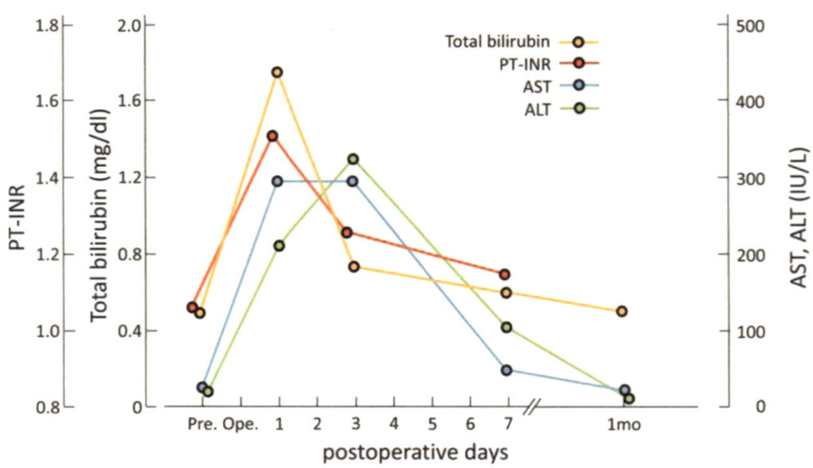

Figure 14. Kinetics of laboratory data in Patient 1 ALT, alanine aminotransferase; AST, aspartate aminotransferase; PT-INR, prothrombin time – international normalized ratio

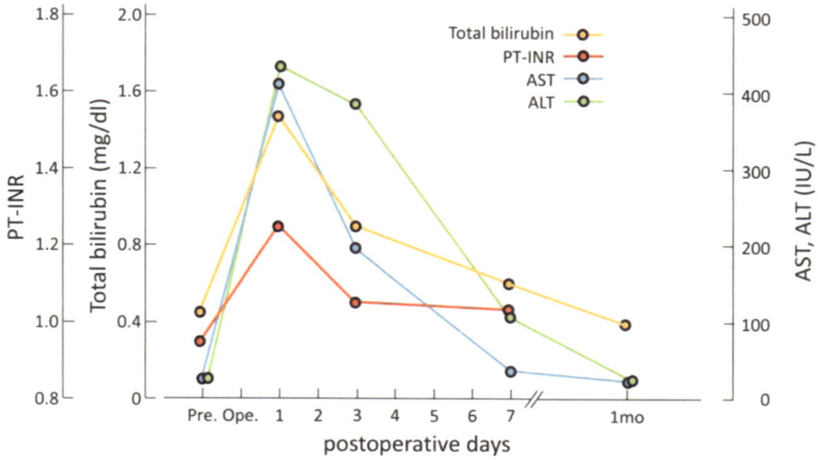

Figure 15. Kinetics of laboratory data in Patient 2 ALT, alanine aminotransferase; AST, aspartate aminotransferase; PT-INR, prothrombin time – international normalized ratio

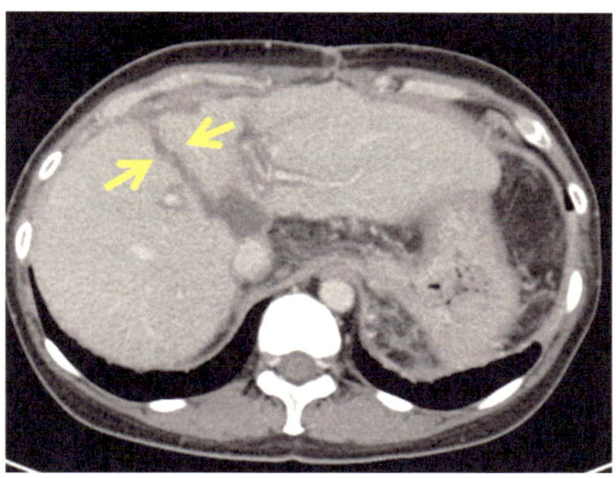

Figure 16. Follow-up CT of Patient 1 two months after the surgery Yellow arrows indicate the dividing plane between the right and left hemilivers.

6. Conclusion

Livers with malignant lesions to be resected are often cirrhotic. Parenchymal transection of cirrhotic liver from the dorsal direction may cause uncontrollable bleeding. The application of hanging maneuvers to an isolated resection of the dorsal sector enables surgeons to safely transect the liver parenchyma only via an anterior approach.

Author details

Hideaki Uchiyama*, Shinji Itoh and Kenji Takenaka
*Address all correspondence to: huchi@surg2.med.kyushu-u.ac.jp
Department of Surgery, Fukuoka City Hospital, Japan

References

[1] Abdalla EK, Vauthey JN, Couinaud, C. The caudate lobe of the liver: implications of embryology and anatomy for surgery. Surg Oncol Clin N Am 2002; 11(4): 835-848.

[2] Asahara T, Dohi K, Hino H, Nakahara H, Katayama K, Itamoto T, Ono E, Moriwaki K, Yuge O, Nakanishi T, Kitamoto M. Isolated caudate lobectomy by anterior approach for hepatocellular carcinoma originating in the paracaval portion of the caudate lobe. J Hepatobiliary Pancreat Surg 1998; 5(4): 416-421.

[3] Chaib E, Ribeiro MA Jr, Souza YE, D'Albuquerque LA. Anterior hepatic transection for caudate lobectomy. Clinics 2009; 64(11): 1121-1125.

[4] Kosuge T, Yamamoto J, Takayama T, Shimada K, Yamasaki S, Makuuchi M, Hasegawa H. An isolated, complete resection of the caudate lobe, including the paracaval portion, for hepatocellular carcinoma. Arch Surg 1994; 129(3): 280-284.

[5] Takayama T, Tanaka T, Higaki T, Katou K, Teshima Y, Makuuchi M. High dorsal resection of the liver. J Am Coll Surg 1994; 179(1): 72-75.

[6] Yanaga K, Matsumata T, Hayashi H, Shimada M, Urata K, Sugimachi K. Isolated hepatic caudate lobectomy. Surgery 1994; 115(6): 757-761.

[7] Utsunomiya T, Okamoto M, Tsujita E, Ohta M, Tagawa T, Matsuyama A, Okazaki J, Yamamoto M, Tsutsui S, Ishida T. High dorsal resection for recurrent hepatocellular carcinoma originating in the caudate lobe. Surg Today 2009;39(9): 829-832.

[8] Yamamoto J, Kosuge T, Shimada K, Yamasaki S, Takayama T, Makuuchi M. Anterior transhepatic approach for isolated resection of the caudate lobe of the liver. World J Surg 1999;23(1): 97-101.

[9] Yamamoto T, Kubo S, Shuto T, Ichikawa T, Ogawa M, Hai S, Sakabe K, Tanaka S, Uenishi T, Ikebe T, Tanaka H, Kaneda K, Hirohashi K. Surgical strategy for hepatocellular carcinoma originating in the caudate lobe. Surgery 2004;135(6): 595-603.

[10] Belghiti J, Guevara OA, Noun R, Saldinger PF, Kianmanesh R. Liver hanging maneuver: a safe approach to right hepatectomy without liver mobilization. J Am Coll Surg 2001; 193(1): 109-111.

[11] Kim SH, Park SJ, Lee SA, Lee WJ, Park JW, Hong EK, Kim CM. Various liver resections using hanging maneuver by three Glisson's pedicles and three hepatic veins. Ann Surg 2007; 245(2): 201-205.

[12] Kim SH, Park SJ, Lee SA, Lee WJ, Park JW, Kim CM. Isolated caudate lobectomy using the hanging maneuver. Surgery 2006; 139(6): 847-850.

[13] López-Andújar R, Montalvá E, Bruna M, Jiménez-Fuertes M, Moya A, Pareja E, Mir J. Step-by-step isolated resection of segment 1 of the liver using the hanging maneuver. Am J Surg 2009; 198(3): e42-48.

[14] Ogata S, Belghiti J, Varma D, Sommacale D, Maeda A, Dondero F, Sauvanet A. Two hundred liver hanging maneuvers for major hepatectomy: a single-center experience. Ann Surg 2007; 245(1): 31-35.

[15] Uchiyama H, Itoh S, Higashi T, Korenaga D, Takenaka K. A two-step hanging maneuver for a complete resection of Couinaud's segment I. Dig Surg 2012; 29(3): 202-205.

Chapter 11

Right Anterior Sectionectomy for Hepatocellular Carcinoma

Hiromichi Ishii, Shimpei Ogino, Koki Ikemoto,
Kenichi Takemoto, Atsushi Toma,
Kenji Nakamura and Tsuyoshi Itoh

Additional information is available at the end of the chapter

http://dx.doi.org/10.5772/51029

1. Introduction

Hepatectomy is an established first-line therapeutic option for hepatocellular carcinoma. Because there is high likelihood of cancer cells from hepatocellular carcinoma spreading throughout the portal venous system, anatomical hepatectomy is effective for eradication of the intrahepatic metastases of hepatocellular carcinoma [1, 2].

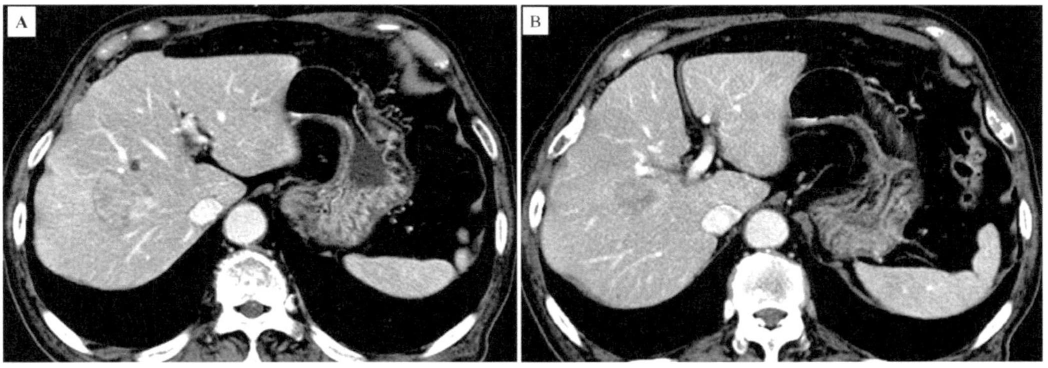

Figure 1. The hepatocellular carcinomais located in segment 8 of the liver (A) and close to the root of the right anterior Glissonean pedicle (B).

For patients with hepatocellular carcinomalocated in the right anterior section or close to the root of the right anterior Glissonean pedicle (Figure 1A, 1B), right anterior sectionectomy has an important advantage, i.e., preservation of nontumorous parenchyma, over conventional hemihepatectomy. Although right anterior sectionectomy is a difficult hepatic resection because of the danger of intraoperative bleeding from the middle and right hepatic veins and risk factor of postoperative bile leakage [3, 4], this surgical procedure is safe and effective in selected patients [5, 6]. Laparoscopic mesohepatectomy is performed at limited institutions [7, 8]; however, the use of this procedure is limited and controversial to date because of the high degree of proficiency required. Herein, we describe techniques of right anterior sectionectomy using theGlissonean pedicle transection method via a conventional open laparotomy approach. The Brisbane 2000 terminology of liver anatomy andresections is used in this manuscript.

2. Surgical technique

Laparotomy is performed through an upper midline incision with right lateral subcostal extension (reversed L-shaped incision). The xiphoid process is excised, the round ligament is ligated and divided, and the falciform ligament is divided along the surface of the liver. We routinely conduct an intraoperative ultrasonography for hepatectomy to define the tumor location and vessels to be manipulated for resection.The right hemiliver is mobilized by dividing the coronary and right triangular ligaments; however, the right adrenal gland is not dissected from the right hemiliver. The ventral surfaces of the root ofthe right and middle hepatic veins are exposed. A cholecystectomy is performed and a 4-Fr. biliary tube is inserted through the cystic duct for a bile leakage test after removing the specimen.

The hepatoduodenal ligament is encircled and taped. The peritoneum of the hepatoduodenal ligament is dissected at the ventral and dorsal sides of the hepatic hilum, the hilar plate is detached blindly and bluntly from the liver parenchyma, and then, the right Glissonean pedicle is encircled extrahepatically using Kelly forceps.To avoid injury to the elements of the caudate lobe, the right Glissonean pedicle should be encircled on the right side of the caudate process branch. After the cystic plate is dissected, the right anterior Glissonean pedicle is identified and encircled extrahepatically[9, 10] (Figure 2). If a large liver tumor is located near the root of the right Glissonean pedicle, it is difficult to approach the Glissonean pedicle extrahepatically; therefore, the anterior branches of the right hepatic artery and right portal vein are encircled separately [11].

After the right anterior Glissonean pedicle is clamped,discoloration of the right anterior section is confirmed, and the demarcation line is then marked by electrocautery (Figure 3).

Using the Pringle maneuver, a parenchymal dissection between the left medial and right anterior sections is performed along the demarcation line from the caudal towardthe cranial direction using an ultrasonic surgical aspirator and the right side of the middle hepatic vein is exposed on the raw surface of the liver. The branches of the middle hepatic vein originating from the anterior section are ligated and divided, and the thick branches should be clamped with vascular clamp forceps, divided and sewn with a continuous suture (Figure 4). At the cranial and caudal ends of the parenchymal dissection, the right side of the middle hepatic vein root and the left side of the right anterior Glissonean pedicle are identified, respectively. The dorsal end point of the parenchymal dissection is the line which connects the root of the middle hepatic vein and the hilar plate.

Using right hemihepatic vascular occlusion [12], a parenchymal dissection between the right anterior and posterior sections is performed along the demarcation line from the caudal toward the cranial direction using anultrasonic surgical aspirator and the left side of the right hepatic vein is exposed on the raw surface of the liver. After the parenchymal dissection is progressed toward the right anterior Glissonean pedicle, the anterior Glissonean pedicle is exposed as distally as possible to avoid biliary injury of the right posterior section (Figure 5) and divided using the stapler or double transfixing sutures (Figure 6). At the cranial end of parenchymal dissection, the left side of the right hepatic vein root is identified.

By retracting the anterior section upward, the parenchymal dissection between the right anterior section and caudate lobe is advanced from the caudal to the cranial direction (Figure 7). Then, the right anterior section is removed (Figure 8).

Hemostasis of the raw surface of the liver is confirmed and the bile leakage test performed. Then, the biliary tube is extracted, and the stump of the cystic duct is ligated.

A closed drain is placed in the raw surface of the liver.

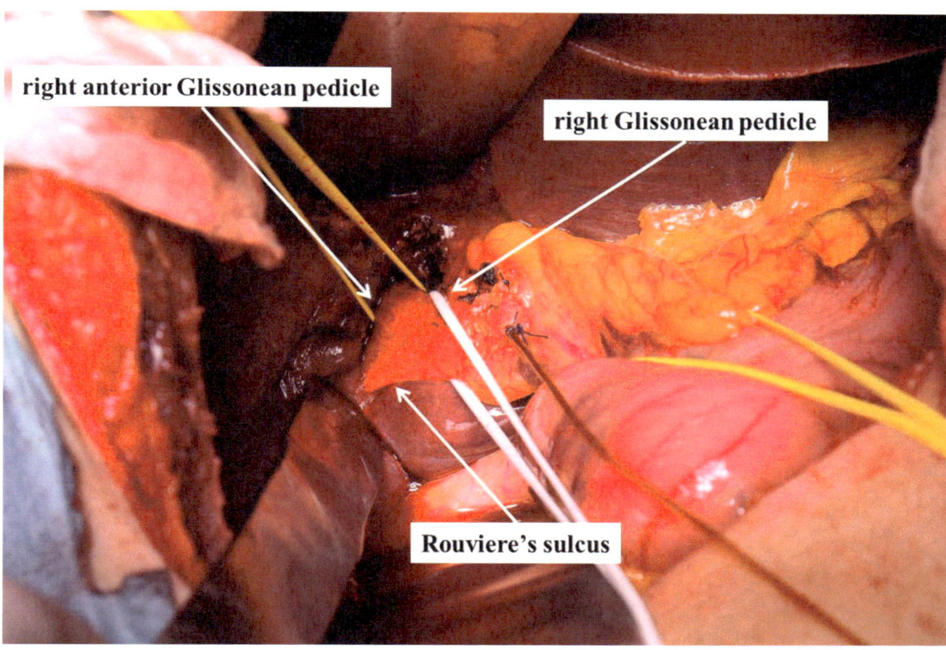

Figure 2. The right and right anterior Glissonean pedicles are encircled extrahepatically.

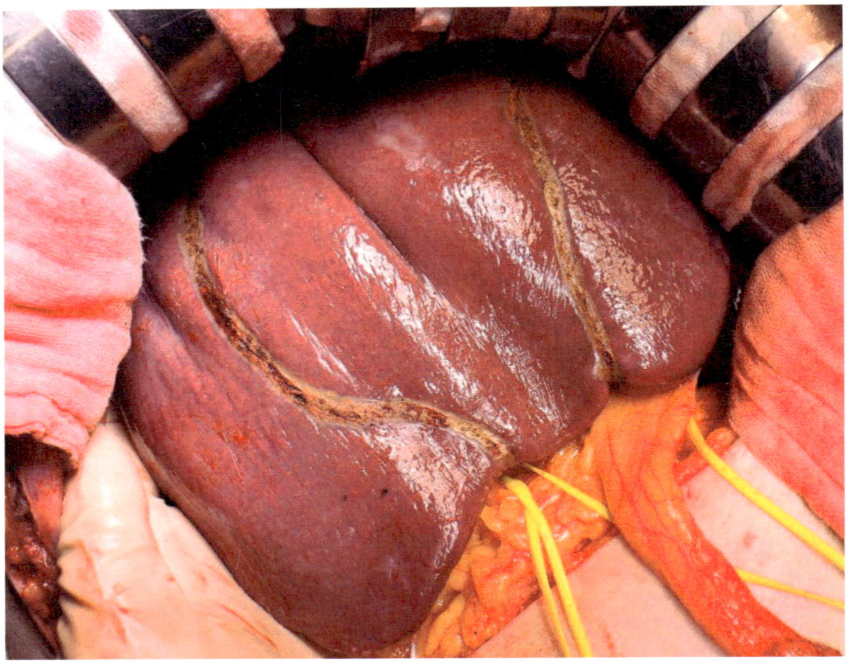

Figure 3. The right anterior section is marked by electrocautery.

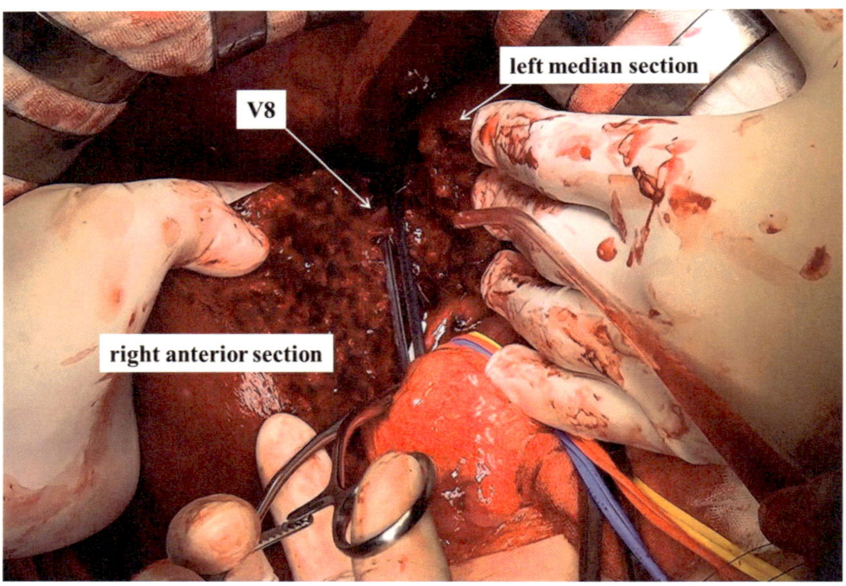

Figure 4. The branch of the middle hepatic vein originating from the anterior section (V8) is clamped with vascular clamp forceps.

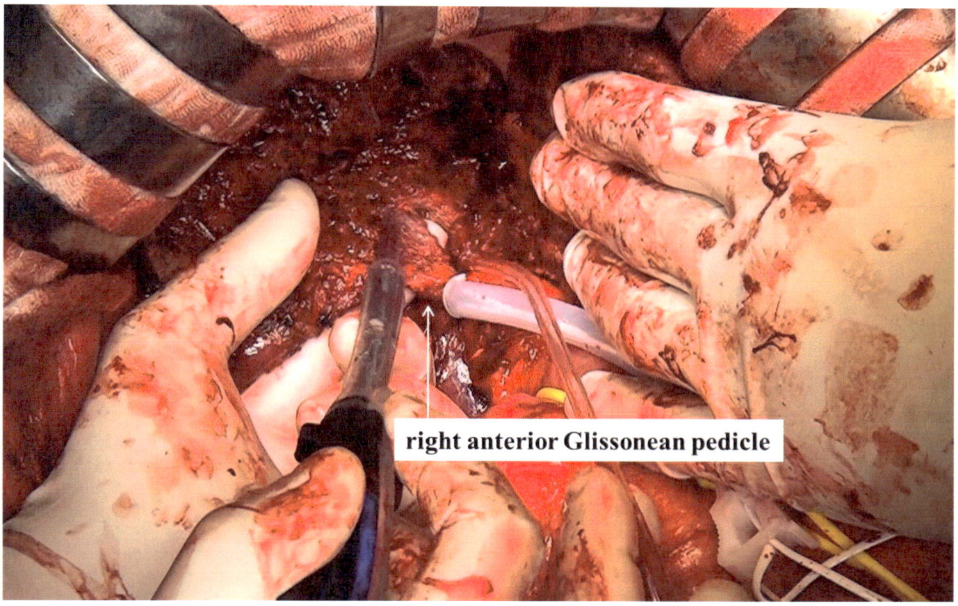

Figure 5. The anterior Glissonean pedicle is exposed as distally as possible.

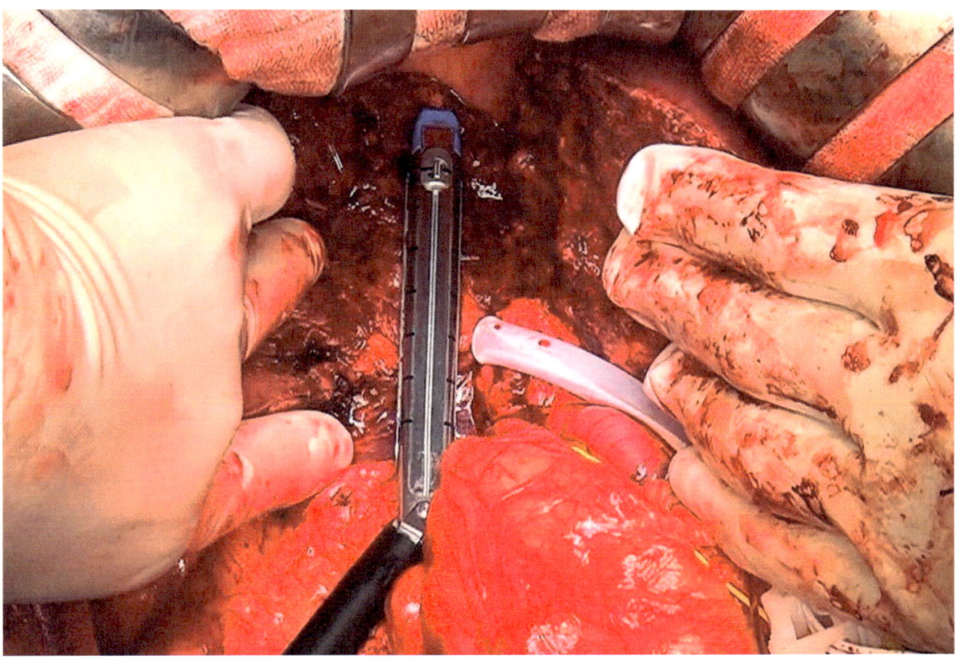

Figure 6. The anterior Glissonean pedicle isdivided using the stapler.

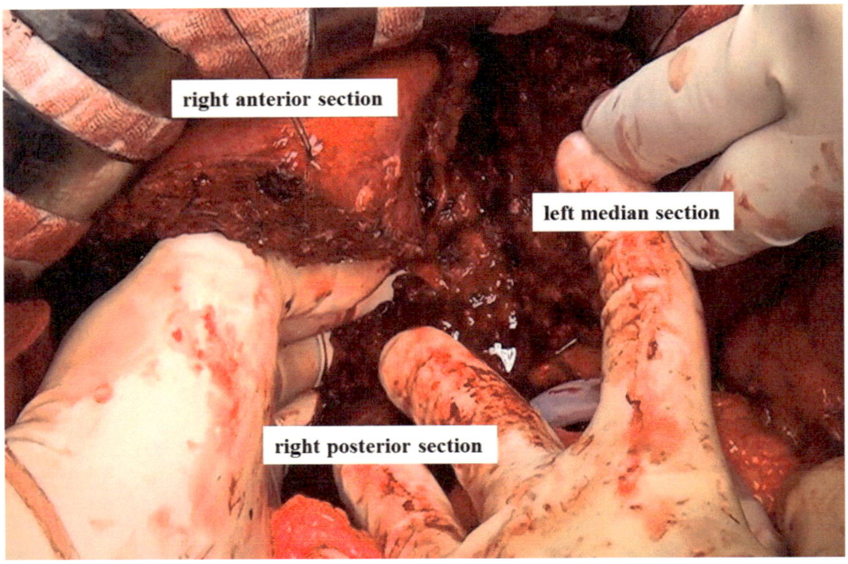

Figure 7. By retracting the anterior section upward, the parenchymal dissection between the right anterior section and caudate lobe is advanced from the caudal to the cranial direction.

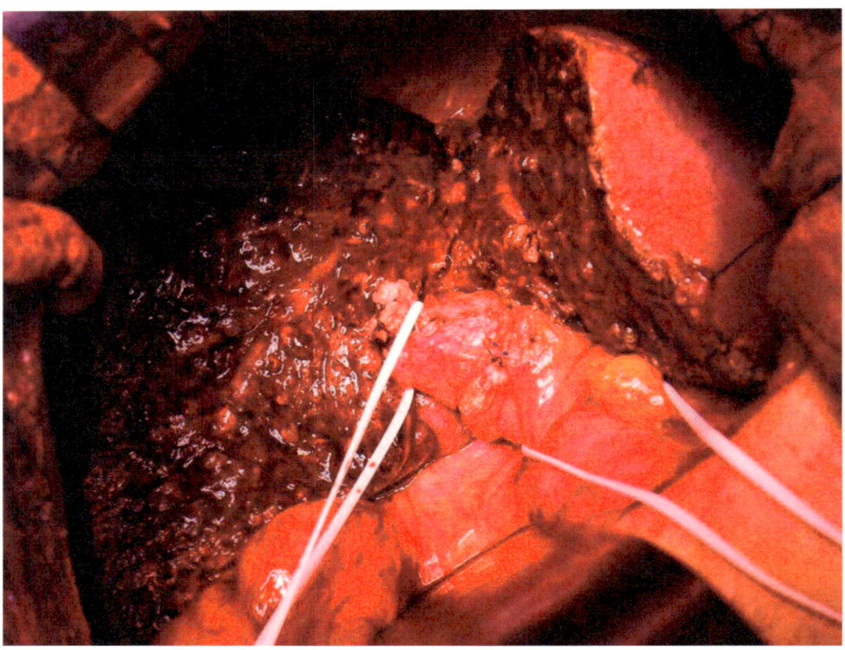

Figure 8. After the right anterior section is removed, the right side of the middle hepatic vein and the left side of the right hepatic vein are exposed on the raw surface of the liver.

3. Comments

Between April 2010 and May 2012, 8 patients underwent a right anterior sectionectomyusing the Glissonean pedicle transection method for hepatocellular carcinoma at our institution. The median surgical time was 323 minutes (range: 227-468 minutes)and the median surgical blood loss was 830.5 ml (range: 180-2009 ml). There was one postoperative complication, i.e., bile leakage, and no mortality.

TheextrahepaticGlissonean pedicle approach is preferable to avoid postoperative lymphatic leakage than separately dividing the arterial and portal branches of the right anterior section. It is important to divide the right anterior Glissonean pedicle as distally as possibleto avoid biliary injury of the right posterior section.

Author details

Hiromichi Ishii[1*], Shimpei Ogino[1], Koki Ikemoto[1], Kenichi Takemoto[1], Atsushi Toma[1], Kenji Nakamura[1] and Tsuyoshi Itoh[1]

*Address all correspondence to: ishii0512h@yahoo.co.jp

1 Division of Surgery, Kyoto Prefectural Yosanoumi Hospital, Japan

References

[1] Hasegawa, K., Kokudo, N., Imamura, H., Matsuyama, Y., Aoki, T., Minagawa, M., Sano, K., Sugawara, Y., Takayama, T., & Makuuchi, M. (2005). Prognostic impact of anatomical resection for hepatocellular carcinoma. *Ann Surg*, 242(2), 252-9.

[2] Arii, S., Tanaka, S., Mitsunori, Y., Nakamura, N., Kudo, A., Noguchi, N., & Irie, T. (2010). Surgical strategies for hepatocellular carcinoma with special reference to anatomical hepatic resection and intraoperative contrast-enhanced ultrasonography. *Oncology*, 78(1), 125-30.

[3] Yamashita, Y., Hamatsu, T., Rikimaru, T., Tanaka, S., Shirabe, K., Shimada, M., & Sugimachi, K. (2001). Bile leakage after hepatic resection. *Ann Surg*, 233(1), 45-50.

[4] Hayashi, M., Hirokawa, F., Miyamoto, Y., Asakuma, M., Shimizu, T., Komeda, K., Inoue, Y., Arisaka, Y., Masuda, D., & Tanigawa, N. (2010). Clinical risk factors for postoperative bile leakage after liver resection. *IntSurg*, 95(3), 232-8.

[5] Hu, R. H., Lee, P. H., Chang, Y. C., Ho, M. C., & Yu, S. C. (2003). Treatment of centrally located hepatocellular carcinoma with central hepatectomy. *Surgery*, 133(3), 251-6.

[6] Kim, K. H., Kim, H. S., Lee, Y. J., Park, K. M., Hwang, S., Ahn, C. S., Moon, D. B., Ha, T. Y., Kim, Y. D., Kim, K. K., Song, K. W., Choi, S. T., Kim, D. S., Jung, D. H., & Lee, S. G. (2006). Clinical analysis of right anterior segmentectomy for hepatic malignancy. *Hepatogastroenterology*, 53(72), 836-9.

[7] Nitta, H., Sasaki, A., Fujita, T., Itabashi, H., Hoshikawa, K., Takahara, T., Takahashi, M., Nishizuka, S., & Wakabayashi, G. (2010). Laparoscopy-assisted major liver resections employing a hanging technique: the original procedure. *Ann Surg*, 251(3), 450-3.

[8] Machado, M. A., & Kalil, A. N. (2011). Glissonian approach for laparoscopic mesohepatectomy. *SurgEndosc*, 25(6), 2020-2.

[9] Couinaud, C. (1985). A simplified method for controlled left hepatectomy. *Surgery*, 97(3), 358-61.

[10] Takasaki, K. (1998). Glissonean pedicle transection method for hepatic resection: a new concept of liver segmentation. *J HepatobiliaryPancreatSurg*, 5(3), 286-91.

[11] Makuuchi, M., Hashikura, Y., Kawasaki, S., Tan, D., Kosuge, T., & Takayama, T. (1993). Personal experience of right anterior segmentectomy (segments V and VIII) for hepatic malignancies. *Surgery*, 114(1), 52-8.

[12] Makuuchi, M., Mori, T., Gunven, P., Yamazaki, S., & Hasegawa, H. (1987). Safety of hemihepatic vascular occlusion during resection of the liver. *SurgGynecolObstet*, 164(2), 155-8.

Chapter 12

Benign Hepatic Neoplasms

Ronald S. Chamberlain and Kim Oelhafen

Additional information is available at the end of the chapter

http://dx.doi.org/10.5772/53848

1. Introduction

Historically benign liver tumors were encountered incidentally during laparotomy or more recently during laparoscopy at which time definitive histological diagnosis can be established. However, with the utilization of advanced imaging modalities hepatic neoplasms have been increasingly identified, with a prevalence rate of up to 50% reported among the general population [1]. Among these incidental lesions, 83% were characterized as benign neoplasms, as outlined in Table 1 [1-3]. Benign hepatic neoplasms represent a diverse group of tumors that develop from either epithelial or mesenchymal cell lines (Table 2), and while the frequency of such lesions is not well documented, more than 50% are classified as hemangiomas [1]. Focal nodular hyperplasia (FNH) and hepatic adenomas represent the next most frequently diagnosed benign tumors. A variety of additional exceedingly rare benign lesions have also been described most of which are sufficiently infrequent enough to be classified as "fascinomas" [1].

Neoplasm	Relative frequency
Hemangioma	52%
Focal nodular hyperplasia	11%
Metastatic tumor (T_xN_xM1)	11%
Hepatocellular adenoma	8%
Focal fatty infiltration	8%
Hepatocellular carcinoma	6%
Extrahepatic process (eg., abscess, adrenal tumor)	3%
Other benign hepatic process	1%

Table 1. Diagnostic frequency of incidentally identified solid liver neoplasms[1,2,9]

Cell of origin	Tumors
Epithelial	
Hepatocellular	Focal nodular hyperplasia (FNH)
	Hepatocellular adenoma (HA)
	Regenerative nodule
Cholangiocellular	Biliary adenoma
	Biliary cystadenoma
Other	Epitheliod leiomyoma
Mesenchymal	
Endothelial	Hemangioma
	Cavernous
	Capillary
	Hemangioendothelioma
	Adult
	Infantile
Mesothelial	Solitary fibrous tumor
	Benign mesothelioma
	Fibroma
Adipocyte	Lipoma
	Myelolipoma
	Angiomyelipoma
Miscellaneous	
Tumors	Biliary hamartoma

Table 2. Benign solid liver neoplasms[1,9]

Most benign tumors are asymptomatic which makes standardizing the work-up difficult. The evaluation of incidental solid hepatic tumors should be individualized based upon the patient's age, sex, past medical history, medications, and associated clinical signs. Although physical examination of the abdomen is typically unremarkable it may rarely reveal localized tenderness and/or a palpable mass. Liver function tests are indicated though are seldom abnormal in asymptomatic patients. Additional laboratory testing such as alpha-fetoprotein (AFP), carcinoembryonic antigen (CEA), carbohydrate antigen (CA) 19-9 and, lactate dehydrogenases may also be ordered depending on the clinical scenario.

Substantial advancements and the widespread availability and use of modern imaging modalities to diagnose and treat abdominal pain, has led to a marked increase in the identification of benign liver tumors. A full discussion of the advantages and disadvantages of

http://dx.doi.org/10.5772/53848

individual imaging techniques is beyond the scope of this chapter but is outlined in Table 3. Briefly, B-mode ultrasonography (US) can effectively differentiate cystic and solid neoplasms and is usually the initial study of choice [4,5]. Contrast-enhanced computed tomography (CT) provides greater sensitivity than US for determination of lesion number, size, and location [5, 6]. Magnetic resonance imaging (MRI) represents the most sensitive and specific study to discriminate between various benign liver lesions, particularly when contrast agents are used [5-7]. Finally, fluorodeoxyglucose positron emission tomography (^{18}FDG-PET) can aid in the differentiation of benign versus malignant tumors based on the metabolic activity of the lesion [8]. Although modern imaging techniques can precisely diagnose the vast majority of incidental benign tumors, laparoscopic or open biopsy is necessary to exclude malignancy when precise diagnosis remains elusive.

Tumor	US	CT	MRI	Tc 99 RBC scan	Tc 99 SC scan
Hemangioma	Hyperechoic Well-demarcated Increased vascular flow Central venous pooling	Highly sensitive **Non-contrast:** Isodense **Contrast:** Hypoense Irregular peripheral enhancement with delayed central filling	Highly sensitive Isodense on T1 Hyperdense on T2 Gadolinium enhanced scan shows similar findings to contrast CT	Blood pooling of radionucleotide	Not indicated
Focal Nodular Hyperplasia (FNH)	Non-specific Hyperechoic	Highly specific **Non-contrast:** isodense **Contrast**: isodense and well-demarcated with central scar	Highly specific Isodense of T1 & T2 Early hyperdense after gadolinium	Not indicated	Takes up Tc99 Tc99 SC contains bile ducts and Kupffer cells
Hepatic Adenoma	Non-specific Hyperechoic Increased blood flow on duplex scanning	Non-specific **Non-contrast:** hypo to isodense **Contrast:** isodense with peripheral enhancement with subsequent centripetal flow	Non-specific Iso- hpointense T1 & T2 Uniform enhancement after gadolinium	Not indicated	Generally does not take Tc99 SC because of the lack of bile ducts and Kupffer cells

US = ultrasonography; CT = computed tomography; MRI = magnetic resonance imaging; T1 = T1-weighted MRI; T2 = T2-weighted MRI; Tc-99m RBC = technetium-99m-labeled red blood cell; Tc-99m SC = technetium-99m sulfur colloid.

Table 3. Radiographic appearance of benign liver neoplasms[1,9]

Accurate diagnosis is essential to the appropriate management of hepatic neoplasms. Although patients may require surgical intervention for diagnostic purposes, few benign tumors require surgical management for symptomatic relief. As such, surgical intervention for benign tumors is primarily indicated (1) for definitive diagnosis when imaging is inconclusive, (2) to prevent malignant transformation, such as in the case of hepatic adenoma, (3) to reduce the risk of rupture and, (4) for the treatment of rare life-threatening complications as a result of rupture or haemorrhage [9].

2. Hemangioma

Hemangioma is the most common benign mesenchymal neoplasm of the liver and occurs in two variants, capillary and cavernous. Hepatic hemangiomas are identified in 0.4% to 20% of all imaging studies preformed [10-14]. Hemangiomas are frequently discovered incidentally on autopsy studies with 60%-80% identified in individuals in their 4th- 6th decade of life [12-16].The precise etiology of hemangiomas is poorly understood but they are generally considered to be benign congenital hamartomas composed of disorganized venous vasculature separated by intervening fibrous tissue [17]. Hemangiomas vary greatly in size from a few millimeters to over 50 cm, with the majority (up to 80%) less than 4 cm [1,12,18]. Although most commonly solitary, up to 40% of patients with hemangiomas have multiple tumors [19].

Capillary hemangiomas are more prevalent than are cavernous hemangiomas [1,20]. However, these hypervascular lesions are typically small (2 cm) and are rarely clinically significant [1]. As such, the management of capillary hemangiomas requires the exclusion of malignancy and patient reassurance that routine surveillance is not necessary in the absence of symptoms [9].

Cavernous hemangiomas are far more often clinically relevant than capillary hemangiomas. The incidence of cavernous hemangiomas is 3 times greater among women than men, with a mean age of 45 years [12,16]. Whether this reflects a true increase in incidence or a result of more frequent imaging amongst females remains unclear as evident by one autopsy series in which there was a nearly equal sex incidence [1,21]. Although no link between oral contraceptive pill (OCP) use and hemangioma incidence has been established, early studies suggest a link between OCP use and increased hemangioma size at initial presentation [18].

3. Clinical presentation

The most frequently reported symptoms of liver hemangiomas include abdominal pain, nausea, vomiting, early satiety, and prolonged fever [1,22]. Most symptoms of hepatic hemangioma are attributable to rapid expansion, thrombosis, or infarction, resulting in inflammation or stretching of Glisson's capsule [1]. Large hemangiomas (> 10 cm) may occasionally present as a non-tender palpable mass in the right upper quadrant, however physical exam more often reveals only vague abdominal tenderness without a mass [1,23]. Occasionally, a bruit maybe detected over the liver. Evidence of intratumoral or intraperitoneal rupture may be reflected by hemoperitoneum and subsequent shock, which requires emergent surgical intervention. Rarely biliary colic, obstructive jaundice, gastric obstruction, torsion of a pedunculated lesion, pulmonary embolism, spontaneous intraperitoneal hemorrhage, and consumptive coagulopathy have been reported [22,24,25]. Kasabach-Merritt syndrome, which was originally used to describe thrombocytopenia and afibrinogenemia associated with hemangiomas on the skin and spleen of infants, is frequently used to define hepatic hemangioma patients with severe thrombocytopenia and concomitant consumptive coagulopathy [26].

4. Pathology

Hemangiomas are typically well demarcated from surrounding hepatic tissue, which often permits surgical enucleation [27]. In tumors not well demarcated, the tumor-parenchymal interface defines the ease with which enucleation versus formal resection is required. Four interface variants between the hemangioma and hepatic parenchyma have been described. The "fibrolamellar" interface is characterized by a capsule-like fibrous ring of various thickness and is the most common [9]. The involved veins parallel the periphery of the hemangioma or traverse the fibrous lamella. The healthy hepatic parenchyma is often atrophic and a plane between the hemangioma and uninvolved liver tissue is well defined. A second variant, the "compression" interface consists of a hemangioma in which the periphery of the neoplasm is well demarcated despite the absence of a fibrous lamella [1]. An "interdigiting" pattern lacks a fibrous lamella and instead is replaced by an ill-defined plane between the vascular channels of the hemangioma and uninvolved hepatic parenchyma [1]. Finally, an "irregular" or "spongy" interface occur when the hemangioma appears to intercalate into the surrounding hepatic parenchyma [1]. Despite the invasive appearance of this variant, hemangiomas do not possess any malignant potential.

The diagnosis of cavernous hemangioma is generally easy to establish with modern imaging techniques. However, in some instances atypical hemangiomas may be confused for other pathology, including but not limited to, hemorrhagic telangiectasia (Osler-Rendu-Weber), hemangioendothelioma, and peliosis hepatis [9]. When diagnosis remains unclear, indeterminate lesions should be managed surgically as percutaneous biopsy may result in uncontrollable hemorrhage [1].

5. Radiographic evaluation

Accurate radiographic diagnosis of hepatic hemangioma is essential since once definitive diagnosis is established no additional intervention is typically required [9]. Radiographic evaluation is largely dictated by clinical presentation as most hemangiomas are discovered incidentally on imaging studies completed for unrelated symptomology and/or pathology. Depending on the initial degree of diagnostic certainty additional imaging maybe superfluous.

B-mode ultrasonography is typically the initial imaging study performed [1]. On US hemangiomas appear as a homogenous hyperechoic mass that is well demarcated from surrounding liver parenchyma [1,28,29]. The addition of duplex US provides additional information regarding peripheral blood flow and central pooling of venous blood [1,28]. As malignant lesions may demonstrate similar acoustic patterns, additional imaging modalities are often required for definitive confirmation. On contrast enhanced compute tomography (CE-CT) hemangiomas initially appear as hypodense masses with a pattern of irregular peripheral nodular enhancement following initial injection of contrast [30,31]. Delayed venous images subsequently demonstrate characteristic central venous filling of the hypodense mass [30,31]. Magnetic resonance imagining (MRI), though rarely needed for diagnosis of most hemangiomas, is the most sensitive and specific modality for the detection and diagnosis of hemangioma [6,32]. T-1 weighted images reveal a smooth well-demarcated homogenous isodense mass, whereas T-2 weighted studies demonstrate a hyperdense pattern [33,34]. The administration of intravenous gadolinium diethylenetriaminepentaacetic acid (Gd-DTPA) contrast results in the pathognomonic pattern of peripheral nodular enhancement with central filling on delayed images [1,35,36]. This enhancement pattern is typical of most hemangiomas > 2 cm [37]. Hemangiomas < 2 cm may demonstrate rapid uniform enhancement which is indistinguishable from hypervascular hepatocellular carcinoma (HCC) [37]. ^{18}F-FDG PET scan may be useful for differentiation between benign and malignant hepatic tumors [38]. Studies have shown that the activity of both glucose-6-phosphatase and glucose transporters are increased in HCC resulting in decreased uptake of ^{18}F-FDG in hemangiomas as compared to HCC [8]. Historically, technetium-99 labeled red blood cells scintigram (Tc-99 RBC scan) was the gold standard for the diagnostic evaluation of hemangiomas, but technological advancements in axial imaging has led to a decline in the reliance on RBC scintigraphy [31,39]. Finally, selective hepatic angiography typically yields a characteristic neovascular "corkscrewing" appearance with rapid central filling from the neovascular periphery described as "cottonwool" [1]. Despite these characteristic findings, the high diagnostic yield of less invasive modalities makes arteriography rarely necessary.

6. Diagnosis & treatment

The majority of hemangiomas are asymptomatic, particularly those lesions < 1.5 cm in size [1]. Although hemangiomas can grow to great sizes, they generally do not compromise liver function and as such liver function tests are often normal. In rare instances thrombosis or intraparenchymal hemorrhage may occur acutely affecting liver function tests. Spontaneous rupture of hepatic hemangiomas is an exceptionally rare event with a review of the literature revealing less than 30 cases of spontaneous rupture since 1898. Given the low yet significant risk of bleeding, fine needle aspiration (FNA) should be avoided [1]. As a rule, biopsy is only indicated if a histologic diagnosis is unclear or will alter planned treatment, thus in the absence of clinical symptoms the most appropriate treatment strategy is careful observation [1].

Surgical resection should be considered in patients with disabling pressure or pain suggestive of extrinsic compression of adjacent structures, in those experiencing acute symptoms related to rupture, or when malignancy cannot be ruled out [22,40]. In general clinical symptoms increase concurrently with tumor size, with most symptomatic tumors having a mean size of 10 ± 8 cm as compared with 6.8 ± 5.8 cm for asymptomatic lesions [41].

Surgical intervention should be approached no differently than for treatment of other hepatic tumors. It is essential that surgeons possess an extensive knowledge of the anatomy and vascular supply of the liver. The extent of hepatic resection required is directly related to the anatomic location of the lesion and its proximity to surrounding vasculature. Thus, the location of the lesion will largely dictate the operative approach hence a full evaluation of the tumor's extent is critical. Large central lesions which border the inferior vena cava, hepatic outflow tract, or the portal vein, may pose an exorbitant surgical risk and as such may not allow for resection [1].

While enucleation is often indicated, formal resection is required in certain instances. Recall it is the histological features of the tumor-parenchymal interface which defines how easily a parenchymal-sparing technique may be utilized. Unlike malignant lesions, resection of hemangiomas does not necessitate removal of a margin of normal tissue with the tumor. Enucleation is carried out by careful dissection within the proper plane between the hepatic parenchyma and tumor. Division and ligation of the principal hepatic artery should be completed early in the operation as this often results in significant tumor decompression thereby facilitating resection [1]. The majority of hemangiomas are contained within a tough fibrous capsule which can be clamped and used for retraction purposes [1]. As hepatic venous branches are encountered extending from the lesion they should be controlled with clips or ties [1]. Presently, mortality outcomes for resection and enucleation are comparable [42].

Hepatic artery ligation for treatment of hemangioma has also been described anecdotally [9]. Although its benefits are likely transient, hepatic artery embolization and/or ligation play a pivotal role only in the temporary management of uncontrolled hemorrhage from rupture [43,44]. Finally, radiation therapy for symptomatic hemangiomas has also been reported. Though data validating the use of radiotherapy is limited, it seems a reasonable approach for symptomatic hemangioma where surgical intervention is clearly contraindicated.

7. Special issue: Hemangioma in children

Hepatic hemangiomas of infancy and childhood differ substantially in their appearance, presentation, and progression than those in adults [1]. These lesions are frequently large and symptomatic. In contrast to adult hemangiomas, the risk of spontaneous rupture in infancy is greater [1]. Similarly, Kasabach-Merritt syndrome occurs more frequently and results more often in death among affected infants. As a result of the numerous venous lakes within these lesions, which serve as siphons for a large proportion of the total cardiac output, severe congestive heart failure and death may result. Initial treatment of high output cardiac failure in children includes oxygen, diuretics, digitalis, corticosteroids, hepatic artery ligation, and radiation therapy [2, 45-48]. Contrary to the conservative management of adult hemangiomas, hemangiomas of infancy and childhood more frequently require life-saving surgical intervention.

8. Focal nodular hyperplasia

Focal nodular hyperplasia (FNH) is the second most common benign hepatic lesion [20]. FNH is found predominately in women (in a ratio of 8-9:1) between the ages of 20-50 years, and has a prevalence of 4 - 8% in the general population [49,50]. Similar to hemangiomas, the prevalence of FNH has markedly increased over the past several decades, which likely reflects the proficiency and widespread use of advanced imaging modalities [1].

Although Klatskin (1977) and Vana (1979) each reported an association between OCP use and the development of FNH, the high frequency of FNH in the absence of OCP use suggests no causal relationship [32,51]. However, enlargement of FNH lesions has been described in the setting of pregnancy and long-term OCP use [52]. While the etiology of these lesions has not yet been clearly delineated, it has been suggested that FNH is a hyperplastic polyclonal response of normal hepatic parenchyma to localized areas of increased arterial perfusion [53]. Expectantly, FNH has been found in association with vascular disorders and malformations including hereditary hemorrhagic telangiectasia, hemihypertrophy Klippel-Trenaunay-Weber syndrome, and congenital absence of the portal vein [49,54-57].

While typically small (< 5 cm), FNH lesions have been reported as large as 19 cm [48,50]. The majority of FNH lesions are solitary in nature (80%-95%), although up to 20% of individuals are reported to have multiple lesions [1, 48, 50]. When multifocal, FNH often occurs in conjuncture with other benign hepatic lesions including hemangiomas [58].

9. Clinical presentation

FNH is frequently asymptomatic with up to 75% of lesions discovered incidentally during radiologic workup, laparotomy, or laparoscopy for unrelated pathology [59]. Similar to hepatic hemangiomas, spontaneous rupture is extremely rare as illustrated by Chamberlain et. al (2003) management of 33 patients with FNH where no ruptures were evident [9]. Large, peripheral, pedunculated lesions may result in a palpable mass associated with abdominal pain and/or fullness, but acute symptoms associated with rupture, necrosis, or infarction are a rarity.

10. Pathology

Macroscopically FNH is a firm pale to red colored lesion with sharp margins. Lesions are typically small, pedunculated, and peripherally located. Unlike hemangiomas and hepatic adenomas, FNH lack a capsule. Histologically FNH appears as regenerative nodules making histopathological differentiation from cirrhosis difficult. Lesions contain normal hepatic elements with a haphazard arrangement of cords and sinusoids [5]. Proliferating bile ducts, fibrous septae, Kupffer cells, and sinusoids are typically present in FNH, and are characteristically absent in hepatocellular adenomas [13,50,59]. Generally FNH contain a large artery with multiple branches radiating through disorganized fibrous septa to the periphery. This radiating arterial pattern produces a spoke and wheel image on angiography and is responsible for the central scar appearance on radiographic imaging studies [60,61].

11. Radiographic imaging

Definitive diagnosis of FNH can be challenging. FNH lesions are well visualized on US but are highly variable and exhibit no distinct characteristic features. Helical CE-CT reveals a well-demarcated lesion that is often isodense [29]. However, during the portal venous phase the pathognomonic central scar may be appreciated. Distinguishing FNH on standard MRI can prove challenging as the lesion is composed of the similar elements as the normal liver parenchyma. FNH may appear isointense with a central scar on T-1 and T-2 weighted imaging [62]. MRI with Gd-DTPA demonstrates a hyperintense lesion early, which becomes isointense with central scar enhancement on delayed imaging [63-65]. The use of reticuloendothelial agents including Ferridex, which is taken up selectively by Kupffer cells, increases the specificity of both CT and MRI imaging [1]. Technetium-99-labeled sulfur colloid scintigraphy may prove helpful in demonstrating the presence of Kupffer cells within the FNH lesion, however this finding is not specific enough for definitive diagnosis [1,66,67]. Angiography, though rarely indicated for the diagnosis of FNH, usually demonstrates a hypervascular mass with a single central artery and enlarged peripheral vessels in a "spoken wheel" appearance [66-68]. Finally, ^{18}F-FDG PET can aid in the differentiation between benign and malignant lesions, but it is neither sensitive nor specific enough for diagnosis of FNH [8,38].

12. Diagnosis & treatment

The natural course of an FNH lesion is generally indolent with minimal risk of rupture or complication. Laboratory testing generally reveals normal liver function tests and alpha-fetoprotein levels, although minor elevations in aspartate and alanine aminotransferase, alkaline phosphatase, and gamma glutamyl transpeptidase may occasionally be seen. Definitive diagnosis of FNH in an asymptomatic patient warrants conservative management and includes close observation with repeat imaging every four to six months [9]. When radiology is equivocal, most surgeons still choose close observation with follow-up studies preformed every three to four months. Biopsy is generally not indicated, as results are seldom diagnostic [69].

Although it may be impossible to distinguish FNH from a well-differentiated HCC without surgical excision, FNH tumors do not undergo malignant transformation. Thus indications for surgical intervention should be limited to those situations where there is a change in the size or number of lesion(s), a change in the intensity of symptoms, or where classic imaging characteristics are absent and diagnostic dilemma remains [70]. Hence, the role of the surgeon is typically limited to patient reassurance and close observation [9].

13. Hepatic adenoma

Hepatic adenomas are identified predominately in women of reproductive age [49]. The estimated prevalence of hepatic adenomas within the general population on postmortem exams is approximately 1% [10]. Etiologically, hepatic adenomas are of epithelial origin. Unlike hepatic hemangiomas and FNH, a clear association between the use of OCPs and hepatic adenomas has been established. First described in 1973, multiple studies have documented a reciprocal relationship between OCP use and adenoma incidence based on estrogen dose and exposure time [71-75]. Approximately 90% of individuals with adenomas have previous OCP exposure [1]. The prevalence of hepatic adenomas is estimated at 1 per 1,000,000 among women who have never used OCP as compared with 30-40 per 1,000,000 amongst long-term OCP users [72,76]. OCPs also affect the course of disease progression as lesions are generally larger, more numerous, and more likely to bleed than tumors in OCP-naïve individuals [32,75,77,78]. Adenoma regression has been observed in patients after discontinuation of OCP with recurrence ensuing during pregnancy and/or OCP re-administration [72,79,-82]. Despite these findings, the mechanism by which estrogen therapy affects the development and course of hepatic adenomas has yet to be clearly elucidated.

Hepatic adenomas are typically small (< 5 cm), soft, solitary lesions but may be multiple in up to 30% of cases [9]. Of note, hepatic adenomatosis disease, defined as the presence of >10 lesions, is a distinct disease entity from that of hepatic adenoma and as such will not be described in further detail [83]. Hepatic adenomas have been associated with type I glycogen storage disease, galactosemia, Klienfelter's syndrome, and Turner's syndrome as well as with androgen, domiphene, danazol and growth hormone use [1,84-86]. Although hepatic adenomas are benign, these lesions have been associated with spontaneous hemorrhage, rupture, and malignant transformation, making prognosis more grave than that of other benign hepatic tumors [5,87].

14. Clinical presentation

Since adenoma and FNH both present in women of reproductive age and have similar radiographic appearances they are frequently confused. Differential diagnosis is critical given that the recommended treatment of each respective lesions differs. Hepatic adenomas are most often diagnosed as a result of imaging done for unrelated pathology or following workup of a palpable abdominal mass (30% patients) [88]. Occasionally episodic pain may be evident as a result of an enlarged liver, intratumoral bleed, or tumor necrosis [9]. Up to 33% of patients with hepatic adenomas present with acute rupture and concomitant intraperitoneal bleeding [1]. The development of acute severe pain associated with hypotension reflects spontaneous rupture and carries a 20% mortality rate if not appropriately identified and treated [32,89-91].

15. Pathology

Grossly hepatic adenomas appear as smooth, soft, and pale yellow tumor on cut surface [1]. These lesions often contain prominent blood vessels that have a high potential for rupture and hemorrhage [1]. As adenomas lack a fibrous capsule intraparenchymal bleeding may occur, which frequently results in a variegated appearance.

Microscopically hepatic adenomas appear as well circumscribed lesions composed of monotonous sheets of hepatocytes laden with glycogen and lipids [5]. These lesions lack normal hepatic architecture and demonstrate thickened trabeculae interspersed with sinusoids and prominent thin walled vessels [1,5]. Biliary ducts and portal tracts are distinctly absent from adenomas.

While the malignant potential of adenomas remains controversial, several authors have reported a low (5%) yet consistent risk of transformation [87]. Histological differentiation between well differentiated HCC and adenoma can be difficult, especially in the presence of fibrolamellar HCC which is also more common in women of reproductive age. This issue is further explained in situations in which HCC and hepatic adenoma have been found adjacent to one another [61,50,89,92,93].

16. Radiological imaging

Although radiographic evaluation is important for complete workup of hepatic adenoma radiographic features are often nonspecific [94]. As such, despite the use of multiple imaging techniques, diagnosis often remains equivocal. Ultrasound exhibits a mixed echogenic pattern with an overall heterogeneous appearance [1,29]. Lesions appear hyperechoic as a result of their high lipid content with a heterogeneous pattern reflecting intratumoral hemorrhage and necrosis [95]. CE-CT imaging is frequently utilized for adenoma visualization and typically demonstrates a hypo- to isodense lesion as a result of low attenuation on non-contrast phase [1]. A variegated appearance with peripheral enhancement during the early contrast phase with subsequent centripetal flow during the venous phase may be apparent, however CT can demonstrate a spectrum of disparate findings [96]. MRI findings for hepatic adenoma are similar to those on CT. Due to the high fat and glycogen content, adenomas are usually well demarcated on MRI imaging [29]. While most adenomas appear iso- to hyperintense on both T-1 and T-2 weighted images, findings are highly variable [1,97]. The administration of contrast agents including gadolinium or gabodenate dimeglumine (Gd-BOPTA) results in early markedly uniform enhancement on arterial phase, which subsequently becomes isodense on the portal venous phase [98]. The use of ^{18}FDG PET scan may also aid in the differentiation of benign versus malignant disease in which where adenomas demonstrate poor uptake of ^{18}FDG as compared to HCC [8,38].

Additional imaging modalities infrequently used include technetium-99 sulfur colloid scanning. This imaging modality is particularly useful in differentiating between hepatic adenoma and FNH, as hepatic adenomas lack bile duct components and frequently appear as a "cold nodules" on imaging [99]. Occasionally however, a minority of lesions do take up the sulfur colloid, rendering them indistinguishable from FNH [99]. Although rarely utilized, angiography typically reveals hypervascular lesions with areas of hemorrhage and necrosis [1,28].

17. Diagnosis & treatment

In the absence of acute hemorrhage, serological tests rarely assist in diagnosis. Liver function tests and tumor makers including CEA, alpha-fetoprotein, and CA 19-9 are invariably normal.

Hepatic adenomas pose a greater risk for rupture (33%) and malignant transformation (5%) than do other benign hepatic lesions [9,87]. As such all patients with suspected or confirmed hepatic adenoma > 3 cm should undergo enucleation or surgical resection [1,100]. The approach to surgical excision should be as previously described. Since all adenomas are suspected to harbor malignancy an adequate margin of normal parenchyma should be taken [1]. When surgical exploration is not feasible angiographic embolization or ligation can provide temporary yet life saving relief.

As a result of the relationship between OCP and adenoma incidence, it is recommended that all individuals suspected of having an adenoma discontinue the use of OCP immediately and indefinitely [1,61]. Patients should also be advised against pregnancy until after adenoma resection, as the growth and rupture risk of hepatic adenomas is highly unpredictable during gestation [101]. Yearly follow-up with imaging is advised among all patients where a causal link between OCP use and adenoma is absent [9]. As a result of improved safety of hepatic resection and the use of minimally invasive techniques in hepatectomy it is suggested that all hepatic adenomas > 3 cm be resected [1,100]. In patients with significant contraindications to surgical intervention, OCP should be discontinued and the patient enrolled in an ongoing surveillance program [9].

18. Additional liver tumors

18.1. Epithelial tumor

Biliary hamartomas

Bile duct adenomas and hamartomas are common tumors. Bile duct adenomas appear as small, white, solitary, subcapsular masses [1]. They are defined histologically by narrow lumen bile ducts surrounded by fibrosis. Hamartomas appear as small gray-white nodules that lie just beneath the capsule of the liver [102]. Biliary hamartomas are frequently multifocal and are characterized microscopically by the presence of dilated mature bile ducts surrounded by fibrous tissue [1]. These lesions are especially important as they are frequently misinterpreted as metastatic tumor by the operating surgeon. This notion heightens the importance of confirmatory diagnosis to rule out malignancy for all hepatic lesions. Precise diagnosis is most important in situations in which the presence of a metastatic liver disease will alter the proceedings of a planned operation.

18.2. Mesenchymal tumors

Solitary fibrous tumor (other names include benign mesothelioma or fibroma)

Solitary fibrous tumors (SFT) are rare mesenchymal tumors that are frequently mistaken for metastatic lesions as a result of their radiographic and intra-operative appearance. Grossly SFT's appear as white-to-gray lesions and can vary greatly in size ranging from 2 – 20 cm in diameter [1]. Despite their large size, most SFT's remain asymptomatic. Histologically, most have a classic short storiform pattern and display an absence of cellular atypia, mitoses, and/or necrosis [1]. However when malignant, SFTs frequently possess a high mitotic rate and marked cellular atypia. Immunohistochemically SFTs display a strong positive staining for vimentin and CD-34 [1]. Since definitive histologic examination is required for diagnosis of either a benign or malignant SFT, surgical resection is indicated in nearly all circumstances.

Lipoma, myelolipoma, or angiomyelipoma

Similar to several other benign hepatic lesions, most benign fatty hepatic tumors are identified at the time of autopsy with only isolated reports of histological diagnosis following operative resection [13]. Multiple variants including angiolipoma, myelolipoma, and angiomyolipoma have been described [13,103]. Additionally, "pseudolipomas" have been described as lesions in which there is an extracapsular fatty tumor with involutional changes. It is probable that this lesion results when a free-floating piece of fat becomes entrapped between diaphragm and liver surface [1,10]. In most situations definitive diagnosis requires surgical resection to exclude malignancy.

Mesenchymal Hamartomas

Mesenchymal hamartomas are exceedingly rare congenital liver tumors which occur most frequently in infants under 1 year of age [9,104]. Microscopically these lesions demonstrate a myxoid background of highly cellular embryonal mesenchyme with haphazard groupings of bile ducts, cysts, and hepatic cells [105]. Generally, the cystic element is the most prominent feature resulting in a characteristic "honeycomb" appearance [106]. In contrast to biliary hamartomas, which are clinically insignificant, mesenchymal hamartomas can significantly impair hepatic function as a result of their large size [106]. Although benign, these lesions can result in death due to mass effect and/or hepatic insufficiency [1]. Thus, all suspected mesenchymal hamartomas should be completely excised when possible. If complete surgical excision cannot be achieved surgical debulking may be sufficient as there have been no reports of recurrence after an incomplete surgical resection to date [107].

Myxoma

Myxomas are exceptionally uncommon benign lesions of the liver. To date fewer than five cases have been reported [9,58,108]. These lesions arise from primitive connective tissue. Histologically myxomas demonstrate a myxoid matrix with scattered proliferation of connective tissue cells [108]. Similar to other types of hepatic tumors described above, surgical resection is generally indicated to exclude malignancy.

Teratoma

Primary teratomas are remarkably rare benign hepatic lesions. A review of the literature revealed only 7 reports to date, with the majority of lesions occurring in children [109]. Secondary hepatic teratomas have been observed following systemic chemotherapy administration for treatment of testicular cancer [1]. Teratomas arise from pluripotent cells and frequently contain components from all three germ layers. Teratomas are typically encapsulated cystic lesions that are easily resectable [1,110]. Imaging characteristics reflect tissue heterogeneity and are often non-specific [110]. Surgical resection of hepatic teratomas is indicated to exclude malignancy.

19. Conclusion

A thorough understanding of the natural history and accurate histologic diagnosis are fundamental to appropriate management of patients with benign liver tumors. Although advancements in imaging have drastically improved the detection and characterization of both benign and malignant liver neoplasms, the ultimate burden of responsibility for diagnosis and treatment remains that of the surgeon. Ongoing improvements in perioperative care and surgical techniques, coupled with increased surgical experience presently permit hepatic resection to be performed with a high level of safety. Despite these developments, a conservative approach including close observation with serial examination and imaging seems most appropriate for asymptomatic patients in which malignancy is not suspected.

Symptomatic patients without medical or anatomic contraindication to a major hepatic resection, as well as patients in whom a malignancy cannot be excluded (including individuals with adenomas > 3 cm), should be considered for surgical intervention. Preoperative needle biopsy is frequently contraindicated due to a high risk of rupture and hemorrhage, and therefore should only be considered after exclusion of hemangioma. Additionally, it is important to note that distinguishing particular lesions (especially adenoma and FNH) on needle biopsy is exceedingly difficult. As such caution should exercised when using this information to make clinical evaluations. Excisional biopsy of small and peripheral lesions and adequate wedge incision biopsy of large lesions should permit the pathologist to make an accurate histologic diagnosis and exclude a malignancy. If doubt remains, formal hepatic resection is indicated.

Author details

Ronald S. Chamberlain[1,2,3] and Kim Oelhafen[3]

1 Department of Surgery, Saint Barnabas Medical Center, Livingston, NJ, USA

2 Department of Surgery, University of Medicine and Dentistry of New Jersey, Newark, NJ, USA

3 Saint George's University School of Medicine, Grenada, West Indies, Grenada

References

[1] Chamberlain RS, DeCorato D, Jarnagin W. Benign liver lesions. In Blumgart L, Fong Y, & Jarnagin W. (ed.) American Cancer Society Atlas of Clinical Oncology Hepatobiliary Cancer. British Colombia: Decker Inc; 2001. p1-30.

[2] Little JM, Kenny J, Hollands MJ. Hepatic incidentaloma: a modern problem. World J Surg 1990;14(4): 448-51.

[3] Little JM, Richardson A, Tait N. Hepatic dyschoma: a five-year experience. HPB Surg 1991;4(4): 291-8.

[4] Izzo F, Cremona F, Ruffolo F, Palaia R, Parisi V, Curley SA. Outcome of 67 patients with hepatocellular cancer detected during screening of 1125 patients with chronic hepatitis. Ann Surg 1998;227(4): 513-8.

[5] Sonnenday C, Welling T, Pelletier S. Hepatic Neoplasms. In Mulholland M & Lillemoe K, et al (5th ed.) Greenfield's Surgery: Scientific Principles & Practice. Philadelphia: Wolter Kluwer/Lippincott Williams & Wilkins; 2011. p934-94.

[6] Yoon SS, Charny CK, Fong Y, Jarnagun WR, Schwartz LH, Blumgart LH et al. Diagnosis, management, and outcomes of 115 patients with hepatic hemangioma. J Am Coll Surg 2003;197(3): 392-402.

[7] Balci NC, Befeler AS, Leiva P, Pilgram TK, Havlioglu N. Imaging of liver disease: comparison between quadruple-phase multidetector computed tomography and magnetic resonance imaging. J Gastroenterol Hepatol 2008;23(10): 1520-7.

[8] Sacks A, Peller P, Surasi D, Chatburn L, Mercier G, Subramaniam RM. Value of PET/CT in the Management of Primary Hepatobiliary Tumors, Part 2. AJR Am J Roentgenol 2011;197(2): W260-5.

[9] Chamberlain RS. Benign Tumors of the Liver: a surgical perspective. In Chamberlain RS & Blumgart LH (ed.) Hepatobiliary Surgery. Texas: Landes Bioscience; 2003. p81-99.

[10] Karhunen PJ. Benign hepatic tumours and tumour like conditions in men. J Clin Pathol 1986;39(2): 183-88.

[11] Lam KY. Autopsy findings in diabetic patients: a 27-yr clinicopathologic study with emphasis on opportunistic infections and cancers. Endocr Pathol 2002;13(1): 39-45.

[12] Gandolfi L, Leo P, Solmi L, Vitelli E, Verros G, Colecchia A. Natural history of hepatic hemangiomas: clinical and ultrasound study. Gut 1991;32(6): 677-80.

[13] Ishak KG, Rabin L. Benign tumors of the lover. Med Clin North Am 1975;59(4): 995-1013.

[14] Gilon D, Slater PE, Benbassat J. Can decisions analysis help in the management of giant hemangioma of the liver? J Clin Gastroenterol 1991;13(3): 255-8.

[15] Edmondson HA. Tumors of the liver and intrahepatic bile duct. In: Atlas of tumor pathology. Section VII, fascicle 25. Washington DC: Armed Forces Institute of Pathology; 1958.

[16] Farges O, Daradkeh S, Bismuth H. Cavernous hemangioma of the liver: are there any indications for resection? World J Surg 1995;19(1): 19-24.

[17] Sewell JH, Weiss K. Spontaneous rupture of hemangioma of the liver. A review of the literature and presentation of illustrative case. Arch Surg 1961;83: 729-33.

[18] Glinkova V, Shevah O, Boaz M, Levine A, Shirin H. Hepatic haemangiomas: possible association with female sex hormones. Gut 2004;53(9): 1352-5.

[19] Little JM. Benign tumors of the liver. In: Terblanche J (ed). Hepatobiliary malignancies: its multidisciplinary management. London: Edward Arnold; 1994. p325-49.

[20] Tait N, Richardson AJ, Muguti G, Little JM. Hepatic cavernous hemangioma: a 10-year review. Aust N Z J Surg 1992;62(7): 521-4.

[21] Dockerty MB, Gray HK, Henson SW. Benign tumors of the liver. II. Hemangiomas. Surg Gynecol Obstet 1965;103(3): 327-31.

[22] Shumacker HB. Hemangioma of the liver: discussion of symptomatology and report of patient treated by operation. Surgery 1942;11: 209-22.

[23] Griecco MB, Miscall BG. Giant hemangioma of the liver. Surg Gyncecol Obstet 1978;147(5): 783-7.

[24] Ochsner JL, Halpert B. Cavernous hemangioma of the liver. Surgery 1958;43(4): 577-82.

[25] Dennis M. Fatal pulmonary embolism due to thrombosis of a hepatic cavernous hemangioma. Med Law 1980;20(4): 287-8.

[26] Hall GW. Kasabach-Merritt syndrome: pathogenesis and management. Br J Haematol 2001;112(4): 851-62.

[27] Baer HU, Dennsion AR, Mouton W, Stain SC, Zimmermann A, Blumgart LH. Enucleation of giant hemangiomas of the liver. Technical and pathologic aspects of a neglected procedure. Ann Surg 1992;216(6): 673-6.

[28] Assy N, Nasser G, Djibre A, Beniashvilli Z, Zidan J. Characteristics of common solid liver lesions and recommendations for diagnostic workup. World J Gastroenterol 2009;15(26): 3217-27.

[29] Madrazo BL. Use of imaging studies to aid in the diagnosis of benign liver tumors. Gastroenterol Hepatol (N Y) 2011;7(10): 683-5.

[30] Trastek VF, van Heerden JA, Sheedy PF II, Adson MA. Cavernous hemangiomas of the liver: resect of observe? Am J Surg 1983;145(1): 49-53.

[31] Foster JH. Evaluation of asymptomatic solitary hepatic lesions. Annu Rev Med 1988;39: 85-93.

[32] Klatskin G. Hepatic tumors: possible relationship to use of oral contraceptives. Gastroenterology 1977;73(2): 386-94.

[33] McFarland EG, Mayo-Smith WW, Saini S, Hahn PF, Goldberg MA, Lee MJ. Hepatic hemangiomas and malignant tumors: improved differentiation with heavily T2-weighted conventional spin-echo MR imaging. Radiology 1994;193(1): 43-7.

[34] Goshima S, Kanematsu M, Kondo H, Yokoyama R, Kajita K, Tsuge Y, et al. Hepatic hemangiomas: a multi-institutional study of appearance on T2-weighted MR findings and apparent diffusion coefficients. Eur J Radiol 2009;70(2): 325-30.

[35] Adam A, Dixon AK, Grainger RG, et al. A Textbook of Medical Imaging. 5th ed. Philadelphia, PA: Churchill Livingston/Elsevier; 2008.

[36] Fulcher AS, Sterling RK. Hepatic neoplasms: computed tomography and magnetic resonance features. J Clin Gastroenterology 2002;34(4): 463-71.

[37] Kim T, Federle MP, Baron RL, Peterson MS, Kawamori Y. Discrimination of small hepatic hemangiomas from hypervascular malignant tumors smaller than 3cm with three-phase helical CT. Radiology 2001;219(3): 699-706.

[38] Kurtaran A, Becherer A, Pfeffel F, Muller C, Traub T, Schmalijohann J, et al. 18F-fluorodeoxyglucose (FDG)-PET features of focal nodular hyperplasia (FNH) of the liver. Liver 2000;20(6): 487-90.

[39] Farlow DC, Chapman RP, Gruenewald SM, Antico VF, Farrell GC, Little JM. Investigation of focal hepatic lesions: is tomographic red blood cell imaging useful? World J Surg 1990;14(4): 463-7.

[40] Alper A, Ariogul O, Emre A, Uras A, Okten A. Treatment of liver hemangiomas by enucleation. Arch Surg 1988;123(5): 660-1.

[41] Charny CK, Jarnagin WR, Schwartz LH, Frommeyer HS, DeMatteo RP, Fong Y, et al. Benign liver tumors: radiologic and surgical management. Br J Surg 2000;88(6): 808-13.

[42] Giuliante F, Ardito F, Vellone M, Giordano M, Ranucci G, Piccoli M, et al. Reappraisal of surgical indications and approach for liver hemangioma: a single center experience on 74 patients. Am J Surg 2011;201(6): 741-8.

[43] Nishida O, Satoh N, Alam AS, Uchino J. The effect of hepatic artery ligation for irresectable cavernous hemangioma of the liver. Am Surg 1988;54(8): 483-6.

[44] DeLorimier AA, Simpson BB, Braum RS, Carlsson E. Hepatic-artery ligation for hepatic hemangiomatosis. N Engl J Med 1967;277(7): 333-7.

[45] Park WC, Phillips R. The role of radiation therapy in the management of hemangiomas of the liver. JAMA 1970;212(9): 1496-8.

[46] Dehner LP, Ishak KG. Vascular tumors of the liver in infants and children. A study of 20 cases and review of the literature. Arch Pathol 1971;92(2): 101-11.

[47] Clatworthy HW, Boles ET, Newton WA. Primary tumors of the liver in infants and children. Arch Dis Child 1960;35: 22–8.

[48] Nguyen L, Shandling B, Ein S, Stephens C. Hepatic hemangioma in childhood: medical management or surgical resection? J Pediatr Surg 1982; 17(5):576-9.

[49] Wanless IR, Mawdsley C, Adams R. On the pathogenesis of focal nodular hyperplasia of the liver. Hepatology 1985;5(6): 1194-200.

[50] Craig J, Peters R, Edmundson H. Tumors of the liver and intrahepatic bile ducts, Fascicle 26. (2nd ed.). Washington DC: DC Armed Forces Institute of Pathology; 1989. p6.

[51] Vana J, Murphy GP, Aronoff BL, Baker HW. Survey of primary liver tumors and oral contraceptive use. J Toxicol Environ Health 1979;5(2-3): 255-73.

[52] Scott LD, Katz AR, Duke JH, Cowan DF, Maklad NF. Oral contraceptives, pregnancy, and focal nodular hyperplasia of the liver. JAMA 1984;251(11): 1461-3.

[53] Poon RT, Fan ST. Assessment of hepatic reserve for indication of hepatic resection: how I do it. J Hepatobiliary Pancreat Surg 2005;12(1): 31-7.

[54] Rebouissou S, Bioulac-Sage P, Zucman-Rossi J. Molecular pathogenesis of focal nodular hyperplasia and hepatocellular adenoma. J Hepatol 2008;48(1): 163-70.

[55] Altavilla G, Guariso G. Focal nodular hyperplasia of the liver associated with portal vein agenesis: a morphological and immunohitsochemical study of one case and review of the literature. Adv Clin Path 1999;3(4): 139-45.

[56] Buscarini E, Danesino C, Plauchu H, de Fazio C, Olivieri C, Brambilla G, et al. High prevalence of hepatic focal nodular hyperplasia in subjects with hereditary hemorrhagic telangiectasia. Ultrasound Med Biol 2004;30(9): 1089-97.

[57] De Gaetano AM, Gui B, Macis G, Manfredi R, Di Stasi C. Congenital absence of the portal vein associated with focal nodular hyperplasia in the liver in a adult woman: imaging and review of the literature. Abdom Imaging 2004;29(4): 455-9.

[58] Mathieu D, Zafrani ES, Anglade MC, Dhumeaux D. Association of focal nodular hyperplasia and hepatic hemangioma. Gastroenterology 1989;97(1): 154-7.

[59] Goodman, ZD. Benign Tumors of the Liver. In: Okuda K, Ihak KD. (ed.) Neoplasms of the Liver. Tokyo: Springer; 1987. p105.

[60] Whelan Jr, Baugh JH, Chandon S. Focal nodular hyperplasia of the liver. Ann Surgery 1973;177(2): 150–8.

[61] Kerlin P, Davis GL, McGill DB, Weiland LH, Adson MA, Sheedy PF 2nd . Hepatic adenoma and focal nodular hyperplasia: clinical, pathologic and radiologic features. Gastroenterology 1983;8(5 Pt 1): 994-1002.

[62] Mattison GR, Glazer GM, Quint LE, Francis IR, Bree RL, Ensminger WD. MR imaging of hepatic focal nodular hyperplasia: characterization and distinction from primary malignant hepatic tumors. ARJ 1987;148(4): 711-5.

[63] Irie H, Honda H, Kaneko K, Kuroiwa T, Fukuya T, Yoshimitsu K, et al. MR imaging of focal nodular hyperplasia of the liver: value of contrast-enhanced dynamic study. Radiat Med 1997;15(1): 29-35.

[64] Mahfouz AE, Hamm B, Taupitz M, Wolf KJ. Hypervascular liver lesions: differentiation of focal nodular hyperplasia from malignant tumors with dynamic gadolinium-enhanced MR imaging. Radiology 1993;186(1): 133-8.

[65] Rummeny E, Weissleder R, Sironi S, Stark DD, Comptom CC, Hahn PF, et al. Central scars in primary liver tumors: MR features, specificity, and pathologic correlation. Radiology 1989;171(2): 323-6.

[66] Mergo PJ, Ros PR. Benign Lesions of the Liver. In The Radiologic Clinics of North America 2nd ed. Philadelphia: WB Saunders; 1998. p319.

[67] Rogers JV, Mack LA, Freeny PC, Johnson ML, Sones PJ. Hepatic focal nodular hyperplasia: angiography, CT, sonography, and scintigraphy. ARJ Am J Roentgenol 1981;137(5): 983-90.

[68] Welch TJ, Sheedy PF 2nd, Johnson CM, Stephens DH, Charboneau JW, Brown ML, et al. Focal nodular hyperplasia and hepatic adenoma: comparisons of the angiography, CT, US, and scintigraphy. Radiology 1985;156(5): 593-5.

[69] Fabre A, Audet P, Vilgrain V, Nguyen BN, Valla D, Belghiti J, et al. Histological scoring of liver biopsy in focal nodular hyperplasia with atypical presentation. Hepatology 2002;35(2): 414-20.

[70] Bonney GK, Gomez D, Al-Mukhtar A, Toogood GJ, Lodge JP, Prasad R. Indication for treatment and long-term outcome of focal nodular hyperplasia. HPB (Oxford) 2007;9(5): 368-72.

[71] Baum JK, Bookstein JJ, Holtz F, Klein EW. Possible association between benign hepatomas and oral contraceptives. Lancet 1973;2(7835): 926-9.

[72] Rooks JB, Ory HW, Ishak KG, Strauss LT, Greenspan JR, Hill AP, et al. Epidemiology of hepatocellular adenoma. The role of oral contraceptive use. JAMA 1979;242(7): 644-8.

[73] Nime F, Pickren JW, Vana J, Aronoff BL, Baker HW, Murphy GP. The histology of liver tumors in oral contraceptive users observed during a national survey by the American College of Surgeons Commission on Cancer. Cancer 1979;44(4): 1481-9.

[74] Rosenberg L. The risk of liver neoplasia in relation to combined oral contraceptive use. Contraception 1991;43(6): 643-52.

[75] Søe KL, Søe M, Gluud C. Liver pathology associated with the use of anabolic-androgenic steroids. Liver 1992;12(2): 73-9.

[76] Reddy KR, Schiff ER. Approach to a liver mass. Semin Liver Dis 1993;13(4): 423-35.

[77] Shortell CK, Schwartz SI. Hepatic adenoma and focal nodular hyperplasia. Surg Gynecol Obstet 1991;173(5): 426-31.

[78] Meissner K. Hemorrhage cause by ruptured liver cell adenoma following long term oral contraceptives: a case report. Hepatogastroenterolog 1998;45(19): 224-5.

[79] Edmondson HA, Reynolds TB, Henderson B , et al. Regression of liver cell adenoma associated with oral contraceptives. Ann Intern Med 1977:86(2): 180-2.

[80] Kawakatsu M, Vilgrain V, Erlinger S, Nahum H. Disappearance of liver cell adenoma: CT and MR imaging. Abdom Imaging 1997;22(3): 274-6.

[81] Aseni P, Sansalone CV, Sammartino C, Benedetto FD, Carrafiello G, Giacomoni A, et al. Rapid disappearance of hepatic adenoma after contraceptive withdrawal. J Clin Gastroenterology 2001;33(3): 234-6.

[82] Norris, S. Drug- and Toxin-Induced Liver Injury. In: Comprehensive Clinical Hepatology, O'Grady, J, Lake, J, Howdle, P. (eds). London: Harcourt Publishers Limited; 2000. p1

[83] Flejou JF, Barge J, Menu Y, Degott C, Bismuth H, Potet F, et al. Liver adenomatosis. An entity distinct from liver adenoma? Gastroenterology 1985;89(5): 1132-8.

[84] Labrune P, Trioche P, Duvaltier I, Chevalier P, Odievre M. Hepatocellular adenomas in glycogen storage disease type I and III: a series of 43 patients and review of the literature. J Pediatr Gastroenterol Nutr 1997;24(3): 276-9.

[85] Espat J, Chamberlain RS, Sklar C, Blumgart LH. Hepatic adenoma associated with recombinant human growth hormone therapy in a patient with Turner's syndrome. Dig Surg 2000;17(6): 640-3.

[86] Carrasco D, Prieto J, Pallardó L, Moll JL, Cruz JM, Munoz C, et al. Multiple hepatic adenomas after long term therapy with testosterone enanthate. Review of the literature. J Hepatol 1985;1(6): 573-8.

[87] Colli A, Fraquelli M, Massironi S, Colucci A, Paggi S, Conte D. Elective surgery for benign liver tumours. Cochrane Database sys Rev 2007;24(1): CD005164.

[88] Molina E, Schiff E. Benign solid lesions of the liver. In: Schiff E, Sorrell M, Maddrey W. (eds). Schiff's Disease of the liver8th ed. Philadelphia: Lippincott-Rave; 1999. p1245.

[89] Leese T, Farges O, Bismuth H. Liver cell adenomas. A 12-year surgical experience from a specialist hepato-biliary unit. Ann Surg 1988; 208(5): 558-64.

[90] Nagorney DM. Benign hepatic tumors: focal nodular hyperplasia and hepatocellular adenoma. World J Surg 1995;19(1): 13-8.

[91] Rubin RA, Mitchell DG. Evaluation of the solid hepatic mass. Med Clin North Am 1996;80(5): 907-28.

[92] Gyorffy EJ, Bredfeldt JE, Black WC. Transformation of hepatic cell adenoma to hepatocellular carcinoma due to oral contraceptive use. Ann Intern Med 1989;110(6): 489-90.

[93] Tesluk H, Lawrie J. Hepatocellular adenoma. Arch Pathol Lab Med 1981;105(6): 296-9.

[94] Mathieu D, Bruneton JN, Drouillard J, Pointreau CC, Vasile N. Hepatic adenomas and focal nodular hyperplasia: dynamic CT study. Radiology 1986;160(1): 53-8.

[95] Golli M, Van Nhieu JT, Mathieu D, Zafrani ES, Cherqui D, Dhumeaux D, et al. Hepatocellular adenoma: color Doppler US and pathologic correlations. Radiology 1994;190(3): 741-4.

[96] Grazoli L, Federle MP, Brancatelli G, Ichikawa T, Olivetti L, Blachar A. Hepatic adenomas: imaging and pathologic findings. Radiographics 2001;21(4): 877-92.

[97] Chung KY, Mayo-Smith WW, Saini S, Rahmouni A, Golli M, Mathieu D. Hepatocellular adenoma: MR imaging features with pathologic correlation. ARJ Am J Roentgenol 1994;163(2): 303-8.

[98] Paulson EK, McClellan JS, Washington K, Spritzer CE, Meyers WC, Baker ME. Hepatic adenoma: MR characteristics and correlation with pathological findings. AJR 1994;163(1): 113-6.

[99] Rubin RA, Lichenstein GR. Hepatic scintigraphy in the evaluation of solitary solid liver masses. J Nucl Med 1993;34(4): 697-705.

[100] Koffron A, Geller D, Gamblin TC, Abecassis M. Laparoscopic liver surgery; Shifting the management of liver tumors. J Hepatology 2006;44(6):1694-700.

[101] Bis KA, Waxman B. Rupture of the liver associated with pregnancy: a review of the literature and report of 2 cases. Obstet Gynecol Surv 1976;31(11); 763-73.

[102] Moran CA, Ishak KG, Goodman ZD. Solitary fibrous tumor of the liver: a clinicopathologic and immunohistochemical study of nine cases. Ann Diagn Pathol 1998;2(1): 19-24.

[103] Pounder DJ. Hepatic angiomyolipoma. Am J Surg Pathol 1982;6(7): 677-81.

[104] Grases PJ, Matos-Villaobos M, Arcia-Romero F, Lecuna-Torres V. Mesenchymal hamartoma of the liver. Gastroenterology 1979;76(6): 1466-9.

[105] Stocker JT, Ishak KG. Mesenchymal hamartoma of the liver: report of 30 cases and review of the literature. Pediatr Pathol 1983;1(3): 245-67.

[106] Klaassen Z, Paragi PR, Chamberlain RS. Adult Mesenchymal hamartoma of the liver: Case report. Case Rep Gastroenterol 2010;4(1):84-92.

[107] Foster JH, Berman M. Solid Liver Tumors. Philadelphia, PA: WB Saunders; 1977.

[108] Yoon GS, Kang GH, Kim OJ. Primary myxoid leiomyoma of the liver. Arch Pathol Lab Med 1998;122(12): 1112-5.

[109] Ukiyama E, Endo M, Yoshida F. Hepatoduodenal ligament teratoma with hepatic artery running inside. Pediatr Surg Int. 2008;24(11): 1239-42.

[110] Prasad SR, Wang H, Rosas H, Menias CO, Narra VR, Middleton WD, et al. Fat-containing lesions of the liver: radiologic-pathologic correlation. Radiographics 2005;25(2): 321-31.

Chapter 13

Surgical Management of Primary Hepatocellular Carcinoma

Kun-Ming Chan and Ashok Thorat

Additional information is available at the end of the chapter

http://dx.doi.org/10.5772/51418

1. Introduction

Hepatocellular carcinoma (HCC) is among the most common malignancy and cause of cancer related death worldwide, with a high prevalence in Asia and south Africa as well as an increasing incidence in the western country. Patients with liver cirrhosis are at highest risk of developing this malignant disease, and the majority of HCC patients will develop the disease on the background of preexisting hepatitis virus infection. It is estimated 50–70% associated with hepatitis C virus in North America and Europe and 70% associated with hepatitis B virus in Asia and Africa [1], and the incidence of HCC is significantly higher in men than in women. However, surveillance programs for HCC in patients with cirrhosis and chronic hepatitis, and the advancement of diagnostic tools are likely to further increase the incidence of HCC and the detection of small lesions in the liver that prompted the proportion of patients diagnosed at a potentially curative stage of disease.

Several staging systems have so far been proposed for aiding assessment of treatment planning for HCC patients, but an overall consensus remains not exist for any of these staging systems.The Tumor-Node-Metastasis staging (TNM) system of the American Joint Committee on Cancer/Committee of the International Union Against Cancer (AJCC/UICC) has been widely used for numerous cancer staging in order to stratify patients into prognostic groups [2], but it is not perfectly applicable for HCC in terms of treatment assessment as the TNM staging does not consider the underlying liver functional reserve and seems only applicable to patients undergoing liver resection or liver transplantation. The Cancer of the Liver Italian Program (CLIP) classifications and the Okuda staging system were introduced not only considering tumor features but also liver functional reserve.The CLIP scoring system considers cirrhotic status in terms of Child-Turcotte-Pugh (CTP) class and several factors related to tumor features including tumor morphology, Alphafeto protein (AFP) level, and portal vein thrombosis [3]. Although the CLIP scoring system is probably helpful to identify patients with a poor prognosis, it might be inadequate to identify patients at early stages of disease. The Okuda system has also been found unsuitable for prognostic stratification of patients at an early stage of disease [4]. Therefore, the Japan Integrated Staging score that combines the CTP class with the Liver Cancer Study Group of Japan TNM stage was formulated to provide better stratification of patients with early HCC than that achieved by the CLIP score and Okuda system [5]. Additionally, the Barcelona Clinic Liver Cancer(BCLC) staging system was suggested as a modification of the Okuda system, and has been validated superior for prognostic stratification of patients with HCC than other staging systems [6-8]. The BCLC staging system involves factors related to underlying liver function, tumor characteristics, and patients' performance status, and was proposed as a means of predicting prognosis and as a guide to selecting appropriate therapy for HCC patients.

Generally, these staging systems was developed aiming to stratify patients into groups with similar prognoses and to serve as a guiding choice of therapy. Current popular treatments for HCC include liver resection, percutaneous ethanol injection (PEI) or radiofrequency ablation (RFA), transcatheter arterial chemoembolization (TACE), liver transplantation, and targeted therapy with novel biologic agent such as sorafenib. The selection of treatment modality for HCC patients should be based on the patient's prognosis, which is complex to assess, as it depends on three factors, namely, the tumor characteristics, the underlying liver functional reserve and the patient's physical condition. At present, only liver resection and liver transplantation are considered the best potential curative therapies. Nonetheless, because of underlying liver dysfunction, lack of liver donor availability, and/or late detection at advanced cancerous stage, only a small proportion of patients are eligible for these curative treatments. This chapter reviews the importance and clinical impact of surgical management in terms of liver resection and transplantation for patients with primary HCC and highlights their relative strengths and weakness.

2. Liver Resection

Liver resection remains the mainstay curative treatment for patients with HCC. However, the majority of HCC patients are often associated with liver cirrhosis due to hepatitis B or C viral infection, which might prohibit from liver resection because of impaired liver function. Moreover, many HCC patients present with advanced tumor stage and only approximately 20–30% of patients are candidates for liver resection on presentation [9-11]. In spite of this situation, the advancement in anesthetic and surgical techniques, as well as a thorough understanding of the liver anatomy, and better perioperative care, have contributed dramatically to the safety and effectiveness of liver resection for HCC.

Since the proposal of the finger fracture technique for hepatic lobectomy in 1953, transection of the hepatic parenchyma has evolved during the last 50 years. By finger fracture technique, the liver tissue is fractured and crushed by the thumb and index finger followed by isolating and ligating the resistant intrahepatic vascular and ductal structures [12]. However, there is some troublesome bleeding from the resection line which makes the surgeons fear for the safety of the finger fracture technique. To overcome this short coming of the finger fracture technique, many special instruments were invented to increase the successful rate and safety of liver resection ever since (Figure 1). Currently, Kelly clamp crushing technique is still one of the most widely used techniques for liver resection. However, in many centers, including the author's center, ultrasonic dissection using the Cavitron Ultrasonic Surgical Aspirator (CUSA) has become the standard technique of liver resection. Today, laparoscopic liver resection has become feasible in experienced centers due to improvement in instruments [13-15]. Additionally, modern concepts including the use of vascular inflow occlusion, anatomic resection, and low central venous pressure anesthesia, and surgical approaches such as the anterior approach and liver hanging maneuver have been developed along with using more effective instruments for transection of hepatic parenchyma [16-18]. As a result, liver resections are increasingly being performed and accepted as a safety procedure.

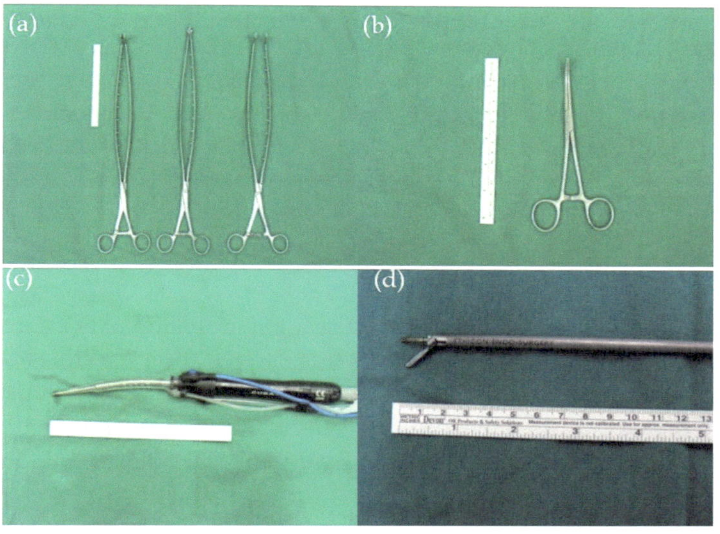

Figure 1. Liver resection instruments. (a). Lin's clamp designed by T.Y. Lin. (b). Kelly clamp. (c). Cavitron Ultrasonic Surgical Aspirator (CUSA). (d). Harmonic scalpel for laparoscopic liver resection.

2.1. Preoperative assessment

The major concern of liver resection in HCC patients is postoperative liver failure, which is particularly worrisome in patients requiring major resections and/or diseased background of cirrhotic liver. Therefore, a thorough evaluating of patients in terms of tumor features of radiologic examination, underlying liver function, and the patient's physical status is very important. Theoretically, a successful liver resection for HCC patients should be weighed against the balance of these three factors.

2.1.1. Evaluation of tumor status

The assessment of tumor status is the essential step for determining resectability and the appropriate type of liver resection. The routine radiologic imaging examination prior to liver resection should include a dynamic liver computed tomography (CT) scan, hepatic angiography, and/or magnetic resonance imaging (MRI) to confirm the diagnosis of HCC as well as tumor status in terms of size, number and location. Additionally, a chest X-ray or contrast CT scan of chest and abdomen could be performed to exclude lung or other extrahepatic metastasis. The CT scan provides important information not only on the tumor size, number, location, and any vascular invasion but also on the relationship between the tumor and major vasculature. Generally, pre-operative biopsy is not necessary as may risk needle track related tumor seeding.

Large HCC—Solitary HCC with diameter of less than 5 cm is the best candidate for liver resection because of favorable patients' outcome in terms of HCC recurrent-free survival [19, 20]. However, numerous patients continue to be diagnosed HCC at an advanced stage that sometimes presented with large tumor with diameter exceed 10 cm. Although liver resection for patients with large tumor can be a great challenge for liver surgeons, liver resection for large HCCs has been shown to be safe and reasonable long-term survival results can be achieved that appear to be much better than any other nonsurgical treatments [21-23]. The 5-year survival rate in patients with tumors larger than 10 cm after liver resection is approximately 21–27.5% [23-25]. Additionally, since liver transplantation and local ablation are not indicated for these patients, surgical resection remains the only treatment of choice that provides potential cure of patients with large HCC.

Multiple HCCs—Multiple HCCs may represent as a manifestation of advanced disease with intrahepatic metastasis or independent tumors that derived from multiple foci of hepatocarcinogenesis, which could be an event associated with a poor prognosis. Patients with multiple HCCs more than 3 nodules have been considered unsuitable for resection. However, it had been shown that liver resection still can provide survival benefits even for patients with multiple tumors in a background of CTP class A cirrhosis, and the overall survival rates can up to 58% at 5 years [26]. Additionally, combined resection and radiofrequency ablation is considered a new strategy to increase the chance of curative treatment for patients with bilobar multiple HCCs. For example, resection of the large tumor in one lobe and ablation of smaller tumors in the other lobe can be performed, or resection of peripheral lesions and ablation of central lesions for patients with multifocal tumors associated with cirrhosis and borderline liver function can be performed [27, 28]. The results showed patients who underwent surgical resection for multiple HCCs had better survival outcomes as compared with those who received nonsurgical therapy. Hence, when clearance of all tumor nodules is feasible and liver function permits, surgical resection or plus effective local ablative therapy should be considered for patients with bilobar or multiple HCCs.

HCC involving major portal and hepatic veins—HCCs with major portal or hepatic veins involvement represent an aggressive tumor behavior and frequently associated with multifocal tumors. Although HCCs with vascular invasion are not considered as favorable surgical candidates, studies from experienced liver surgical groups have shown that surgical resection for such tumors seems justified as it still results in better survival rates as compared with that of nonsurgical treatment [29, 30]. The overall survival rates at 5 years were ranged from 23% to 42% in selected patient who has no liver cirrhosis or impaired liver function.

2.1.2. *Evaluation of liver function*

Preoperative proper assessment of liver function is fundamental to the safe of liver resection for HCC patients, but there is no individual test accurately predicting liver function.The CTP classification is the most common measure to assess liver function, and it combines different parameters and provides a rough evaluation of the gross synthetic and excretory capacity of the liver. Generally, patients with CTP class A are considered good candidates for liver resection. Patients with CTP class B may be only suitable for minor liver resection such as wedge resection or single segmentectomy [31], whereas patients with CTP class C are contraindicated for resection. The risk of death after liver resection increases with each CTP class. However, this classification is a crude measure and has proven insufficient to stratify the surgical risk of patient with liver cirrhosis.

Portal hypertension is usually defined by that the portal venous pressure is greater than 10 mmHg, in which the normal value ranges from 5 to 8 mmHg. Patients with portal hypertension undergoing liver resection may lead to severe complications, such as variceal bleeding, endotoxemia, and even hepatic failure in the postoperative period [32]. However, measurement of portal venous pressure prior to liver resection is difficult, and portal hypertension could only be roughly assessed by clinical and radiologic signs including splenomegaly, abdominal collaterals, thrombocytopenia with platelet count less than 100,000/mm^3, or esophagogastric varices. Although portal hypertension is considered a relatively contraindication of liver resection, study had shown that liver resection is also capable of providing survival benefits to patients with a background of portal hypertension [26]. Additionally, patients with abnormal elevation of liver function tests in terms of serum aspartate and alanine aminotransferase levels might have a higher risk of postoperative complication and mortality rates, and are considered to be poor candidates for major liver resection [33, 34]. Therefore, patients with abnormal liver function tests should be carefully assessed and selected prior to liver resection.

Additionally, several hepatobiliary centers have employed more sophisticated quantitative liver function tests, such as the lidocaine monoethylglycinexylidide test, aminopyrine breath test, galactose elimination capacity, and indocyanine green (ICG) clearance test to evaluate the hepatic metabolic function and to predict the risk of postoperative liver failure [35-37]. However, these specific tests reflect the function of the whole liver, whereas the risk of postoperative liver failure relies on the liver function reserve of the remnant liver. Among the various methods, the ICG test is the most widely used to assess liver function prior to liver resection. The ICG is an organic dye that is taken up by the hepatocytes and excreted via the bile in an adenosine triphosphate (ATP) dependent manner without been metabolized and undergoing enterohepatic circulation. Thus, the clearance of ICG from systemic circulation is merely a measure of hepatic blood flow and function. This test evaluates the retention ratio of ICG from the peripheral blood at definitive time point after injection of 0.5 mg ICG/kg (usually 15 minutes, ICG-15), and Makuuchi et al. have incorporated the ICG-15 and two clinical features in terms of serum bilirubin level and the presence of ascites into an algorithm of liver resection (Figure 2) [38]. In patients with bilirubin levels less than 1.0mg/dL and the absence of ascites, ICG-15 is used to predict the extent of liver segments that can be safely removed. In general, an ICG-15 of 10–20% is usually considered a safety upper limit for major liver resection. Accordingly, the algorithm has been validated toward zero surgical mortality after liver resection by several hepatobiliary centers [39, 40].

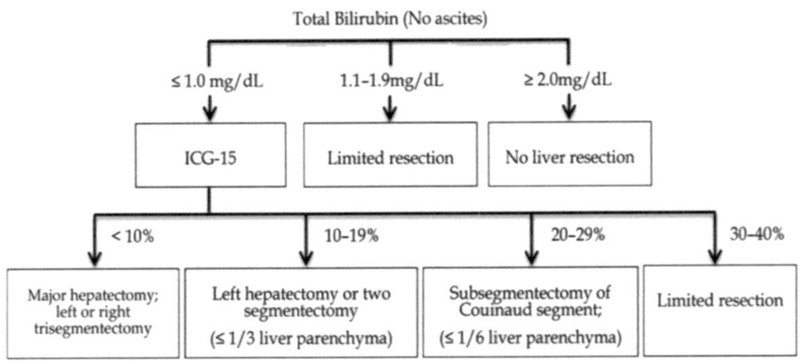

Figure 2. Makuuchi's algorithm for liver resection in patients with HCC [38]. Limited resection means enucleation of the tumor (usually ≤ 5cm) and less than 1 cm of liver tissue surrounding the tumor was removed.

ICG-15 (%)	Safe resection ratio of liver volume
0	< 63.3%
~ 5	< 53.4%
~ 10	<43.5%
~ 15	<33.6%
~ 20	<23.7%
~ 25	<13.8%
~ 30	<3.9%
≥ 32	0%

Table 1. The safe resection ratio of liver volume based on the ICG test [43].

Although the assessment of hepatic function and liver volume to be resected is crucial for a safe liver resection, volumetric analysis of the future liver remnant (FLR) has also been suggested. The FLR can be measured directly by computer-assisted models of contrast-enhanced spiral CT. However, it remains controversial regarding which index of the FLR volume should be used. Some surgeons use the actual total liver volume minus liver volume to be removed on CT images as the FLR volume, while others use the estimated ideal liver volume that is calculated by a formula based on body surface area as a standard for calculation of the FLR. Nonetheless, the exactly number of the adequate FLR volume in cirrhotic patients is also no consensus, and at least an FLR of 40% is recommended in patients with chronic liver disease [41, 42]. In the authors' center, we have established an equation to reveal the relationship between the ratio of FLR volume and ICG-15 values as well as references for determining a safe resection ratio of the liver volume (Table 1)[43].

2.2. Preoperative therapy

Since not all patients with HCC are amenable to surgical resection, several strategies such as preoperative TACE that might be used to downsize large HCC or portal vein embolization (PVE) to increase the FLR have been suggested. However, the efficacy of these preoperative approaches in terms of HCC oncologic viewpoint remains the subject of debate.

2.2.1. Portal vein embolization

The concept of PVE was introduced on the basis of the idea that an increase in the FLR will reduce the risk of liver failure after major liver resection for hilar bile duct carcinoma in 1982 [44]. By occluding portal venous branch of the tumor-bearing liver, PVE induces atrophy of the resection part and hypertrophy of the FLR. Although the ability of liver regeneration in cirrhotic liver is impaired, PVE may induce clinically sufficient hypertrophy in these patients as well.Currently, PVE could be considered for patients with liver cirrhosis when the FLR is expected less than 40% of the total liver volume [45, 46]. PVE may also be used as a dynamic liver function test, in which inadequate hypertrophy of the FLR or intolerance of the patient after PVE indicate that major liver resection is contraindicated. In general, PVE is a relatively safe procedure, and it may increase the resectability of initial unresectable HCC and reduce the risk of post hepatectomy liver failure. Additionally, it seems no adverse effect on the oncologic outcome of HCC patients undergoing major liver resection [47, 48]. However, the potential for progression of the primary tumor after PVE remains a major concern, whereas a combination of TACE as a complementary procedure to PVE could be considered in order to improve the outcome of HCC patients [49].

2.2.2. Preoperative transcatheter arterial chemoembolization (TACE)

The use of TACE as a neoadjuvant treatment for HCC was proposed in a variety of settings such as palliative treatment for unresectable HCC, to improve the resectability of intial unresectable HCC, to downstage the primary tumor for liver transplantation or for delay surgery. The major goal of TACE is aimed at inducing tumor necrosis and shrinkage as well as preventing the dissemination of the primary tumor (Figure 3). Theroretically, the use of neoadjuvant TACE in the setting of resectable HCC might be capable of improving survival by reducing tummor recurrences. Nonethelesss, the fact is that most studies show conflict outcomes of TACE as a neoadjuvant therapy and do not support routine use of preoperative TACE before liver resection [50-53]. Moreover, preoperative TACE for resectable large HCC is not recommended because it does not provide complete necrosis of the large tumor andmay actually result in progression of the primary tumor owing to delay surgery and complicate the operation during the process of liver mobilization due to the presence of perihepatic adhesions after TACE.

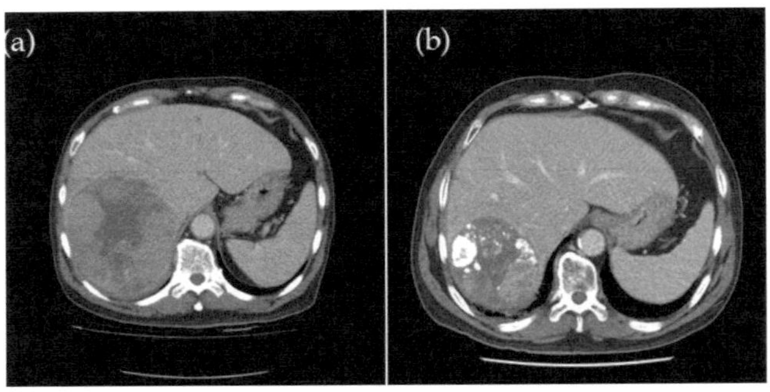

Figure 3. TACE induces remarkable shrinkage of tumor mass. (a) A huge liver tumor around 15 cm in size located at right lobe liver. (b) The tumor was decreased by half in size after three courses of TACE. (4 months after HCC diagnosed)

Clinically, spontaneous tumor rupture accompanied by hemorrhaging has been seen in small portion of patients with HCC at initial presentation, which might lead to a life-threatening condition depending on the severity of hemorrhage. Transcatheter arterial embolization (TAE) should be performed for ruptured HCC to control tumor bleeding as well as stabilizing clinical condition of patients. Liver resection then can be evaluated after the patient has recovery from shock status and post-TAE damage of the liver according to the criteria of liver resection. Generally, TAE followed by staged liver resection of tumor seems to be a rational treatment strategy for patients with ruptured HCC and hemorrhage if the lesion is resectable, and long-term survival could be expected [54, 55].

2.3. Outcome of liver resection

The operative mortality of liver resection has been reduced to less than 5% with some centers approaching to zero mortality in recent years [39, 40, 56]. The improvement is primarily resulting from advances in surgical techniques, perioperative management, and more cautious patient selection. However, the postoperative morbidity rate remains high that ranges from 25 to 50% even in experienced centers [11, 57, 58]. Ascites and pulmonary complications are the most common complications, but serious complications such as liver failure, postoperative hemorrhage, bile leakage, and intra-abdominal sepsis are less frequent nowadays. Apart from that, the long-term survival after resection of HCC have much improvedlately, but HCC recurrence remains a major concern for patients undergoing liver resection.

2.3.1. HCC recurrence

The high incidence of postoperative recurrence, estimated excess of 70% at 5 years, is the greatest frustration in treating patient with HCC. Recurrent HCCs are mostly intrahepatic that accounts for approximately 80–90% of cases after liver resection. There are two peaks of HCC recurrence after liver resection:The first peak occurs at approximately 1 year posthepatectomy and about 40% of recurrence within the period, in which metastatic dissemination of the primary tumor is mainly responsible for this early peak. The second peak is observed at the 4th postoperative year with a 35% of recurrent rate per year, and the majority of the second peak is more likely attributable to new tumors development related to the carcinogenic effect of underlying chronic liver disease [59].

Currently, there is no well-established adjuvant therapy to reduce the risk of recurrence after curative liver resection. Although numerous studies have demonstrated the efficacy of some new modalities including acyclic retinoid, polyprenoic acid [60], intra-arterial iodine-131-labelled lipiodol [61], and adoptive immunotherapy [62] as adjuvant therapy in the prevention of HCC recurrence after liver resection, the sample size of these individual studies was rather small and further validated by randomized trials with large sample size is required. Additionally, interferon has been proposed as adjuvant therapy in patients with HCC and viral hepatitis after liver resection and shown beneficial for reducing recurrence and prolonging survival [63, 64]. Nonetheless, a more recent cohort study based on a phase III randomized trial of adjuvant interferon alfa-2b in HCC after curative resection does not support the benefit of interferon in reducing postoperative recurrence of viral hepatitis-related HCC [65]. Apart from that, another potential approach is to use molecular targeted therapy such as sorafenib that is applied for advanced HCC and may inhibit HCC cell proliferation and angiogenesis. However, further trial is indicated to test the efficacy of these targeting drugs as adjuvant therapy after resection of HCC.

Compared with the development of postoperative adjuvant therapy, the risk factors for HCC recurrence after liver resection have been extensively explored and established. The risk factors for tumor recurrence can be categorized into three core groups, related to host factors, tumor factors, and surgical factors [66]. The tumor factors including vascular invasion, satellite nodules, large tumor, elevation of AFP, poor differentiated histologic grade, tumor rupture, and advanced tumor stage are frequently reported risk factor for HCC recurrence after liver resection. The host factors are the patient's characteristics and underlying liver diseases such as cirrhosis and viral hepatitis. Both tumor and host factors are determined before operation, and the surgeon can only control surgical factors including negative resection margin, anatomic resection, meticulous liver mobilization, and less blood transfusion.

The treatment strategy for HCC recurrence after liver resection should be the same as that for primary HCC. Although repeat hepatectomy could be a difficulty owing to perihepatic adhesion related to first operation, surgical resection remains a preferred treatment whenever the tumor is considered to be resectable [67-69].

2.3.2. *Survival of patients*

Despite the high incidence of postoperative HCC recurrence, current strategy of aggressive multimodality treatments for recurrent tumors using TACE, RFA, or liver transplantation has largely improved the overall outcomes of patients even after the development of recurrent HCC. Moreover, surgical resection of recurrent HCC presenting as extrahepatic metastases could be considered in selected patients who are with isolated extrahepatic metastases and has otherwise good performance status, good hepatic functional reserve, and well-treated intrahepatic HCC, and a survival benefit can be expected from this aggressive approach [70]. Generally, the overall 5-year survival after resection of HCC reported in the literature from large series is mostly near 50% or even better in recent years (Table 2).

Authors (Years)	Study period	Subgroups	No. of patients	5-year RFS/OS
Hanazaki et al. (2000) [71]	1983–1997		386	23.3%/34.4%
Zhou et al. (2001) [58]	1967–1998	size≤5cm	1000	—/62.7%
		size>5cm	1366	—/37.1%
Wang et al. (2010) [72]	1991–2004		438	—/43.3%
Fan et al. (2011) [73]	1989–2008	1989–1998	390	24%/42.1%
		1999–2008	808	34.8%/54.8%
Sakamoto et al. (2011) [74]	1988–2010	Caudate lobe	46	44%/76%
		Other sites	737	40%/64%
Nara et al. (2012) [75]	1990–2007	SM>1mm	374	40.0%/72.2%
		SM≤1mm	165	28.1%/63.5%
		SM-postive	31	7.4%/36%
Chan et al. (2012) [76]	2001–2005		651	33.9%/51.7%
Giuliante et al. (2012) [77]	1992–2008	Tumor ≤3cm	588	32.4%/52.8%
Shrager et al. (2012) [78]	1992–2008	Non-cirrhosis	206	39%/46.3%
		cirrhosis	462	—/—
Altekruse et al. (2012) [79]	1998–2008	SEER–13	1348	—/47%

Table 2. Long-term survival of patients undergoing liver resection for HCC reported from large series in recent years. RFS, recurrence-free survival; OS, overall survival; SM, surgical margin; SEER-13, Surveillance Epidemiology and End Results of USA.

3. Liver transplantation

Recurrence remains a major problem after liver resection for HCC even after margin-negative resection. Most of the patients with HCC have underlying cirrhosis that provides potential field for development of hepatocellular carcinoma. Since majority hepatic malignancies are HCC and almost 80% of them have underlying cirrhosis, resection is option in only small number of patients and in such patients, recurrence rate is high after resection. Liver transplantation practically offers greater chance of cure by removing underlying liver cirrhosis and HCC. Also, HCC is multifocal especially with hepatitis C, and total hepatectomy removes the source of potential possibility of later-developing tumors whereas partial hepatic resection does not.

However, liver transplantation for HCC did not yield satisfactory results initially. Recurrence rates were up to 80% and long term survival rates were unacceptably below that of patients who underwent liver transplantation for non-malignant causes. These recurrences usually appeared within 2 years of transplant, most common site being liver allograft that led to a decline in enthusiasm and a serious concern about using precious donor livers for treatment [80].It was Bismuth who initially reported good outcomes with liver transplantation for small HCC [81] and subsequently, Mazzaferro et al introduced the Milan criteria reporting liver transplantation for HCC with equivalent outcomes to non-HCC patients[82].

Liver transplantation has become now potential curative treatment and it is presently the treatment of choice for patients with CTP class B or C cirrhosis and early hepatocellular carcinoma. Compared with surgical resection, liver transplantation is associated with better overall and recurrence-free survival in well selected patients [83-85]. The improved overall-results after liver transplantation are thought to be due to better patient selection and the emergence of various locoregional therapies for HCC that prevent tumor progression while patient is waitlisted for liver transplantation, thus preventing drop out.

3.1. Patient selection criteria

A major goal of liver transplant team is to select the patients with HCC and cirrhosis at earlier stage of their disease in order to achieve survival duration comparable with that of other patients with benign liver disease receiving transplants, so as to justify or prioritize the allocation of a liver graft. Liver transplant candidates with HCC must meet the Milan criteria to qualify for exceptional HCC waiting list consideration. Also, several other extended criteria such as UCSF (University of California at San Francisco) criteria are used for patient selection in highly specialized transplant centres.

3.1.1. Milan's criteria

In 1996, a prospective cohort study defined restrictive selection criteria that led to superior survival for transplant patients in comparison with any other previous experience with transplantation or other options for HCC. Since then, these selection criteria have become universally known as the Milan criteria in recognition of their origin (Table 3) [82]. These criteria have been widely applied in the selection of patients with HCC for liver transplantation.In North America as well as in many other world regions, patients within Milan criteria HCC are given priority to liver transplantation. Generally, a 4-year overall and recurrence-free survival rates of 85% and 92%, respectively, can be achieved using this selection criteria.

Criteria of liver transplantation for patients with HCC
Single lesion ≤5 cm.
Up to three separate lesions, none larger than 3 cm.
No evidence of gross vascular invasion.
No regional nodal or distant metastases.

Table 3. Milan's criteria for liver transplantation.

3.1.2. Extended Criteria

Considerable interest has arisen in expansion of usual transplant criteria in highly specialized centres to offer liver transplantation to broader group of patients with HCC as investigators argued that Milan's criteria are too restrictive and limit liver transplantation at the time when incidence of HCC is on the rise. Using explant pathologic data, Yao and co-workers at the University of California, San Francisco (UCSF) reported 5-year post-transplantation survival of 75% in patients with tumors as large as 6.5 cm and cumulative tumor burden ≤8 cm (Table 4)[86].

Extended criteria of liver transplantation for patients with HCC
Solitary tumor up to 6.5 cm.
A maximum of 3 tumor nodules each up to 4.5 cm.
A total tumor diameter not exceeding 8 cm.
No regional nodal or distant metastases.

Table 4. UCSF criteria for liver transplantation.

The UCSF criteria have been shown to be associated with long -term survival similar to Milan criteria when based on explant pathology [87, 88]. However, because of the small sample size and use of retrospective explant tumor pathology, the results of these studies were challenged and also several groups advised caution in expanding the criteria.

Additionally, a recent multicentre study led by the Milan's group had retrospectively reviewed patients who underwent transplantation for HCC in order to explore the survival of patients with tumors that exceed the Milan criteria. Accordingly, a prognostic model of overall survival based on tumor characteristics in terms of size and number was derived, and an expanded criterion termed "up-to-seven criteria" was introduced [89]. Patients who fell within the criteria that the sum of the largest tumor size and the number of tumors does not exceed seven could achieve a 5-year overall survival of 71.2% after liver transplantation enabling more patients to qualify as transplant candidates.

3.2. Prognostic Indicators

Several studies have identified patient and tumor-related variables associated with prognosis following liver transplantation for HCC. The majority of prognostic factors are similar to that of liver resection for patients with HCC.

3.2.1. Tumor related factors

Important prognostic factors in most of scientific studies include tumor number, size, and location (especially bilobar distribution). The most consistent association is with tumor size. Other factors are histologic grade of differentiation, stage of disease according to the American Liver Tumor Study Group (ALTSG) modification of the TNM staging criteria, the presence of macrovascular and microvascular invasion, absolute level of serum AFP, and extrahepatic spread. Tumor size predicts both the likelihood of vascular invasion and tumor grade, but the relationship is nonlinear and a significant proportion of small tumors have unfavourable histology, whereas some larger ones do not [90, 91].

3.2.2. Patient related factors

Patients with HCV infection tend to have severe underlying liver disease and more advanced HCC at presentation as compared to HBV infection and underlying alcoholic cirrhosis. Hence, the recurrence of HCC is more common among the HCV recipients and thus reduced survival [92]. The immunosuppressive treatment after liver transplantation is associated with increased risk of tumor recurrence. Thus, immunosuppressant should be reduced to minimum effective levels. Several studies have shown lower recurrence with sirolimus which is attributed to its anti-proliferative effects on HCC [93-95]. But there is need for large randomized controlled trials to conclude sirolimus as most appropriate immunosuppressant for patients undergoing liver transplantation for HCC.

3.3. Deceased Donor Liver Transplantation (DDLT)

3.3.1. Graft Allocation

The shortage of donor livers has necessitated the development of allocation system, whereby priority for donor organs is given to the most severely ill patients. The prolonged waiting period frequently results in tumor progression to an extent beyond the transplantable criteria, leading to a patient's removal or dropout from the waiting list [96]. Allocation of deceased donor livers for both adults and children is based upon the "model for end stage liver disease" or MELD score, a statistical model based upon predicted survival in patients with cirrhosis.As a result of the high dropout rate for patients with HCC, the Organ Procurement and Transplantation Network (OPTN) of the U.S. has reconsidered the priority of liver graft allocation. While waiting list priority was determined primarily by liver disease severity based on the Model for End-Stage Liver Disease (MELD) score, patients with HCC that fulfilled the Milan criteria were registered with an adjusted score and were subsequently assigned additional scores at regular intervals to reflect their risk for dropout as a result of tumor progression.

3.3.2. Listing Criteria of transplantation candidates

In an attempt to ensure that preoperative assessment is as accurate as possible, UNOS provides a set of specific requirements for listing patients with HCC for orthotopic liver transplantation.

I. The diagnosis must be confirmed by thorough assessment by imaging modalities such as ultrasound, dynamic CT and /or MRI. Tumor numbers, size, presence or absence of extrahepatic disease and major vascular disease must be documented.

II. Patient must have one of the following:

1. An Alfa fetoprotein level > 200 ng/mL.
2. Celiac angiography showing tumor blush corresponding to the site shown by CT/MRI/ultrasonography.
3. A biopsy confirming HCC
4. History of RFA, TACE or other locoregional therapy.

III. Must be within Milan's criteria.

IV. Continued documentation of the tumor is required every three months by CT or MRI to ensure continued eligibility for liver transplantation.

Patients will be given priority MELD score depending upon the state of underlying disease. Prioritization scores for patients with HCC are based upon tumor size and number. With this new organ allocation policy, waiting time for the patients with HCC to receive a deceased-donor liver has decreased significantly.

3.4. Living Donor Liver Transplantation (LDLT)

The shortage of organs from deceased donors has curtailed the adoption of living donor liver transplantation. Living donors can potentially provide an essentially unlimited source of liver grafts for a planned transplant operation as soon as the diagnosis of HCC is made, thus decreasing the uncertainty of long waiting periods and reducing possibility of tumor progression [97]. The living donor can be from adult-to-adult or adult-to-child. In children mostly left lateral segment of the liver harvested and donors are usually ABO-compatible parents. While in adult-to-adult, right or left liver can be harvested that depends upon pretransplant evaluation of donor and CT volumetry of liver. The GRWR (graft to recipient weight ratio) must be more than 0.8%. Donor not meeting these criteria is rejected for the fear of small-for-size syndrome and subsequent graft failure [98, 99].

Because a live donor graft is a dedicated gift that is directed exclusively to a particular recipient, there is no need for an objective allocation system based on a prioritization scheme. Presently LDLT comprises almost >90% of liver transplants in Asia as compared to <5% in

US. Unlike in the U.S., where recipients with malignancies receive extra prioritization in the deceased donor organ allocation scheme, HCC patients in Asia do not. HCC patients in Asia have a dismal chance of receiving a deceased donor graft and LDLT is often the only option.

3.5. Pretransplant locoregional therapies

Pretransplant locoregional therapy has been adopted by the liver transplant community worldwide. This concept, known as "bridging therapy" is meant to limit tumor progression and dropout rate while patients are on the transplant wait list. The most popular techniques include TACE, transarterial drug-eluting beads, transarterial radio-embolizationand RFA.In the transplant setting, TACE is currently the most popular neo-adjuvant treatment. It is indicated in Child–Pugh A or B cirrhotic patients to downstage tumors into the Milan criteria or to prevent tumor progression. For patients with small HCC confined to the liver, recent data also indicate that transplantation when used with multimodal therapy using locoregional procedures and neoadjuvant systemic chemotherapy, results in improved recurrence-free survival [100, 101]. Apart from that, it is also important to know the wait list dropout rate and bridging therapy-associated complication rate, because the benefit of preventing wait list dropout should outweigh the risk of bridging therapy.Patient-individualized treatment strategy should be based on the performance status, hepatic reserve, tumor burden, and tumor vascularity pattern.

3.6. Outcome of liver transplantation

To date, orthotopic liver transplantation is no doubt the best therapeutic option for early, unresectable HCC, although it is limited by graft shortage and the need for appropriate patient selection. Since the introduction of the milan's criteria, the liver transplantation for primary HCC is on rise with promising recurrence-free survival and overall survival. Excellent 5-year post-transplant patient survival of at least 70% has been reported from many centers [102]. Furthermore, better definition of the prognostic factors and more rigorous patient selection have resulted in significant improvement in 5-year survival for patients receiving transplants for HCC in the past decade.

However, a tendency for higher HCC recurrence has been reported for patients who underwent LDLT than patients who underwent DDLT [103, 104]. The reasons for this difference are not completely answered by current studies. Possible explanations can be related to the selection bias for clinical characteristics associated with aggressive tumor behavior, elimination of natural selection during the waiting period, and enhancement of tumor growth and invasiveness by small-for-size graft injury and regeneration [105, 106]. Additionally, more clinical studies with long-term follow-up are needed to evaluate the role of LDLT for early HCC. At present, if a suitable and willing donor is identified, LDLT is a reasonable alternative to waiting 6 to 12 months for a deceased donor graft in patients with HCC who are otherwise eligible for liver transplantation.

Although liver transplantation is the only option for the cure in majority of the patients with HCC complicated by underlying cirrhosis precluding resection, identification of prognostic factors and refinement of selection criteria will improve the outcomes of liver transplantation for this otherwise fatal disease. Nonetheless, liver transplantation may also pose a risk of post transplant lymphoproliferative disorders and other de novo malignacy associated with long term immunosuppression.

4. Conclusion

The management of patients with HCC remains complex and challenging. Although liver resection and liver transplantation are the curative treatments for HCC at present, there is considerable controversy as to whether patients with HCC are better served with liver transplantation versus liver resection. Liver transplantation removes HCC with underlying cirrhosis and thus sounds best option; however, technical challenges associated with transplantation and/or immunosuppression should be taken into consideration for selecting transplant cadidates. Currently, most studies suggest that liver resection should be a priority in patients who are candidates for either liver resection or transplantation [102, 107]. Despite a better cancer cure rate for liver transplatation, liver resection remains superior for patients in terms of limited organ availability and transplantation-associated morbidity and mortality. Therefore, the optimal treatment for patients with preservd liver function should always be resection whenever the tumor is resectable, and liver transplantation could be reserved as a salvage therapy for patients who encounter HCC recurrence after primary liver resection. Theoretically, this strategy will not only improve patient survival but relieve the growing demand of available donor livers.

Author details

Kun-Ming Chan* and Ashok Thorat*

*Address all correspondence to: chankunming@adm.cgmh.org.tw

Division of Liver and Organ Transplantation Surgery, Department of General Surgery, Chang Gung Memorial Hospital at Linkou, Chang Gung University College of Medicine, Taiwan, Republic of China

References

[1] Forner, A., Llovet, J. M., & Bruix, J. (2012). Hepatocellular Carcinoma. *Lancet*, 379(9822), 1245-1255.

[2] Sobin, L. H., Gospodarowicz, M. K., & wittekind, C. (2009). Tnm Classification of Malignant Tumours. *John Wiley & Sons.*

[3] Anonymous. (1998). NewA.PrognosticSystem.forHepatocellular.CarcinomaA Retrospective Study of 435 Patients: The Cancer of the Liver Italian Program (Clip) Investigators. *Hepatology*, 28(3), 751-755.

[4] Okuda, K., Ohtsuki, T., Obata, H., Tomimatsu, M., Okazaki, N., Hasegawa, H., Nakajima, Y., & Ohnishi, K. (1985). Natural History of Hepatocellular Carcinoma and Prognosis in Relation to Treatment. Study of 850 Patients. *Cancer*, 56(4), 918-928.

[5] Kudo, M., Chung, H., & Osaki, Y. (2003). Prognostic Staging System for Hepatocellular Carcinoma (Clip Score): Its Value and Limitations, and a Proposal for a New Staging System, the Japan Integrated Staging Score (Jis Score). *J Gastroenterol*, 38(3), 207-215.

[6] Llovet, J. M., Bru, C., & Bruix, J. (1999). Prognosis of Hepatocellular Carcinoma: The Bclc Staging Classification. *Semin Liver Dis*, 19(3), 329-338.

[7] Marrero, J. A., Fontana, R. J., Barrat, A., Askari, F., Conjeevaram, H. S., Su, G. L., & Lok, A. S. (2005). Prognosis of Hepatocellular Carcinoma: Comparison of 7 Staging Systems in an American Cohort. *Hepatology*, 41(4), 707-16.

[8] Bruix, J., & Llovet, J. M. (2009). Major Achievements in Hepatocellular Carcinoma. *Lancet*, 373(9664), 614-616.

[9] Cance, W. G., Stewart, A. K., & Menck, H. R. (2000). The National Cancer Data Base Report on Treatment Patterns for Hepatocellular Carcinomas: Improved Survival of Surgically Resected Patients, 1985-1996. *Cancer*, 88(4), 912-920.

[10] Liu, C. L., & Fan, S. T. (1997). Nonresectional Therapies for Hepatocellular Carcinoma. *Am J Surg*, 173(4), 358-365.

[11] Fong, Y., Sun, R. L., Jarnagin, W., & Blumgart, L. H. (1999). An Analysis of 412 Cases of Hepatocellular Carcinoma at a Western Center. *Ann Surg*, 229(6), 790-799, discussion 9-800.

[12] Lin, T. Y. (1974). A Simplified Technique for Hepatic Resection: The Crush Method. *Ann Surg*, 180(3), 285-290.

[13] Buell, J. F., Thomas, M. T., Rudich, S., Marvin, M., Nagubandi, R., Ravindra, K. V., Brock, G., & Mc Masters, K. M. (2008). Experience with More Than 500 Minimally Invasive Hepatic Procedures. *Ann Surg*, 248(3), 475-486.

[14] Cherqui, D., Husson, E., Hammoud, R., Malassagne, B., Stephan, F., Bensaid, S., Rotman, N., & Fagniez, P. L. (2000). Laparoscopic Liver Resections: A Feasibility Study in 30 Patients. *Ann Surg*, 232(6), 753-762.

[15] Vibert, E., Perniceni, T., Levard, H., Denet, C., Shahri, N. K., & Gayet, B. (2006). Laparoscopic Liver Resection. *Br J Surg*, 93(1), 67-72.

[16] Lai, E. C., Fan, S. T., Lo, C. M., Chu, K. M., & Liu, C. L. (1996). Anterior Approach for Difficult Major Right Hepatectomy. World J Surg discussion 8., 20(3), 314-317.

[17] Wang, W. D., Liang, L. J., Huang, X. Q., & Yin, X. Y. (2006). Low Central Venous Pressure Reduces Blood Loss in Hepatectomy. *World J Gastroenterol*, 12(6), 935-939.

[18] Wu, T. J., Wang, F., Lin, Y. S., Chan, K. M., Yu, M. C., & Lee, W. C. (2010). Right Hepatectomy by the Anterior Method with Liver Hanging Versus Conventional Approach for Large Hepatocellular Carcinomas. *Br J Surg*, 97(7), 1070-1078.

[19] Dahiya, D., Wu, T. J., Lee, C. F., Chan, K. M., Lee, W. C., & Chen, M. F. (2010). Minor Versus Major Hepatic Resection for Small Hepatocellular Carcinoma (Hcc) in Cirrhotic Patients: A 20-Year Experience. *Surgery*, 147(5), 676-685.

[20] Wayne, J. D., Lauwers, G. Y., Ikai, I., Doherty, D. A., Belghiti, J., Yamaoka, Y., Regimbeau, J. M., Nagorney, D. M., Do, K. A., Ellis, L. M., Curley, S. A., Pollock, R. E., & Vauthey, J. N. (2002). Preoperative Predictors of Survival after Resection of Small Hepatocellular Carcinomas. *Ann Surg*, 235(5), 722-730, discussion 30-1.

[21] Ng, K. K., Vauthey, J. N., Pawlik, T. M., Lauwers, G. Y., Regimbeau, J. M., Belghiti, J., Ikai, I., Yamaoka, Y., Curley, S. A., Nagorney, D. M., Ng, I. O., Fan, S. T., & Poon, R. T. (2005). Is Hepatic Resection for Large or Multinodular Hepatocellular Carcinoma Justified? Results from a Multi-Institutional Database. *Ann Surg Oncol*, 12(5), 364-373.

[22] Regimbeau, J. M., Farges, O., Shen, B. Y., Sauvanet, A., & Belghiti, J. (1999). Is Surgery for Large Hepatocellular Carcinoma Justified? *J Hepatol*, 31(6), 1062-1068.

[23] Yeh, C. N., Lee, W. C., & Chen, M. F. (2003). Hepatic Resection and Prognosis for Patients with Hepatocellular Carcinoma Larger Than 10 Cm: Two Decades of Experience at Chang Gung Memorial Hospital. *Ann Surg Oncol*, 10(9), 1070-1076.

[24] Huang, J. F., Wu, S. M., Wu, T. H., Lee, C. F., Wu, T. J., Yu, M. C., Chan, K. M., & Lee, W. C. (2012). Liver Resection for Complicated Hepatocellular Carcinoma: Challenges but Opportunity for Long-Term Survivals. J Surg Oncol. (In press)

[25] Poon, R. T., Fan, S. T., & Wong, J. (2002). Selection Criteria for Hepatic Resection in Patients with Large Hepatocellular Carcinoma Larger Than 10 Cm in Diameter. *J Am Coll Surg*, 194(5), 592-602.

[26] Ishizawa, T, Hasegawa, K, Aoki, T, Takahashi, M, Inoue, Y, Sano, K, Imamura, H, Sugawara, Y, Kokudo, N, & Makuuchi, M. (2008). Neither Multiple Tumors nor Portal Hypertension Are Surgical Contraindications for Hepatocellular Carcinoma. *Gastroenterology*, 134(7), 1908-1916.

[27] Choi, D., Lim, H. K., Joh, J. W., Kim, S. J., Kim, M. J., Rhim, H., Kim, Y. S., Yoo, B. C., Paik, S. W., & Park, C. K. (2007). Combined Hepatectomy and Radiofrequency Ablation for Multifocal Hepatocellular Carcinomas: Long-Term Follow-up Results and Prognostic Factors. *Ann Surg Oncol*, 14(12), 3510-3518.

[28] Liu, C. L., Fan, S. T., Lo, C. M., Ng, I. O., Poon, R. T., & Wong, J. (2003). Hepatic Resection for Bilobar Hepatocellular Carcinoma: Is It Justified? *Arch Surg*, 138(1), 100-104.

[29] Pawlik, T. M., Poon, R. T., Abdalla, E. K., Ikai, I., Nagorney, D. M., Belghiti, J., Kianmanesh, R., Ng, I. O., Curley, S. A., Yamaoka, Y., Lauwers, G. Y., & Vauthey, J. N. (2005). Hepatectomy for Hepatocellular Carcinoma with Major Portal or Hepatic Vein Invasion: Results of a Multicenter Study. *Surgery*, 137(4), 403-410.

[30] Minagawa, M., Makuuchi, M., Takayama, T., & Ohtomo, K. (2001). Selection Criteria for Hepatectomy in Patients with Hepatocellular Carcinoma and Portal Vein Tumor Thrombus. *Ann Surg*, 233(3), 379-384.

[31] Kuroda, S., Tashiro, H., Kobayashi, T., Oshita, A., Amano, H., & Ohdan, H. (2011). Selection Criteria for Hepatectomy in Patients with Hepatocellular Carcinoma Classified as Child-Pugh Class B. *World J Surg*, 35(4), 834-841.

[32] Bruix, J., Castells, A., Bosch, J., Feu, F., Fuster, J., Garcia-Pagan, J. C., Visa, J., Bru, C., & Rodes, J. (1996). Surgical Resection of Hepatocellular Carcinoma in Cirrhotic Patients: Prognostic Value of Preoperative Portal Pressure. *Gastroenterology*, 111(4), 1018-1022.

[33] Noun, R., Jagot, P., Farges, O., Sauvanet, A., & Belghiti, J. (1997). High Preoperative Serum Alanine Transferase Levels: Effect on the Risk of Liver Resection in Child Grade a Cirrhotic Patients. World J Surg discussion 5., 21(4), 390-394.

[34] Poon, R. T., Fan, S. T., Lo, C. M., Liu, C. L., Ng, I. O., & Wong, J. (2000). Long-Term Prognosis after Resection of Hepatocellular Carcinoma Associated with Hepatitis B-Related Cirrhosis. *J Clin Oncol*, 18(5), 1094-1101.

[35] Ercolani, G., Grazi, G. L., Calliva, R., Pierangeli, F., Cescon, M., Cavallari, A., & Mazziotti, A. (2000). The Lidocaine (Megx) Test as an Index of Hepatic Function: Its Clinical Usefulness in Liver Surgery. *Surgery*, 127(4), 464-471.

[36] Merkel, C., Gatta, A., Zoli, M., Bolognesi, M., Angeli, P., Iervese, T., Marchesini, G., & Ruol, A. (1991). Prognostic Value of Galactose Elimination Capacity, Aminopyrine Breath Test, and Icg Clearance in Patients with Cirrhosis. Comparison with the Pugh Score. *Dig Dis Sci*, 36(9), 1197-21103.

[37] Redaelli, C. A., Dufour, J. F., Wagner, M., Schilling, M., Husler, J., Krahenbuhl, L., Buchler, M. W., & Reichen, J. (2002). Preoperative Galactose Elimination Capacity Predicts Complications and Survival after Hepatic Resection. *Ann Surg*, 235(1), 77-85.

[38] Makuuchi, M., Kosuge, T., Takayama, T., Yamazaki, S., Kakazu, T., Miyagawa, S., & Kawasaki, S. (1993). Surgery for Small Liver Cancers. *Semin Surg Oncol*, 9(4), 298-304.

[39] Imamura, H., Seyama, Y., Kokudo, N., Maema, A., Sugawara, Y., Sano, K., Takayama, T., & Makuuchi, M. (2003). One Thousand Fifty-Six Hepatectomies without Mortality in 8 Years. *Arch Surg*, 138(11), 1198-206, discussion 206.

[40] Torzilli, G., Makuuchi, M., Inoue, K., Takayama, T., Sakamoto, Y., Sugawara, Y., Kubota, K., & Zucchi, A. (1999). No-Mortality Liver Resection for Hepatocellular Carcinoma in Cirrhotic and Noncirrhotic Patients: Is There a Way? A Prospective Analysis of Our Approach. *Arch Surg*, 134(9), 984-992.

[41] Kubota, K., Makuuchi, M., Kusaka, K., Kobayashi, T., Miki, K., Hasegawa, K., Harihara, Y., & Takayama, T. (1997). Measurement of Liver Volume and Hepatic Functional Reserve as a Guide to Decision-Making in Resectional Surgery for Hepatic Tumors. *Hepatology*, 26(5), 1176-1181.

[42] Shirabe, K., Shimada, M., Gion, T., Hasegawa, H., Takenaka, K., Utsunomiya, T., & Sugimachi, K. (1999). Postoperative Liver Failure after Major Hepatic Resection for Hepatocellular Carcinoma in the Modern Era with Special Reference to Remnant Liver Volume. *J Am Coll Surg*, 188(3), 304-309.

[43] Lee, C. F., Yu, M. C., Kuo, L. M., Chan, K. M., Jan, Y. Y., Chen, M. F., & Lee, W. C. (2007). Using Indocyanine Green Test to Avoid Post-Hepatectomy Liver Dysfunction. *Chang Gung Med J*, 30(4), 333-338.

[44] Makuuchi, M., Thai, B. L., Takayasu, K., Takayama, T., Kosuge, T., Gunven, P., Yamazaki, S., Hasegawa, H., & Ozaki, H. (1990). Preoperative Portal Embolization to Increase Safety of Major Hepatectomy for Hilar Bile Duct Carcinoma: A Preliminary Report. *Surgery*, 107(5), 521-527.

[45] Farges, O., Belghiti, J., Kianmanesh, R., Regimbeau, J. M., Santoro, R., Vilgrain, V., Denys, A., & Sauvanet, A. (2003). Portal Vein Embolization before Right Hepatectomy: Prospective Clinical Trial. *Ann Surg*, 237(2), 208-217.

[46] Kokudo, N., & Makuuchi, M. (2004). Current Role of Portal Vein Embolization/ Hepatic Artery Chemoembolization. *Surg Clin North Am*, 84(2), 643-657.

[47] Seo, D. D., Lee, H. C., Jang, M. K., Min, H. J., Kim, K. M., Lim, Y. S., Chung, Y. H., Lee, Y. S., Suh, D. J., Ko, G. Y., Lee, Y. J., & Lee, S. G. (2007). Preoperative Portal Vein Embolization and Surgical Resection in Patients with Hepatocellular Carcinoma and Small Future Liver Remnant Volume: Comparison with Transarterial Chemoembolization. *Ann Surg Oncol*, 14(12), 3501-3509.

[48] Siriwardana, R. C., Lo, C. M., Chan, S. C., & Fan, S. T. (2012). Role of Portal Vein Embolization in Hepatocellular Carcinoma Management and Its Effect on Recurrence: A Case-Control Study. *World J Surg*, 36(7), 1640-6.

[49] Yoo, H., Kim, J. H., Ko, G. Y., Kim, K. W., Gwon, D. I., Lee, S. G., & Hwang, S. (2011). Sequential Transcatheter Arterial Chemoembolization and Portal Vein Embolization Versus Portal Vein Embolization Only before Major Hepatectomy for Patients with Hepatocellular Carcinoma. *Ann Surg Oncol*, 18(5), 1251-1257.

[50] Wu, C. C., Ho, Y. Z., Ho, W. L., Wu, T. C., Liu, T. J., & P'Eng, F. K. (1995). Preoperative Transcatheter Arterial Chemoembolization for Resectable Large Hepatocellular Carcinoma: A Reappraisal. *Br J Surg*, 82(1), 122-126.

[51] Yamasaki, S., Hasegawa, H., Kinoshita, H., Furukawa, M., Imaoka, S., Takasaki, K., Kakumoto, Y., Saitsu, H., Yamada, R., Oosaki, Y., Arii, S., Okamoto, E., Monden, M., Ryu, M., Kusano, S., Kanematsu, T., Ikeda, K., Yamamoto, M., Saoshiro, T., & Tsuzuki, T. (1996). A Prospective Randomized Trial of the Preventive Effect of Pre-Opera-

tive Transcatheter Arterial Embolization against Recurrence of Hepatocellular Carcinoma. *Jpn J Cancer Res*, 87(2), 206-211.

[52] Zhang, Z., Liu, Q., He, J., Yang, J., Yang, G., & Wu, M. (2000). The Effect of Preoperative Transcatheter Hepatic Arterial Chemoembolization on Disease-Free Survival after Hepatectomy for Hepatocellular Carcinoma. *Cancer*, 89(12), 2606-2612.

[53] Zhou, W. P., Lai, E. C., Li, A. J., Fu, S. Y., Zhou, J. P., Pan, Z. Y., Lau, W. Y., & Wu, M. C. (2009). A Prospective, Randomized, Controlled Trial of Preoperative Transarterial Chemoembolization for Resectable Large Hepatocellular Carcinoma. *Ann Surg*, 249(2), 195-202.

[54] Hwang, T. L., Chen, M. F., Lee, T. Y., Chen, T. J., Lin, D. Y., & Liaw, Y. F. (1987). Resection of Hepatocellular Carcinoma after Transcatheter Arterial Embolization. Reevaluation of the Advantages and Disadvantages of Preoperative Embolization. *Arch Surg*, 122(7), 756-759.

[55] Liu, C. L., Fan, S. T., Lo, C. M., Tso, W. K., Poon, R. T., Lam, C. M., & Wong, J. (2001). Management of Spontaneous Rupture of Hepatocellular Carcinoma: Single-Center Experience. *J Clin Oncol*, 19(17), 3725-3232.

[56] Grazi, G. L., Ercolani, G., Pierangeli, F., Del Gaudio, M., Cescon, M., Cavallari, A., & Mazziotti, A. (2001). Improved Results of Liver Resection for Hepatocellular Carcinoma on Cirrhosis Give the Procedure Added Value. *Ann Surg*, 234(1), 71-78.

[57] Wei, A. C., Tung-Ping, Poon. R., Fan, S. T., & Wong, J. (2003). Risk Factors for Perioperative Morbidity and Mortality after Extended Hepatectomy for Hepatocellular Carcinoma. *Br J Surg*, 90(1), 33-41.

[58] Zhou, X. D., Tang, Z. Y., Yang, B. H., Lin, Z. Y., Ma, Z. C., Ye, S. L., Wu, Z. Q., Fan, J., Qin, L. X., & Zheng, B. H. (2001). Experience of 1000 Patients Who Underwent Hepatectomy for Small Hepatocellular Carcinoma. *Cancer*, 91(8), 1479-1486.

[59] Imamura, H., Matsuyama, Y., Tanaka, E., Ohkubo, T., Hasegawa, K., Miyagawa, S., Sugawara, Y., Minagawa, M., Takayama, T., Kawasaki, S., & Makuuchi, M. (2003). Risk Factors Contributing to Early and Late Phase Intrahepatic Recurrence of Hepatocellular Carcinoma after Hepatectomy. *J Hepatol*, 38(2), 200-207.

[60] Muto, Y., Moriwaki, H., Ninomiya, M., Adachi, S., Saito, A., Takasaki, K. T., Tanaka, T., Tsurumi, K., Okuno, M., Tomita, E., Nakamura, T., & Kojima, T. (1996). Prevention of Second Primary Tumors by an Acyclic Retinoid, Polyprenoic Acid, in Patients with Hepato cellular Carcinoma. Hepatoma Prevention Study Group. *N Engl J Med*, 334(24), 1561-1567.

[61] Lau, W. Y., Leung, T. W., Ho, S. K., Chan, M., Machin, D., Lau, J., Chan, A. T., Yeo, W., Mok, T. S., Yu, S. C., Leung, N. W., & Johnson, P. J. (1999). Adjuvant Intra-Arterial Iodine-131-Labelled Lipiodol for Resectable Hepatocellular Carcinoma: A Prospective Randomised Trial. *Lancet*, 353(9155), 797-801.

[62] Takayama, T., Sekine, T., Makuuchi, M., Yamasaki, S., Kosuge, T., Yamamoto, J., Shimada, K., Sakamoto, M., Hirohashi, S., Ohashi, Y., & Kakizoe, T. (2000). Adoptive Immunotherapy to Lower Postsurgical Recurrence Rates of Hepatocellular Carcinoma: A Randomised Trial. *Lancet*, 356(9232), 802-807.

[63] Huang, J. F., Yu, M. L., Huang, C. F., Chiu, C. F., Dai, C. Y., Huang, C. I., Yeh, M. L., Yang, J. F., Hsieh, M. Y., Hou, N. J., & LinChenWangChuang, Z. Y.S. C.L. Y.W. L. (2011). The Efficacy and Safety of Pegylated Interferon Plus Ribavirin Combination Therapy in Chronic Hepatitis C Patients with Hepatocellular Carcinoma Post Curative Therapies- a Multicenter Prospective Trial. *J Hepatol*, 54(2), 219-26.

[64] Shen, Y. C., Hsu, C., Chen, L. T., Cheng, C. C., Hu, F. C., & Cheng, A. L. (2010). Adjuvant Interferon Therapy after Curative Therapy for Hepatocellular Carcinoma (Hcc): A Meta-Regression Approach. *J Hepatol*, 52(6), 889-894.

[65] Chen, L. T., Chen, M. F., Li, L. A., Lee, P. H., Jeng, L. B., Lin, D. Y., Wu, C. C., Mok, K. T., Chen, C. L., Lee, W. C., Chau, G. Y., Chen, Y. S., Lui, W. Y., Hsiao, C. F., Whang-Peng, J., & Chen, P. J. (2012). Long-Term Results of a Randomized, Observation-Controlled, Phase Iii Trial of Adjuvant Interferon Alfa-2b in Hepatocellular Carcinoma after Curative Resection. *Ann Surg*, 255(1), 8-17.

[66] Tung-Ping, Poon. R., Fan, S. T., & Wong, J. (2000). Risk Factors, Prevention, and Management of Postoperative Recurrence after Resection of Hepatocellular Carcinoma. *Ann Surg*, 232(1), 10-24.

[67] Itamoto, T., Nakahara, H., Amano, H., Kohashi, T., Ohdan, H., Tashiro, H., & Asahara, T. (2007). Repeat Hepatectomy for Recurrent Hepatocellular Carcinoma. *Surgery*, 141(5), 589-597.

[68] Lee, P. H., Lin, W. J., Tsang, Y. M., Hu, R. H., Sheu, J. C., Lai, M. Y., Hsu, H. C., May, W., & Lee, C. S. (1995). Clinical Management of Recurrent Hepatocellular Carcinoma. *Ann Surg*, 222(5), 670-676.

[69] Wu, C. C., Cheng, S. B., Yeh, D. C., Wang, J., & P'Eng, F. K. (2009). Second and Third Hepatectomies for Recurrent Hepatocellular Carcinoma Are Justified. *Br J Surg*, 96(9), 1049-1057.

[70] Chan, K. M., Yu, M. C., Wu, T. J., Lee, C. F., Chen, T. C., Lee, W. C., & Chen, M. F. (2009). Efficacy of Surgical Resection in Management of Isolated Extrahepatic Metastases of Hepatocellular Carcinoma. *World J Gastroenterol*, 15(43), 5481-5488.

[71] Hanazaki, K., Kajikawa, S., Shimozawa, N., Mihara, M., Shimada, K., Hiraguri, M., Koide, N., Adachi, W., & Amano, J. (2000). Survival and Recurrence after Hepatic Resection of 386 Consecutive Patients with Hepatocellular Carcinoma. *J Am Coll Surg*, 191(4), 381-388.

[72] Wang, J., Xu, L. B., Liu, C., Pang, H. W., Chen, Y. J., & Ou, Q. J. (2010). Prognostic Factors and Outcome of 438 Chinese Patients with Hepatocellular Carcinoma Underwent Partial Hepatectomy in a Single Center. *World J Surg*, 34(10), 2434-2441.

[73] Fan, S. T., Mau, Lo. C., Poon, R. T., Yeung, C., Leung, Liu. C., Yuen, W. K., Ming, Lam. C., Ng, K. K., & Ching, Chan. S. (2011). Continuous Improvement of Survival Outcomes of Resection of Hepatocellular Carcinoma: A 20-Year Experience. *Ann Surg*, 253(4), 745-758.

[74] Sakamoto, Y., Nara, S., Hata, S., Yamamoto, Y., Esaki, M., Shimada, K., & Kosuge, T. (2011). Prognosis of Patients Undergoing Hepatectomy for Solitary Hepatocellular Carcinoma Originating in the Caudate Lobe. *Surgery*, 150(5), 959-967.

[75] Nara, S., Shimada, K., Sakamoto, Y., Esaki, M., Kishi, Y., Kosuge, T., & Ojima, H. (2012). Prognostic Impact of Marginal Resection for Patients with Solitary Hepatocellular Carcinoma: Evidence from 570 Hepatectomies. *Surgery*, 151(4), 526-536.

[76] Chan, K. M., Lee, C. F., Wu, T. J., Chou, H. S., Yu, M. C., Lee, W. C., & Chen, M. F. (2012). Adverse Outcomes in Patients with Postoperative Ascites after Liver Resection for Hepatocellular Carcinoma. *World J Surg*, 36(2), 392-400.

[77] Giuliante, F., Ardito, F., Pinna, A. D., Sarno, G., Giulini, S. M., Ercolani, G., Portolani, N., Torzilli, G., Donadon, M., Aldrighetti, L., Pulitano, C., Guglielmi, A., Ruzzenente, A., Capussotti, L., Ferrero, A., Calise, F., Scuderi, V., Federico, B., & Nuzzo, G. (2012). Liver Resection for Hepatocellular Carcinoma </=3 Cm: Results of an Italian Multicenter Study on 588 Patients. *J Am Coll Surg.*

[78] Shrager, B., Jibara, G., Schwartz, M., & Roayaie, S. (2012). Resection of Hepatocellular Carcinoma without Cirrhosis. *Ann Surg*, 255(6), 1135-1143.

[79] Altekruse, S. F., McGlynn, K. A., Dickie, L. A., & Kleiner, D. E. (2012). Hepatocellular Carcinoma Confirmation, Treatment, and Survival in Surveillance, Epidemiology, and End Results Registries, 1992-2008. *Hepatology*, 55(2), 476-482.

[80] Pichlmayr, R. (1988). Is There a Place for Liver Grafting for Malignancy? *Transplant Proc*, 20(1, 1), 478-482.

[81] Bismuth, H., Chiche, L., Adam, R., Castaing, D., Diamond, T., & Dennison, A. (1993). Liver Resection Versus Transplantation for Hepatocellular Carcinoma in Cirrhotic Patients. *Ann Surg*, 218(2), 145-151.

[82] Mazzaferro, V., Regalia, E., Doci, R., Andreola, S., Pulvirenti, A., Bozzetti, F., Montalto, F., Ammatuna, M., Morabito, A., & Gennari, L. (1996). Liver Transplantation for the Treatment of Small Hepatocellular Carcinomas in Patients with Cirrhosis. *N Engl J Med*, 334(11), 693-9.

[83] Onaca, N., Davis, G. L., Goldstein, R. M., Jennings, L. W., & Klintmalm, G. B. (2007). Expanded Criteria for Liver Transplantation in Patients with Hepatocellular Carcinoma: A Report from the International Registry of Hepatic Tumors in Liver Transplantation. *Liver Transpl*, 13(3), 391-399.

[84] Takada, Y., Ito, T., Ueda, M., Sakamoto, S., Haga, H., Maetani, Y., Ogawa, K., Ogura, Y., Oike, F., Egawa, H., & Uemoto, S. (2007). Living Donor Liver Transplantation for

Patients with Hcc Exceeding the Milan Criteria: A Proposal of Expanded Criteria. *Dig Dis*, 25(4), 299-302.

[85] Toso, C., Asthana, S., Bigam, D. L., Shapiro, A. M., & Kneteman, N. M. (2009). Reassessing Selection Criteria Prior to Liver Transplantation for Hepatocellular Carcinoma Utilizing the Scientific Registry of Transplant Recipients Database. *Hepatology*, 49(3), 832-838.

[86] Yao, F. Y., Ferrell, L., Bass, N. M., Watson, J. J., Bacchetti, P., Venook, A., Ascher, N. L., & Roberts, J. P. (2001). Liver Transplantation for Hepatocellular Carcinoma: Expansion of the Tumor Size Limits Does Not Adversely Impact Survival. *Hepatology*, 33(6), 1394-1403.

[87] Sotiropoulos, G. C., Molmenti, E. P., Omar, O. S., Bockhorn, M., Brokalaki, E. I., Lang, H., Frilling, A., Broelsch, C. E., & Malago, M. (2006). Liver Transplantation for Hepatocellular Carcinoma in Patients Beyond the Milan but within the Ucsf Criteria. *Eur J Med Res*, 11(11), 467-470.

[88] Yao, F. Y., Ferrell, L., Bass, N. M., Bacchetti, P., Ascher, N. L., & Roberts, J. P. (2002). Liver Transplantation for Hepatocellular Carcinoma: Comparison of the Proposed Ucsf Criteria with the Milan Criteria and the Pittsburgh Modified Tnm Criteria. *Liver Transpl*, 8(9), 765-774.

[89] Mazzaferro, V., Llovet, J. M., Miceli, R., Bhoori, S., Schiavo, M., Mariani, L., Camerini, T., Roayaie, S., Schwartz, M. E., Grazi, G. L., Adam, R., Neuhaus, P., Salizzoni, M., Bruix, J., Forner, A., De Carlis, L., Cillo, U., Burroughs, A. K., Troisi, R., Rossi, M., Gerunda, G. E., Lerut, J., Belghiti, J., Boin, I., Gugenheim, J., Rochling, F., Van Hoek, B., & Majno, P. (2009). Predicting Survival after Liver Transplantation in Patients with Hepatocellular Carcinoma Beyond the Milan Criteria: A Retrospective, Exploratory Analysis. *Lancet Oncol*, 10(1), 35-43.

[90] Klintmalm, G. B. (1998). Liver Transplantation for Hepatocellular Carcinoma: A Registry Report of the Impact of Tumor Characteristics on Outcome. *Ann Surg*, 228(4), 479-490.

[91] Pawlik, T. M., Delman, K. A., Vauthey, J. N., Nagorney, D. M., Ng, I. O., Ikai, I., Yamaoka, Y., Belghiti, J., Lauwers, G. Y., Poon, R. T., & Abdalla, E. K. (2005). Tumor Size Predicts Vascular Invasion and Histologic Grade: Implications for Selection of Surgical Treatment for Hepatocellular Carcinoma. *Liver Transpl*, 11(9), 1086-1092.

[92] Roayaie, S., Haim, M. B., Emre, S., Fishbein, T. M., Sheiner, P. A., Miller, C. M., & Schwartz, M. E. (2000). Comparison of Surgical Outcomes for Hepatocellular Carcinoma in Patients with Hepatitis B Versus Hepatitis C: A Western Experience. *Ann Surg Oncol*, 7(10), 764-770.

[93] Kneteman, N. M., Oberholzer, J., Al Saghier, M., Meeberg, G. A., Blitz, M., Ma, M. M., Wong, W. W., Gutfreund, K., Mason, A. L., Jewell, L. D., Shapiro, A. M., Bain, V. G., & Bigam, D. L. (2004). Sirolimus-Based Immunosuppression for Liver Transplan-

tation in the Presence of Extended Criteria for Hepatocellular Carcinoma. *Liver Transpl*, 10(10), 1301-1311.

[94] Toso, C., Meeberg, G. A., Bigam, D. L., Oberholzer, J., Shapiro, A. M., Gutfreund, K., Mason, A. L., Wong, W. W., Bain, V. G., & Kneteman, N. M. (2007). De Novo Sirolimus-Based Immunosuppression after Liver Transplantation for Hepatocellular Carcinoma: Long-Term Outcomes and Side Effects. *Transplantation*, 83(9), 1162-1168.

[95] Zimmerman, M. A., Trotter, J. F., Wachs, M., Bak, T., Campsen, J., Skibba, A., & Kam, I. (2008). Sirolimus-Based Immunosuppression Following Liver Transplantation for Hepatocellular Carcinoma. *Liver Transpl*, 14(5), 633-638.

[96] Yao, F. Y., Bass, N. M., Nikolai, B., Davern, T. J., Kerlan, R., Wu, V., Ascher, N. L., & Roberts, J. P. (2002). Liver Transplantation for Hepatocellular Carcinoma: Analysis of Survival According to the Intention-to-Treat Principle and Dropout from the Waiting List. *Liver Transpl*, 8(10), 873-883.

[97] Lo, C. M., & Fan, S. T. (2004). Liver Transplantation for Hepatocellular Carcinoma. *Br J Surg*, 91(2), 131-3.

[98] Dahm, F., Georgiev, P., & Clavien, P. A. (2005). Small-for-Size Syndrome after Partial Liver Transplantation: Definition, Mechanisms of Disease and Clinical Implications. *Am J Transplant*, 5(11), 2605-2610.

[99] Emond, J. C., Renz, J. F., Ferrell, L. D., Rosenthal, P., Lim, R. C., Roberts, J. P., Lake, J. R., & Ascher, N. L. (1996). Functional Analysis of Grafts from Living Donors. Implications for the Treatment of Older Recipients. *Ann Surg*, 224(4), 544-552, discussion 52-4.

[100] Yao, F. Y., Kerlan, R. K., Jr, Hirose, R., Davern, T. J., 3rd, Bass, N. M., Feng, S., Peters, M., Terrault, N., Freise, C. E., Ascher, N. L., & Roberts, J. P. (2008). Excellent Outcome Following Down-Staging of Hepatocellular Carcinoma Prior to Liver Transplantation: An Intention-to-Treat Analysis. *Hepatology*, 48(3), 819-827.

[101] Chan, K. M., Yu, M. C., Chou, H. S., Wu, T. J., Lee, C. F., & Lee, W. C. (2011). Significance of Tumor Necrosis for Outcome of Patients with Hepatocellular Carcinoma Receiving Locoregional Therapy Prior to Liver Transplantation. *Ann Surg Oncol*, 18(9), 2638-2646.

[102] Rahbari, N. N., Mehrabi, A., Mollberg, N. M., Muller, S. A., Koch, M., Buchler, M. W., & Weitz, J. (2011). Hepatocellular Carcinoma: Current Management and Perspectives for the Future. *Ann Surg*, 253(3), 453-469.

[103] Fisher, R. A., Kulik, L. M., Freise, C. E., Lok, A. S., Shearon, T. H., Brown, R. S., Jr., Ghobrial, R. M., Fair, J. H., Olthoff, K. M., Kam, I., & Berg, C. L. (2007). Hepatocellular Carcinoma Recurrence and Death Following Living and Deceased Donor Liver Transplantation. *Am J Transplant*, 7(6), 1601-1608.

[104] Poon, R. T., Fan, S. T., Lo, C. M., Liu, C. L., & Wong, J. (2007). Difference in Tumor Invasiveness in Cirrhotic Patients with Hepatocellular Carcinoma Fulfilling the Mi-

lan Criteria Treated by Resection and Transplantation: Impact on Long-Term Survival. *Ann Surg*, 245(1), 51-58.

[105] Jonas, S., Bechstein, W. O., Steinmuller, T., Herrmann, M., Radke, C., Berg, T., Settmacher, U., & Neuhaus, P. (2001). Vascular Invasion and Histopathologic Grading Determine Outcome after Liver Transplantation for Hepatocellular Carcinoma in Cirrhosis. *Hepatology*, 33(5), 1080-1086.

[106] Yang, Z. F., Poon, R. T., Luo, Y., Cheung, C. K., Ho, D. W., Lo, C. M., & Fan, S. T. (2004). Up-Regulation of Vascular Endothelial Growth Factor (Vegf) in Small-for-Size Liver Grafts Enhances Macrophage Activities through Vegf Receptor 2-Dependent Pathway. *J Immunol*, 173(4), 2507-2515.

[107] Koniaris, L. G., Levi, D. M., Pedroso, F. E., Franceschi, D., Tzakis, A. G., Santamaria-Barria, J. A., Tang, J., Anderson, M., Misra, S., Solomon, N. L., Jin, X., Di Pasco, P. J., Byrne, M. M., & Zimmers, T. A. (2011). Is Surgical Resection Superior to Transplantation in the Treatment of Hepatocellular Carcinoma? *Ann Surg*, 254(3), 527-537, discussion 37-8.

Chapter 14

Liver Resection for Hepatocellular Carcinoma

Mazen Hassanain, Faisal Alsaif,
Abdulsalam Alsharaabi and Ahmad Madkhali

Additional information is available at the end of the chapter

http://dx.doi.org/10.5772/54175

1. Introduction

Hepatocellular carcinoma (HCC), an epithelial tumor derived from hepatocytes, accounts for 80% of all primary liver cancers and ranks globally as the fourth leading cause of cancer-related deaths. Annual mortality rates of HCC remain comparable to its yearly incidence, making it one of the most lethal varieties of solid-organ cancer. Well-established risk factors for the development of HCC include hepatitis B carrier state, chronic hepatitis C infection, hereditary hemochromatosis, and cirrhosis of any etiology, as well as certain environmental toxins. HCC treatment is a multidisciplinary and a multimodal task with surgery in the form of liver resection and liver transplantation representing the only potentially curative modalities. Here we going to discuss the liver resection as treatment modality for HCC in detail.

1.1. Pathology of HCC

Three gross morphologic types of HCC have been identified: nodular, massive and diffuse. Nodular HCC is often associated with cirrhosis and is characterized by well-circumscribed nodules. The massive type of HCC, usually associated with a non-cirrhotic liver, occupies a large area with or without satellite nodules in the surrounding liver. The less common diffuse type is characterized by diffuse involvement of many small indistinct tumor nodules throughout the liver. *Histologically*, six growth forms of HCC can be differentiated. The most common form is the trabecular type, usually comprising highly differentiated carcinomas with polygonal tumor cells similar to hepatocytes; they grow in multilayered trabeculae and enclose blood spaces lined with endothelium (usually without Kupffer cells). The pseudoglandular type is generally found in combination with the trabecular form. It is characterized by the formation of gland-like structures containing detritus and bile or liquid material. The scirrhous type shows excessive deposits of sclerosed connective tissue, which is relatively low in cells. The

Surgical: Liver resection Liver transplantation
Locoregional: - Ablation: Radiofrequency ablation (RFA) Percutaneous ethanol injection (PEI) Cryotherapy - Embolization: Bland embolization Transarterial chemoembolization (TACE) Radioembolization
Systemic treatment: Sorafenib
External beam radiation therapy and stereotactic radiotherapy

Table 1. Different treatment modality of HCC

moderately differentiated tumor cells lie between the septa, which resemble connective tissue. This type is mostly found after chemotherapy or radiation therapy. The solid type is an undifferentiated HCC, with the tumor cells displaying considerable cellular polymorphism; the trabecular tissue pattern has disappeared. The tumor is compact due to compression of the sinusoids. Differentiation is, however, only possible in rare cases, since there is often considerable heterogenicity within the tumor, i.e. different tissue types may be found in the same HCC. Fibrolamellar HCC is rare; it consists of solid cell trabeculae with connective-tissue septation and a capsule. Spindle cell-like differentiated HCC is likewise a very rare histological form with a fascicular-sarcomatous growth pattern. Prognosis is significantly poorer than with other forms of HCC.

1.2. Preoperative evaluation

The preoperative evaluation for resection of HCC should focus on the likelihood of disease being confined to the liver, and whether the anatomical location of the tumor and the underlying liver function will permit resection (table 2).

Preoperative checklist for HCC patient		
Chick points		**Remark**
History:		
	Age	
	Comorbidities	
	Liver disease	Symptom of liver cirrhosis
	Alcohol /smoking	

	Medication (warfarin, aspirin)	
	Previous surgery	
	Physical status	
Examination:		
	Stigmata of liver disease	
	Chest /CVS/abdomen	
	Nutritional assessment	
Laboratory:		
	CBC	Platelet level is an indirect reflection of portal hypertension in cirrhosis.
	LFT	Bilirubin level for synthetic liver function and for Child Pugh score
	Coagulation	PT/INR for synthetic liver function and for Child Pugh score
	Chemistry	For electrolyte imbalance in cirrhotic patient and assessment of renal function
	Albumin	Liver synthetic function, nutritional status and Child Pugh score
	AFP	Tumor marker for HCC
	Hepatitis screen	HBV and HCV
Radiology:		
	US	Screening image for high risk patient It evaluate liver lesion and liver parenchyma
	CT and /or MRI	- Number and size of lesion and it's relation to major vessel - If it is classic HCC appearance by one image no need to be supported by another imaging. - Assessment of future liver remnant - Role out metastasis
	Portal Portal vein pressure	If patient cirrhotic and he is candidate for surgery with questionable portal hypertension
	Portal vein embolization	If future liver remnant small
Biopsy:		
	Core biopsy (tumor)	If CT and /or MRI are not classical for HCC
	Liver biopsy	If cirrhosis is not clear and sometime to know the cause of cirrhosis
Others:		
	Child Pugh score	If patient cirrhotic
	ICG	For assessment of adequate liver reserve before major resection (in some centers)
	Pre anesthesia evaluation	

Table 2. Preoperative checklist for HCC patient

1.3. Determining the extent of tumor involvement

Anatomic delineation of tumor extent is best achieved with dynamic multiphase CT or MRI scanning. Arterial phase imaging detects 30 -40 % more tumor nodules than conventional CT and may be the only phase to demonstrate the tumor in 7 -10 % of cases. Typical picture of HCC on CT will be an enhanced lesion on arterial phase (figure 1(a)) and early washout of contrast on venous phase (figure 1(b)).

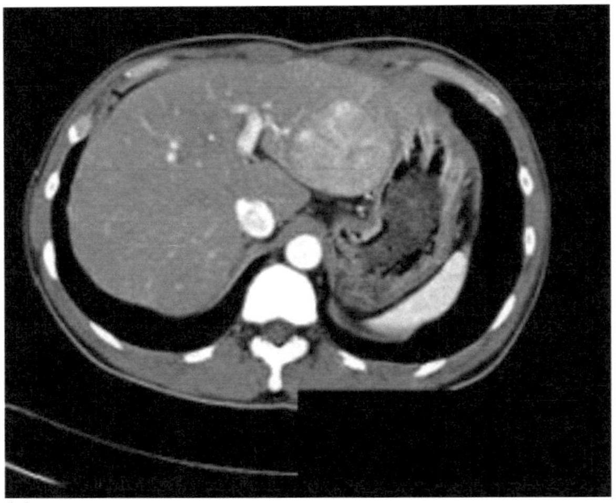

(a)

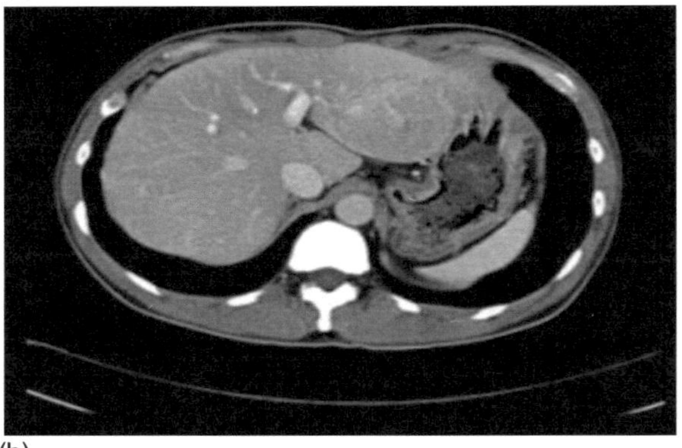

(b)

Figure 1. (a) Enhanced lesion on arterial phase in HCC (b) Early washout of contrast on venous phase in HCC

There is no general rule regarding tumor size for selection of patients for resection. Certainly, patients with smaller tumors are less likely to harbor occult vascular invasion and have a better outcome after therapy. Size alone is not a contraindication for resection of multinodular HCC.

Lymph node metastases are uncommon overall (between 1 - 8 %), but their presence portends a worse outcome. Preoperative detection of nodal metastases is limited by the frequent

http://dx.doi.org/10.5772/54175

presence of benign nodal enlargement, most often involving the porta hepatis and portacaval space, in patients with cirrhosis. Highly suspicious nodes based on enhancement similar to the intrahepatic HCC lesions indicate the need for biopsy in a patient being considered for resection. However, involved nodes are not a contraindication to surgery for fibrolamellar HCC; these patients should have a formal lymph node dissection.

A chest CT is recommended to complete the staging evaluation and bone scan if suspicious bone pain or hypercalcemia. HCC has lower FDG accumulation in well-differentiated and low-grade tumors than in high-grade tumors. In a study by *Khan et al*, the sensitivity of PET in diagnosis of HCC was 55% compared with 90% for CT scanning, although some tumors (15 %) were detected by PET only (including distant metastases). So, PET imaging may help assess tumor differentiation and may be useful in the diagnosis, staging and prognostication of HCC as an adjunct to CT. However, the utility of PET scanning for detection primary and occult distant metastatic disease is uncertain, need to be explored further and not recommended in guidelines from the National Comprehensive Cancer Network (NCCN).

1.4. Assessment of hepatic reserve

Operative mortality is related to the severity of the underlying liver disease; it is 7- 25% in cirrhotic and less than 3% in non-cirrhotic patients. In patients with cirrhosis, surgical resection is most safely performed in those with Child-Pugh class A (table 3) disease who has a normal bilirubin and well preserved liver function. However, even Child-Pugh class A patients may develop rapid hepatic decompensation following surgery due to limited functional hepatic reserve.

CHILD – PUGH SCORE			
Clinical and laboratory parameter	**Scores**		
	1	**2**	**3**
Encephalopathy (grade)	None	1-2	3-4
Ascites	None	Slight	Moderate
Albumin (g/dL)	> 3.5	2.8-3.5	< 2.8
Prothrombin time prolonged (sec)	1-4	4-6	6
Bilirubin (mg/dL)	< 2	2-3	> 3
For primary biliary cirrhosis	< 4	4-10	> 10

Class A = 5–6 points; Class B = 7–9 points; Class C = 10–15 points.

Class A: Good operative risk

Class B: Moderate operative risk

Class C: Poor operative risk

Table 3. Child Pugh score

Although helpful, the Child-Pugh classification and other tools for assessing underlying liver disease, such as the Model for End-stage Liver Disease (MELD) score, are not adequate to select patients with sufficient hepatic reserve for major resection.

Multiple studies have demonstrated that a normal serum bilirubin level and the absence of clinically significant portal hypertension (i.e., hepatic venous pressure gradient <10 mm Hg) are the best available indicators of acceptably low risk of postoperative liver failure after liver resection. In the absence of an elevated serum bilirubin and portal hypertension, survival after PH can exceed 70% at 5 years. Survival after liver resection in patients with significant portal hypertension alone decreases to < 50% at 5 years. However, in patients with both an elevated serum bilirubin and significant portal hypertension, survival drops to < 30% at 5 years, regardless of Child-Pugh score. Direct measurement of portal pressure is not necessary in patients with clinical signs of severe portal hypertension, including esophageal varices, ascites, or splenomegaly associated with a platelet count less than 100,000/mL.

In many centers the Child-Pugh score may be supplemented by specialized investigations such as the indocyaninegreen (ICG) retention test, especially in marginal cases (e.g. Child-Pugh B, possible mild portal hypertension). ICG retention of 14% at 15 min is widely accepted (in Asia Pacific area) as a reflection of adequate functional reserves for major resection (defined as resection of > 2 Couinaud segments) (figure 2).

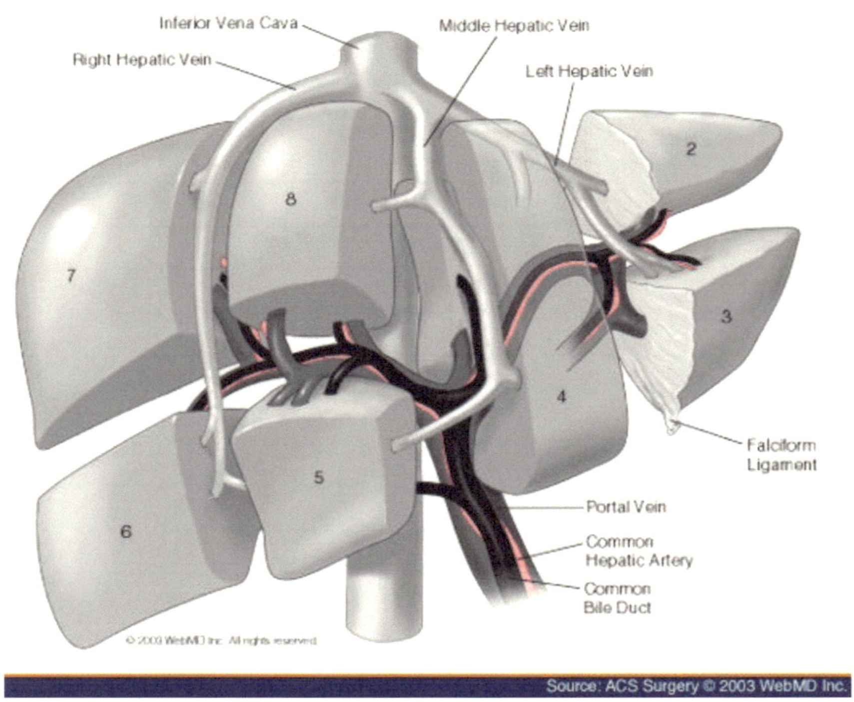

Figure 2. Couinaud liver segments

http://dx.doi.org/10.5772/54175

Assessment of the volume and function of residual liver should also be addressed by CT volumetry, particularly since portal vein embolization can be a valuable tool to increase the liver remnant volume and function prior to major hepatic resection, particularly for right sided tumors.

1.5. Portal vein embolization

Preoperative portal vein embolization (PVE) is a valuable adjunct to major liver resection. PVE can initiate hypertrophy of the anticipated future liver remnant to enable an extended resection in a patient with normal liver or major resection in a well compensated cirrhotic patient that would otherwise leave a remnant liver insufficient to support life following partial hepatectomy.

There are potential benefits to use of PVE:

- Reduce post-operative morbidity and mortality,
- Convert unresectable tumor due insufficient future liver remnant to resectable for potential cure.
- Subclinical disease or rapid progression may be detected prior to definitive surgery on post-embolization imaging studies, thus sparing the patient an unnecessary operation.
- The absence of compensatory hypertrophy identify patient with impaired liver regeneration,for that decrease post liver resection failure by preclude them from major liver resection.

The success of PVE was addressed by *Abulkhir A et al,* in a meta-analysis of data from 37 published series of PVE prior to liver resection. Four weeks after PVE, there was an overall increase in liver volume of between 10 and 12 % that was independent of technique, and 85 % of patients underwent planned laparotomy for attempted major hepatectomy. Following resection, only 23 patients had transient liver failure (2.5 %), and seven patients died of acute liver failure (0.8 %).

Liver regeneration usually peaks within the first 2 weeks after PVE. Studies in swine have shown that regeneration peaks within 7 days of PVE, with 14% of hepatocytes undergoing replication. Regeneration rates reported for humans are comparable to those found in animals. Non-cirrhotic livers demonstrate the fastest regeneration: 12–21 cm^3 /day at 2 weeks after PVE, approximately 11 cm^3 /day at 4 weeks, and 6 cm^3 /day at 32 days. Livers in patients with cirrhosis or diabetes regenerate more slowly (approximately 9 cm^3 /day at 2 weeks). Biliary obstruction, diabetes, chronic ethanol consumption, nutritional status, male gender, old age, and hepatitis all limit regeneration. Controlling these factors where possible is essential to maximize liver hypertrophy.

Two techniques can be utilized for PVE:

- The TIPE procedure is performed via a minilaparotomy and requires general anesthesia.
- The percutaneous approach (PTPE), which is more commonly used, can be performed in the radiology suite with local anesthesia and conscious sedation.

Volumetric assessment of the liver volume with CT imaging should be done before PVE and again before surgery. A standardized technique for measuring the future liver remnant, to select patients for PVE prior to a planned extended hepatectomy (trisegmentectomy) or hemihepatectomy in the setting of underlying liver disease, is strongly recommended. In considering the need for PVE, the ratio of future liver remnant and total estimated liver volume should be calculated. If the future liver remnant is < 20% in a patient with a normal liver or 40% in a patient with a cirrhotic liver, PVE should be considered.

Some reports have shown accelerated tumor growth in the liver after PVE. Problems with tumor growth are not seen when all of the tumor-bearing areas of the liver are embolized.

Transarterial chemoembolization (TACE) has been proposed as a complementary procedure prior to PVE in patients with HCC. TACE not only eliminates the arterial blood supply to the tumor, but it also embolizes potential arterioportal shunts in cirrhotic livers that attenuate the effects of PVE. Most reserve the "double embolization" procedure for patients with HCC in patients with liver disease who require right hepatectomy.

2. Surgery

Liver resection is a potentially curative therapy for patients with early-stage HCC (solitary tumor ≤5 cm in size, or ≤3 tumors each ≤3 cm in size and no evidence of gross vascular invasion) in a Child-Pugh class A score and no evidence of portal hypertension (although a minor resection could be considered in some patients with portal hypertension) $_{\text{Table 4}}$. However, in highly selected cases, patients with a Child-Pugh class B score may be considered for limited liver resection, particularly if liver function tests are normal and no portal hypertension.

Optimal tumor characteristics for liver resection are solitary tumors without major vascular invasion. Although no limitation on the size of the tumor is specified for liver resection, the risk of vascular invasion and dissemination increases with size. However, in one study by *Pawlik TM*, no evidence of vascular invasion was seen in approximately one-third of patients with single HCC tumors of 10 cm or larger. Nevertheless, the presence of macro- or microscopic vascular invasion is considered to be a strong predictor of HCC recurrence.

Liver resection is controversial in patients with limited and multifocal disease as well as those with major vascular invasion. Multifocality is associated with lower survival, but does not exclude a good outcome in selected patients. In several studies, resection of multifocal HCC is associated with five-year survival rates of approximately 24 %. Patients with multinodular HCC who appear to benefit from resection are those with sufficient liver reserve to tolerate resection, without extrahepatic disease and without major vascular invasion. Liver resection in patients with major vascular invasion should only be performed in highly selected situations by experienced teams.

Despite even aggressive surgical approaches, most patients have HCC or liver disease too advance to permit treatment with "curative" intent. In high-incidence regions of the world, only 10 to 15 % of newly diagnosed patients are candidates for standard resection, whereas in low incidence areas, between 15 and 30 % of patients are potentially resectable. Furthermore, only one-half of patients referred for surgery actually have resectable tumors. Among the reasons for unresectability are the extent of intrahepatic disease, extrahepatic extension, inadequate functional hepatic reserve, and involvement of the confluence of the portal or hepatic veins.

Indication for liver resection:
Indicated:
- Solitary tumor ≤5 cm in size or ≤3 tumors each ≤3 cm in size and no evidence of gross vascular invasion.
- Solitary tumors (any size) without major vascular invasion.
Patient should be in a Child-Pugh class A and no evidence of portal hypertension
Controversial:
- Multifocal disease
- Major vascular invasion
- Child-Pugh class B score and no portal hypertension

Table 4. Indications for liver resection in hepatocellular carcinoma

2.1. Intraoperative staging

Laparoscopy and intraoperative ultrasound (IOUS) may improve the selection of patients for potentially curative resection. IOUS can accurately determine the size of the primary tumor and detect portal or hepatic vein involvement, which precludes curative resection. Another benefit of IOUS is the identification of major intrahepatic vascular structures, which can be used to guide segmental or non-anatomic resections.

2.2. Technique

In non-cirrhotic liver, an anatomical resection should be performed. Up to two-thirds of the functional parenchyma can be removed safely depending upon the age of the patient and his liver's regenerative capacity. However, for cirrhotic patients, because the capacity for liver regeneration is impaired in these patients, resection is generally limited to less than 25% of functional parenchyma. to maintain postoperative liver function. However, some patients maintain adequate functional hepatic reserve even after a formal hemi-hepatectomy, particularly if preoperative portal vein embolization (PVE) is used to induce compensatory hypertrophy in the future liver remnant. Both anatomic and wedge resection are acceptable, though some studies suggest portal-oriented resections enable longer overall and disease-free survival when feasible which might be because of the pattern of intrahepatic spread of liver cancer cells along segmental portal vein pedicle, so segmental resection may improve the chance of tumor clearance compared with a non-anatomical wedge resection.

Surgical outcomes in cirrhotic patients have improved over the past decade as a result of advances in surgical techniques, in particular the techniques that help to reduce bleeding during liver parenchyma transection and perioperative support. One of the most important advances is the thorough understanding of the segmental anatomy of the liver, which can be delineated using intraoperative ultrasound during operation. The delineation of a proper transaction plane is important not only for adequate tumor-free margin in resection of liver tumors but also to avoid inadvertent injuries to major intrahepatic vessels or bile duct pedicles. Use of the Pringle maneuver for vascular inflow occlusion as an alternative to total vascular occlusion has decrease deleterious effect on liver. Intermittent Pringle occlusion is well tolerated by cirrhotic patients for up to 60 minutes and is better tolerated than continuous clamping. The use of low CVP (less than 5mm Hg) anesthesia and newer instruments such as the ultrasonic dissector, hydrojet and vascular stapling devices has also significantly improved visualization, limited blood loss and decreased operative times.

2.3. Anterior technique

Some surgeons have advocated an anterior or "no touch" technique to resection of these tumors. This approach utilizes initial transection of the liver parenchyma to the inferior vena cava (IVC), and ligation of the inflow and outflow vessels before mobilization of the right liver lobe. The advocates of this technique hypothesize that separation of the right liver and the tumor from the IVC before mobilization avoids prolonged rotation and displacement of the hepatic lobes, therefore reducing the risk of vascular rupture. In addition, division of the vessels before tumor manipulation theoretically minimizes the potential for tumor cell dissemination caused by tumor compression.

2.4. Centrally located tumors

Surgical management of centrally located tumors (i.e., those in segments IV, V, and VIII) is especially problematic. Extended right or left hemi-hepatectomy is the treatment of choice if potentially curative surgery can be undertaken safely. An alternative segment-oriented approach, meso-hepatectomy (also called central hepatectomy), has been proposed in which the central liver segments IV and/or V, and VIII (with or without segment I) are removed and the lateral sectors remain intact.

While randomized trials have not been conducted, the available data suggest that meso-hepatectomy is a reasonable alternative to extended resection for centrally located tumors, providing acceptable oncologic outcomes with less hepatic parenchymal loss. However, in some centers, meso-hepatectomy is seldom used, partly because it is a complex and technically demanding procedure that requires two hepatic resection planes and bilateral biliary reconstruction. This results in a higher risk of bile leak and bleeding as well as long-term biliary stricture and biliary dysfunction. In addition, some data suggest that portal vein embolization followed by major hepatectomy might be safer.

2.5. Minimally invasive surgery

The success of minimally invasive resection of benign hepatic tumors has led to interest in laparoscopic approaches to surgery for HCC. The available literature is limited by the lack of prospective trials and the paucity of information on long-term oncologic outcomes.

Looking to the available literature, laparoscopic resection is feasible and safe in experienced hands. It is also highly technically demanding and should be undertaken only in high volume centers.

2.6. Tumor rupture

Approximately 10% of HCC spontaneously rupture. The clinical picture is that of acute abdominal pain and distension with drop in the hematocrit and hypotension. Initially, these patients' hemodynamic should be stabilized followed by trans-arterial embolization for control of bleeding. If unsuccessful, emergency surgery may be required.

Although the presence of a tumor rupture suggests a high likelihood of peritoneal seeding and usually a poor outcome from resection, this is not inevitable. If bleeding can be controlled (arterial embolization is recommended), a formal staging evaluation should be undertaken, followed by laparoscopic exploration and a subsequent attempt at resection, if feasible. Several retrospective series suggest a low, but defined long-term survival rate following resection in such situations.

In the largest series from Hong Kong by *Liu CL et al*, 154 of 1716 patients who were newly diagnosed with HCC between 1989 and 1998 presented with spontaneous rupture. The 30-day mortality rate following tumor rupture was 38 %. After initial stabilization and clinical evaluation, 33 underwent hepatic resection. Although the median survival after hepatectomy was worse in ruptured as compared to non-ruptured cases (26 *versus* 49 months) and the rate of extra-hepatic recurrence was higher (46 *versus* 26 %), 8 patients (24 %) remained alive without recurrent disease after a median follow-up period of 45 months.

2.7. Postoperative management

Postoperative management is primarily supportive. Those patients should be monitored in ICU with great attention to hydration status, not over or under hydrated with CVP monitor. The extent of postoperative morbidity is related to the extent of operative resection. Major postoperative complications include bile leak in 8% and pleural effusion in 7%, which are usually treated conservatively.

2.8. Perioperative mortality

The 30-day operative mortality rate in modern series of HCC resection ranges widely from 1 -24 %. Fewer than 10 % of perioperative deaths are due to uncontrolled intraoperative hemorrhage; most are due to postoperative liver failure. The presence of cirrhosis is the most important predictor of post-resection liver failure and death. The 30-day postoperative mortality for cirrhotic patients ranges from 14 -24 %, compared to 0.8 -7 % for non-cirrhotics.

Two additional factors influence the development of postoperative liver failure in cirrhotic patients are intraoperative blood loss of >1500 ml and postoperative infection of any type. Mortality can also be reduced by appropriate selection of patients and meticulous surgical technique, with the inclusion of preoperative volumetry and portal vein embolization when appropriate.

Consensus is growing that 30-day operative mortality is an inadequate indicator of risk, particularly of postoperative hepatic insufficiency and failure. Using an approach similar to liver transplantation reporting, 90-day mortality reporting appears to be a more valuable indicator of outcome of liver resection, especially in the cases of extended resection and resection in patients with diseased livers. This relates to the late development of slowly progressive jaundice, ascites, and eventual death, which typically occurs outside the hospital and well after 30 postoperative days in patients with marginal or inadequate liver remnants (post resection liver failure will be discussed in detail at end of this chapter).

2.9. Fast track surgery

Surgical pathway and 'fast-track' (FT) programs are structured interdisciplinary strategies that have been introduced to optimize perioperative care and accelerate post-operative recovery. The main aim of the FT protocol is to reduce the metabolic and inflammatory response to surgical stress and preserve vital functions. A review done by *Lidewij et al* showed primary hospital stay was significantly reduced after FT care in two out of the three studies. In one study, median hospital stay was 6 days in the FT group compared with 8 days in the control group ($P < 0.001$). In the other study, primary hospital stay was reduced from 11 days to 7 days ($P < 0.01$). There were no significant differences in rates of readmission, morbidity and mortality between FT and control groups. One trial found a significantly shorter time to successful resumption of a normal diet in the FT group (1 post-operative day for FT patients vs. 3 days for the control group).

3. Long-term outcomes

Results of large retrospective studies have shown 5-year survival rates of over 50% for patients undergoing liver resection for HCC, and some studies suggest that in carefully selected patients having no vascular invasion by tumor, solitary lesions without intrahepatic metastasis, tumor diameter ≤5 cm, and a negative surgical margin of >1 cm, five-year survival rates up to 78 %. However, HCC tumor recurrence rates at 5 years following liver resection have been reported up to 70%.

Palavecino M et al reported series of 54 patients with advanced HCC and significant tumor burden who were treated with PVE plus major hepatectomy, the five-year overall survival was 72 % and the five-year disease-free survival was 56 %.

3.1. Tumor-related prognostic factors

The most important tumor-related prognostic factors are presence and degree of vascular invasion, tumor number and size, and surgical margin status. Other poor prognostic indicators are absence of a tumor capsule, preoperative alpha fetoprotein (AFP) levels >10,000 ng/ml, and poor histologic grade of differentiation.

Both intrahepatic and extra-hepatic spread of HCC is more common with tumors >5 cm, particularly when associated with venous invasion. In a report by Zhou XD compared 1000 patients with tumors ≤5 cm and 1366 patients having tumors >5 cm, all of whom underwent hepatectomy over the same period, five-year survival rates were significantly better for patients with smaller tumors (63 %versus 37 %, respectively). Nevertheless, several series indicate five year survival rates ranging from 25 to 35 percent in selected patients undergoing resection for single HCC ≥10 cm. However, although increasing tumor size is associated with increased risk for vascular invasion, large, solitary tumors without vascular invasion have the same prognosis as small solitary tumors without vascular invasion.

The importance of wide resection margins is debated. In study by *Ozawa K* of 225 patients with HCC who underwent resection, three-year survival was significantly better when a >1 cm tumor-free margin was achieved (77 % *versus* 21%, respectively). However, larger series by *Poon RT* suggest that a negative margin of <1 cm is acceptable.

Gross or microscopic invasion of branches of the portal or hepatic veins is associated with a lower probability of survival following resection.

3.2. Underlying liver dysfunction

Preoperative liver dysfunction and cirrhosis are important negative prognostic factors. *Yamanaka N* reported a series of 295 patients undergoing resection of HCC, the four-year survival was more than twofold higher for non-cirrhotic compared to cirrhotic patients (81% versus 35 %). This difference in outcome may be related in part to the higher frequency of multicentric HCC in cirrhotic patients.

In patients with cirrhosis related to HBV infection, active hepatitis is also a poor prognostic factor. As a general rule, the severity of cirrhosis, rather than the presence of a small, early stage HCC, limits long-term survival in cirrhotic patients with HCC. Chronic liver disease provides a field that contributes to the development of second primary HCCs and a persisting risk of HCC-related death beyond five years.

3.3. Recurrences

Treatment of recurrence is a poorly investigated area. Solitary recurrence might benefit from repeat resection, but in most patients recurrence will be multifocal.It has been suggested, retrospective analyses, that patients with recurrence might be candidates for salvage transplantation.. Most of the recurrences and specially those that appear early during follow-up are due to tumor dissemination and have a more aggressive biological pattern as compared to primary tumors. Hence, only those patients in whom recurrence is due to de novo oncogenesis can be expected to benefit from salvage transplantation or repeated resection. While the most accurate predictors of recurrence due to dissemination (vascular invasion, satellites) may be identified on pathology, and since the results of transplantation in these patients is good, some authors have proposed that this category of patients should be listed immediately after resection. This might be more effective than waiting for recurrence to develop with excessive tumor burden possibly excluding liver transplantation. Organ allocation policies might have to be modified to take these findings into account. Other treatment modalities can provide disease control (i.e., trans-arterial arterial embolization of chemoembolization, radiofrequency ablations, sorafenib).

Fewer than 20 % of disease recurrences have an extra-hepatic with overall poor prognosis, and the benefit of systemic therapy is modest, at best.

3.4. Surveillance

Although data on the role of surveillance in patients with resected HCC are very limited, recommendations are based on the consensus that earlier identification of disease may facilitate patient eligibility for investigational studies or other forms of treatment. The NCCN panel recommends high-quality cross-sectional imaging every 3-6 months for 2 years, then every 6-12 months. AFP levels, if initially elevated, should be measured every 3 months for 2 years, then every 6-12 months. Re-evaluation according to the initial work-up should be considered in the event of disease recurrence.

3.5. Survival

Liver resection is a potentially curative therapy for patients with early-stage HCC (solitary tumor ≤5 cm in size, or ≤3 tumors each ≤3 cm in size and no evidence of gross vascular invasion). 5-year survival rates of over 50% for patients undergoing liver resection for HCC, and some studies suggest that for selected patients with preserved liver function and early stage HCC, liver resection can achieve a 5-year survival rate of about 70%. However, HCC tumor recurrence rates at 5 years following liver resection have been reported to exceed 70%.

3.6. Post-Resection Liver Failure (PRLF)

PRLF is a devastating complication that is resource intensive and carries with it considerable morbidity and mortality. The reported incidence of PRLF ranges between 0.7 - 9.1%. An inadequate quantity and/or quality of residual liver mass are key events in its pathogenesis. Major risk factors are the presence of comorbid conditions, pre-existent liver disease and small Remnant Liver Volume (RLV). It is essential to identify these risk factors during the pre-operative assessment that includes evaluation of liver volume, anatomy and function.

There is no uniformity concerning the definition of PRLF. In general, PRLF is characterized as failure of one or more of the hepatic synthetic and excretory functions that include hyper-bilirubinemia, hypo-albuminemia, prolonged prothrombin time, elevated serum lactate and/or different grades of hepatic encephalopathy (HE). PRLF is defined by the so-called 50–50 criteria, which describe PRLF as prothrombin index less than 50% (equal to an international

http://dx.doi.org/10.5772/54175

standardized ratio more than1.7) and serum bilirubin more than 50 mmol/L (2.9 mg/dL) on post-operative day 5. When these 50–50 criteria were fulfilled, patients had a 59% risk of mortality compared with 1.2% when they were not met (sensitivity 69.6% and specificity 98.5%). This rarely occurs in isolation and is often coupled with failure of multiple organs and/or features of sepsis.

3.7. Pathophysiology of PRLF

After resection of various amounts of functional liver mass, both death and regeneration of the remaining hepatocytes occur. Physiologically, regeneration outweighs hepatocyte death and both liver mass and function are restored rapidly. For example, during the first 10 days after right hepatectomy for living donor liver transplantation, restoration of liver mass up to 74% of the initial volume has been reported. This regeneration is triggered by an increased metabolic demand placed upon remnant hepatocytes. The ability of the liver remnant to surmount the effect of surgical resection depends on its capacity to limit hepatocyte death, to resist metabolic stress, to preserve or recover an adequate synthetic function and to enhance its regenerative power. These factors rely on both the quality and the quantity of remaining liver parenchyma. A variety of intraoperative as well as post-operative hits identified that may attribute to the development of PRLF. These include hepatic parenchymal congestion, ischemia–reperfusion injury (IRI) and reduced phagocytosis capacity. Liver failure could be defined as either ''cholestatic'' (characterized by regeneration of hepatocytes and fibrosis) or ''non-regenerative'' (characterized by pronounced apoptosis of hepatocytes).

3.8. Hepatic parenchymal congestion

Partial liver resection leads to a relatively augmented sinusoidal perfusion, leading to shear–stress and congestion of hepatic parenchyma and resulting in vascular and parenchymal damage similar to small-for-size syndrome after liver transplantation, although less severe. Moreover, inadequate venous drainage of the liver remnant induces hepatic venous congestion and functional hepatic volume loss. Hepatic parenchymal congestion may be less severe in patients with cirrhosis of the liver with preexisting portacaval collaterals.

3.9. Hepatic ischemia–reperfusion injury

Hepatic ischemia–reperfusion injury follows massive bleeding or hepatic in- or outflow occlusion during liver surgery. Although the resistance of the liver to warm ischemia is relatively high, hepatic ischemia and reperfusion activate a complex cascade that triggers the innate immune response by recruitment and activation of Kupffer cells, endothelial cells and the complement system. These express pro-inflammatory proteins [nuclear factor kB, tumour necrosis factor-a, interleukin-6], reactive oxygen species, chemokines, complement factors and vascular cell adhesion molecules. Subsequently, polymorphonuclear neutrophils are activated, which aggravate hepatic injury. Although these processes are primarily intended to maintain homoeostasis, unrestrained activation may become destructive.

3.10. Reduced phagocytosis capacity

Infection complicates the course of PLF either as a precipitant or during later stages. Partial hepatectomy reduced the phagocytosis capacity of the hepatic reticuloendothelial system. Nevertheless, the liver remnant has to clear bacteria and their products following bacterial translocation or intra-abdominal infection. Diminished hepatic clearance of bacteria might enhance the susceptibility for the development infections and PRLF.

3.11. Risk factors of PRLF

The extent of resection correlates most closely with rates of PRLF and death; and the incidence increases with the number of segments resected. The incidence of PLF is < 1 % in patients with no underlying parenchymal disease when 1-2 segments are resected, around 10 % when 4 segments are resected, and 30 % when5 segments or more are resected. However, the exact amount of residual liver mass required to preserve sufficient liver function is unknown. In general, an RLV ≥ 25–30% in otherwise healthy livers is consistent with a good post-resectional outcome. RLV below 25% in normal livers predicted PRLF with a positive predictive value of 90% (95% CI 68–99%) and a specificity of 98% (95% CI 92–100%). When liver function is restricted, RLV should be as high as 40% to guarantee adequate remnant liver function.

The use of vascular occlusive techniques and significant intraoperative blood loss can exacerbate the level of dysfunction. Vascular occlusive techniques induce ischemia in the liver remnant. These effects are greatest following total vascular exclusion (inflow + outflow occlusion), but also occur after prolonged intermittent inflow occlusion.

Intraoperative blood loss (> 1–1.2 liters) and the need for blood transfusion increase the risk of PLF and sepsis. This may relate to the immunosuppressive effects of blood transfusion or the initiation of the inflammatory response that accompanies significant hemorrhage.

Vascular reconstruction following *in situ en bloc* liver and inferior vena cava resection or *ex vivo* liver resection is associated with increased rates of PRLF. *Ex vivo* resection and reimplantation is associated with an unacceptably high mortality rate. Biliary reconstruction is associated with increased morbidity and mortality after liver resection but does not independently predict PRLF.

Underlying parenchymal disease reduces the functional and regenerative capacity of the liver remnant. In patients with cirrhosis but no functional impairment or portal hypertension, resection of up to 50 % is safe. In patients with Child–Pugh grade B or C disease, even small resections can result in PRLF. The high risk of developing PLF in patients with cirrhosis can be explained by the wide range of comorbid conditions like portal hypertension, diabetes mellitus, jaundice, malnutrition, hypersplenism and coagulopathy as well as frequent impaired preoperative liver function and hepatic functional reserve. Furthermore, patients with cirrhosis have an impaired hepatic regenerative capacity. NAFLD (non alcoholic fatty liver disease) represents a spectrum of disease ranging from steatosis to steatohepatitis (non-alcoholic steatohepatitis, NASH), fibrosis and cirrhosis. The grade of steatosis, correlates with rates of PRLF and death following major Resection. The presence of steatosis is hypothesized to be associated with impaired hepatic microcirculation, decreased resistance to ischemia–reperfusion injury, increased intrahepatic oxidative stress and dysfunction in mitochondrial adenosine triphosphate synthesis. Chemotherapy-induced liver injury is increasingly prevalent as more patients receive chemotherapy for colorectal liver metastases before liver resection. Cholestasis reduces both hepatic metabolic and regenerative capacities, and increases rates of liver dysfunction after major resection.

Other patient-based factors that predict PRLF are age, malnutrition, diabetes mellitus and male sex. Elderly patients (≥65) suffer frequently from comorbid conditions and have reduced regenerative capacity of hepatocytes. Approximately 65–90% of patients with advanced liver disease suffer from protein–calorie malnutrition. Malnutrition is associated with an altered immune response, reduced hepatic protein synthesis and a reduction in hepatocyte regenerative capacity. Diabetes mellitus is associated with increased morbidity and mortality after liver resection. This may be due to immune dysfunction or because insulin absence or resistance reduces regenerative capacity. PRLF is more common in males as testosterone may have immune-inhibitory effects, predisposing to septic complications.

3.12. Prevention of PRLF

Diabetes mellitus should be screened for and treated before surgery. Nutrition should be evaluated and consideration given to preoperative oral carbohydrate loading in order to reduce postoperative insulin resistance. There is no evidence to support delaying liver resection for a period of nutritional optimization, unless the patient is severely malnourished. It has been hypothesized that the nutritional status of depleted patients should be corrected via oral, enteral or parenteral methods before surgery. A meta-analysis on the effect of total parenteral nutrition compared with enteral nutrition on morbidity and mortality after liver resection revealed no superiority of either form of nutrition. However, a beneficial effect of additional parenteral nutrition has been demonstrated in a subgroup of patients who had cirrhosis and underwent major hepatectomy.

The risk of PRLF may be reduced by strategies to increase parenchymal volume and protect against parenchymal damage. Strategies available for volume manipulation for HCC patients include portal vein embolization alone or in combined with locoregional treatment (RFA or TAE). Portal vein embolization induces apoptosis in the ipsilateral lobe, and proliferation and growth of the contralateral lobe. This increases the functional capacity of the liver remnant, limits the effects of hepatic hyperperfusion that may occur in a small-for-size remnant, and predicts the regenerative response in the future remnant. Failure to proliferate after portal vein embolization can be used to select patients with impaired regenerative capacity in which major resection would not be tolerated. The primary concern over portal vein embolization is that it may increase tumor growth owing to an ipsilateral surge in hepatic arterial flow. Locoregional treatment can be used in combination with Portal vein embolization to control tumor load before resection.

In order to limit parenchymal damage and optimize regenerative capacity, a series of hepatoprotective measures may be employed (intermittent portal clamping, ischemic preconditioning and hypothermic liver preservation). Total vascular occlusion should be avoided unless resection cannot be undertaken without it (for example a tumor at the cavohepatic intersection). If resection without vascular occlusion is not possible, inflow occlusion is preferable to total vascular exclusion. Intermittent portal clamping with intervals allowed for reperfusion is preferred to continuous clamping, usually applying a 15-min clamp–5-min release regimen. Ischemic preconditioning increases tolerance to prolonged hepatic ischemia and adenosine 5 -triphosphate depletion by exposing the parenchyma to short intervals of ischemia and reperfusion intraoperatively before resection. This downregulates ischemia–reperfusion injury and results in less hepatic injury. Ischemic preconditioning reduces the histological effects of ischemia–reperfusion injury, however, without improving clinical outcome. Hypothermic liver preservation in conjunction with total vascular exclusion attenuates ischemia–reperfusion injury. The future remnant is infused with a preservative fluid and surrounded by crushed ice to maintain the liver at 4 °C.

Data from living liver donors suffering from biopsy proven moderate steatosis revealed that a body weight reduction of 5% or intervention with a low-fat, high protein diet and exercise significantly improved hepatic steatosis. However, weight reduction before surgery may not be feasible because of time deficit and the often pre-existent malnutrition.

Patients with cirrhosis of the liver are more susceptible to the development of PRLF in case of resection of comparable tumor volumes. However, cirrhosis of the liver cannot be prevented and, therefore, prevention of PRLF in these patients can only be achieved by careful patient selection, adequate nutritional support and the use of an appropriate surgical technique.

3.13. Manifestation

PRLF reflects deregulation of the synthetic, excretory and detoxifying capacities of the liver remnant. In addition, the majority of patients suffering from PRLF will also meet the criteria of the systemic inflammatory response syndrome and experience multiple organ failure. Unfortunately, a substantial number of patients suffering from PRLF deteriorate, leading to a fatal outcome in approximately 80%. However, PRLF is a potentially reversible disorder because of the regenerative capacity of the liver remnant.

3.13.1. Liver

The clinical consequences of PRLF are jaundice, coagulopathy, ascites, edema and/or HE.

Ascites occurs as a result of surgery (portal hypertension, dissection, gross fluid overload), and may be difficult to assess it in the immediate postoperative period.

Data from Suc *et al.* and Balzan *et al.* concerning liver function on different days after uncomplicated hepatic resection showed an initial increase of serum bilirubin and a decrease of prothrombin time before normalization of these values on the seventh post-operative day.

3.13.2. Circulation

Circulatory failure occurring during PRLF resembles the circulatory failure of patients with sepsis. The pathophysiological changes usually observed are enhanced vascular permeability, diffuse intravascular coagulation and peripheral vasodilatation that are clinically represented by reduced peripheral resistance and hemodynamic instability.

3.13.3. Kidneys

Post-hepatic resection renal dysfunction can either result from perioperative disturbances in renal circulation inducing acute tubular necrosis or accompany PRLF. It is characterized by azotemia or oliguria and may cause ascites formation; pleural effusion and fluid overload requiring diuretics or hemofiltration. There is a distinct chance of reversibility of renal failure when there is recovery of PRLF. Furthermore, it can be hypothesized that the pivotal role of the kidney in ammonia excretion is impaired, leading to hyperammonemia and HE in patients suffering from PRLF.

3.13.4. Lung

Although moderate pulmonary edema seems to be a normal finding after partial hepatic resection owing to general hemodynamic alterations, this usually does not impair oxygen exchange. Severe remote lung injury, pulmonary edema and acute respiratory distress syndrome can develop as part of the multiple organ dysfunction syndromes that accompanies PRLF.

3.13.5. Hepatic encephalopathy

Hepatic encephalopathy is a potentially reversible neuropsychiatric disorder, characterized by varying degrees of confusion and disorientation. Hyperammonemia plays a central role in its development and has a direct toxic effect on neurotransmission and astrocyte function. Although hepatic encephalopathy are important markers for liver failure, altered mental state may occur in response to drugs such as opiates and may be difficult to assess it in the immediate postoperative period.

3.13.6. Treatment of PRLF

Large, randomized trials concerning the treatment of PRLF are lacking, and therefore, recommendations for treatment modalities are difficult to make. Management principles resemble those applied to patients with acute liver failure, acute-on-chronic liver failure or sepsis and focus on support of liver and end-organ function. Goal-directed therapy should be provided for circulatory disturbances, renal and ventilatory dysfunction, coagulopathy, malnutrition and HE (table 5). Patients should undergo clinical and laboratory assessment after liver resection, with the frequency of monitoring and level of care stratified according to risk.

It is normal for serum bilirubin levels and INR to rise in the first 48–72 h postresection. However, bilirubin concentration above 50 μmol/l (3 mg/dl) or INR greater than 1 7 beyond 5 days is unusual and usually reflects liver dysfunction. Serum bilirubin remains the most sensitive predictor of outcome in PLF. PT and INR are also valuable, but interpretation may be compromised if the patient has received clotting factors. Serum albumin, although an indicator of hepatic synthetic function, will vary in response to inflammation and administration of intravenous fluids. Increased levels of liver enzymes are common after liver resection and do not predict outcome. C-reactive protein levels are dampened after major liver resection, and day 1 levels inversely correlate with PRLF indices. Serum lactate has a prognostic value in severe sepsis and ALF, with a serum lactate level above 3 0 mmol/l after fluid resuscitation predicting death in ALF.

The systemic inflammatory response syndrome (SIRS) is present in more than 50 % of patients with ALF and predicts a negative outcome.The incidence of SIRS in patients with PLF has not been evaluated formally, but as in ALF it is likely to be implicated in sepsis, encephalopathy and end-organ dysfunction. Several studies have examined the role of postoperative functional assessment of the liver. The ICG15 predicts PRLF, but its value diminishes once liver failure is established because changes in hepatic blood flow also influence ICG15. Although PRLF is a potentially reversible condition, mortality rates remain high and currently there is little scope for therapeutic intervention.

Management of PRLF must be undertaken in conjunction with critical care, hepatology, infectious disease and radiology services. The pattern of organ dysfunction that occurs as a result of PRLF is similar to that in sepsis. Cardiovascular failure is characterized by reduced systemic vascular resistance and capillary leak. Acute lung injury, pulmonary oedema and acute respiratory distress syndrome may ensue. Acute kidney injury can progress rapidly in PRLF. Fluid balance should be managed judiciously with avoidance of salt and water overload. Identifying and treating underlying sepsis is a key in managing patients with PRLF. Sepsis may exacerbate PRLF, and bacterial infection is present in 80 % of patients with PRLF and in 90 % of those with ALF. Any acute deterioration should be attributed to sepsis until proven otherwise. Management of sepsis should be in accordance with the surviving sepsis guidelines. A trial of prophylactic antibiotics after liver resection failed to show a reduction in liver dysfunction or infective complications. However, the administration of antibiotics in patients suffering from acute liver failure is associated with a significant decrease in infectious complications and this may also be advantageous in patients suffering from PRLF. In critically ill patients with PRLF, chest radiography and cultures of blood, urine, sputum and drain site/ascetic fluid should be performed. Current guidelines for ALF propose that broad spectrum antibiotics should be administered empirically to patients with progression to grade 3 or 4 hepatic encephalopathy, renal failure and/or worsening SIRS parameters.

Coagulopathy may occur transiently after major resections and is found in all patients with PRLF. As in ALF, coagulation parameters can be used to chart the progress of PRLF, provided blood products have not been given. In a multinational review of fresh frozen plasma given for transient coagulopathy after resection, there was no consensus for its use. In the absence of bleeding it is not necessary to correct clotting abnormalities, except for invasive procedures or when coagulopathy is profound. The level at which a coagulopathy should be corrected before an interventional procedure in ALF has yet to be defined (the commonly used threshold for correction is an INR above 1 5). Vitamin K may be given, but this is not supported by clinical trials. Thrombocytopenia may complicate liver failure. Indications for platelet transfusion in ALF include bleeding, profound thrombocytopenia (< 20×10^{6} /L), or when an invasive procedure is planned. A platelet count above 70×10^{6} / L is deemed safe for interventional Procedures. Recombinant factor VIIa (rFVIIa) has been used to treat coagulopathy in patients with ALF.In a large controlled trial of rFVIIa following major liver resection, no reduction in bleeding events was observed. Its role in PRLF is yet to be defined.

Gastrointestinal hemorrhage is a recognized complication of liver failure. In ALF, H_2-receptor blockers and proton pump inhibitors (PPIs) reduce gastrointestinal hemorrhage in mechanically ventilated patients. In the non-ventilated patient an oral or sublingual PPI or oral H_2 -receptor blocker is likely to protect against gastrointestinal hemorrhage. High risk patients or patients with established PRLF should therefore receive prophylaxis. Large-volume ascites may also complicate PRLF. As in ALF, when this causes severe abdominal discomfort and/or respiratory compromise, consideration should be given to therapeutic paracentesis with simultaneous volume replacement with a plasma expander (ideally 20 % salt-poor albumin solution). The ratio for replacement is 6-8 gram 20% albumin per liter ascites drained. Nutrition is important and supplementation should be established early in patients with liver failure. Enteral nutrition is the preferred route as it improves gut function and restores normal intestinal flora. Parenteral nutrition can be used when enteral feeding is not tolerated, but should be introduced with caution owing to the risk of infection. In critically ill patients ensuring euglycemia improves survival and reduces morbidity.

The role of imaging in PRLF is to assess hepatic blood flow, identify reversible causes of liver failure and locate sites of infection. Hepatic blood flow can be evaluated using non-invasive imaging. Doppler ultrasonography may identify portal vein, hepatic artery and hepatic vein thrombosis. Contrast CT or MRI can be used to establish hepatic blood flow, provide more details of vascular abnormalities and identify sites of infection. If patency of hepatic vessels is still in doubt on cross-sectional imaging, angiography is the 'gold standard'. Vascular disorders may complicate liver resection and induce PRLF, but are rare. Longitudinal exposure of hepatic veins and the use of ultrasonic dissection may lead to hepatic vein thrombosis. Portal vein thrombosis has also been implicated in the development of PRLF. In these rare cases of inflow and outflow thrombosis with PRLF, a decision must be made regarding the benefit of surgical or radiological thrombectomy or dissolution *versus* anticoagulation.

Cerebral edema and intracranial hypertension may occur as a result of PRLF. Cerebral edema is unlikely in patients with grade 1 or 2 hepatic encephalopathy. With progression to grade 3, a head CT should be performed to exclude intracranial hemorrhage or other causes of declining mental status. In patients with established ALF and encephalopathy, enteral lactulose might prevent or treat cerebral edema, although the benefits remain unproven. Progression to grade 3/4 encephalopathy warrants ventilation and may require intracranial pressure monitoring.

Stress ulcer	**Proton pump inhibitor**
Nutrition	Enteral energy supply of 2000 kcal/day Enteral preferred over total parenteral nutrition Maintain euglycemia
Sepsis	Serial chest X-ray, sputum, urine and blood culture Ascetic fluid from drain site Consider CT abdomen Broad spectrum antibiotic if progression of encephalopathy, renal failure or worsening SIRS parameters
Circulatory disturbances	CVP 8–12 mmHg MAP 70 mmHg Hematocrit >30% Pulmonary capillary wedge pressure ≤ 12–15 mmHg
Ventilatory dysfunction	Arterial oxygen saturation > 93% Central venous oxygen saturation > 70%
Renal dysfunction	Urine output > 0.5 mL/kg/hour
Coagulopathy	Correct if bleeding or interventional procedure (INR<1.5)
Thrombocytopenia	Correct if bleeding, profound thrombocytopenia (<20 × 10^6/L) or interventional procedure planned (<70 × 10^6/L)
Vascular inflow/outflow (thrombosis)	Doppler ultrasound CT/MR angiography If evidence of inflow/outflow occlusion consider anticoagulation/revascularization
Ascites	Paracentesis if severe pain/respiratory impairment
Encephalopathy	Lactulose If progression to grade 3–4 encephalopathy, CT head, ventilate and consider ICP monitoring

** ICP: IntraCranial Pressure, INR: International Normalized Ratio, MAP: Mean Arterial Pressure MR: Magnetic Resonance CT: Computed Tomography, CVP: Central Venous Pressure, SIRS: Systemic Inflammatory Response Syndrome

Table 5. Management of post resection liver failure.

The concept of hepatocyte transplantation has been investigated as a strategy to boost residual liver function. Intrahepatic hepatocyte transplantation has been used successfully to treat patients with metabolic disorders of the liver. The efficacy of orthotopic liver transplantation for PRLF has only recently been reported. However, no criteria are available for the selection of patients who will benefit from emergency liver transplantation for PRLF. Patient who have favorable tumor characteristics (i.e. R0 resection, low T and negative N status, HCC within Milan criteria and absence of extra-hepatic disease), without comorbid conditions and without a limited life expectancy because of other medical conditions considered to be good candidate for emergency transplantation.

Extracorporeal liver support (ELS) devices fall into two categories: artificial and bioartificial systems. Artificial devices use combinations of hemodialysis and adsorption over charcoal or albumin to detoxify plasma. Bioartificial devices use human or xenogenic hepatocytes maintained within a bioreactor to detoxify and provide synthetic function. These systems have not been evaluated extensively in patients with PRLF. A recent meta-analysis and systematic review showed that ELS might improve survival in patients with ALF, but not acute-on-chronic liver failure, in comparison with standard medical therapy.

Abbreviation

ALF Acute liver faliure

ICG Indocyaninegreen

HCC Hepatocellular carcinoma

FT Fast Track

RFA Radiofrequency ablation

PEI Percutaneous ethanol injection

SIRS Systemic Inflammatory Response Syndrome

PLRF Post-resection liver failure

TACE Transarterial chemoembolization

Author details

Mazen Hassanain*, Faisal Alsaif, Abdulsalam Alsharaabi and Ahmad Madkhali

*Address all correspondence to: mhassanain@ksu.edu.sa

Department of surgery, College of Medicine, Liver Disease Research Centre, King Saud University, Riyadh, Saudi Arabia

References

[1] Jordi Bruix, and Morris Sherman. Management of Hepatocellular Carcinoma: An Update. HEPATOLOGY, (2011). , 53(3)

[2] Peter Abrams, J. Wallis Marsh. Current Approach to Hepatocellular Carcinoma. Surg Clin N Am (2010). , 90(2010), 803-816.

[3] Erwin Kuntz. Malignant liver tumor. HEPATOLOGY TEXTBOOK AND ATLAS (2008). Part DOI:, 4, 795-835.

[4] Khan, M. A, Combs, C. S, Brunt, E. M, et al. Positron emission tomography scanning in the evaluation of hepatocellar carcinoma. J Hepatol (2000). , 32, 792-7.

[5] Hepatobiliary Cancers. National comprehensive cancer network 2.(2012). www.nccn.org

[6] Steven Curley, Carlton Barnett, Eddie Abdalla. Surgical resection for hepatocellular carcinoma.uptodate Feb.2. (2012). www.uptodate.com

[7] Pierce Kah-Hoe ChowResection for hepatocellular carcinoma: Is it justifiable to restrict this to the American Association for the Study of the Liver/Barcelona Clinic for Liver Cancer criteria? *REVIEW*. Journal of Gastroenterology and Hepatology (2012). , 27(2012), 452-457.

[8] Pawlik, T. M, Delman, K. A, Vauthey, J. N, et al. Tumor size predicts vascular invasion and histologic grade: Implications for selection of surgical treatment for hepatocellular carcinoma. Liver Transpl. (2005). Sep; , 11(9), 1086-92.

[9] Yokoyama, Y, Nagino, M, & Nimura, Y. Mechanisms of Hepatic Regeneration Following Portal Vein Embolization and Partial Hepatectomy: A Review.World J Surg ((2007).

[10] Abbdalla, E, Hicks, M, & Vauthey, J. Portal vien embolization: rational,technique and future prospect.British Journal of Surgery (2011). , 2011(88), 165-175.

[11] Eddie, K. Abdalla.Portal Vein Embolization Prior to Major Hepatectomy: The Evidence.*Venous Embolization of the Liver*.(2011). part , 6, 293-305.

[12] David, C. Transhepatic Portal Vein Embolization: Anatomy, Indications, and Technical Considerations. RadioGraphics (2002). , 22, 1063-1076.

[13] Abulkhir, A, Limongelli, P, Healey, A. J, et al. Preoperative portal vein embolization for major liver resection: a meta-analysis. Ann Surg. (2008).

[14] Liu, C. L, Fan, S. T, Lo, C. M, et al. Management of spontaneous rupture of hepatocellular carcinoma: single-center experience. J Clin Oncol. (2001).

[15] Lidewij Spelt *et al*Fast-track programmes for hepatopancreatic resections: where do we stand?.*Review*. HPB (2011). , 2011(13), 833-838.

http://dx.doi.org/10.5772/54175

[16] De-Xin Lin *et al*Implementation of a Fast-Track Clinical Pathway Decreases Postoperative Length of Stay and Hospital Charges for Liver Resection. Cell Biochem Biophys ((2011).

[17] Zhou, X. D, Tang, Z. Y, Yang, B. H, et al. Experience of 1000 patients who underwent hepatectomy for small hepatocellular carcinoma. Cancer. (2001).

[18] Ozawa, K, Takayasu, T, Kumada, K, et al. Experience with 225 hepatic resections for hepatocellular carcinoma over a year period. Am J Surg. (1991). , 4.

[19] Poon, R. T, Fan, S. T, Ng, I. O, & Wong, J. Significance of resection margin in hepatectomy for hepatocellular carcinoma: A critical reappraisal. Ann Surg. (2000).

[20] Poon, R. T, Fan, S. T, Ng, I. O, & Wong, J. Significance of resection margin in hepatectomy for hepatocellular carcinoma: A critical reappraisal. Ann Surg. (2000).

[21] Giuseppe GarceaG. J. Maddern. Liver failure after major hepatic resection. J Hepatobiliary Pancreat Surg ((2009).

[22] Hammond, J. S. *et al*. Prediction, prevention and management of postresection liver failure. *British Journal of Surgery* (2011). , 98, 1188-1200.

[23] Maartje, A. J. van den Broek. Liver failure after partial hepatic resection: definition, pathophysiology, risk factors and treatment. Liver International ((2008).

[24] Suc, B, Panis, Y, Belghiti, J, & Fekete, F. Natural history' of hepatectomy. Br J Surg (1992). , 79, 39-42.

[25] Balzan, S, Belghiti, J, Farges, O, et al. The ''50-50 criteria'' on postoperative day 5: an accurate predictor of liver failure and death after hepatectomy. Ann Surg (2005). , 242, 824-8.

Chapter 15

Transplantation for Hepatocellular Carcinoma

Ahmad Madkhali, Murad Aljiffry and
Mazen Hassanain

Additional information is available at the end of the chapter

http://dx.doi.org/10.5772/54174

1. Introduction

Hepatocellular carcinoma (HCC) is the third leading cause of cancer mortality worldwide, accounting for more than 500,000 deaths annually. Major risk factors include chronic liver disease and liver cirrhosis due to hepatitis B and C viral infections, alcoholic liver disease and non-alcoholic steatohepatitis (NASH). Surgical resection and liver transplantation are the only potentially curable options for patients with HCC. While surgical resection is the treatment of choice in patients with good hepatic function, it is contraindicated in those with moderate to severe cirrhosis (Child class B or C), leaving these patients with liver transplantation as the only option. Moreover, transplantation is the optimal treatment even for small, otherwise resectable disease. This is a reflection of a number of factors. Liver transplantation will most likely result in a microscopically negative resection, which is the most effective oncologic treatment. Most HCCs are multifocal especially in the background of cirrhosis, though pre-neoplastic lesions may not be visible on perioperative evaluation; they are likely to continue to evolve into new primary HCCs. Furthermore, transplantation eliminates cirrhosis and restores normal hepatic function. However, limited organ availability mandates the restriction of liver transplantation to patients with early stage tumors who are not candidates for resection.

2. Organ allocation

In an effort to prioritize liver transplant candidates according to the highest short-term risk of mortality from end stage cirrhosis, the model for end-stage liver disease (MELD) scoring system was implemented in 2002 (table 1). To impart more urgent access to liver transplantation for patients with small HCCs, additional points within the scoring system were allotted to these patients. This is done to equilibrate their risk of death in comparison with the mortality of end-stage cirrhosis. The original scoring exception included lesions smaller than 2 cm, which resulted in an over distribution of donor livers to patients with HCC (with many expected small tumors turning out not to be HCC on explanted pathology). Therefore, the scoring exception was modified later by reducing the upgrade for Stage II tumors and eliminating it for Stage I tumors. Using the American Liver Tumor Study Group Modified TNM staging system, current UNOS guidelines do not allow upgrading of candidates with Stage I disease, irrespective of biopsy confirmation; only candidates with Stage II HCC disease are upgraded on the waiting list to a MELD score of 22 (equivalent to a 15% probability of candidate death within 3 months) with the intent to shorten their waiting time. From 2002-2007 in UNOS database, patients with an "HCC MELD-exception" had similar survival to patients without HCC.

MELD score component, calculation and mortality prediction	
Serum bilirubin (mg/dL)	
Serum creatinine (mg/dL)	
INR	
MELD = 3.8[Ln serum bilirubin (mg/dL)] + 11.2[Ln INR] + 9.6[Ln serum creatinine (mg/dL)] + 6.4	
* If a patient has had 2 or more hemodialysis treatments or 24 hours of CVVHD in the week prior to the time of the scoring, Creatinine will be set to 4 mg/dL	
MELD score	Mortality in 3 months
- <9	1.9 %
- 10–19	6.0 %
- 20–29	19.6 %
- 30–39	52.6 %
- >40	71.3%

Table 1. MELD score component, calculation and mortality prediction

3. Criteria for transplantation

Retrospective study by *Mazzaferro* and colleagues established that favorable results could be achieved in patients with cirrhosis with either a solitary HCC ≤5 cm or with up to 3 nodules ≤3 cm, criteria that came to be called "the Milan criteria (Table3)." The 5-year survival of these early-stage patients exceeded 70%. Recipient age, gender, type of viral infection, or Child-Pugh score (table 2) did not affect survival after transplantation. In a multivariate analysis by *Marsh JW* and colleagues, found that independent predictors of tumor-free survival included lymph node status, depth of vascular invasion, greatest tumor dimension, lobar distribution, and tumor number.

The strict application of the Milan criteria by UNOS for MELD upgrades allocation disadvantages patients with HCC with tumor profiles exceeding the criteria's maximal size or multifocal

CHILD – PUGH SCORE			
Clinical and laboratory parameter	**Scores**		
	1	2	3
Encephalopathy (grade)	None	1-2	3-4
Ascites	None	Slight	Moderate
Albumin (g/dL)	> 3.5	2.8-3.5	< 2.8
Prothrombin time prolonged (sec)	1-4	4-6	6
Bilirubin (mg/dL) · For primary biliary cirrhosis	< 2 < 4	2-3 4-10	> 3 > 10
Class A = 5–6 points; Class B = 7–9 points; Class C = 10–15 points. Class A: Good operative risk Class B: Moderate operative risk Class C: Poor operative risk			

Table 2. Child Pugh score

parameters but in whom favorable outcomes after liver transplantation have been demonstrated. There is an ongoing debate within the liver transplantation community regarding whether to expand indications for liver transplantation as primary therapy for HCC. For patients with HCC disease beyond Milan criteria in whom there is no macroscopic evidence of vascular invasion or extrahepatic spread, the survival rates after liver transplantation are generally comparable with patients transplanted for disease within the criteria. Most groups report a 5-year survival of more than 50% in patients transplanted for HCC beyond Milan, which many investigators have argued is the minimum acceptable survival rate. In 2001*Yao* and colleagues at the University of California, San Francisco (UCSF) defined an expanded set of HCC criteria (solitary tumor ≤ 6.5 cm, or ≤ 3 nodules with the largest tumor ≤ 4.5 cm and total tumor diameter ≤ 8 cm)(table3) for which 1 and 5-year survival rates after LT were 90% and 75%, respectively. Retrospectively evaluating post- liver transplantation survival for patients with tumors beyond Milan criteria but within "UCSF" expanded criteria by pre-transplantation imaging and explant pathology, the group at the University of California, Los Angeles (UCLA) confirmed acceptable 1,3-, and 5-year survival rates of 82%, 65%, and 52%, respectively. Moreover, the difference in 5-year recurrence-free survival after liver transplantation for HCC in the UCLA study did not reach statistical significance between Milan criteria and UCSF expanded criteria tumor groups (74% vs 65%, P =.09). Liver transplantation in such candidates is controversial and widely adopted. The short-term outcomes are similar to those who are transplanted within the Milan criteria.

Group from Edmonton have study Total Tumor Volume (TTV) in patients with HCC who had liver transplant based on Milan or UCSF criteria in 3 centers and they found TTV < 115 cm^3 has lower recurrence rate than TTV > 115 cm^3. In same study they also found that patients beyond Milan but within TTV < 115 cm^3 had survivals similar to those of patients within Milan. On the contrary, patients with TTV >115 cm^3 demonstrated lower survival than those within TTV <115 cm^3 when pathology (5-year: 47% versus 79%, $P < 0.001$) and radiology staging (5-year: 53% versus 76%, $P < 0.1$) was used.

Milan criteria:
- Single lesion ≤ 5 cm or
- ≤3 nodules each ≤ 3 cm
Without vascular invasion.
"UCSF" expanded criteria:
- Single lesion ≤ 6.5 cm or
- ≤ 3 nodules with the largest tumor ≤ 4.5 cm and total tumor diameter ≤ 8 cm
Without vascular invasion.

Table 3. Criteria for liver transplantation

4. Pre-transplant treatment for HCC

The major limitation for liver transplantation as therapy for early-stage HCC is the insufficient number of donor livers. There is always a waiting period between candidate listing and transplantation. If the waiting period extends over a sufficient length of time, the tumor will grow and eventually hinders transplantation. In a study by *Yao* and colleagues of patients with HCC on the waiting list, a 6-month waiting period for liver transplantation was associated with a 7.2% cumulative dropout probability, increasing to 37.8% and 55.1% at 12 and 18 months, respectively. In this setting the treatment of HCC prior to liver transplantation has three potential goals: (a) controlling tumor growth and vascular invasion during the waiting time and therefore decrease dropouts from the waiting list; (b) carrying out neoadjuvant therapy to improve the post-transplant outcome by reducing the risk of postoperative recurrence, and (c) downstaging the HCC burden to make a patient eligible for transplantation.

Followups for patients on waiting list are required every three months by CT or MRI to ensure continued eligibility for liver transplantation.

5. Percutaneous ablation therapy

5.1. Bridging therapy

Bridge therapy is used to decrease tumor progression and the dropout rate from the liver transplantation waiting list. It is considered for patients who meet the transplant criteria. A number of studies have investigated the role of locoregional treatment as a bridge to liver transplantation in patients on a waiting list. These studies included radiofrequency ablation (RFA), transarterial chemoembolization (TACE), surgical resection, conformal radiation therapy, and sorafenib as "bridge" therapies.

5.1.1. TACE

The rationale for using TACE as a bridge therapy prior to OLT is to control tumor growth while the patient awaits an organ. In addition, TACE could cause significant tumor necrosis, which may reduce tumor dissemination, making it a potential neoadjuvant therapy. TACE can also be used to learn more about the natural history and behavior of a particular tumor prior to liver transplantation. *Decaens et al.* failed to demonstrate survival benefit in a retrospective case-control study comparing 100 patients who underwent TACE prior to liver transplantation (median 1 session/patient) versus 100 matched controls without prior treatment. Mean waiting time was 4.2 months, and 5-year post-LT survival rates were 69% versus 63% (p = ns); dropout was not analyzed. *Yao et al.* retrospectively studied 168 HCC patients who underwent liver transplantation, 88 of whom received TACE (in most cases immediately prior to LT). For patients with HCC within the Milan criteria, 5-year recurrence-free survival was 96% for the TACE group versus 87% for controls ($p = 0.12$), but for HCC beyond the Milan criteria the difference was statistically significant (86% vs. 51%, $p = 0.05$). *Roayaie et al.* reported a 46% dropout rate, but only advanced HCC (>5 cm) were included in this study. *Graziadei et al.* found no dropout from the waiting list in patients treated wit TACE meeting Milan criteria and the mean waiting time was only 178 days. Furthermore, the monitoring protocol of repeat staging and the criteria for dropout was not specified. In view of this study and others, the dropout rate ranged from 15 to 46%. The rate of dropout was related to the tumor state and to the duration in the waiting list, the higher rate (46%) being observed in more advanced HCC and when the mean waiting time was 340 days. A systematic review of bridging therapy with TACE by *Lesurtel et al.* concluded that there was insufficient good quality evidence to demonstrate that TACE either improved post-LT survival, altered post-LT complication rates, or impacted on waitlist drop out.

Although pre-liver transplantation TACE does not influence post-LT overall survival and disease-free survival, it remains indicated in context of clinical trial when the period on the waiting list is more than 6 months.

5.1.2. Percutaneous ablation therapy

Patients with small tumors can have ablation either by percutaneous ethanol injection, radiofrequency or any other technique. Pre-transplant RFA ablation for HCC as a strategy to reduce dropout has been addressed in view studies. More than 80% of patients were in the Milan criteria with approximately 1 year on the waiting list. The dropout rate ranged from 0 to 14%. In a nonrandomized series from Toronto of 74 patients bridged using ablation compared with 79 non-bridged patients, the analysis of dropout for tumor progression identified a difference ($p < 0.005$) that became apparent only with prolonged waiting time superior to 300 days.

The main concern with this approach is seeding due to tumor puncture as has been reported for diagnostic biopsy. However, puncture-related seeding is usually a case of poorly differentiated tumors and to peripheral tumors that cannot be approached through a rim of non-tumoral liver.

In conclusion, due to small size of these studies and the heterogeneous nature of the study populations, as well as the absence of randomized clinical trials evaluating the utility of bridge therapy for reducing the liver transplantation waiting list dropout rate, limit the conclusions that can be drawn. Therefore, if liver transplantation can be done without significant delay (i.e. within 6 month) would the optimum. However, in patients whose waiting time is predicted to be prolonged, an RCT of TACE and/or ablation as bridging therapy to decrease dropout of transplantation could be justified.

5.2. Liver resection

Advances in liver surgery have significantly improved the safety of resection. Resection can be used as a treatment for HCC prior to liver transplantation in three different settings. First, resection can be used as a primary therapy, and liver transplantation reserved as a ''salvage'' therapy for patients who develop recurrence or liver failure. A second justification for resection prior to transplantation is that it helps refine the selection process. Resection, indeed, gives access to detailed pathological examination of the tumor and the surrounding liver parenchyma. Important prognostic information can be obtained from the entire resected tumor, including differentiation (which proved to be heterogeneous within the tumor), satellite nodules, microvascular invasion, and capsular effraction. As a result, resection may help deny transplantation in patients with tumors apparently within the Milano criteria but with histological features of especially poor prognosis (undetected macrovascular invasion in particular). On the other hand, resection may help decide transplantation in patients with tumors slightly outside the Milano criteria but with histological features of good prognosis. Third, resection can be used as a ''bridge'' therapy for patients who have already been enlisted for liver transplantation. Resection as the first line treatment for patients with small HCC with preserved liver function, followed by salvage transplantation only for recurrence or liver failure is an attractive option. Initial resection with negative margins, gives rapid access to an effective therapy, without the need for a donor, and offers 5-year survival rates exceeding 50% with a good quality of life. The main obstacle to this strategy is the risk of ''loss of chance'' in case of rapid and extensive recurrence not amendable to salvage liver transplantation. At the time of recurrence, salvage liver transplantation is only applicable in patients with a tumor within the Milan criteria. Initial data showed that patients with HCV infection who developed recurrence after partial resection had multifocal tumors and/or vascular invasion at the time of recurrence.

Although limited resection appears to be sufficient in this setting, it is associated with increased risk of post resection liver failure and is only appropriate for patients with peripheral tumors and Child A cirrhosis and no portal hypertension. As disadvantage for this approach the subsequent liver transplantation would be more difficult due to increase operative time and blood loss.

The use of laparoscopic approaches for peripheral tumors may further contribute to expand this strategy by minimizing technical difficulties during the transplant procedure.

5.3. Tumor dowenstaging

The role of downstaging of tumors before liver transplantation has been explored. Downstaging is done using HCC directed therapy that aims at reducing the size and/or number of HCC lesions. *Graziadei et al.* achieved downstaging to within Milan using TACE in 15/36 patients (41%). Among those downstaged, four dropped out prior to LT, one remained waiting, and 10 underwent LT; there were six deaths including three HCC recurrences, and 4- year post-transplant survival of 41%. *Yao et al.* reports successful downstaging in 21/30 patients with HCC beyond UCSF using a multimodality approach including resection in four cases. There were two deaths related to downstaging treatment (one postresection). Among 16 patients transplanted there was one death and no recurrence, but follow-up was limited (median 16 months). Recent prospective studies have demonstrated that downstaging (prior to transplant) with percutaneous ethanol injection (PEI), RFA, TACE and transarterial radioembolization (TARE) with yttrium 90 microspheres improves disease-free survival following transplant. However, such studies have used different selection criteria for the downstaging therapy and different transplant criteria after successful downstaging. In some studies response to locoregional therapy has been associated with good outcomes after transplantation. Further validation is needed to define the end-points for successful downstaging prior to transplant.

6. Living donor transplantation

Efforts to address the large waiting list of liver transplantation candidates and to decrease the dropout rate have included several strategies such as living donor LT, domino LT, split LT, the use of extended criteria donors, and donors after cardiac death. Living donor LT appears to be an effective option for patients with HCC within the Milan criteria, essentially equivalent in terms of survival to OLT, and it is cost effective if waiting times exceed 7 months. There are few data to support the use of living donor LT for patients with HCC who exceed the Milan criteria, although its use for this purpose is becoming increasingly common.

7. Immunsupression

Immunsupresion is used post liver transplantation to reduce graft rejection but, especially in transplantation for HCC, is associated with a risk of tumor growth. While results of liver transplantation including survival and rates of rejection were dramatically improved in cyclosporine treated patients compared with "historical controls", a high incidence of neoplasm and its aggressive phenotype were found to be due to cyclosporine and its activation of transforming growth factor-beta (TGFβ). *Vivarelli* and colleagues reported an increase in 5-year recurrence free survival in patients treated with smaller cumulative doses of cyclosporine in the first year following liver transplantation for HCC. Furthermore, they observed a significantly higher mean cyclosporine level in patients with HCC recurrence. Tacrolimus, another calcineurin inhibitor was also found to promote cell cycle progression by an increase in cdk4 kinase activity and thus was linked to increased tumor recurrence.

On the other hand, the calcineurin-independent immunosuppressive agent sirolimus, a binder of mTOR, inhibits tumor growth in cell lines, and it inhibits primary and metastatic tumor growth *in vivo*. In a study by *Wang Z et al*, looking at HCC in mouse model of human HCC, they identify that sirolimus induces cell cycle arrest and blocke proliferation of an HCC cell line, also sirolimus found to prevent tumor growth and metastatic progression by down-regulating the mRNA expression of VEGF and HIF-1α.

Several retrospective reports suggest a lower risk of post-transplant tumor recurrence in patients with HCC with the use of sirolimus as compared to other types of immunosuppressive agents (such as the calcineurin inhibitors tacrolimus and cyclosporine). However, these reports are limited by small size and uncertainty as to whether the observed benefits were due to a specific antitumor effect or an impact on liver transplant in general.

8. Surveillance

There is no consensus as to the optimal approach for post-transplant surveillance. Guidelines from the National Comprehensive Cancer Network (NCCN) suggest the follow up after liver transplant with triphasic CT every 3-6 months for 2 years, then every 6-12 months. AFP levels every 3 months for 2 years, if initially elevated, then every 6-12 months.

9. Survival

There is a clear survival benefit and low recurrence rate after transplantation for hepatocellular carcinoma. When surgeons adhere to Milan criteria, 5-year survival rates after transplantation range from 70% to 80%, and tumor recurrence rates are approximately 10%. Since the initial report by Yao and colleagues that demonstrated acceptable survival rates using the UCSF criteria (90% 1-year survival rates and 75% 5-year survival rates) and showed no survival deference from Milan criteria in 1,3 and 5 years, long-term survival need to be further identified.

10. Recurrence

Tumor recurrence remains a main limitation to the long-term survival of patients following liver transplantation for HCC. While the majority of patients recur in the first two years after transplantation, late recurrence is not infrequent. Most common sites of recurrence are liver graft, lung, bone, abdominal lymph nodes, adrenal glands and peritoneum. The incidence of recurrent HCC following transplantation has been reported to vary, ranging from 6-56%. However, in cases in which the Milan selection criteria were adopted, risk of recurrence decreased to 10–15% at 5 years. While several recipient and tumor specific factors are prognostically important, primary tumor size, number of lesions, grade of tumor and presence of vascular invasion have been noted to be the most significan clinical risk factors for both recurrence and survival. De-novo tumor development from recurrent hepatitis and cirrhosis in the liver graft can occur, however presence of microscopic foci of disease in lymph nodes or distant organs at the time of transplantation, as well as hematogenous or peritoneal tumor dissemination during transplantation, are mechanisms attributed to disease recurrence. Recurrent disease following liver transplantation for HCC may involve an extrahepatic site in 10-43% of patients.

Successful surgical salvage has been reported for intrahepatic and/or confined extrahepatic HCC metastases. In a study by *Regalia et al*, involving several Italian centers, 7 out of 21 patients (30%) underwent salvage resection of recurrent HCC of the liver (2), lung (2), bone (1), skin or other sites (2). Surgical resection was associated with a survival of 15.5 months, which was better than the 5.5 months noted among patients treated with a non-surgical approach. *Schlitt et al*. reported on 39 patients with recurrent disease, 9 intrahepatic recurrences, 15 extrahepatic disease and 15 had both intra and extrahepatic recurrence. Eleven of these patients were able to undergo complete removal of the recurrent disease, including 5 patients with an intrahepatic recurrence; 7 (63%) were alive at 4.3 years of follow-up. As with HCC of the native liver, the utilization of resection versus ablation to treat recurrence in the allograft is dependent on surgical judgment, as well as the size and location of the tumor. While resection may be more applicable to more superficial and larger tumors, ablative techniques may be sufficient and appropriate in the setting of smaller and more deeply situated tumors. Although liver resection for intrahepatic HCC recurrence has been reported by several centers, most series are limited by a small sample size.

Reports of repeat liver transplantation as a treatment of recurrent intrahepatic HCC are limited to a few very select case series and is not the standard of care.

Another potential approach to intrahepatic HCC recurrence is the utilization with TACE and RFA. *Ko et al*, reported on 28 patients with recurrent HCC who underwent one or more cycles of TACE after transplantation (mean, 2.5 cycles). In this study, the targeted tumor reduced in size by ≥25% in 19 of the 28 study patients (68%). However, intrahepatic or extrahepatic metastasis occurred in 21 of the 28 patients (75%) during the 3-month follow-up period and mean survival was only 9 months.

Systemic therapeutic options for recurrent HCC are limited. While cytotoxic agents have traditionally had marginal effect in the treatment of HCC, systemic therapy with molecular targeted therapy has been shown to prolong survival in recent trials. Sorafenib, a multi-targeted kinase inhibitor, demonstrated a significant overall survival benefit in patients with advanced or metastatic HCC when compared with placebo in two separate Phase 3 trials. These studies were carried out in patients who presented initially with advanced disease (mostly liver confined disease), and did not include patients who had previously undergone curative-intent therapy, such as surgical resection or liver transplantation. A number of retrospective studies have reported acceptable safety data for sorafenib in liver transplant patients, with very few unexpected toxicities or interaction with immunosuppressive medications. The numbers in these studies are small, and there is clearly a need for a prospective trial to fully assess the potential survival benefit of sorafenib in this setting.

Radiation therapy is another option for patients with recurrent unresectable HCC. Three dimensional conformal radiation, as well as stereotactic body radiation therapy and radioembolization, have been utilized in the treatment of primary unresectable HCC. In addition, radiation therapy is a treatment option for symptomatic palliation of extrahepatic disease. *Yamashi et al*, reported on 28 patients with metastatic HCC involving the portal and/or peripancreatic lymph nodes who were treated with radiation therapy. A total of 18 (64%) and five (18%) patients achieved partial responses and complete responses, respectively. The 1- and 2-year overall survival rates were 53% and 33%, respectively. In one study, *Seong et al.* investigated the effectiveness of palliative radiation therapy for HCC bone metastasis. In this study, 51 patients received radiation therapy for 77 bony metastatic lesions, with a median total dose of 30 Gy. There was pain relief in 56 lesions (73%), however, median and 1 year survival were only 5 months and 15%, respectively. In aggregate, these studies suggest that recurrent metastatic HCC may be sensitive to palliative radiation therapy. Therefore, radiation therapy should be considered for palliation of metastatic HCC lesions.

Abbreviation

HCC Hepatocellular carcinoma

HIF-1α Hypoxia-inducible factor 1, alpha

MELD Model for end-stage liver disease

RFA Radiofrequency ablation

PEI Percutaneous ethanol injection

TACE Transarterial chemoembolization

TGFβ Transforming growth factor-beta

TNM Classification of Malignant Tumors (Tumor, lymph Node, Metastasis)

VEGF Vascular endothelial growth factor

UNOS United Network for Organ Sharing

UCSF University of California, San Francisco

Author details

Ahmad Madkhali[1], Murad Aljiffry[2] and Mazen Hassanain[1,3]

1 Department of surgery, College of Medicine, King Saud University, Riyadh, Saudi Arabia

2 Department of surgery, College of Medicine, King Abdulaziz University, Jeddah, Saudi Arabia

3 College of Medicine, Liver Disease Research Centre, King Saud University, Riyadh, Saudi Arabia

References

[1] Jordi Bruix, and Morris Sherman. Management of Hepatocellular Carcinoma: An Update. HEPATOLOGY, Vol. 53, No. 3, 2011.

[2] Peter Abrams, J. Wallis Marsh. Current Approach to Hepatocellular Carcinoma.Surg Clin N Am 90 (2010) 803–816

[3] Mazzaferro V, Regalia E, Doci R et al. Liver transplantation for the treatment of small hepatocellular carcinomas in patients with cirrhosis. N Engl J Med 1996; 334: 693–699.

[4] Marsh JW, Dvorchik I, Bonham CA, et al. Is the pathologic TNM staging system for patients with hepatoma predictive of outcome? Cancer 2000; 88(3):538–43.

[5] Yao FY, Bass NM, Nikolai B, et al. A follow-up analysis of the pattern and predictors of dropout from the waiting list for liver transplantation in patients with hepatocellular carcinoma: implications for the current organ allocation policy. Liver Transpl 2003;9(7):684–92.

[6] Duffy JP, Vardanian A, Benjamin E, et al. Liver transplantation criteria for hepatocellular carcinoma should be expanded: a 22-year experience with 467 patients at UCLA. Ann Surg 2007;246(3):502–9.

[7] Toso C, Trotter J, Wei A.et al. Total tumor volume predicts risk of recurrence following liver transplantation in patients with hepatocellular carcinoma. Liver Transpl. 2008 Aug;14(8):1107-15.

[8] Hepatobiliary Cancers .National comprehensive cancer network 2.2012.www.nccn.org

[9] George Tsoulfas, Steven A Curley, Eddie K Abdalla, et *al*.Liver transplantation for hepatocellular carcinoma.uptodate 21 may 2012.www.uptodate.com

[10] Decaens T, Roudot-Thoraval F, Bresson-Hadni S et al. Impact of pretransplantation transarterial chemoembolization on survival and recurrence after liver transplantation for hepatocellular carci- noma. Liver Transpl 2005; 11: 767–775.

[11] Yao FY, Kinkhabwala M, LaBerge JM et al. The impact of pre- operative loco-regional therapy on outcome after liver transplan- tation for hepatocellular carcinoma. Am J Transplant 2005; 5: 795– 804.

[12] Roayaie S, Frischer JS, Emre SH et al. Long-term results with multimodal adjuvant therapy and liver transplantation for the treat- ment of hepatocellular carcinomas larger than 5 centimeters. Ann Surg 2002; 235: 533–539.

[13] Graziadei IW, Sandmueller H, Waldenberger P et al. Chemoem- bolization followed by liver transplantation for hepatocellular car- cinoma impedes tumor progression while on the waiting list and leads to excellent outcome. Liver Transpl 2003; 9: 557–563.

[14] M.Lesurtel, B.Mu llhaupt, B.C.Pestalozzi. et al. Transarterial Chemoembolization as a Bridge to Liver Transplantation for Hepatocellular Carcinoma: An Evidence-Based Analysis. *American Journal of Transplantation 2006; 6: 2644–2650*

[15] J. Belghiti, B. I. Carr, P. D. Greig. Treatment before Liver Transplantation for HCC. Annals of Surgical Oncology 15(4):993–1000

[16] A. James Hanje and Francis Y. Yao. Current approach to downstaging of hepatocellular carcinoma prior to liver transplantation. Curr Opin Organ Transplant 13:234–240

[17] Cheow PC, Al-Alwan A, Kachura J, et al. Ablation of hepa- toma as a bridge to liver transplantation reduces drop-out from prolonged waiting time. Hepatology 2005; 42:333A.

[18] Shin Hwang ,Sung Gyu Lee and Jacques Belghiti.Liver transplantation for HCC: its role.Eastern and Western perspectives. J Hepatobiliary Pancreat Sci (2010) 17:443–448

[19] Vivarelli M, Cucchetti A, Piscaglia F, La Barba G, Bolondi L, Cavallari A, et al. Analysis of risk factors for tumor recurrence after liver transplantation for hepatocellular carcinoma: key role of immunosuppression. Liver Transpl 2005;11:497-503.

[20] Wang Z, Zhou J, Fan J, Tan CJ, Qiu SJ, Yu Y, et al. Sirolimus inhibits the growth and metastatic progression of hepato- cellular carcinoma. J Cancer Res Clin Oncol 2009;135:715- 722.

[21] Schlitt HJ, Neipp M, Weimann A, et al. Recurrence patterns of hepatocellular and fibrolamellar carcinoma after liver transplantation. J Clin Oncol 1999;17:324–331.

[22] Ko HK, Ko GY, Yoon HK, Sung KB: Tumor response to transcatheter arterial chemoembolization in recurrent hepatocellu- lar carcinoma after living donor liver transplantation. Korean J Radiol 2007;8:320–327.

[23] Michael A. Zimmerman, *et al*. Recurrence of Hepatocellular Carcinoma Following Liver Transplantation. A Review of Preoperative and Postoperative Prognostic Indicators. Arch Surg. 2008;143(2):182-188

[24] Ali Zarrinpar, Fady Kaldas and Ronald W Busuttil. Liver transplantation for hepatocellular carcinoma:an update. Hepatobiliary Pancreat Dis Int ,Vol 10,No 3 .June 15 , 2011

[25] G. C. Sotiropoulos, *et al*. META-ANALYSIS OF TUMOR RECURRENCE AFTER LIVER TRANSPLANTATION FOR HEPATOCELLULAR CARCINOMA BASED ON 1,198 CASES. Eur J Med Res (2007) 12: 527-534

[26] Sasan Roayaie, *et al*. Recurrence of Hepatocellular Carcinoma After Liver Transplant: Patterns and Prognosis. Liver Transplantation, Vol 10, No 4 (April), 2004: pp 534–540

[27] Myron Schwartz, Sasan Roayaie, Josep Llovet.How should patients with hepatocellular carcinoma recurrence after liver transplantation be treated?. J Hepatol. 2005 Oct; 43(4):584-9

[28] Peter J. Kneuertz, *et al*.Multidisciplinary Management of Recurrent Hepatocellular Carcinoma Following Liver Transplantation. J Gastrointest Surg (2012) 16:874–881

[29] Enrico Regalia ,*et al*. Pattern and management of recurrent hepatocellular carcinoma after liver transplantation. J Hep Bil Pancr Surg (1998) 5:29–34

[30] Yamashita H, Nakagawa K, Shiraishi K, et al Radiotherapy for lymph node metastases in patients with hepatocellular carcinoma: retrospective study. J Gastroenterol Hepatol 2007;22:523–527.

[31] Seong J, Koom WS, Park HC: Radiotherapy for painful bone metastases from hepatocellular carcinoma. Liver Int 2005;25:261– 265

Chapter 16

Secondary Liver Tumors

Hesham Abdeldayem, Amr Helmy, Hisham Gad,
Essam Salah, Amr Sadek, Tarek Ibrahim,
Elsayed Soliman, Khaled Abuelella, Maher Osman,
Amr Aziz, Hosam Soliman, Sherif Saleh,
Osama Hegazy, Hany Shoreem, Taha Yasen,
Emad Salem, Mohamed Taha, Hazem Zakaria,
Islam Ayoub and Ahmed Sherif

Additional information is available at the end of the chapter

http://dx.doi.org/10.5772/51766

1. Introduction

The liver is a common site of metastases. The most relevant metastatic tumor of the liver to the surgeon is colorectal cancer because of the well-documented potential for long-term survival after complete resection. However, a large number of other tumors commonly metastasize to the liver, including cancers of the upper gastrointestinal system (stomach, pancreas, biliary), genitourinary system (renal, prostate), neuroendocrine system, breast, eye (melanoma), skin (melanoma), soft tissue (retroperitoneal sarcoma), and gynecologic system (ovarian, endometrial, cervix). [1]

The high frequency of liver metastases is caused by: [2]

1. The liver's vast blood supply, which originates from portal and systemic systems.
2. The fenestrations of the hepatic sinusoidal endothelium may facilitate penetration of malignant cells into the hepatic parenchyma.
3. Humoral factors that promote cell growth and cellular factors, such as adhesion molecules, favor metastatic spread to the liver.
4. The liver's geographic proximity to other intra-abdominal organs may allow malignant infiltration by direct extension.

Not so long ago, oncologists were so pessimistic about the appearance of hepatic metastases that "no treatment" was often the recommendation. Advancing technology and improved surgical techniques now offer potential therapeutic options for patients with such lesions. Patient selection is the most important aspect of surgical therapy for metastatic disease in the liver and clinical follow-up of resected patients has identified those most and least likely to benefit. Therefore, realistic expectations and honest patient education is an important aspect of treatment. [1]

1.1. Clinical presentation

The clinical presentation of patients with liver metastases is variable and subtle. Most patients are asymptomatic; a minority may report abdominal pain, jaundice, or pruritus. Hepatic metastases from gastrointestinal carcinoid tumors are associated with release of vasoactive peptides and serotonin into the systemic circulation. Symptoms of the carcinoid syndrome, specifically flushing, sweats, and diarrhea, frequently occur in this setting. Liver metastases from neuroendocrine tumors can lead to significant symptoms caused by the production of functioning hormones. [1]

Physical examination may reveal hepatomegaly, a friction rub over hepatic metastases, or ascites caused by hepatic venous obstruction or peritoneal carcinomatosis. [2]

1.2. Histopathology

The histologic appearances of metastatic deposits in the liver may resemble those of the primary tumors; however, there can be marked differences. These differences exist because metastatic foci are derived from a select subpopulation of tumor cells. Cells that are capable of successful metastasis are believed to have specific characteristics, such as high motility, resistance to immune-mediated destruction, and a high concentration of matrix receptors or matrix-degrading enzymes.

Because the metastatic cell population may not be representative of the primary tumor, it can be difficult to determine the site of origin based on the histologic appearance of the metastases alone.

The initial light-microscopic findings can be used to categorize the tissue into one of three groups:

1. poorly differentiated carcinoma or adenocarcinoma,
2. well-differentiated adenocarcinoma, and
3. squamous carcinoma.

In most cases, immunohistochemical studies further differentiate these metastases. (Table 1) [3]

http://dx.doi.org/10.5772/51766

Tumor	Antigens
Colonic adenocarcinoma	CEA
Pancreatic carcinoma	CEA, pancreatic carcinoma-associated antigen
Lung carcinoma	CEA, cytokeratin, neuron-specific enolase
Breast carcinoma	CEA, milk-fat globulin, hCG
Thyroid carcinoma	Thyroglobulin
Prostate carcinoma	Prostate-specific acid phosphatase, PSA
Melanoma	S-100, vimentin, neuron-specific enolase
Carcinoid	Chromogranin, neuron-specific enolase
Lymphoma and leukemia	CLA
Sarcoma	
Smooth muscle	Type IV collagen, vimentin, desmin
Skeletal muscle	Myoglobin, vimentin, desmin
Neurogenic	S-100, myelin basic protein
Cartilage	S-100, vimentin
Bone	Vimentin
Germ cell tumors	α-fetoprotien, α1-antitrypsin
Trophoblastic tumors	hCG, α-Fetoprotein

Table 1. Immunohistochemical antigens for the identification of primary tumors.

Abbreviations: CEA, carcinoembryonic antigen; CLA, common leukocyte antigen; hCG, human chorionic gonadotropin; PSA, prostate-specific antigen.

1.3. Biochemical Laboratory Tests

The laboratory tests that are available for liver function assessment are not very sensitive. CEA remains the most sensitive test for metastatic colon cancer, but even this test can be normal in the presence of liver metastases, especially with minimal hepatic disease.

1.4. Imaging Techniques

The choice among the various techniques, and the sequence with which they are used, should be guided primarily by the clinical indication, taking into account the primary type and the different possible treatments, which also depend on the general status of clinical history of the patient. Dedicated liver imaging is not needed in patients diagnosed with disseminated, inoperable disease. [4]

1.4.1. Ultrasonography

1.4.1.1. Transabdominal ultrasonography (US)

US presents several advantages, including low cost, absence of irradiation, wide availability, and portability. Transabdominal ultrasound generally has a lower sensitivity for tumor detection than does CT scan or MR imaging, especially for lesions less than 2 cm in size. US is most commonly used for screening for metastases because of its wide availability. Hepatic metastases may be hypoechoic, hyperechoic, cystic, or of mixed echogenicity on ultrasound. Hyperechoic masses are observed more commonly in vascular tumors, such as renal cell and islet cell tumors. Hypovascular lesions, such as lymphoma, appear as hypoechoic masses. [5]

1.4.1.2. Contrast-enhanced US

Contrast-enhanced US, using intravascular microbubble contrast agents, has shown similar accuracy compared to CT and MR. An advantage of contrast-enhanced US is the potential for characterization of liver lesions based on morphologic evaluation as well as temporal vascular enhancement pattern. During the portal venous phase, benign lesions typically enhance more than the liver, whereas malignant lesions enhance less. [6]

1.4.1.3. Endoscopic ultrasound (EUS)

EUS is a well-established tool for diagnosing and staging various gastrointestinal tumors, especially pancreatic cancer; however, it is not used often for hepatic imaging. A few reports in the literature address the use of EUS in the evaluation of hepatic metastases. EUS can detect lesions that are not seen on conventional CT scanning and allows for tissue sampling using fine-needle aspiration. [4]

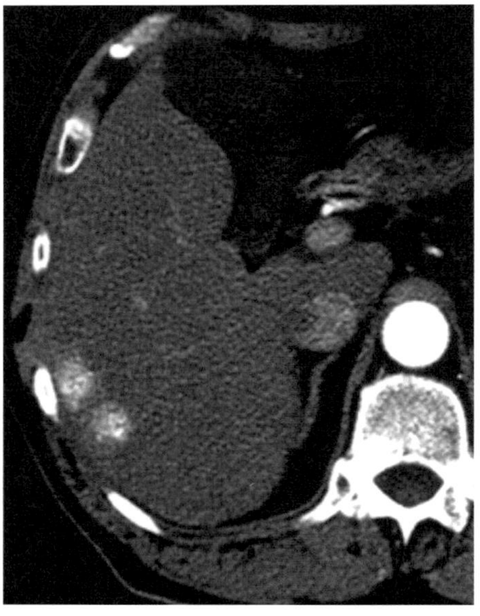

Figure 1. Computed tomography of hypervascular liver metastases from a renal primary tumor at the arterial phase.

1.4.1.4. Intraoperative US (IOUS)

IOUS involves a direct scan of the liver, allowing the use of higher-frequency transducers with higher resolution. IOUS can also be useful at detecting small, deep hepatic metastases not palpable. IOUS is more accurate than conventional CT scanning or MR imaging for delineating liver lesions and is regarded as an important tool in determining resectability and prognosis. [7]

1.4.2. Computed Tomography

1.4.2.1. Noncontrast Computed Tomography

Contrast CT is sometimes not possible because of contrast allergic reactions or renal impairment. Although the sensitivity and specificity of noncontrast CT is far reduced as compared to contrast CT, it may help in identifying hypervascular metastases (especially carcinoid tumors, islet cell tumors, and renal cell carcinomas) or visualizing calcifications or hemorrhage. Noncontrast CT often fails to distinguish hypovascular tumors from the liver parenchyma. Nonenhanced blood vessels may also appear as low-attenuation masses and be confused with metastases. [4]

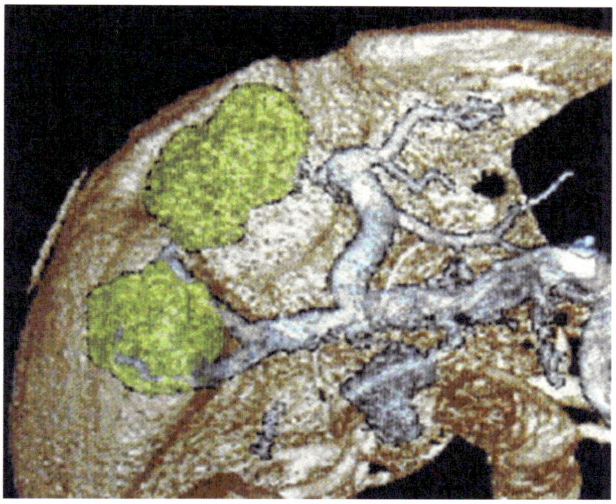

Figure 2. Computed tomography 3-D reconstruction before surgical showing liver metastases (http://c2i2.digithalamus.com/winter2003/Imaging%20update%20in%20metastatic%20liver%20disease.asp).

1.4.2.2. Contrast Computed Tomography

The CT appearance of liver metastases varies according to the pathologic type of the primary tumor. Most lesions are seen best in the portal venous phase, and some lesions are best seen in delayed venous and occasionally arterial phases. Metastases from melanomas, sarcomas, neuroendocrine tumors, and renal cell carcinomas (fig. 1) are hypervascular and there-

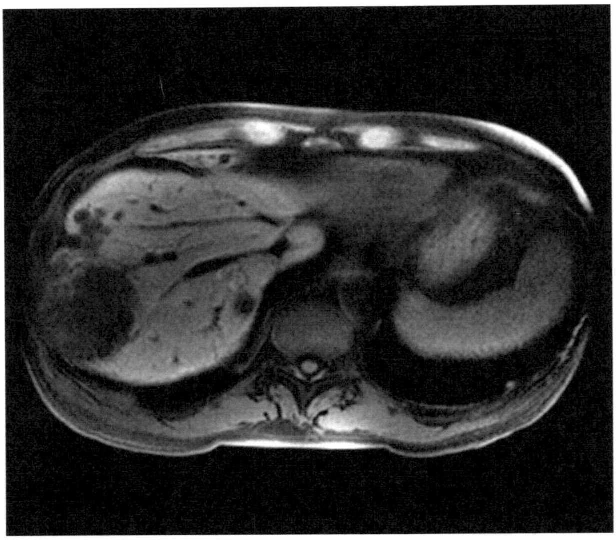

Figure 3. Liver metastases after Mn DPPD or mangafodipir injection.

fore better visualized during the hepatic arterial phase. Metastases from colorectal cancer are hypovascular and therefore better visualized during the portal venous phase. [8]

1.4.3. Magnetic Resonance Imaging (MRI)

T1-weighted images generally show hepatic metastases as low-intensity lesions, whereas T2-weighted images show these lesions to be areas of increased signal intensity. Dynamic, breath-hold MR imaging with a gadolinium-based contrast material is considered to be the most sensitive MR technique for detection of hepatic metastases (fig. 3). Similar to CT, MR angiography can be used as a noninvasive method to evaluate hepatic vasculature. Novel MR contrast agents have the potential for improving detection of liver metastases. [8, 9]

1.4.4. Positron Emission Tomography (PET)

PET, in which a radioactively labeled tracer is administered to the patient and the scanner collects the emitted positron radioactivity to generate an image, allows imaging of cellular processes (such as cellular proliferation (18F-labeled thymidine), hypoxia (18F-labeled Miso), and blood flow ([15O]water) to be visualized. The majority of clinical experience relies on the uptake and use of glucose in human cells. 18F-Fluorodeoxyglucose 18FDG, the most commonly used marker in PET imaging, is an analogue of glucose in which a carbon atom is replaced by a radioactive fluorine isotope. 18FDG is transported into cells, where it accumulates to create an intense signal on PET imaging. Malignant lesions typically have increased 18FDG uptake because of the increased expression of glucose transporter proteins and elevated levels of glycolysis. [10, 11]

http://dx.doi.org/10.5772/51766

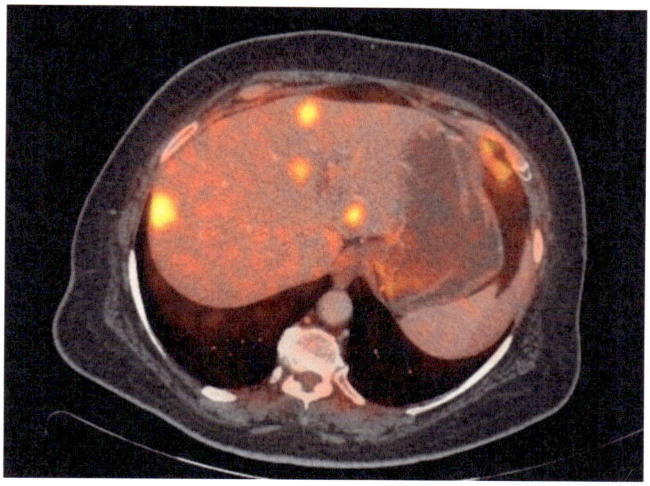

Figure 4. PET/CT Cancer pancreas with liver metastases (http://www.radrounds.com/photo/petct- -2context).

1.4.5. PET/CT (fig. 4)

Despite excellent clinical results with FDG PET, the technique is intrinsically limited by the lack of precise and reliable anatomic information. Foci of increased uptake that are clearly located in the liver parenchyma are readily identified and usually correspond to metastases, but the bowel uptake is highly variable and may be focally increased in regions close to the liver, and therefore be mistaken with peripheral liver lesions. Combined PET/CT scanners allow the precise localization of the abnormal areas of uptake. Modern PET/CT devices are equipped with high-end CT scanners, fully capable of performing full diagnostic CT studies. [11]

2. Colorectal Liver Metastases (CLM)

The liver is the most common site for hematogenous metastasis from colorectal cancers (CRC). A quarter of patients with primary colorectal carcinoma are found to have synchronous hepatic metastasis. Nearly half of patients who undergo resection of the colorectal primary eventually develop metachronous liver metastasis. [2]

CRC principally spreads through two mechanisms:

1. Via portal venous drainage.
2. To regional lymph nodes and then through central lymphatics into the systemic circulation or

2.1. Prognostic Variables and Staging Systems

All patients with colorectal metastases by definition are grouped as stage IV in the TNM staging system, but considerable diversity exists within this group. The prognosis of a patient with a solitary liver metastasis found years after resection of a node-negative right colon cancer is different from the prognosis of a patient with synchronously discovered diffuse bilateral liver metastases at the time of operation for a perforated node- positive colon cancer. A classification system that can discriminate between these patients and provide meaningful prognostic information is essential. This classification system must enable the comparison of patients from diverse publications and facilitate patient selection for adjuvant therapy or clinical trials. [2, 12]

2.1.1. Independent predictors of prognosis include [2]

1. the presence of extrahepatic disease,
2. a positive resection margin,
3. nodal metastases from primary cancer,
4. a short disease-free interval,
5. largest tumor greater than 5 cm,
6. more than one liver metastasis, and
7. CEA greater than 200 ng/mL.

- The first two parameters are data that are determined intraoperatively only because preoperative evidence of extrahepatic disease and inability to obtain negative margins would be relative contraindications to surgery. There is no role for surgical debulking in this setting.
- Using the last five criteria, a preoperative clinical risk score (CRS) system was created with each positive criterion counting as 1 point.
- This CRS is a simple, easily remembered staging system for classifying patients with liver-exclusive metastatic colorectal cancer

2.1.2. Prognostic Scoring System for Hepatic Colorectal Metastases: Clinical risk score (CRS)

- Node-positive primary tumor
- Disease-free interval <12 mo between colon resection and appearance of metastases
- Size of largest lesion >5 cm
- >1 tumor
- CEA >200 ng/dL

Sum of points with 1 point assigned for each positive criterion

- The presence of any one of these characteristics still was associated with a 5-year survival.
- No single criterion can be considered a contraindication to resection.
- The total score out of 5 is highly predictive of outcome.

- A score of 2 or less places a patient in a good prognostic group, for whom resection is ideal.
- For scores of 3 or 4, outcome is less favorable, and patients should be considered for aggressive trials of adjuvant therapy.
- For a score of 5, long-term disease-free survivors rarely are encountered, and resections in this high-risk group should be accompanied by trials of adjuvant therapy.
- This CRS proved useful in selection of patients for neoadjuvant therapy and ablative therapies and in stratification of patients enrolled in clinical trials
- A high CRS has been associated with sufficiently high incidence of occult metastatic disease that fluorodeoxyglucose positron emission tomography (FDG PET) can be justified as a preoperative test
- The yield from laparoscopy in the preoperative staging of patients with hepatic colorectal metastases also has been correlated with the CRS.
- For patients with a high CRS, a laparoscopy can save patients with disseminated disease from having a laparotomy, minimizing morbidity and hospital stay, whereas patients with a low CRS can avoid the added anesthesia and operating room time associated with a negative laparoscopy. [2, 12]

2.1.3. Molecular Determinants of Outcome

There are reports that molecular characteristics that predict response to chemotherapy, such as tumor thymidylate synthase levels or levels of the transcription factor E2F-1, are important in predicting the outcome It is likely that these and other molecular determinants will be incorporated into postoperative prognostic scales in the future. [2]

2.2. Medical Treatment

Over the past 3 decades, the most widely used chemotherapeutic agent in the treatment of metastatic CRC has been 5-fluorouracil (5-FU), used either alone or in combination with other chemotherapies. [13]

Now, the most commonly used regimens are: FOLFOX, FOLFIRI, and FOLFOXIRI.

2.2.1. FOLFOX is a made up of the drugs

- FOL – Folinic acid (leucovorin), a vitamin B derivative used as a "rescue" drug for high doses of the drug methotrexate and that modulates/potentiates/reduces the side effects of fluorouracil;
- F – Fluorouracil (5-FU) fluorouracil (5-FU), a pyrimidine analog and antimetabolite which incorporates into the DNA molecule and stops synthesis; and
- OX – Oxaliplatin (Eloxatin) A platinum-based drug, usually classified as alkylating agents, although it is not actually alkylating groups (functions by a similar mechanism)

This regimen is recommended for 12 cycles, every 2 weeks. The recommended dose schedule given every two weeks is as follows:

- Day 1: Oxaliplatin 85 mg/m^2 IV infusion in 250-500 mL D5W and leucovorin 200 mg/m^2 IV infusion in D5W both given over 120 minutes at the same time in separate bags using a Y-line, followed by 5-FU 400 mg/m^2 IV bolus given over 2-4 minutes, followed by 5-FU 600 mg/m^2 IV infusion in 500 mL D5W (recommended) as a 22-hour continuous infusion.
- Day 2: Leucovorin 200 mg/m^2 IV infusion over 120 minutes, followed by 5-FU 400 mg/m^2 IV bolus given over 2-4 minutes, followed by 5-FU 600 mg/m^2 IV infusion in 500 mL D5W (recommended) as a 22-hour continuous infusion.FOLFOX4 regime.

Premedication with antiemetics, including 5-HT3 blockers with or without dexamethasone, is recommended.

FOLFOX4				
drug	dose	administration	time	term
Oxaliplatin	85 mg/m^2	IV infusion	2 h	day 1
Folinic acid	200 mg/m^2	IV infusion	2 h	day 1 + 2
Fluorouracil	400 mg/m^2	IV bolus	2 min	day 1 + 2
Fluorouracil	600 mg/m^2	IV infusion	22 h	day 1 + 2

Table 2.

2.2.2. FOLFIRI is is made up of the following drugs:

- FOL – folinic acid (leucovorin).
- F – fluorouracil (5-FU); and
- IRI – irinotecan (Camptosar), a topoisomerase inhibitor, which prevents DNA from uncoiling and duplicating.

The dosage consists of: Irinotecan (180 mg/m^2 IV over 90 minutes) concurrently with folinic acid (400 mg/m^2 [or 2 x 250 mg/m^2] IV over 120 minutes).

Followed by fluorouracil (400-500 mg/m^2 IV bolus) then fluorouracil (2400-3000 mg/m^2 intravenous infusion over 46 hours).

This cycle is typically repeated every two weeks. The dosages shown above may vary from cycle to cycle.

FOLFOX and FOLFIRI are widely considered to be equivelent in the metastatic setting and are generally selected according to the toxicity profile. The FOLFOX regimen is characterized by a higher rate of grade 3 and 4 neurotoxicity and neutropenia. The FOLFIRI is associated with more nasuea and vomiting, mucositis, and alopecia.

2.2.3. Folfoxiri

- irinotecan, oxaliplatin, fluorouracil, and folinate

FOLFOXIRI has been shown to have better results than FOLFIRI and FOLFOX in several studies.

2.2.4. Cetuximab (Erbitux) and panitumumab (Vectibix)

Both are monoclonal antibodies against the epidermal growth factor receptor (EGFR) and are now an important part of the treatment algorithm for unresectable colorectal metastases. Cetuximab is a chimeric monoclonal antibody approved for treatment of metastatic CRC in combination with irinotecan in patients with disease refractory to irinotecan or as a single agent in patients who cannot tolerate irinotecan or oxaliplatin. Panitumumab is a fully humanized monoclonal antibody and therefore appears to have a lower rate of serious infusion reactions compared with cetuximab. Like cetuximab, panitumumab is approved for single-agent therapy in patients who have progressed on standard chemotherapy. [2]

2.3. Regional treatment for metastatic colorectal cancer

The rationale for a regional approach to what normally would be thought of as a systemic process is based on the concept that tumor cells from gastrointestinal malignancies, especially colorectal cancer, spread hematogenously via the portal circulation, making the liver the first site of metastasis in most patients. This stepwise spread of cancer from primary site to liver and from there to other organs provides an opportunity to prevent dissemination of tumor to other sites by direct treatment of hepatic metastases. In this way, metastatic colorectal cancer differs from most other metastatic malignancies. In addition, the remarkable ability of the liver to regenerate after hepatic resection has enabled aggressive surgical options for hepatic metastases. There is no doubt that surgery alone can cure a subset of patients. [14]

Liver resection has become the standard treatment for metastatic lesions from colorectal primaries. With many series reporting long-term survival for these patients, even before the era of modern chemotherapy, 5-year, 10-year, and 20-year survivals with hepatic resection can be expected to reach 40%, 25%, and 20%. [2]

2.3.1. Preoperative evaluation

All patients with CLM benefit from evaluation by a multidisciplinary team comprising physicians (surgeons, medical oncologists, radiologists, pathologists), nurses, social workers, and research coordinators. The central tenets in the preoperative evaluation of patients for potential surgical resection of CLM are:

1. establishing the diagnosis,
2. anatomically defining the liver lesion for diagnosis and surgical planning, and
3. staging to rule out extrahepatic disease.
4. evaluation of the patient's fitness for operation;

5. estimation of an individual's tumor biology.

Preoperative biopsy of CLM is rarely indicated or beneficial for assessment of CLM, and has been associated with tumor dissemination and decreased survival. Preoperative biopsy may have usefulness for confirmation of extrahepatic disease when a change in therapy is planned based on the biopsy results. [1]

2.3.1.1. Evaluation of Fitness for Operation

A careful evaluation of a patient's physiologic capability to tolerate hepatic resection is necessary to ensure favorable outcomes after hepatectomy. History, physical examination, and routine laboratory studies (complete blood count, liver function testing, and coagulation studies) are relied on to screen for underlying liver dysfunction.The criteria for patient operability are similar to the criteria considered for any major laparotomy. A history of cardiac and pulmonary disease must be investigated because these patients are at significant risk for perioperative complications. Any previous liver disease that might have impaired hepatic function should be evaluated because this determines the volume of liver than can be resected safely. [2, 14]

2.3.1.2. Anatomic and Functional parameters

Determination of resectability is primarily based on preoperative imaging. High-quality cross-sectional imaging is critical for gauging the extent of disease, response to preoperative therapy, and for operative planning (The role of preoperative imaging was discussed above). [14]

Patients should be routinely reimaged after any course of systemic therapy; preferably within 4 weeks of planned resection. Meticulous preoperative attention to the relationships of CLM to arterioportal inflow, biliary drainage, and hepatic venous outflow is necessary and allows for an informed and efficient hepatectomy. Preoperative imaging may also help to identify the presence of concomitant parenchymal disease (eg, fibrosis/cirrhosis, portal hypertension, steatohepatitis) or extrahepatic disease. [2]

Resectability of CLM has been well defined by the American Hepato-Pancreato-Biliary Association (AHPBA)/Society of Surgery of the Alimentary Tract (SSAT)/Society of Surgical Oncology (SSO) in a 2006 consensus statement as an expected margin-negative (R-0) resection resulting in preservation of at least 2 contiguous hepatic segments with adequate inflow, outflow, and biliary drainage with a functional liver remnant (FLR) volume of more than 20% (for healthy liver). [1, 14]

2.3.1.3. Tumor biology

Careful evaluation of all patients in a multidisciplinary setting allows for better identification of those patients most likely to benefit from surgical resection as opposed to those who would benefit more from nonoperative therapies, given their particularly aggressive disease. Consideration of this question is far from an exact science, but valuable information can be gleaned from factors such as [1]

1. the stage of primary disease,

http://dx.doi.org/10.5772/51766

2. number and distribution of CLM,
3. tumor histology,
4. response to chemotherapy,
5. rate of growth of CLM on serial imaging,
6. rate of increase in serum carcinoembryonic antigen (CEA).

2.3.1.4. Diagnostic laparoscopy

Diagnostic laparoscopy has a role in staging those patients in whom preoperative imaging or high-risk scores suggest a high likelihood for finding intra-abdominal extrahepatic disease or for patients with indeterminate intrahepatic lesions that may be best characterized by IOUS. Laparoscopy is useful at identifying peritoneal disease or the involvement of periportal lymph nodes not apparent on preoperative imaging. When laparoscopy is employed, laparotomy can be avoided in patients with unresectable disease. [1, 2]

2.3.2. Operative technique

The goal should be a safe R-0 hepatectomy allowing for preservation of adequate FLR volume to avoid hepatic insufficiency. Given the significant decrease in survival between R-0 and R-1/2 resections, the ability to achieve R-0 resection, is paramount. The optimal width of resection margin is unclear, with no clear minimum margin established. A predicted margin width of less than 1 cm should not be used as an exclusion to resection. The extent of resection depends on the number and location of metastases relative to the portal triads and hepatic veins. Anatomic resections, which are facilitated by intraoperative ultrasound, are preferred to wedge resections. Anatomic resections permit excision of parenchymal areas distal to the tumor, where vascular micrometastases tend to occur, and, most importantly they are less likely to have positive margins. [14, 15]

The principles of hepatic resection are no different for colorectal metastases than for any other hepatic surgery. Technical details of liver mobilization and various anatomic hepatectomies have been well described elsewhere in this book. Most procedures can be divided into distinct stages: [1, 2, 14, 15]

1. exploration,
2. liver mobilization,
3. intraoperative ultrasonography,
4. inflow control,
5. outflow control,
6. parenchymal transection, and

7. hemo- and biliostasis.

The abdomen must be explored thoroughly for evidence of extrahepatic metastases. In particular, the celiac axis and portocaval and hilar lymph nodes must be palpated, and any suspicious nodes should be removed and examined by frozen section.

Most surgeons routinely use intraoperative ultrasound after mobilization of the liver. IOUS can delineate better the interior anatomy of the liver, including intrahepatic vessels, and hepatic resection can be performed more safely and in a more anatomically oriented fashion. In addition to the initial planning, the operation can be monitored by the repeated use of IOUS because the resection line is displayed in relation to the lesion and blood vessels. [14, 15]

2.3.3. Follow-up

Patients after hepatic resection usually are monitored in an attempt to identify early recurrence that may be amenable to further resection. Currently, most patients undergo serial physical examination, serum CEA level, annual chest x-ray, and CT of the abdomen and pelvis every 3 to 4 months for the first 2 years and then every 6 months for the next 5 years. [16]

2.3.3.1. Adjuvant Chemotherapy

1- Adjuvant Systemic Chemotherapy

Although the use of oxaliplatin-based or irinotecan-based chemotherapies in this setting is common, there are no clear data from comparative studies supporting such practice. [17]

2- Adjuvant Hepatic Arterial Infusion Chemotherapy

Regional chemotherapy, via the hepatic artery, is a theoretically attractive mode of adjuvant therapy, because the liver is the most common site for tumor recurrence after liver resection and is the sole site of recurrence in 40% of patients.

The rationale for HAI of chemotherapy is based on the concept that most metastatic liver tumors preferentially derive their blood supply from the hepatic artery, whereas normal hepatic tissue relies on the portal venous blood supply.

The ability of the hepatic parenchyma to extract and metabolize chemotherapy drugs to nontoxic metabolites offers a unique opportunity to administer highly toxic drug levels to tumor cells, while minimizing systemic toxicity. The most extensively studied agent is 5-fluorouracil-2-deoxyuridine (FUDR), an analogue of 5-FU that can be concentrated 100-fold to 400-fold in the liver because of a 95% hepatic extraction ratio. [17, 18, 19, 20]

2.4. Controversial issues

2.4.1. Downstaging of unresectable tumor and neoadjuvant chemotherapy.

Potential benefits of prehepatectomy chemotherapy include [2, 20]

1. the potential to render formerly unresectable patients resectable i.e. the possibility for downstaging liver metastases,
2. in vivo testing of chemotherapeutic efficacy,
3. identification of occult intra- or extrahepatic metastases, and
4. early exposure of subclinical microscopic metastases to systemic therapy.
5. with prudent monitoring and attention to comorbidities, allows for improved patient selection

Patients with tumor progression during preoperative chemotherapy have a significantly worse outcome CLM. Potential downsides of preoperative chemotherapy are largely related to hepatic toxicities that may be clinically relevant. Oxaliplatin has been linked to steatohepatitis and sinusoidal obstruction; irinotecan has been associated with steatohepatitis and periportal inflammation. A preoperatively treated liver is more fibrotic, often with perivascular adhesions. The planes of resection are difficult to dissect, making the procedure more challenging overall. Despite the operative complexity, the perioperative morbidity and mortality in the trials of resection after neoadjuvant chemotherapy do not seem to be higher than series of de novo hepatic resection. [1, 2]

One controversial issue is the treatment of a patient with a *complete clinical response* to neoadjuvant chemotherapy. When there is no visible tumor left to resect, should a blind resection, based on the site of previous metastasis, be undertaken? Suggested practice is to use intraoperative ultrasound to attempt to identify the lesion, and if this is not possible a hepatic resection of the area previously involved with tumor is performed. This is not, however, a universally accepted practice. [1, 2, 20]

Patients who present with liver lesions that are potentially resectable for cure should be offered a surgical resection because there are no definite data supporting a neoadjuvant chemotherapeutic approach.

2.4.2. Repeated resection for recurrent tumor

In the absence of extrahepatic disease and in a patient with a good performance status and adequate hepatic reserve, a repeat hepatectomy may be considered. Approximately one third of recurrence is amenable to further resection The presence of adhesions and the altered anatomy of the liver, particularly the position of the vasculature and biliary system, make this technically challenging.

There is a higher likelihood of further recurrence, however, and the study of adjuvant therapy should be encouraged in these patients. [21]

2.4.3. Synchronous Metastases

Synchronous CLM are noted in 20% to 30% of patients at the time of initial colorectal cancer diagnosis. Surgical management of this group of early metastases has been debated in terms of disease biology, operative approach (staged vs. simultaneous colorectal and liver resection), the order of resection, and timing of chemotherapy. [2, 22]

Some suggests that synchronous diagnosis of metastases portends a worse prognosis, perhaps as a result of a failure to detect micrometastatic foci in the liver. Delaying hepatic resection may increase survival in the surgically resected group by selecting out the patients with aggressive tumor biology who would be unlikely to derive a survival benefit from resection. Although delayed resection does not seem to impair survival, it does increase the volume of resected liver, a factor that is predictive of postoperative complications. [22]

Potential benefits of simultaneous CLM resection include [2]

1. avoidance of morbidity of a second laparotomy and anesthesia, and
2. decreased time to initiation of chemotherapy.

Risks of simultaneous resection are related to the magnitude and complexity of the combined operation.

A selective approach to synchronous CLM should be based on careful consideration of the technical complexity and risks for the colorectal and liver resections, as well as judicious intraoperative decision making. Good judgment is required in selection of patients for a simultaneous or a staged resection in close coordination with medical oncologists and collaborating surgeons. [1]

2.4.4. Bilobar Metastases

Bilobar metastases are no longer an absolute contraindication to resection. Possible options include:

1. Extended hepatectomy,
2. 2-stage hepatectomy,
3. Combined hepatic resection and ablation.
4. For patients with insufficient FLR, portal vein embolization (PVE) may be a useful adjunct to increase the size of the FLR and allow for safe extended hepatectomy.

Two-stage hepatectomy for patients with bilobar metastases involves an initial hepatectomy with contralateral portal vein ligation or postoperative PVE, followed by chemotherapy. After restaging, a second hepatectomy is performed based on response to PVE/chemotherapy and ability to achieve resection with an adequate FLR. A proportion of patients will not be eligible for second hepatectomy because of disease progression, inadequate FLR, or perioperative or chemotherapy-associated complications. [23, 24]

http://dx.doi.org/10.5772/51766

2.4.5. Extrahepatic Colorectal Metastases

In the past, extrahepatic disease has been labeled an absolute contraindication to resection of CLM. However, with the advent of more effective systemic therapies, a growing body of literature supports R-0 resection of CLM and extrahepatic metastases. [25]

- An assessment of tumor biology is critical to selecting patients for resection of CLM as well as extrahepatic metastases. For patients found to have extrahepatic metastases preoperatively, a short course of preoperative chemotherapy followed by reimaging is prudent to better define the disease biology.
- Intraoperative decision for previously unrecognized intra-abdominal extrahepatic metastases is difficult. The following should be considered:

1. the complexity and extent of the R-0 hepatic resection,
2. the complexity of resection of the R-0 extrahepatic metastases,
3. the physiologic age of the patient,
4. availability of postoperative chemotherapeutic options, and
5. the patient's risk of rapid progression with the additional finding of extrahepatic metastases.

3. Neuroendocrine Liver Metastases (NLMs)

The liver is the most common site of metastatic disease for neuroendocrine tumors. Nonoperative therapies for advanced neuroendocrine malignancies are associated with minimal response rates, short durations of disease stability, and no clear survival benefit. [26]

3.1. Pathology and Classification

Most NLMs are of gastrointestinal or pancreatic origin, or so-called gastroenteropancreatic (GEP) tumors GEP neuroendocrine tumors historically are divided into two broad types: carcinoid and noncarcinoid. Either type may or may not be associated with hormone production causing a clinical endocrinopathy (functional or nonfunctional). [26, 27]

Traditionally, gastrointestinal carcinoids have been classified by their site of origin—foregut (lung, thymus, stomach, duodenum, pancreas, bile duct, gallbladder, and liver), midgut (small intestine, appendix, and proximal colon), and hindgut (distal colon and rectum)—because of the various biologic and biochemical features shown within these groups. Pancreatic neuroendocrine tumors have been classified by whether they are functional or not. [26, 28]

Regardless of origin, neuroendocrine tumors are similar histopathologically. Many histologic and morphologic features may be shared by benign and malignant tumors. Histologically, neuroendocrine tumors typically are well differentiated, and atypia and mitoses are rare.

Neuroendocrine tumors stain positive for chromogranin A, neuron-specific enolase, and synaptophysin, which confirms neuroendocrine cell origin. Neuroendocrine tumors also stain positively for one or more endocrine hormones immunohistochemically. [27]

Morphologically, neuroendocrine tumors can be solitary or multiple and solid or cystic. Tumor size alone is not a reliable indicator of malignancy. Neuroendocrine tumors greater than 2 cm throughout the GEP tract have a greater probability of malignant behavior, however, than tumors less than 2 cm. Gross or microscopic vascular invasion may occur for any GEP neuroendocrine tumors, although major vascular invasion is most typical of pancreatic NECs. Only the confirmed presence of metastases confers an unequivocal diagnosis of malignancy. [28]

Regardless of whether NECs are classified as carcinoid or noncarcinoid, the natural history of patients with unresected or unresectable hepatic metastases generally has been similar. Overall, patients with unresected hepatic metastases from NEC have an approximately 30% 5-year survival The presence of liver metastases alone is the most significant factor adversely affecting outcome Five-year survival with and without liver metastases from NECs is approximately 30% to 40% and 90% to 100%. [26]

3.2. Treatment of NLMs

3.2.1. Liver resection

The treatment of hepatic metastases from NECs is aimed at reduction of the mass of malignant tissue (cytoreduction) chiefly for two reasons. [29]

First, metastatic gastrointestinal neuroendocrine tumors are usually indolent and slow growing because most are low-grade malignancies (WHO classification). Chemotherapeutic and radiotherapeutic regimens targeted at rapidly dividing cells are relatively ineffective, targeting only a paucity of the total population of malignant cells.

Second, symptoms secondary to expression and secretion of biologically active peptides by these tumors are directly related to overall mass of tumor, although production of peptides may be heterogeneous among individual metastases. Similarly, pain and debilitating decrease in performance status may have a negative impact on quality of life for nonfunctional NECs metastatic to the liver. Cytoreduction of the tumor is the most direct and immediately effective method to provide symptomatic relief.

These reasons, coupled with improved safety for hepatic resection, have prompted hepatic resection as a primary therapeutic option for patients with functional and nonfunctional metastatic GEP NECs. Currently, hepatic resection of NLMs is recommended if the primary tumor and regional disease are resectable or resected, and greater than 90% of hepatic metastases are resectable or ablatable.

The concept of hepatic resection for NLMs has grown because of several clinical observations: [30]

1. the protracted natural history of NECs compared with other gastrointestinal tract cancers,

http://dx.doi.org/10.5772/51766

2. the often prolonged duration of intrahepatic disease before evidence of extrahepatic progression,
3. the clinical impression that the severity of clinical endocrinopathies correlates with the intrahepatic volume of metastatic disease,
4. the frequent resectability of the primary and regional neuroendocrine tumors despite metastatic disease, and
5. the rarity of underlying concomitant hepatic disease (fibrosis or cirrhosis).

3.2.1.1. Debulking strategy

When complete resection of gross liver disease is not feasible or in the presence of unresectable extrahepatic disease, resection as a tumor debulking strategy should be considered in patients with extreme hormonal symptoms refractory to other treatments or with tumors in locations that would affect short-term quality of life, such as large lesions abutting the hepatic hilum (resulting in biliary obstruction) or the colon/duodenum (resulting in gastrointestinal obstruction). [31, 32]

3.2.1.2. Subsequent plan for treatment of recurrence. [26, 33]

1. For solitary recurrences, either resection or ablation is appropriate. Percutaneous ablative approaches often are preferable.
2. Repeat hepatic resection is advised for lesions in sites that preclude safe radiofrequency ablation (RFA) (i.e., surface metastases adjacent to bowel, near bile ducts, or near diaphragm).
3. Sequential ablation or resection is undertaken as recurrence is recognized until precluded by extent of recurrence within the liver.
4. Extensive recurrent intrahepatic metastases are treated by embolization or chemoembolization with or without systemic chemotherapy in the absence of extrahepatic disease and chemotherapy in the presence of extrahepatic disease.

3.2.2. Liver transplantation

Liver transplantation (OLT) has been employed increasingly to treat metastatic NEC. OLT may be indicated if the primary and regional NEC has been resected, and distal metastases have been excluded. While transplantation has the benefits of removing all hepatic disease burden, rapid disease recurrence is near universal. Long-term actuarial survival among patients transplanted for NLM is poor compared with overall patient and graft survival rates for all indications. At present, liver transplantation cannot be considered a viable option for unresectable NLM. OLT should be considered as an investigative treatment alternative in specialty centers. [34]

3.2.3. Radiofrequency Ablation

Radiofrequency ablation (RFA) can provide local control and short-term symptomatic relief from NLM when resection is not possible. Successful ablation typically occur in the treatment of small metastases (<5 cm). [35-38]

3.2.4. Ethanol Ablation

Percutaneous ethanol injection permits ablation of metastases located adjacent to structures at risk of damage by RFA. It can be performed on metastases located adjacent to vital structures (e.g., the hepatic flexure of the colon); adjacent to large vessels vulnerable to the heat-sink effect; and adjacent to central bile ducts, where subsequent biliary stricture may occur. [61]

3.2.4.1. Guidelines for Ablation

General guidelines in the ablation of liver metastases are analogous to the treatment of hepatocellular carcinoma and colorectal metastases. [35-38]

There are three clinical scenarios for ablation of neuroendocrine hepatic metastases:

1. adjunct to concurrent surgical resection of hepatic metastases,
2. treatment of limited hepatic metastases in patients unfit for operation, and
3. primary therapy when clinical expertise or intraoperative circumstances preclude safe resection.

3.2.5. Hepatic arterial therapy

Because neuroendocrine tumors usually are highly vascular lesions that predominantly derive blood supply from the hepatic artery (as opposed to the normal hepatic parenchyma that derive the majority of blood supply from the portal vein), opportunities exist for selected ischemia of NLM and/or delivery of directed chemotherapy via hepatic artery therapy. Hepatic arterial embolization with cyanoacrylate, gel foam particles, polyvinyl alcohol, and microspheres have all been used to achieve distal embolization without surgical ligation of the hepatic artery. Chemoembolization provides an intratumoral concentration of chemotherapy that is 10 to 20 times higher than systemic administration.

Complete response and long-term survival are not common after hepatic arterial therapy, as the periphery of the tumor is spared from ischemia or chemotherapy. Thus, embolization of lesions close to the hepatic hilum is generally unsuccessful, as the periphery of the tumor will still cause mass-effect associated symptoms. [39, 40]

The morbidity of embolization approaches include liver abscess, transient liver failure, pleural effusion, and postembolization syndrome, the latter consisting of fever, abdominal pain, leukocytosis, and a transient increase in liver enzymes and/or bilirubin. Multiple sessions of therapy are often needed with varying intervals between sessions. Contraindications to hepatic arterial therapy include hepatic failure, portal vein occlusion, uncorrectable coagulopathy, and renal failure. [40]

http://dx.doi.org/10.5772/51766

3.2.6. Medical treatment

A- Somatostatin Analogues

Short-acting somatostatin analogue therapy is used to prevent or to treat the carcinoid crisis periprocedurally for any intervention, including resection, transplantation, ablation, or embolization. Somatostatin analogue treatment generally is well tolerated. Steatorrhea, diarrhea, abdominal discomfort, and biliary sludge or gallstones can develop, but rarely preclude continued use. [41]

B- Chemotherapy

Systemic chemotherapy generally is reserved for patients with advanced or progressive disease in whom other treatment efforts have failed Streptozocin-based combinations with 5-FU and doxorubicin have resulted in objective responses. Carcinoid tumors may be less sensitive to cytotoxic agents because of the preponderance of low-grade malignant (well-differentiated) histology and low proliferation index. [24]

C- Interferon Alfa

Systemic interferon alfa may be used to treat advanced NEC. The mechanism of interferon alfa is mediated through direct inhibitors of the cell cycle (G1/S phase) and of protein and hormone production, through antiangiogenesis, and indirectly through increased immune stimulation. Adverse reactions to interferon alfa are common. Chronic fatigue and hematologic cytopenias are the most common side effects. [42]

3.3. Primary hepatic neuroendocrine tumors

NECs may arise primarily within the liver. The diagnosis presumes a thorough search and exclusion of an extrahepatic NEC. The cell of origin is unknown. Pancreatic heterotopia has been postulated as a source of these tumors. Some tumors may arise from intrahepatic biliary tract radicles because carcinoids of the extrahepatic biliary tract are more common. Primary hepatic neuroendocrine tumors may be metastases from an occult primary NEC or a primary NEC that had spontaneously regressed. [24]

4. Non-colorectal Non-neuroendocrine Liver Metastases (NCNNLM)

Except for gastrointestinal primaries, the liver is not the primary filter for venous blood. In other words, liver metastases from nongastrointestinal cancers indicate systemic tumor spread; this makes selection of patients a crucial factor to offer hepatic resection to patients who may benefit the most.

Tumor biologies among NCNNLM vary widely, and their treatment requires dedicated multidisciplinary teams with expertise in diverse areas including hepatic surgery, surgical oncology, medical oncology, radiation oncology, diagnostic imaging, and interventional radiology. Patient care must be individualized, especially in the absence of data to clearly guide therapy. [43]

4.1. Treatment options

4.1.1. Resectional treatment

The potential utility of surgery in NCNNLM relates to several factors:

1. advances in chemotherapy have led to effective control of extra hepatic disease for certain tumor types, supporting a rationale for surgical resection of LM in the presence of presumed or de facto systemic disease;
2. improvements in patient preparation for surgery, surgical technique and perioperative care have reduced the perioperative risk of hepatic resection, tipping the risk–benefit ratio in favor of surgical resection in selected cases;
3. the increased emphasis on multimodality treatment approaches has improved patient selection and strengthened the role of hepatic resection as a key component of integrated multidisciplinary care in selected patients with NCNNLM.

Although it might appear that patients with isolated liver metastases can benefit from hepatic resection, the proper selection of patients that may potentially benefit from treatment remains the most critical issue. Patient selection criteria depend on the primary tumor type. After selection based on patient performance status and evaluation of comorbidities, staging studies are required not only to assess the overall disease status of the patient but also to characterize liver lesions and their precise location relative to intrahepatic vascular structures. Assessment of the liver volume that will remain after resection is an equally important component of surgical planning for extensive hepatectomy. [43, 45]

Patient selection and oncologic outcome of metastasectomy depends fundamentally on complete resection of all disease. Preoperative studies are essential in defining both the extent and the limits of surgical resection. Hepatic volumetry to assess the planned future liver remnant (FLR) volume is a critical tool for the selection of patients who will undergo major hepatic resection If the future liver remnant is of inadequate volume, preoperative portal vein embolization can be used to induce hypertrophy of the future liver remnant to allow safe resection. Liver tumors are deemed resectable if preoperative evaluation shows that complete resection of the tumor-bearing liver leaves an adequate remnant volume with adequate vascular inflow, outflow, and biliary drainage. The treatment of each individual tumor type requires expertise in staging, systemic therapy, and hepatic surgery. [43, 45]

4.1.2. Nonresectional treatment

Percutaneous and intraoperative ablative techniques may play a role in the treatment of many types of liver tumors because the therapy

1. can be performed percutaneously or with minimally invasive approaches,

2. is associated with low morbidity and mortality, and

3. can help preserve liver parenchyma in selected patients.

The role of nonresectional ablative approaches for NCNNLM is not well defined. Data and experience are still accruing, and for now such treatment should be considered only in those centers that can provide the full spectrum of therapies for liver metastases. [43]

4.1.3. Hepatic arterial therapies

The utility of hepatic arterial therapies in the treatment of NCNNLM is not well understood. TACE, TAE, and hepatic artery infusion are not considered standard therapy for NCNNLM. For certain tumor subtypes, including unresectable soft tissue sarcomas (STS) and gastrointestinal stromal tumors (GIST), these approaches hold promise. [43, 45]

4.2. Specific tumor types

4.2.1. Gastrointestinal tumors

Overall reported survival rates for patients with NCNNLM from gastrointestinal tumors (esophageal, stomach, duodenum, pancreas, and small bowel) are worse than for those with nongastrointestinal LM.

4.2.1.1. Esophagus and stomach

Currently, there are no accepted indications for resection of esophageal cancer LM, either for palliation or cure. The justification for resection of gastric cancer liver metastases remains controversial. A few published series from Japan and Korea, where the incidence of gastric cancer is high, specifically address gastric cancer LM. Currently, hepatic resection for gastric adenocarcinoma cannot be recommended as standard of care. Data supporting hepatic resection in highly selected patients need confirmation by additional clinical studies. [43]

4.2.1.2. Small bowel

Metastases from small bowel adenocarcinoma are most often widespread and associated with a dismal outcome regardless of treatment. There currently are no data to support resection of small bowel LM except in highly selected cases. [43]

4.2.1.3. Anus

Liver metastases from anal adenocarcinoma are very uncommon, and a meaningful discussion of the indications for resection is difficult. [43]

4.2.2. Bile ducts and pancreas

4.2.2.1. Gallbladder, hilar bile ducts, and ampulla

There currently are no generally accepted indications for hepatic resection in patients with gallbladder cancer, cholangiocarcinoma, or ampullary carcinoma. Judicious recommendations should be made on a case-by-case basis. [43, 45]

4.2.2.2. Pancreas

Even for pancreatic carcinoma patients without LM, the overall survival is poor. LM from pancreatic adenocarcinoma occurs nearly always in the setting of disseminated systemic disease.. In the majority of cases, benefit cannot be expected from hepatic resection for this disease. [43, 45]

4.2.3. Breast

Although it has not been formally proven that liver resection prolongs survival for selected patients with liver metastases of breast cancer, recent studies suggest that with careful patient selection, resection of breast LM can produce long-term survival. Some authors also suggest that patients first should undergo systemic chemotherapy, and that only patients who do not progress should undergo liver resection. [45]

4.2.4. Genitourinary

4.2.4.1. Kidney

In patients with hepatic metastases of renal tumors in whom a complete resection seems possible, surgical exploration may be justified. The number of studies evaluating renal tumors including Wilms' tumors, renal cell adenocarcinomas, and nephroblastomas are few, and the cohorts of patients are small. [43, 45]

4.2.4.2. Testicle

Effective chemotherapeutic regimens are available for most reproductive tumors. Treatment with chemotherapy can lead to complete responses. Surgical resection is considered a necessary salvage treatment in the absence of complete radiographic response to systemic therapy, because residual teratomas have been known to degenerate into invasive carcinoma. [43]

"Salvage" hepatic resection may be considered because

1. resection is the only way to confirm a complete response in the residual liver masses,

2. teratomas may progress to malignant transformation in 30% of cases,

3. mortality and morbidity from hepatic resection is low, and

4. if feasible, concomitant resection of liver metastases and residual retroperitoneal disease is associated with favorable outcome.

http://dx.doi.org/10.5772/51766

Because of the small number of published cases, however, no general conclusions can be drawn.

4.2.4.3. *Uterus and ovary*

The concept of hepatic resection for LM from ovarian cancer has evolved from the fact that cytoreductive surgery can significantly alter the natural history of ovarian cancer metastatic to the peritoneum. Resection of ovarian LM may be considered in carefully selected patients that are candidates for complete cytoreduction after evaluation by a multidisciplinary team. [43]

4.2.5. *Melanoma*

Most patients with liver metastases of melanoma have unresectable disease owing to extrahepatic disease or disseminated hepatic metastases. Isolated liver metastasis from cutaneous melanoma is uncommon. Uveal melanoma is a distinct entity that seems to have a different tumor biology, and it commonly spreads to the liver.. Hepatic resection has been performed in both populations, although outcomes differ based on the primary site of origin. Hepatic resection for uveal or cutaneous melanoma should only be considered in a multidisciplinary setting and by experienced hepatic surgeons. [43, 45]

4.2.6. *Adrenal*

Hepatic resection can provide acceptable results in selected patients with limited adrenal metastases, particularly for palliation of symptoms in patients with secreting hepatic tumors. For patients with symptomatic disease who are not candidates for surgery, ablative therapy such as RFA may be an effective alternative therapy for symptom control. [43]

4.2.7. *Soft tissue sarcoma and gastrointestinal stromal tumor*

Hepatic resection for STS metastases is indicated for disease confined to the liver. Patients with retroperitoneal and intra-abdominal visceral STS and those with leiomyosarcomas are more likely to have liver-only metastatic disease than are patients with extra-abdominal STS.

The treatment strategy for patients with liver metastases from gastrointestinal stromal tumors has changed since the development of the targeted agent imatinib mesylate, which achieves dramatic tumor response rates. Imatinib is now the first-line treatment. Therapy with imatinib has revolutionized the treatment of patients with GIST and has been used alone and in conjunction with hepatic resection for GIST LM. "Complete" radiographic response assessed by CT or PET, including cystic changes after imatinib treatment of GIST, are not necessarily equivalent to complete pathologic response. Because hepatic lesions contain viable tumor in >85% of cases after chemotherapy and biologic therapy, the goal of surgical treatment is complete removal of all residual disease including small residual cystic lesions and "scars." [43, 45]

4.2.8. Squamous cell carcinoma

Because the dataset is so heterogeneous, standard recommendations cannot be made, except that careful patient selection for hepatic resection is mandatory. [43]

4.2.9. Lung cancer

Resection of liver metastases of lung cancer has been reported, and in selected patients long-term survival has been achieved. [43]

4.2.10. Unknown primary cancer

Patients presenting with liver metastases from an unknown primary tumor are a challenge to manage because median overall survival is approximately 5 months. The treatment plan for these patients should be individualized and discussed in a multidisciplinary team. [43, 45]

Author details

Hesham Abdeldayem*, Amr Helmy, Hisham Gad, Essam Salah, Amr Sadek, Tarek Ibrahim, Elsayed Soliman, Khaled Abuelella, Maher Osman, Amr Aziz, Hosam Soliman, Sherif Saleh, Osama Hegazy, Hany Shoreem, Taha Yasen, Emad Salem, Mohamed Taha, Hazem Zakaria, Islam Ayoub and Ahmed Sherif

*Address all correspondence to: habdeldayem64@hotmail.com

Department of Surgery, National Liver Institute, Egypt

References

[1] Kemeny, N., & Kemeny, M. L. (2008). Dawson Liver Metastases. *From: Abeloff: Abeloff's Clinical Oncology, 4th ed. / Chapter 59Liver Abeloff: Abeloff's Clinical Oncology, 4th ed.*, Copyright © 2008 Churchill Livingstone, An Imprint of Elsevier.

[2] Winter, J., & Auer, R. A. C. (2012). Metastatic malignant liver tumors Colorectal cancer Chapter 81A. *From: Jarnagin & Blumgart: Blumgart's Surgery of the Liver, Pancreas and Biliary Tract, 5th ed. / Chapter 81A- Metastatic malignant liver tumors*, Copyright © 2012 Saunders, An Imprint of Elsevier.

[3] Haskell, C. M., Cochran, A. J., Barsky, S. H., & Steckel, R. J. (2008). Metastasis of unknown origin. *Curr Probl Cancer*, 12, 5-58.

[4] Faingold, R., Albuquerque, P. A. B., & Carpineta, L. (2011). *Hepatobiliary Tumors Radiol Clin N Am*, 49-679, doi:10.1016/j.rcl.2011.05.002.

[5] Bipat, S., Leeuwen, M. V., Comans, E., et al. (2005). Colorectal liver metastases: CT, MR imaging, and PET for diagnosis-meta-analysis. *Radiology*, 237, 123-131.

[6] Krix, M., & Kiesslink, F. (2004). Low mechanical index contrast-enhanced ultrasound better reflects high arterial perfusion of liver metastases than arterial phase computed tomography. *Invest Radiol*, 39, 216-222.

[7] Rydzewski, B., Dehdashti, F., Gordon, B. A., et al. (2002). Usefulness of intraoperative sonography for revealing hepatic metastases from colorectal cancer in patients selected for surgery after undergoing FDG PET. *Am J Roentgenol*, 178, 353-358.

[8] Voroney, J. J., Brock, K. K., Eccles, C., et al. (2006). Prospective comparison of CT and MRI for liver cancer delineation using deformable image registration. *Int J Radiat Oncol Biol Phys*, 66, 780-791.

[9] Das, C. J., Dhingra, S., Gupta, A. K., et al. (2009). Imaging of paediatric liver tumors with pathological correlation. Clin Radiol the, 64, 1015-25.

[10] Takahashi, S., Kuroki, Y., Nasu, K., et al. (2006). Positron emission tomography with F-18 fluorodeoxyglucose in evaluating hepatic metastases down staged by chemotherapy. *Anticancer Res*, 26, 4705-4711.

[11] Hustinx, R., Witvrouw, N., & Tancredi, T. (2008). *Liver Metastases PET Clinics- 32-CopyrightSaunders*, An Imprint of Elsevier.

[12] Nordlinger, B., Guiguet, M., Vaillant, J. C., et al. (1996). Surgical resection of colorectal carcinoma metastases to the liver. A prognostic scoring system to improve case selection, based on 1568 patients. *Association Fran?aise de Chirurgie. Cancer*, 77, 1254-1262.

[13] Adam, R., Aloia, T., Figueras, J., et al. (2006). Liver Met Survey: analysis of clinicopathologic factors associated with the efficacy of preoperative chemotherapy in 2,122 patients with colorectal liver metastases. *In 2006 ASCO Annual Meeting. Atlanta, Georgia*, USA, Am Soc Clin Oncol.

[14] Hao, C. Y., & Ji, J. F. (2006). Surgical treatment of liver metastases of colorectal cancer: strategies and controversies in 2006. *Eur J Surg Oncol*, 32, 473-483.

[15] Abdalla, E. K., Vauthey, J. N., Ellis, L. M., et al. (2004). Recurrence and outcomes following hepatic resection, radiofrequency ablation, and combined resection/ablation for colorectal liver metastases. *Ann Surg*, 239, 818-827.

[16] Pozzo, C., Basso, M., Quirino, M., et al. (2006). Long-term followup of colorectal cancer (CRC) patients treated with neoadjuvant chemotherapy with irinotecan and fluorouracil plus folinic acid (5FU/FA) for unresectable liver metastases. *In: 2006 ASCO Annual Meeting. Atlanta, Georgia*, USA, American Society of Clinical Oncology, 3576.

[17] Huitzil-Melendez, F., Capanu, M., Haviland, D., & Kemeny, N. E. (2007). Evaluation of the impact of systemic (SYS) neoadjuvant chemotherapy (neoadj) in patients (pts) with resectable liver metastasis (mets) from colorectal carcinoma (CRC) treated with

adjuvant hepatic arterial infusion (HAI) and SYS chemotherapy. *In: 2007 Gastrointestinal Cancers Symposium. Orlando, Florida*, USA, American Society of Clinical Oncology, 14503.

[18] Mentha, G., Majno, P. E., Andres, A., et al. (2006). Neoadjuvant chemotherapy and resection of advanced synchronous liver metastases before treatment of the colorectal primary. *Br J Surg*, 93, 872-878.

[19] Kemeny, N. E., Jarnagin, W., Gonen, M., et al. (2005). Phase I trial of hepatic arterial infusion (HAI) with floxuridine (FUDR) and dexamethasone (DEX) in combination with systemic oxaliplatin (OXAL), fluorouracil (FU) + leucovorin (LV) after resection of hepatic metastases from colorectal cancer. *In: 2005 ASCO Annual Meeting. Orlando, Florida* , USA, American Society of Clinical Oncology.

[20] Adam, R., Delvart, V., Pascal, G., et al. (2004). Rescue surgery for unresectable colorectal liver metastases downstaged by chemotherapy: a model to predict long-term survival. *Ann Surg*, 240, 644-658.

[21] Petrowsky, H., Gonen, M., Jarnagin, W., et al. (2002). Second liver resections are safe and effective treatment for recurrent hepatic metastases from colorectal cancer: a bi-institutional analysis. *Ann Surg*, 235, 863-871.

[22] Tanaka, K., Shimada, H., Matsuo, K., et al. (2004). Outcome after simultaneous colorectal and hepatic resection for colorectal cancer with synchronous metastases. *Surgery*, 136, 650-659.

[23] Bolton, J. S., & Fuhrman, G. M. (2000). Survival after resection of multiple bilobar hepatic metastases from colorectal carcinoma. *Ann Surg*, 231, 743-751.

[24] Kornprat, P., Jarnagin, W. R., Gonen, M., et al. (2007). Outcome after hepatectomy for multiple (4 or more) colorectal metastases in the era of effective chemotherapy. *Ann Surg Oncol*, 14, 1151-1160.

[25] Headrick, J. R., Miller, D. L., Nagorney, D. M., et al. (2001). Surgical treatment of hepatic and pulmonary metastases from colon cancer. *Ann Thorac Surg*, 71, 975-990.

[26] Khan, S., Nagorney, D. M., & Que, F. G. (2012). *Metastatic malignant liver tumors : Neuroendocrine Chapter 81B- Jarnagin & Blumgart: Blumgart's Surgery of the Liver, Pancreas and Biliary Tract* (5th ed), Copyright © 2012 Saunders, An Imprint of Elsevier.

[27] Sutcliffe, R., Maguire, D., Ramage, J., et al. (2004). Management of neuroendocrine liver metastases. *Am J Surg 187*, 39-46.

[28] Clary, B. (2006). Treatment of isolated neuroendocrine liver metastases. *J Gastrointest Surg 10*, 332-334.

[29] Que, F., Sarmiento, J. M., & Nagorney, D. M. (2002). Hepatic surgery for metastatic gastrointestinal neuroendocrine tumors. *Cancer Control*, 9, 67-79.

[30] Guruswamy, K. S., Ramamoorthy, R., Sharma, D., et al. (2009). Liver resection versus other treatments for neuroendocrine tumours in patients with resectable liver metastases. Cochrane Database Syst Rev 2. CD007060.

[31] Touzios, J. G., Kiely, J. M., Pitt, S. C., et al. (2005). Neuroendocrine hepatic metastases: does aggressive management improve survival? *Ann Surg 241*, 776-785.

[32] Sarmiento, J. M., Heywood, G., Rubin, J., et al. (2003). Surgical treatment of neuroendocrine metastases to liver: a plea for resection to increase survival. *J Am Coll Surg 197*, 29-37.

[33] Sarmiento, J. M., & Que, F. G. (2003). Hepatic surgery for metastases from neuroendocrine tumors. *Surg Oncol Clin N Am 12*, 231-242.

[34] van Vilsteren, F. G. I., Baskin-Bey, E. S., Nagorney, D. M., et al. (2006). Liver transplantation for gastroenteropancreatic neuroendocrine cancers: defining selection criteria to improve survival. *Liver Transpl 12*, 448-456.

[35] Henn, A. R., Levine, E. A., Mc Nulty, W., & Zagoria, R. J. (2003). Percutaneous radiofrequency ablation of hepatic metastases for symptomatic relief of neuroendocrine syndromes. *Am J Roentgenol*, 181, 1005-1010.

[36] Wettstein, M., Vogt, C., Cohnen, M., et al. (2004). Serotonin release during percutaneous radiofrequency ablation in a patient with symptomatic liver metastases of a neuroendocrine tumor. *Hepatogastroenterology*, 51, 830-832.

[37] Gilliams, A., Cassoni, A., Conway, G., et al. (2005). Radiofrequency ablation of neuroendocrine liver metastases: the Middlesex experience. *Abdom Imaging*, 30, 435-441.

[38] Mazzaglia, P. J., Berber, E., Milas, M., et al. (2007). Laparoscopic radiofrequency ablation of neuroendocrine liver metastases: a 10year experience evaluating predictors of survival. *Surgery*, 142, 10-19.

[39] Osborne, D. A., Zervos, E. E., Strosberg, J., et al. (2006). Improved outcome with cytoreduction versus embolization for symptomatic hepatic metastases of carcinoid and neuroendocrine tumors. *Ann Surg Oncol*, 13, 572-581.

[40] Guruswamy, K. S., Pamecha, V., Sharma, D., et al. (2009). Palliative cytoreductive surgery versus other palliative treatments in patients with unresectable liver metastases from gastro-entero-pancreatic neuroendocrine tumours. Cochrane Database Syst Rev 1. CD007118.

[41] Pasieka, J. L., Mc Ewan, A. J. B., & Rorstad, O. (2004). The palliative role of 131I-MIBG and 111In-octreotide therapy in patients with metastatic progressive neuroendocrine neoplasms. *Surgery*, 136, 1218-1226.

[42] Faiss, S., Pape, U. F., Bohmig, M., et al. (2003). Prospective, randomized, multicenter trial on the antiproliferative effect of lanreotide, interferon alfa, and their combination for therapy of metastatic neuroendocrine gastroenteropancreatic tumors-the International Lanreotide and Interferon Alfa Study Group. *J Clin Oncol*, 21, 2689-2696.

[43] Jürgen, Weitz., Ronald, P., & De Matteo, . (2012). Noncolorectal nonneuroendocrine metastases Chapter 81C- Jarnagin & Blumgart: Blumgart's Surgery of the Liver, Pancreas and Biliary Tract, 5th ed. Copyright © 2012 Saunders, An Imprint of Elsevier.

[44] Adam, R., Chiche, L., Aloia, T., et al. (2006). Hepatic resection for noncolorectal nonendocrine liver metastases: analysis of 1,452 patients and development of a prognostic model. *Ann Surg*, 244, 524-535.

[45] Reddy, S. K., Barbas, A. S., Marroquin, C. E., et al. (2007). Resection of noncolorectal nonneuroendocrine liver metastases: a comparative analysis. *J Am Coll Surg*, 204, 372-382.

Chapter 17

The Assessment and Management of Chemotherapy Associated Liver Injury

S. M. Robinson, J. Scott, D. M. Manas and S. A. White

Additional information is available at the end of the chapter

http://dx.doi.org/10.5772/53915

1. Introduction

Historically chemotherapy for the treatment of colorectal cancer consisted of the thymidylate synthase inhibitor 5-FU (Adrucil®, Fluouracil®, Efudex®, Fluoroplex®), or more recently it's oral pro-drug Capecitabine (Xeloda®), in combination with Folinic acid. Alone these agents were associated with overall tumour response rates in the order of 20%.[10] In the last decade newer agents such as Oxaliplatin and Irinotecan have emerged on the market. These agents are not administered alone but normally in combination with a thymidylate synthase inhibitor. These combinations have seen the reported objective response to chemotherapy rise to typical rates of 50%.[11-13]

In parallel with the development of these conventional chemotherapeutics a new class of biological agents, i.e. antibody based therapies, have emerged. These agents are used to tackle specific pathways in tumour growth and development such as angiogenesis (e.g. anti-VEGFA antibody Bevacizumab) or cellular proliferation (e.g. the anti-epidermal growth factor antibodies Cetuximab and Panitumumab). When these agents are added to Oxaliplatin or Irinotecan based chemotherapy a further 10-15% increase in overall tumour response rate can be obtained.[14-17]

This improvement in response rates has led to a resurgence of interest in utilising chemotherapy as a means of down-sizing metastatic disease to enable subsequent surgical resection – so called conversion chemotherapy.[18] This approach was initially described in 1996 in a series of 330 patients with inoperable colorectal liver metastases of whom 53 (16%) were able to undergo a subsequent liver resection with curative intent after receiving systemic chemotherapy. The five year survival for these patients was 40% which compared favourably to patients with operable disease treated with surgery alone during the same period.[19] In 2004 the same group reported the outcome of 1104 patients with initially unresectable colorectal liver metastases who were treated primarily with systemic chemotherapy over an 11 year period from 1988 – 1999. Of this cohort 138 patients had a sufficient response to chemotherapy to permit subsequent curative intent surgery with an overall 5 year survival of 33% being achieved.[20]

In a small phase II trial of 42 patients with inoperable colorectal liver metastases Alberts et al reported that systemic treatment with 5-FU/Oxaliplatin was associated with a tumour response rate of around 60% with 14 patients (33%) having a sufficient response to permit a liver resection with curative intent.[21] Similar results have been reported with a 5-FU/Irinotecan regimen by Nuzzo et al with 15 out of 42 patients (36%) with inoperable disease being able to undergo subsequent surgical treatment.[22] In an attempt to determine the most appropriate regimen for use as conversion chemotherapy the GERCOR trial randomised patients with inoperable metastatic colorectal cancer to receive either 5-FU/Irinotecan until disease progression or unacceptable toxicity and then 5-FU/Oxaliplatin or the reverse sequence (n=113 per arm). Those patients receiving first line Oxaliplatin demonstrated a higher resection rate (n=24; 22%) than those receiving first line Irinotecan (n=10; 9%) and as such this is the approach most commonly applied in UK practice.[23]

More recently studies have been designed to determine the role of the biological agents in conversion therapy. In the phase II uncontrolled BOXER trial 46 patients with inoperable colorectal liver metastases were treated with Capecitabine/Oxaliplatin in combination with Bevacizumab. 35 of these patients experienced an objective tumour response with 18 (40%) able to undergo a liver resection with curative intent. In addition 5 patients (11%) experienced a complete radiological response to systemic therapy.[24] The CRYSTAL trial randomised patients with inoperable metastatic disease to Irinotecan/5-FU either alone or in combination with Cetuximab and found that the addition of Cetuxmiab was more likely to result in patients undergoing subsequent R0 liver resection with curative intent (Odds Ratio 3.02; p=0.002).[17] It is important to note that the response to Cetuximab is primarily determined by KRAS mutation status. In the Crystal trial there was no evidence of benefit in patients with mutant KRAS who received Cetuximab as compared to those who received 5-FU/Irinotecan alone.[25]

For those patients who receive successful conversion chemotherapy and are subsequently considered for liver resection with curative intent it is important to be aware of what the likely long term outcome will be. Adam et al. reported a series of 184 patients with initially inoperable disease who underwent hepatectomy after systemic therapy. In these patients a 5 year overall survival rate of 33% was obtained although it is important to note that a significant proportion of patients in this study underwent 2 or more surgical procedures, often interspersed with further chemotherapy, before long lasting disease control was obtained.[26]

Whilst the role of conversion chemotherapy is widely accepted in the HPB community more recently the question has been asked about what role systemic therapy may play in the management of patients presenting with operable disease from the outset i.e. true neoadjuvant chemotherapy. The EPOC trial was a multicentre randomised controlled trial which allocated such patients to receive either surgery alone or 6 cycles of 5-FU/Oxaliplatin prior to surgery followed by a further 6 cycles of therapy after surgery (n=182 per arm). Of those patients randomised just over 80% of patients in both arms underwent a curative intent liver resection. When the results of this study were analysed on an intention to treat basis there was a non-significant trend to improved 3 year overall survival in the chemotherapy arm (35.4% vs. 28.1%; p=0.058) although statistical significance was only achieved when the analysis was limited to only those who underwent resection (42.4% vs. 33.2%; p=0.025).[27] The difficulty in interpretation of the EPOC trial is that it is impossible to know whether the benefits of peri-operative chemotherapy were primarily a result of the neoadjuvant or adjuvant treatment or if both are required. This important question remains, at present, unanswered.

At present most authors would agree that there is insufficient evidence to consider all patients with operable disease candidates for systemic therapy prior to surgery although it may play a role in those with poor prognostic features such as multiple tumour deposits, a large tumour size or extra-hepatic disease.[28, 29] What is clear however is that an ever increasing number of patients are presenting for surgical resection on the background of multiple cycles of chemotherapy.[30] As experience of managing this patient cohort has increased there has been a growing recognition that the use of chemotherapy can be associated with a toxic injury to the liver parenchyma.[31] The nature of this liver injury and its implication for the surgical approach to these patients will form the subject of the remainder of this chapter.

2. Chemotherapy associated liver injury

2.1. Steatosis/steatohepatitis

The presence of fatty change within the liver is increasingly prevalent in the general adult population where it is commonly associated with the presence of obesity and insulin resistance (i.e. the metabolic syndrome). Fatty liver disease represents a spectrum of changes within the liver ranging from simple steatosis through to steatohepatitis and in extreme cases cirrhosis.[32] Steatohepatitis differs from simple steatosis in that significant inflammatory infiltrates are present in the liver commonly in association with ballooning degeneration of hepatocytes.[33]

The link between chemotherapy use and fatty liver disease was first reported in the literature in 1998. In a series of 21 patients with colorectal liver metastases treated with systemic 5-FU Peppercorn et al. reported that 48% (n=10) of patients had developed radiological evidence of steatosis on follow-up imaging.[34] In a later series Pawlik et al. reported the histological findings in the liver parenchyma of 334 patients who had undergone resection of colorectal liver metastases, 153 of whom had received pre-operative chemotherapy. In this study steatosis ≥ 30% (i.e. steatosis affecting more than 30% of hepatocytes) was present in 18.4% of patients who received pre-operative chemotherapy as compared to only 3.4% of patients who were chemotherapy naive (p=0.004). In particular the authors observed that steatosis was most strongly associated with Irinotecan based chemotherapy (27.3% of patients; p<0.001) than 5-FU monotherapy (14.9%; p=0.03) and lastly Oxaliplatin based chemotherapy

(9.6%; $p=0.04$) suggesting that the nature of the chemotherapy regimen may be important in determining liver toxicity.[35]

In contrast however a separate series of 406 patients who underwent resection of colorectal liver metastases failed to demonstrate any association between the administration of pre-operative chemotherapy and the subsequent development of steatosis ≥ 30%. In those receiving Irinotecan based chemotherapy (n=94) there was however a dramatic increase in the incidence of steatohepatitis as compared to those patients who were chemotherapy naive (20.2% vs. 4.4%; $p=0.001$), a finding which was in contrast to the smaller study described above.[35, 36]

To more accurately determine the nature of the association between chemotherapy use and the development of fatty change within the liver our group undertook a systematic review and meta-analysis of the published literature. In this analysis it was not possible to demonstrate any association with chemotherapy use overall (Relative Risk 1.25; 95% confidence interval 0.99 – 1.57; $p=0.15$) or Oxaliplatin based chemotherapy (Relative Risk 0.98; 95% confidence interval 0.59 – 1.63; $p=0.95$) and the development of steatosis ≥ 30%. In the case of Irinotecan based chemotherapy there was a strong trend to an increased risk of steatosis > 30% (Relative Risk 2.51; 95% Confidence Interval 0.79 – 7.90; $p=0.12$) which was not statistically significant as a consequence of the heterogeneity within the included studies. In contrast there was a strong association between Irinotecan based chemotherapy and steatohepatitis (Relative Risk 3.45; 95% Confidence Interval 1.12 – 10.62; $p=0.03$) which was not demonstrated with other regimens.[37]

2.2. Sinusoidal obstruction syndrome

Sinusoidal obstruction syndrome (SOS; previously known as hepatic veno-occlusive disease) represents a microvascular injury to the liver characterised by the histological findings of dilatation of the hepatic sinusoids and associated atrophy of the surrounding hepatocytes. In more advanced SOS these changes are accompanied by the development of regenerative nodules within the liver and ultimately peri-sinusoidal liver fibrosis.[38] Historically SOS was described as a condition occurring after ingestion of pyrrolizidine alkaloids, a group of compounds found in plants used in traditional African herbal remedies.[39, 40] Furthermore SOS has been reported to occur in up to 50% of patients receiving myeloablative chemotherapy prior to bone marrow transplantation.[41, 42]

In a seminal paper in 2004 Rubbia-Brandt published a report of histological changes in the liver parenchyma of 153 patients who had undergone resection of colorectal liver metastases. In this study it was reported that 44 out of 87 patients treated with pre-operative chemotherapy had histological features of SOS, the majority of whom had received treatment with Oxaliplatin based regimens.[38] Similar results were reported by Vauthey et al who demonstrated a significantly increased incidence of SOS in patients receiving Oxaliplatin based chemotherapy as compared to those who were chemotherapy naive (18.9% vs. 1.9%; $p<0.001$) where as no such association was demonstrated with other chemotherapy regimens.[36] In our systematic review of the published literature we demonstrated a strong association between Oxaliplatin based chemotherapy and SOS (Relative Risk 2.78; 95%

http://dx.doi.org/10.5772/53915

Confidence Interval 1.35 – 5.69; p=0.0007) which again was not replicated in patients receiving alternative chemotherapy regimens.[37] The typical appearances of an Oxaliplatin injured liver, as encountered at laparotomy, are shown in Figure 1.

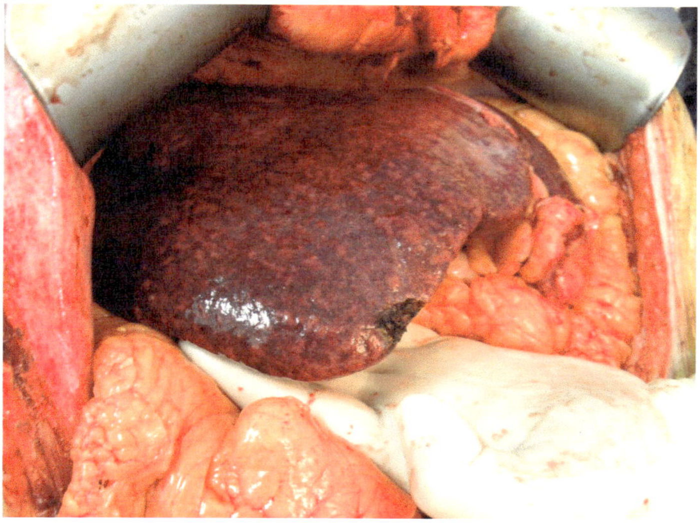

Figure 1. The classical appearance of the Oxaliplatin injured liver with SOS – commonly described as a "blue liver"

It is therefore clear from this discussion that the nature of liver injury following administration of chemotherapy to patients with colorectal liver metastases is dependent on the nature of the regimen administered. Irinotecan based regimens are primarily associated with the development of hepatic steatosis/steatohepatitis whereas Oxaliplatin based regimens are associated with the development of SOS. The assessment of the severity of this liver injury and its implications for the surgical management of these patients forms the discussion in the remainder of this chapter.

3. Assessment of the post-chemotherapy liver

Post hepatectomy liver failure (PHLF) is a feared complication of major liver resection and was recently defined as "a postoperatively acquired deterioration in the ability of the liver to maintain its synthetic, excretory and detoxifying functions"[43] whose presence is associated with a dramatic increase in the risk of post-operative mortality.[44, 45]

A key risk factor for the development of PHLF is the presence of background liver disease or injury. Belghiti et al reported, in a series of 747 patients undergoing liver resection, that the presence of either cirrhosis or steatosis affecting more than 30% of hepatocytes (n=253) was associated with a post-operative mortality of 9.5% as compared to only 1% in those with a normal liver parenchyma.[46] In a series of 406 patients undergoing resection of colorectal liver metastases Vauthey et al reported that those patients with steatohepatitis (n=34) experienced an increase in both 90 day mortality (14.7% vs. 1.6% p = 0.001) and post hepatectomy liver failure (5.8% vs. 0.8%; p=0.01).[36] The findings from these case series have been supported by a meta-analysis of the published literature which demonstrated that the presence of hepatic steatosis > 30% was associated with an increased risk of peri-operative complications (risk ratio 2.01; p<0.0001) and mortality (risk ratio 2.79; p=0.02).[47] Similarly the presence of SOS has been associated with an increased incidence of PHLF in a series of 51 patients undergoing resection of CRLM, 38 of whom had histologically proven SOS (68% vs. 23%; p=0.004)[48]

The other factor that is pivotal in determining the risk of PHLF is the volume of liver which will remain following surgery, commonly referred to as the future liver remnant or FLR, which can often be estimated pre-operatively by CT volumetry.[49] In 2003 Shoup et al reported a series of 126 patients who had undergone a liver resection to treat colorectal liver metastases. In those patients with a FLR of ≤ 25% (n=20) 90% developed PHLF as compared to 19% of those with an FLR > 25%. Logistic regression analysis demonstrated that the presence of an FLR<25% tripled the risk of PHLF (Odds Ratio 3.09; p<0.0001). Similarly in a study of 119 patients with a normal liver parenchyma undergoing major liver resection (i.e. resection of 3 or more Couinaud segments) the median FLR in the 7 patients who developed PHLF was 29.6% as compared to 42.5% in those who did not (p=0.009).[50] As a consequence of this evidence the minimum safe FLR in patients with an otherwise normal liver undergoing resection of CRLM is 25%.[51]

In those patients presenting for surgery on the background of multiple cycles of pre-operative chemotherapy it is pivotal, particularly when an extensive liver resection is planned, to minimise the risk of PHLF. When significant parenchymal injury is present it may be necessary for the FLR to be as high as 40% and this may have a significant impact on the surgical strategy employed.[52] Careful pre-operative assessment of the liver is therefore essential in these patients and the techniques which can be employed for doing this are discussed in more detail below.

3.1. Clinical/biochemical markers of chemotherapy induced liver injury

Identifying those patients at risk of steatohepatitis following Irinotecan based chemotherapy is particularly difficult not least because a significant proportion of patients in the background community will have a fatty liver as a consequence of either the metabolic syndrome, other underlying liver disease or lifestyle. This is reflected in the study of Ryan et al. which analysed histological changes in the liver of 334 patients undergoing resection of colorectal metastases. Only 8 patients in this study had histologically defined steatohepatitis the presence of which, on multivariate analysis, was found to be independently associated with a BMI > 30kg/m^2 but not the use of chemotherapy.[53] The study of Vauthey et al. reported that, in 94 patients treated with Irinotecan, the incidence of steatohepatitis was 12.1% in those with a BMI of < 25kg/m^2 but 24.6% in those with a BMI of ≥ 25kg/m^2. This study did not however undertake a multivariate analysis to identify independent risk factors associated with the presence of steatohepatitis.[36] It has been proposed that elevated serum transaminases may be of use in determining simple steatosis from steatohepatitis in patients with non-alcoholic fatty liver disease but it is not know whether this observation also holds true in those with chemotherapy associated steatohepatitis.[54-56]

Whilst one might intuitively expect that there would be a direct correlation between the number of cycles of chemotherapy received and the presence of liver injury this relationship is in fact less than clear cut. In the study of Vauthey et al. which reported the presence of liver injury in 406 patients undergoing resection of colorectal metastases there was no association between the number of cycles of chemotherapy administered and the incidence of steatohepatitis or SOS.[36] On the other hand Kishi et al., in a series of 219 patients who were treated pre-operatively with Oxaliplatin based chemotherapy, reported that SOS was present more frequently in those who received 9 or more cycles of chemotherapy than those who did not (42% vs. 26%; p=0.017).[57] Similarly the study of Aloia et al. reported that the incidence of SOS in those receiving greater than 12 cycles of chemotherapy was 50% as compared to 25% in those receiving 6-12 cycles and 10% in those who received less than 6 cycles (p=0.01).[58] Several studies have undertaken multivariate analysis to identify independent risk factors associated with the development of chemotherapy induced liver injury. Nakano et al demonstrated that the presence of SOS was independently associated with receiving 6 or more cycles of Oxaliplatin based chemotherapy (Relative Risk 3.2; p=0.048).[59] In contrast however 3 other studies have failed to demonstrate any such independent association between the number of cycles of Oxaliplatin administered and the development of SOS.[48, 60, 61] This raises the question of whether other variables, such as the presence of underlying liver disease, also make a significant contribution to the development of chemotherapy induced liver injury.

Some authors have suggested that tumour related factors may play a role in determining the development of SOS. On a univariate analysis of 78 patients treated with pre-operative Oxaliplatin based chemotherapy Soubrane et al. reported that those with SOS tended to have a larger tumour size (7.8cm vs. 5.2cm; p = 0.004) although this was not identified as an independent risk factor on multivariate analysis.[48] Tamandl et al. were able to confirm this observation in a separate study and on this occasion they were able to demonstrate that a tumour size > 5cm was independently associated with the development of SOS on multivariate analysis (Hazard Ratio 4.42; p = 0.012).[61] This clinical data is supported by experimental data from our group which suggests that the presence of tumour within the liver of mice treated with Oxaliplatin based chemotherapy accelerates changes in gene expression associated with the development of SOS.[62]

The role of various haematological and biochemical parameters to predict the presence of SOS has also been explored in several studies. Soubrane et al. reported on univariate analysis that an elevated AST (p=0.0009), ALT (p=0.02) and a low platelet count (p<0.0001) were all suggestive of the presence of SOS. On multivariate analysis they demonstrated that a high AST to platelet count ratio (APRI score) was an independent predictor for the presence of SOS (Odds Ratio 5; p<0.005).[48] Similarly a multivariate analysis from Nakano et al. demonstrated an independent association between an elevated AST and the presence of SOS (Relative Risk 3.86; p=0.044). [59] Tamandl et al. reported that on multivariate analysis on multivariate analysis an elevated alkaline phosphatase or γGT was an independent predictor of SOS (Hazard Ratio 4; p=0.038) although this was not true for AST or ALT.[61]

Whilst none of these studies have demonstrated a single factor that is reliably able to predict the presence of chemotherapy induced liver injury it is possible to begin to develop a picture of the patient characteristics which may lead to a raised index of suspicion and prompt a more thorough assessment of the liver parenchyma prior to surgery.

3.2. Radiological assessment of chemotherapy induced liver injury

The volume of data on the radiological assessment of fatty liver disease is vast and this is a reflection of the high incidence of non-alcoholic fatty liver disease in the general population. The consequence of this is that the appearances of fatty liver disease on each of the 3 main imaging modalities of the liver have been well described and is summarised in Table 1. It should be pointed out that on CT scanning hepatic steatosis is best detected on unenhanced images which are often not performed routinely in most imaging protocols in order to minimise patient radiation exposure.[63] A recent systematic review and meta-analysis of the published literature concluded that MRI represented the most accurate method for determining the extent of hepatic steatosis with a reported sensitivity of 97.4% and specificity of 76.1% for the detection of steatosis >30%.[64]

Imaging Modality	Characteristic features hepatic steatosis
Ultrasound	Intracellular fat accumulation leads to an increase in liver echogenicity [63]
Computed Tomography	Steatosis leads to a decrease in attenuation of the liver parenchyma [63, 65]
Magnetic Resonance Imaging	A loss of liver signal intensity occurs on T1 weighted gradient echo (GRE) opposed images[63, 65]

Table 1. Appearances of hepatic steatosis on the main liver imaging modalities

Several studies have attempted to identify the utility of pre-operative cross sectional imaging to identify hepatic steatosis specifically in patients undergoing liver resection. The first of these was published in 2008 by Cho et al. who conducted a retrospective analysis of 131 patients undergoing partial hepatectomy over a 4 year period who had one of either a non-contrast CT scan (n=26), contrast enhanced CT scan (n=74) or a gradient opposed MRI (n=32) with a median interval between imaging and surgery of 17 Days. The ability of these imaging modalities to predict histologically defined steatosis > 30% was determined. The authors demonstrated that of the two CT methods studied only non-contrast CT was of any utility in determining the presence of hepatic steatosis with a high degree of specificity (100%) but had low sensitivity (33%) with a corresponding positive predictive value (PPV) of 100% and negative predictive value (NPV) of 83%. In contrast MRI fared much better in excluding the presence of hepatic steatosis with an NPV of 94% but a PPV of only 44% with a sensitivity of 88% and specificity of 63%. The conclusion of this study was that cross-sectional imaging alone was not consistently able to determine the presence of hepatic steatosis and was therefore of limited utility for this purpose.[66]

In 2009 O'Rourke et al. reported a prospective study of n=37 patients undergoing resection of colorectal liver metastases who received pre-operative liver specific MRI. Again this study demonstrated a much better performance for MRI in determining the presence of hepatic steatosis > 30% with a PPV of 100%, NPV of 87% a sensitivity of 63% and a specificity of 100%.[67] A subsequent retrospective study by Marsman et al compared the ability of non-contrast enhanced CT (n=32) and MRI (n=36) to detect the presence of histologically defined steatosis > 33% in patients undergoing resection of colorectal liver metastases after receiving pre-operative chemotherapy. In this study MRI by far out performed CT in terms of sensitivity (78% vs. 70%), specificity (100% vs. 86.4%); PPV (100% vs. 70%) and NPV (93.1% vs. 86.4%) suggesting that this is the imaging modality of choice.[68]

On the basis of the currently available evidence it appears that MRI is the imaging modality of choice to assess the extent of hepatic steatosis in patients with colorectal liver metastases prior to surgery. It must be highlighted that cross-sectional imaging is not able to differentiate between simple steatosis and steatohepatitis which can only be achieved with histological assessment of the liver. Furthermore a 'normal' imaging study does not exclude the presence of hepatic steatosis and in those cases where there is a high level of clinical suspicion a further evaluation of the liver must be undertaken.

The role of cross-sectional imaging in detecting the presence of SOS is much less clear cut as compared to hepatic steatosis. It has been proposed that the development of splenomegaly on post-chemotherapy imaging may serve as a surrogate marker for the presence of SOS. Overman et al conducted a study in patients who received either 5-FU/Oxaliplatin (n=96) or 5-FU alone (n=40) as adjuvant therapy following resection of a colonic primary and compared spleen size on pre-operative imaging to that 6 weeks after the final cycle of chemotherapy. They demonstrated that the median increase in spleen size was 22% for those patients receiving 5-FU/Oxaliplatin whereas there was no increase in size in those receiving 5-FU alone (p<0.001). The authors went on to look at a subgroup of patients (n=63) who underwent a liver resection after 5-FU/Oxaliplatin and demonstrated, on multivariate analysis, that a greater than 50% increase in spleen size following chemotherapy was independently able to predict the presence of SOS (Odds Ratio 2.34; p=0.02) with a sensitivity of 43%, and specificity of 90%.[60]

Several authors have explored the utility of various MRI protocols to predict the presence of SOS. Ward et al. reported a study of 60 patients with colorectal liver metastases who underwent superparamagnetic iron oxide (SPIO) enhanced MRI prior to liver resection. Following SPIO administration SOS is characterised by reticular hyperintensity on $T2^*$-gradient response echo weighted MRI images the presence of which the authors graded on a scale of 0 – 3 (summarised in Table 2) with a score of 2 or greater indicating the presence of SOS. Using this technique 24 of the 60 patients were thought to have SOS on the basis of MRI the presence of which was subsequently confirmed histologically in 20 patients. Of the 36 patients thought not to have SOS on the basis of MRI 3 were subsequently found to have histological features of SOS. This means that SPIO enhanced MRI, in this study, had a sensitivity of 87%, specificity of 89%, PPV of 83% and NPV of 92% for the presence of SOS.[69] In contrast to these findings however O'Rourke et al. in their study of 37 patients found that SPIO enhanced MRI had a high specificity (100%) and PPV (100%) for the presence of severe SOS but a low sensitivity (11%) with a NPV of 78% suggesting that this technique may fail to identify a significant proportion of patients with SOS.[67]

Grade	Description
0	Absent
1	Fine reticulations on a minority of sections
2	Diffuse reticulations or localised coalescent areas of high signal
3	Diffuse reticulations present on all sections or densely coalescent areas of high signal on multiple sections

Table 2. Grading of reticular hyperintensity on SPIO enhanced MRI to determine the presence of SOS[69]

Shin et al. explored the ability of Gadoxetic acid disodium (EOB-MRI; Primavist®) enhanced MRI to detect the presence of SOS prior to resection of colorectal metastases. On EOB-MRI the presence of SOS appears as reticular hypointensity which the authors graded on a scale of 1-5 with a score of 4 (probably present) or 5 (definitely present) being considered diagnostic of SOS. Of the 42 patients included in this study all 12 MRI identified cases of SOS had the diagnosis confirmed histologically and of the 30 MRI negative cases 4 had histological evidence of SOS. This resulted in a sensitivity of 75%, specificity of 100%, PPV of 100% and a NPV of 87%. The images in this study were independently reviewed by a radiological resident with a good level of agreement (weighted kappa 0.765) suggesting that this technique is subject to minimal interobserver variability.[70]

The small number of patients in these studies make it difficult to recommend the routine use of any of these MRI protocols for the sole purpose of detecting pre-operative SOS. The presence of splenomegaly on pre-operative imaging, particularly in patients who have received multiple cycles of Oxaliplatin based chemotherapy, should raise suspicion about the presence of SOS and prompt a thorough assessment of the liver parenchyma if extended resection is to be performed.

3.3. Functional assessment of the future liver remnant

A variety of techniques have been described which aim to quantitatively assess the functional reserve of the liver and thereby provide a means to determine the minimum safe FLR that is required to avoid the risk of PHLF. Perhaps the most widely described of these techniques is the Indocyanine Green (ICG) retention test. Following injection ICG is transported in the systemic circulation bound to albumin and does not leave the serum until it reaches the liver where it is taken up by hepatocytes. These hepatocytes then clear ICG by excreting the compound into the biliary system in an ATP dependent manner. ICG does not enter the portal circulation nor is it metabolised by hepatocytes prior to its excretion and therefore the clearance of ICG provides a direct measure of hepatocyte function.[71]

Typically the retention of ICG at 15 minutes is measured in a serum sample (ICGR-15) and this value is used as a measure of hepatic functional reserve with a value of <10% being considered normal. Based on their experience of using this test in a series of 1429 patients Imamura et al. described the maximum extent of liver resection they thought could be safely performed according to the ICGR-15 value (see Table 3).[72] Others however view this ICGR-15 value as too conservative and state that a cut off of <14% should be used to identify those patients in whom it is safe to perform major liver resection.[73] The use of ICG retention as a pre-operative assessment of liver function is however predominantly limited to Asia where the majority of liver resections are performed for hepatocellular carcinoma and therefore the data regarding the validity of this test in patients with colorectal liver metastases is limited.

ICGR-15 Value	Typical Safe Liver Resection
<10%	Right/Left Trisectionectomy
10 – 19%	Left hepatectomy / Right sectorectomy
20 – 29%	Segmentectomy
≥ 30%	Limited non-anatomical resection

Table 3. Typical safe liver resection volumes as recommended by Imamura et al based on ICGR-15 values[72]

Nakano et al reported the outcome of 36 patients who underwent major hepatectomy (>3 Couinaud segments) 20 of whom had histologically proven SOS and 16 who had a normal liver parenchyma. The presence of SOS in these patients was independently associated with an ICGR-15 of >10%. It is of note that these patients experienced an increased risk of peri-operative complications (40% vs. 6.3%; p=0.026) and a longer mean hospital stay (17 days vs. 11 days; p = 0.006).[59] Experimental studies have also suggested that ICGR-15 may be a useful measure of hepatocyte function in the context of hepatic steatosis.[74] In a series of 101 patients undergoing liver resection for colorectal metastases Klinger et al reported that the use of preoperative chemotherapy (n=83; all regimens) was associated with a longer ICGR-15 (7.3% vs. 3.5%; p = 0.005). Similarly those who had received pre-operative chemotherapy were more likely to have an ICGR-15 ≥ 10% (27.7% vs. 0%; p=0.011) and this was associated with an increased rate of post-operative complications (39.1% vs. 12.8%; p=0.005). No attempt was made in this study to correlate ICGR-15 values with histological changes within the liver parenchyma.[75]

The LiMAx test has recently been described as an alternative means of assessing the hepatic functional reserve. This test measures the cytochrome P450 mediated metabolism of ^{13}C labelled methacetin into acetaminophen and $^{13}CO_2$ which is exhaled. The test measures changes in the ratio of exhaled $^{13}CO_2$: $^{12}CO_2$ over a 60 minute period – the greater the $^{13}CO_2$ excretion the greater the functional reserve of the liver.[76] The authors have demonstrated that low post-operative LiMAx values (<80µg/kg/h) are correlated with an unacceptable risk of post-operative morbidity. On the basis of this they have proposed an algorithm to determine the safety of liver surgery based upon pre-operative measurement of the LiMAx to calculate the likely post-operative LiMAx using CT volumetric calculations of the FLR. This strategy has not however been proven in an independent prospective cohort and therefore cannot currently be recommended for routine clinical use.[77]

A final technique for assessing the functional reserve of the liver is hepatobiliary scintigraphy using ^{99m}Tc-mebrofenin. Following injection ^{99m}Tc-mebrofenin is taken up by hepatocytes and excreted directly into the biliary system without prior intracellular metabolism in a similar manner to ICG. The hepatic uptake and excretion of ^{99m}Tc-mebrofenin is determined using images obtained with a gamma camera and from this it is possible to determine the total liver uptake, corrected for body surface area, as a %/min/m^2 of the total injected dose (referred to as the total liver function or TL-F). In addition the FLR uptake function (FLR-F) can be calculated as a function of the TL-F based on uptake in the calculated.[78]

De Graaf et al. reported a series 55 patients judged to be at high risk of post-operative complications following liver resection assessed with ^{99m}Tc-mebrofenin scintigraphy prior to liver resection. They demonstrated that TL-F was significantly reduced in those patients with background parenchymal disease (7.4 vs. 8.5 %/min/m^2; p=0.007). In addition the FLR-F was significantly lower in those patients who developed PHLF as compared to those who did not (2.2 vs. 4.3%/min/m^2; p=0.001).[79] Whilst this technology needs further evaluation in prospective studies it is likely that the emerging ability to perform single photon emission computed tomography (SPECT) thereby enabling quantification of tracer compound activity in combination with standard CT will lead to renewed interest in the technique.

At present none of these technologies have been adequately characterised in patients with colorectal metastases undergoing liver resection. Whilst they undoubtedly have potential merit in identifying those patients with an impaired hepatocyte mass it is not known whether the information they add is superior to that obtained standard clinical and radiological assessment. This must be established before the routine integration of these technologies into the assessment of this cohort of patients can be recommended.

4. Surgical management of the chemotherapy injured liver

When either clinical suspicion or pre-operative imaging suggest the presence of a chemotherapy induced injury to the liver it may no longer be possible to resect all metastatic disease whilst maintaining an adequate FLR to avoid the risk of liver failure. In this situation two key surgical strategies have been described to reduce the risk of surgery i.e. pre-operative portal vein embolisation and two-stage hepatectomy and these are discussed in more detail below.

http://dx.doi.org/10.5772/53915

4.1. Pre-operative portal vein embolisation

Portal vein embolisation (PVE) is a particularly useful technique in patients who have disease which is technically resectable in a single operation but where so doing would lead to a compromised FLR. As early as 1920 Rous and Larimore observed that if they ligated a single branch of the portal vein in a rabbit there was atrophy of the ipsilateral lobe and hypertrophy of the contralateral lobe.[80] As a clinical technique PVE was initially described by Kinoshita et al. in 1986 as a means of limiting the extension of tumour thrombus in patients with hepatocellular carcinoma.[81] Subsequently in 1990 Makuuchi et al. demonstrated the safety and efficacy of this technique as a means of increasing the FLR in a series of 14 patients undergoing resection of hilar cholangiocarcinoma.[82] In a prospective study Farges et al. performed CT volumetry on patients undergoing pre-operative PVE and demonstrated that in those patients with no underlying parenchymal disease the typical increase in FLR was 16% whereas in those with chronic liver disease the typical increase in FLR was 9%.[83]

In 2010 Wicherts et al. reported a retrospective series of 67 patients who underwent liver resection for colorectal metastases after pre-operative PVE with a cohort of 297 patients who did not receive PVE. The authors observed that those patients treated with pre-operative PVE demonstrated a significantly higher complication rate (55.5% vs. 41.1%; $p = 0.035$) although there was no difference in surgical mortality between groups. Whilst this difference in morbidity is striking it is difficult to interpret since whilst all patients in the study underwent a major hepatectomy (≥3 Couinaud segments) 54% of those in the PVE group underwent a right trisectionectomy as compared to only 28% in the control group. What was striking in this study however was that 32 of the patients treated with PVE did not proceed to surgery and amongst these patients there were no 3 year survivors as compared to a 3 year survival rate of 44% in those who did undergo surgery.[84]

A similarly designed study by Pamecha et al. compared the outcome of 36 patients treated with pre-operative PVE with 65 patients who did not receive PVE all of whom had a diagnosis of colorectal metastases. Of the 36 patients treated with PVE 12 did not progress to surgery and had a median survival of 14 months as compared to 42 months in those who did progress to surgery ($p<0.0001$). Again there was a tendency to higher morbidity in the PVE group (36% vs. 20%) but in a similar manner to the study of Wicherts et al. more of these patients had undergone a right trisectionectomy (22% vs. 11%).[85]

The most important finding in both of these series is that nearly a third of all patients selected to undergo pre-operative portal vein embolisation do not undergo subsequent surgery and this is primarily a consequence of disease progression.[84, 85] It is likely that the most important factor driving this disease progression is the compensatory increase in arterial blood flow which occurs in the embolised lobe.[86] The blood supply of colorectal metastases is predominantly derived from the hepatic artery[87] and it is probable that the increase in arterial flow results in increased oxygen and nutrient supply to the tumour. In addition following PVE there is an increase in the hepatic production of a wide variety of cytokines, growth factors and other humoral factors that mediate liver regeneration and it may be that these also contribute to the progression of metastatic disease.[88, 89]

In summary PVE is a potentially useful technique for increasing the FLR in patients in whom this is likely to be compromised there is a significant risk that the procedure will result in disease progression rendering the patient inoperable and therefore must not be embarked upon lightly.

4.2. Two-stage hepatectomy

For a proportion of patients presenting with bilobar disease it is not possible to clear the entire tumour burden by an extended resection alone (e.g. right trisectionectomy) but rather it is necessary to combine an anatomical resection (e.g. or the right lobe) with multiple metastectomies from the contralateral lobe potentially resulting in an insufficient FLR, particularly in patients with a background liver injury (Figure 2). In such circumstances a PVE alone would not be appropriate because of the significant risk of tumour progression in the FLR and therefore a two stage resection should be considered. In the scenario described above this would typically consist of an initial operation to clear the left liver of tumour using multiple metastectomies followed several weeks later by a right hepatectomy. If it was felt at the time of the primary operation that the hypertrophy induced by surgery alone would not leave an adequate FLR for the second operation then it may be desirable to perform either intra-operative ligation of the right portal vein or post-operative percutaneous portal vein embolisation.[90] In this situation it is the authors preference to perform the latter procedure thereby avoiding unnecessary dissection of the hilum prior to right hepatectomy.

Wicherts et al. reported the outcomes of 59 patients considered to be inoperable using a single stage procedure who were selected for a two stage approach. All of these patients underwent a primary surgical procedure which in the majority of cases consisted of a minor hepatectomy (<3 Couinaud segments resected) the aim of which was to clear the left liver of tumour. Subsequently 42 patients underwent a second procedure which was typically a major hepatic resection (≥3 Couinaud segments) and typically this took place 3 months after the initial surgical procedure. It is of note that 17 patients selected for this approach did not undergo a second procedure primarily as a consequence of disease progression. The overall 5 year survival in this series was 31% when analysed on an intention to treat basis and this did not differ, in a statistically significantly manner, from patients undergoing a single stage hepatectomy over the same period in the authors unit.[91]

More recently Narita et al. reported the outcome of 79 patients treated using a two stage approach. After the initial surgical procedure 75 of these patients were considered appropriate to proceed to the second operation although the majority (92%) were thought to require portal vein embolisation to facilitate this. Of that cohort of patients 61 (78% of the original cohort) eventually underwent a successful second operation. The main reasons for patients not proceeding to a second procedure were tumour progression in 10 cases and insufficient regeneration of the FLR in a further 5 cases. It is of note that almost 1:6 of the patients who underwent a second surgical procedure were found to have new disease in the previously cleared FLR although this was dealt with at the time of surgery in all cases. In those patients who underwent a successful two stage resection the overall 5 year survival was 32%. Of the 61 patients who were treated successfully by a two stage approach 11 went on to have a subsequent resection of lung metastases although this had no effect on overall survival when compared to the 50 patients who did not.[92]

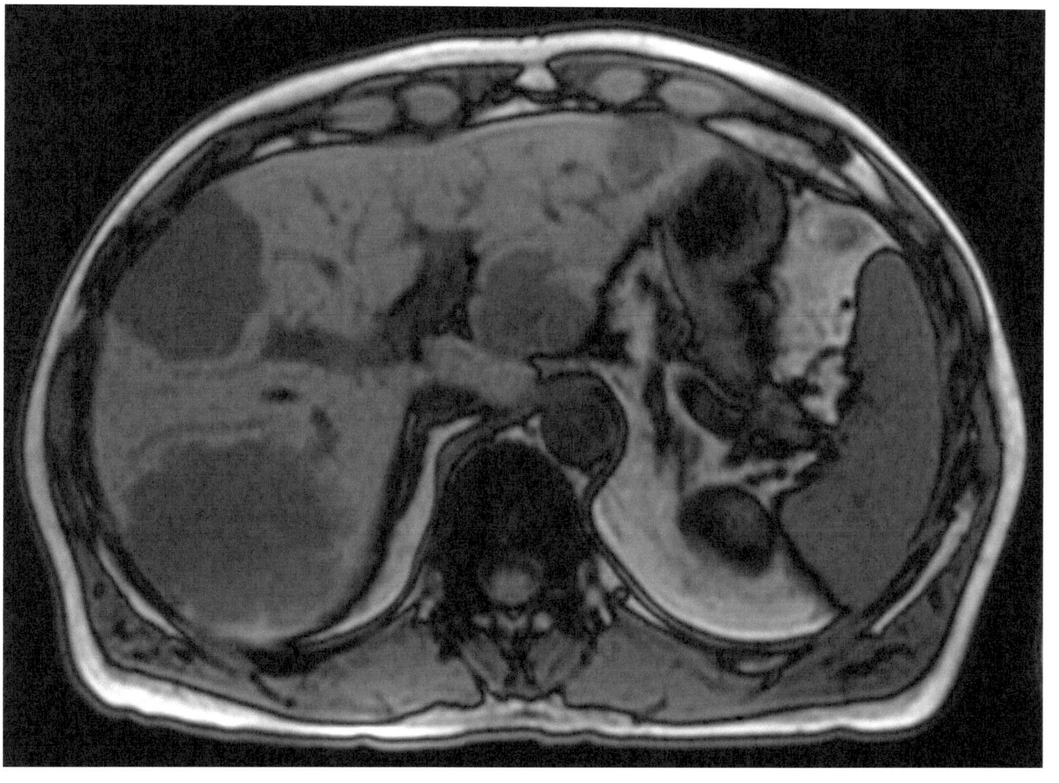

Figure 2. Typical MRI scan of patient with bilobar disease who would be considered suitable for a two staged approach to liver resection. With this distribution of disease a one stage approach would not leave an adequate FLR.

In a similar manner to PVE alone a two stage hepatectomy is a major undertaking and before embarking on this both surgeon and patient should be aware that there is a significant risk of not being able to complete the planned course of treatment. Despite this it does provide an opportunity to achieve a meaningful long term survival in selected patients with advanced disease.

5. The long term consequences of chemotherapy associated liver injury

Whilst the primary focus of this chapter is on the effects of chemotherapy associated liver injury on the surgical management of patients with colorectal liver metastases it would not be complete without some mention of the emerging evidence that this injury may have an effect on long term disease specific outcomes. Tamandl et al. have suggested that the presence of the histological features of SOS within the resected liver of patients with colorectal liver metastases may have a negative impact on long term disease specific survival. In particular patients with SOS demonstrated a significantly poorer 3 year progression free survival (6.7% vs. 22.7%; p=0.006) a finding which was upheld on multivariate analysis (Hazard Ratio 2.20; p=0.006). Specifically patients with SOS demonstrated a higher rate of intra-hepatic recurrence following surgery (66.7% vs. 30.5%; p=0.003) and not surprisingly this was associated with an increased risk of early all cause mortality on multivariate analysis (Hazard Ratio 2.90; p<0.001).[61]

A major criticism of the study of Tamandl et al. is that it includes only small numbers of patients (n=20 with SOS) and therefore it is difficult to draw definitive conclusions.[61] None the less a recent paper by Vreuls et al. has reported that the development of SOS may be associated with a poorer tumour response to Oxaliplatin based chemotherapy which the authors propose may be a consequence of tissue hypoperfusion leading to diminished leading to impaired delivery of chemotherapy to the tumour.[93] An alternative explanation may be that SOS is associated with increased expression of the chemokine CCL20 within the liver which is known to act as a chemo-attractant for colorectal cancer cells.[94] At the same time as this is occurring within the liver Oxaliplatin chemotherapy also results in increased expression of the CCL20 receptor CCR6 within colorectal liver metastases thereby increasing the migration and proliferation of tumour cells in response to CCL20.[95, 96] It may therefore be that the presence of SOS leads to the establishment of an autocrine signalling loop which favours the further growth and development of colorectal liver metastases.[97]

This emerging evidence is clearly a cause for concern and, if proven to be true, would add further impetus to the drive to develop strategies for the prevention of liver injury in patients being treated with systemic chemotherapy.

6. Conclusion

Advances in chemotherapy over the last decade or so have revolutionised the care for patients with colorectal liver metastases with the end result that patients who historically would have been considered inoperable are now able to undergo potentially curative surgical resection. The pay off for this advance has been the development of a chemotherapy associated injury to the liver the nature of which is determined the specific regimens used.

There is no specific test that is able to reliably detect the presence of an injured liver parenchyma and ultimately surgeons must maintain a high index of suspicion for its presence particularly in patients who have received multiple cycles of chemotherapy over a prolonged period of time. When a liver injury is present it is important that the surgical approach is considered carefully and makes allowances for the possibility of an impaired FLR with a subsequent risk of post operative liver failure. In those situations where there is a high risk of an insufficient FLR it may be appropriate to utilise techniques such as PVE or two stage hepatectomy although there is a risk with both these techniques of treatment failure as a consequence of disease progression.

http://dx.doi.org/10.5772/53915

Author details

S. M. Robinson[1], J. Scott[2], D. M. Manas[3] and S. A. White[3]

*Address all correspondence to: s.m.robinson@newcastle.ac.uk

1 Institute of Cellular Medicine, Newcastle University, Framlington Place, Newcastle upon Tyne, UK

2 Department of Radiology, Freeman Hospital, Newcastle upon Tyne, UK

3 Department of HPB Surgery, Freeman Hospital, Newcastle upon Tyne, UK

References

[1] Cancer Research UK. CancerStats - Bowel Cancer. Cancer Research UK; 2011 (updated 2011; cited 13/11/2011); Available from: http://info.cancerresearchuk.org/cancerstats/types/bowel/.

[2] Leporrier J, Maurel J, Chiche L, Bara S, Segol P, Launoy G. A population-based study of the incidence, management and prognosis of hepatic metastases from colorectal cancer. Br J Surg. 2006 Apr;93(4):465-74.

[3] Kopetz S, Chang GJ, Overman MJ, Eng C, Sargent DJ, Larson DW, et al. Improved survival in metastatic colorectal cancer is associated with adoption of hepatic resection and improved chemotherapy. J Clin Oncol. 2009 Aug 1;27(22):3677-83.

[4] Pawlik TM, Abdalla EK, Ellis LM, Vauthey JN, Curley SA. Debunking dogma: surgery for four or more colorectal liver metastases is justified. J Gastrointest Surg. 2006 Feb;10(2):240-8.

[5] Scheele J, Stangl R, Altendorf-Hofmann A. Hepatic metastases from colorectal carcinoma: impact of surgical resection on the natural history. Br J Surg. 1990 Nov;77(11): 1241-6.

[6] Poston G, Adam R, Vauthey JN. Downstaging or downsizing: time for a new staging system in advanced colorectal cancer? J Clin Oncol. 2006 Jun 20;24(18):2702-6.

[7] Brouquet A, Vauthey JN, Contreras CM, Walsh GL, Vaporciyan AA, Swisher SG, et al. Improved survival after resection of liver and lung colorectal metastases compared with liver-only metastases: a study of 112 patients with limited lung metastatic disease. J Am Coll Surg. 2011 Jul;213(1):62-9; discussion 9-71.

[8] Neeff H, Horth W, Makowiec F, Fischer E, Imdahl A, Hopt UT, et al. Outcome after resection of hepatic and pulmonary metastases of colorectal cancer. J Gastrointest Surg. 2009 Oct;13(10):1813-20.

[9] Pawlik TM, Schulick RD, Choti MA. Expanding criteria for resectability of colorectal liver metastases. Oncologist. 2008 Jan;13(1):51-64.

[10] Van Cutsem E, Twelves C, Cassidy J, Allman D, Bajetta E, Boyer M, et al. Oral capecitabine compared with intravenous fluorouracil plus leucovorin in patients with metastatic colorectal cancer: results of a large phase III study. J Clin Oncol. 2001 Nov 1;19(21):4097-106.

[11] Giacchetti S, Perpoint B, Zidani R, Le Bail N, Faggiuolo R, Focan C, et al. Phase III multicenter randomized trial of oxaliplatin added to chronomodulated fluorouracil-leucovorin as first-line treatment of metastatic colorectal cancer. J Clin Oncol. 2000 Jan;18(1):136-47.

[12] de Gramont A, Figer A, Seymour M, Homerin M, Hmissi A, Cassidy J, et al. Leucovorin and fluorouracil with or without oxaliplatin as first-line treatment in advanced colorectal cancer. J Clin Oncol. 2000 Aug;18(16):2938-47.

[13] Saltz LB, Cox JV, Blanke C, Rosen LS, Fehrenbacher L, Moore MJ, et al. Irinotecan plus fluorouracil and leucovorin for metastatic colorectal cancer. Irinotecan Study Group. N Engl J Med. 2000 Sep 28;343(13):905-14.

[14] Hochster HS, Hart LL, Ramanathan RK, Childs BH, Hainsworth JD, Cohn AL, et al. Safety and efficacy of oxaliplatin and fluoropyrimidine regimens with or without bevacizumab as first-line treatment of metastatic colorectal cancer: results of the TREE Study. J Clin Oncol. 2008 Jul 20;26(21):3523-9.

[15] Hurwitz H, Fehrenbacher L, Novotny W, Cartwright T, Hainsworth J, Heim W, et al. Bevacizumab plus irinotecan, fluorouracil, and leucovorin for metastatic colorectal cancer. New England Journal of Medicine 2004 Jun 3;350(23):2335-42.

[16] Bokemeyer C, Bondarenko I, Makhson A, Hartmann JT, Aparicio J, de Braud F, et al. Fluorouracil, leucovorin, and oxaliplatin with and without cetuximab in the first-line treatment of metastatic colorectal cancer. J Clin Oncol. 2009 Feb 10;27(5):663-71.

[17] Van Cutsem E, Kohne CH, Hitre E, Zaluski J, Chang Chien CR, Makhson A, et al. Cetuximab and chemotherapy as initial treatment for metastatic colorectal cancer. N Engl J Med. 2009 Apr 2;360(14):1408-17.

[18] Khatri VP, Chee KG, Pertrelli NJ. Modern multimodality approach to hepatic colorectal metastases: Solutions and controversies. Surgical Oncology. 2007;16:71-83.

[19] Bismuth H, Adam R, Levi F, Farabos C, Waechter F, Castaing D, et al. Resection of nonresectable liver metastases from colorectal cancer after neoadjuvant chemotherapy. Ann Surg. 1996 Oct;224(4):509-20; discussion 20-2.

[20] Adam R, Delvart V, Pascal G, Valeanu A, Castaing D, Azoulay D, et al. Rescue surgery for unresectable colorectal liver metastases downstaged by chemotherapy: a model to predict long-term survival. Ann Surg. 2004 Oct;240(4):644-57; discussion 57-8.

[21] Alberts SR, Horvath WL, Sternfeld WC, Goldberg RM, Mahoney MR, Dakhil SR, et al. Oxaliplatin, fluorouracil, and leucovorin for patients with unresectable liver-only metastases from colorectal cancer: a North Central Cancer Treatment Group phase II study. Journal of Clinical Oncology. 2005;23(36):9243-9.

[22] Nuzzo G, Giuliante F, Ardito F, Vellone M, Pozzo C, Cassano A, et al. Liver resection for primarily unresectable colorectal metastases downsized by chemotherapy. J Gastrointest Surg. 2007 Mar;11(3):318-24.

[23] Tournigand C, Andre T, Achille E, Lledo G, Flesh M, Mery-Mignard D, et al. FOLFIRI followed by FOLFOX6 or the reverse sequence in advanced colorectal cancer: a randomized GERCOR study. J Clin Oncol. 2004 Jan 15;22(2):229-37.

[24] Wong R, Cunningham D, Barbachano Y, Saffery C, Valle J, Hickish T, et al. A multicentre study of capecitabine, oxaliplatin plus bevacizumab as perioperative treatment of patients with poor-risk colorectal liver-only metastases not selected for upfront resection. Ann Oncol. 2011 Sep;22(9):2042-8.

[25] Van Cutsem E, Kohne CH, Lang I, Folprecht G, Nowacki MP, Cascinu S, et al. Cetuximab plus irinotecan, fluorouracil, and leucovorin as first-line treatment for metastatic colorectal cancer: updated analysis of overall survival according to tumor KRAS and BRAF mutation status. J Clin Oncol. May 20;29(15):2011-9.

[26] Adam R, Wicherts DA, de Haas RJ, Oriana C, Levi F, Paule B, et al. Patients with Initially Unresectable Colorectal Liver Metastases: Is There a Possibility of Cure. Journal of Clinical Oncology. 2009;27(11):1829-935.

[27] Nordlinger B, Sorbye H, Glimelius B, Poston GJ, Schlag PM, Rougier P, et al. Perioperative chemotherapy with FOLFOX4 and surgery versus surgery alone for resectable liver metastases from colorectal cancer (EORTC Intergroup trial 40983): a randomised controlled trial. Lancet. 2008 Mar 22;371(9617):1007-16.

[28] Fong Y, Fortner J, Sun RL, Brennan MF, Blumgart LH. Clinical score for predicting recurrence after hepatic resection for metastatic colorectal cancer: analysis of 1001 consecutive cases. Ann Surg. 1999 Sep;230(3):309-18; discussion 18-21.

[29] Adam R, Bhangui P, Poston G, Mirza D, Nuzzo G, Barroso E, et al. Is Perioperative Chemotherapy Useful for Solitary, Metachronous, Colorectal Liver Metastases. Annals of Surgery. 2010;252(5):774-87.

[30] Adam R, Frilling A, Elias D, Laurent C, Ramos E, Capussotti L, et al. Liver resection of colorectal metastases in elderly patients. Br J Surg. 2010 Mar;97(3):366-76.

[31] Nordlinger B, Benoist S. Benefits and risks of neoadjuvant therapy for liver metastases. Journal of Clinical Oncology. 2006;24(31):4954-5.

[32] Anstee QM, McPherson S, Day CP. How big a problem is non-alcoholic fatty liver disease? BMJ. 2011;343:d3897.

[33] Kleiner DE, Brunt EM, Van Natta M, Behling C, Contos MJ, Cummings OW, et al. Design and validation of a histological scoring system for nonalcoholic fatty liver disease. Hepatology. 2005 Jun;41(6):1313-21.

[34] Peppercorn PD, Reznek RH, Wilson P, Slevin ML, Gupta RK. Demonstration of hepatic steatosis by computerized tomography in patients receiving 5-fluorouracil-based therapy for advanced colorectal cancer. Br J Cancer. 1998 Jun;77(11):2008-11.

[35] Pawlik TM, Olino K, Gleisner AL, Torbenson M, Schulick R, Choti MA. Preoperative chemotherapy for colorectal liver metastases: impact on hepatic histology and postoperative outcome. J Gastrointest Surg. 2007 Jul;11(7):860-8.

[36] Vauthey JN, Pawlik TM, Ribero D, Wu TT, Zorzi D, Hoff PM, et al. Chemotherapy regimen predicts steatohepatitis and an increase in 90-day mortality after surgery for hepatic colorectal metastases. Journal of Clinical Oncology. 2006;24(13):2065-72.

[37] Robinson SM, Wilson CH, Burt AD, Manas DM, White SA. Chemotherapy Associated Liver Injury in Patients with Colorectal Liver Metastases : A Systematic Review and Meta-Analysis. Annals of Surgical Oncology. 2012.

[38] Rubbia-Brandt L, Audard V, Sartoretti P, Roth AD, Brezault C, Le Charpentier M, et al. Severe hepatic sinusoidal obstruction associated with oxaliplatin-based chemotherapy in patients with metastatic colorectal cancer. Ann Oncol. 2004 Mar;15(3): 460-6.

[39] Willmot FC, Robertson GW. Senecio disease, or cirrhosis of the liver due to senecio poisoning. Lancet. 1920;2:848-9.

[40] DeLeve LD, Shulman HM, McDonald GB. Toxic injury to hepatic sinusoids: sinusoidal obstruction syndrome (veno-occlusive disease). Semin Liver Dis. 2002 Feb;22(1): 27-42.

[41] McDonald GB, Hinds MS, Fisher LD, Schoch HG, Wolford JL, Banaji M, et al. Veno-occlusive disease of the liver and multiorgan failure after bone marrow transplantation: a cohort study of 355 patients. Ann Intern Med. 1993 Feb 15;118(4):255-67.

[42] Hasegawa S, Horibe K, Kawabe T, Kato K, Kojima S, Matsuyama T, et al. Veno-occlusive disease of the liver after allogeneic bone marrow transplantation in children with hematologic malignancies: incidence, onset time and risk factors. Bone Marrow Transplant. 1998 Dec;22(12):1191-7.

[43] Rahbari NN, Garden OJ, Padbury R, Brooke-Smith M, Crawford M, Adam R, et al. Posthepatectomy liver failure: A definition and grading by the International Study Group of Liver Surgery (ISGLS). Surgery. 2011 Jan 13.

[44] Mullen JT, Ribero D, Reddy SK, Donadon M, Zorzi D, Gautam S, et al. Hepatic insufficiency and mortality in 1,059 noncirrhotic patients undergoing major hepatectomy. J Am Coll Surg. 2007 May;204(5):854-62; discussion 62-4.

[45] Reissfelder C, Rahbari NN, Koch M, Kofler B, Sutedja N, Elbers H, et al. Postoperative course and clinical significance of biochemical blood tests following hepatic resection. Br J Surg. 2011 Jun;98(6):836-44.

[46] Belghiti J, Hiramatsu K, Benoist S, Massault P, Sauvanet A, Farges O. Seven hundred forty-seven hepatectomies in the 1990s: an update to evaluate the actual risk of liver resection. J Am Coll Surg. 2000 Jul;191(1):38-46.

[47] de Meijer VE, Kalish BT, Puder M, Ijzermans JN. Systematic review and meta-analysis of steatosis as a risk factor in major hepatic resection. Br J Surg. 2010 Sep;97(9): 1331-9.

[48] Soubrane O, Brouquet A, Zalinski S, Terris B, Brezault C, Mallet V, et al. Predicting high grade lesions of sinusoidal obstruction syndrome related to oxaliplatin-based chemotherapy for colorectal liver metastases: Correlation with post-hepatectomy outcome. Annals of Surgery. 2010;251(3):454-60.

[49] Karlo C, Reiner CS, Stolzmann P, Breitenstein S, Marincek B, Weishaupt D, et al. CT- and MRI-based volumetry of resected liver specimen: comparison to intraoperative volume and weight measurements and calculation of conversion factors. Eur J Radiol. 2010 Jul;75(1):e107-11.

[50] Ferrero A, Vigano L, Polastri R, Muratore A, Eminefendic H, Regge D, et al. Postoperative liver dysfunction and future remnant liver: where is the limit? Results of a prospective study. World J Surg. 2007 Aug;31(8):1643-51.

[51] Garden OJ, Rees M, Poston GJ, Mirza D, Saunders M, Ledermann J, et al. Guidelines for resection of colorectal cancer liver metastases. Gut. 2006 Aug;55 Suppl 3:iii1-8.

[52] Kubota K, Makuuchi M, Kusaka K, Kobayashi T, Miki K, Hasegawa K, et al. Measurement of liver volume and hepatic functional reserve as a guide to decision-making in resectional surgery for hepatic tumors. Hepatology. 1997 Nov;26(5):1176-81.

[53] Ryan P, Nanji S, Pollett A, Moore M, Moulton CA, Gallinger S, et al. Chemotherapy-induced liver injury in metastatic colorectal cancer: semiquantitative histologic analysis of 334 resected liver specimens shows that vascular injury but not steatohepatitis is associated with preoperative chemotherapy. American Journal of Surgical Pathology. 2010;34(6):784-91.

[54] Anty R, Iannelli A, Patouraux S, Bonnafous S, Lavallard VJ, Senni-Buratti M, et al. A new composite model including metabolic syndrome, alanine aminotransferase and cytokeratin-18 for the diagnosis of non-alcoholic steatohepatitis in morbidly obese patients. Aliment Pharmacol Ther. Dec;32(11-12):1315-22.

[55] Boza C, Riquelme A, Ibanez L, Duarte I, Norero E, Viviani P, et al. Predictors of non-alcoholic steatohepatitis (NASH) in obese patients undergoing gastric bypass. Obes Surg. 2005 Sep;15(8):1148-53.

[56] Neuschwander-Tetri BA, Clark JM, Bass NM, Van Natta ML, Unalp-Arida A, Tonascia J, et al. Clinical, laboratory and histological associations in adults with nonalcoholic fatty liver disease. Hepatology. Sep;52(3):913-24.

[57] Kishi Y, Zorzi D, Contreras CM, Maru DM, Kopetz S, Ribero D, et al. Extended preoperative chemotherapy does not improve pathologic response and increases postoperative liver insufficiency after hepatic resection for colorectal liver metastases. Annals of Surgical Oncology. 2010;17(11):2870-6.

[58] Aloia T, Sebagh M, Plasse M, Karam V, Levi F, Giacchetti S, et al. Liver histology and surgical outcomes after preoperative chemotherapy with fluorouracil plus oxaliplatin in colorectal cancer liver metastases.[see comment]. Journal of Clinical Oncology. 2006 Nov 1;24(31):4983-90.

[59] Nakano H, Oussoultzoglou E, Rosso E, Casnedi S, Chenard-Neu MP, Dufour P, et al. Sinusoidal injury increases morbidity after major hepatectomy in patients with colorectal liver metastases receiving preoperative chemotherapy. Annals of Surgery. 2008;247(1):118-24.

[60] Overman MJ, Maru DM, Charnsangavej C, Loyer EM, Wang H, Pathak P, et al. Oxaliplatin-mediated increase in spleen size as a biomarker for the development of hepatic sinusoidal injury. Journal of Clinical Oncology. 2010;28(15):2549-55.

[61] Tamandl D, Klinger M, Eipeldauer S, Herberger B, Kaczirek K, Gruenberger B, et al. Sinusoidal obstruction syndrome impairs long-term outcome of colorectal liver metastases treated with resection after neoadjuvant chemotherapy. Ann Surg Oncol. 2011 Feb;18(2):421-30.

[62] Robinson SM, Mann J, Burt AD, Manas DM, Mann DA, White SA. Does a pro-thrombotic environment contribute to the development of chemotherapy associated liver injury in patients with colorectal liver metastases? British Journal of Surgery. 2012;99(S4).

[63] Schwenzer NF, Springer F, Schraml C, Stefan N, Machann J, Schick F. Non-invasive assessment and quantification of liver steatosis by ultrasound, computed tomography and magnetic resonance. J Hepatol. 2009 Sep;51(3):433-45.

[64] Bohte AE, van Werven JR, Bipat S, Stoker J. The diagnostic accuracy of US, CT, MRI and 1H-MRS for the evaluation of hepatic steatosis compared with liver biopsy: a meta-analysis. Eur Radiol. Jan;21(1):87-97.

[65] Robinson PJ. The effects of cancer chemotherapy on liver imaging. Eur Radiol. 2009 Jul;19(7):1752-62.

[66] Cho CS, Curran S, Schwartz LH, Kooby DA, Klimstra DS, Shia J, et al. Preoperative radiographic assessment of hepatic steatosis with histologic correlation. J Am Coll Surg. 2008 Mar;206(3):480-8.

[67] O'Rourke TR, Welsh KFS, Tekkis PP, Mustajab A, John TG, Peppercorn D, et al. Accuracy of liver-specific magnetic resonance imaging as a predictor of chemotherapy-

associated hepatic cellular injury prior to liver resection. European Journal of Surgical Oncology. 2009;35(10):1085-91.

[68] Marsman HA, Van Der Pool AE, Verheij J, Padmos J, Ten Kate FJW, Dwarkasing RS, et al. Hepatic steatosis assessment with CT or MRI in patients with colorectal liver metastases after neoadjuvant chemotherapy. Journal of Surgical Oncology.104(1): 10-6.

[69] Ward J, Guthrie JA, Sheridan MB, Boyes S, Smith JT, Wilson D, et al. Sinusoidal obstructive syndrome diagnosed with superparamagnetic iron oxide-enhanced magnetic resonance imaging in patients with chemotherapy-treated colorectal liver metastases. Journal of Clinical Oncology. 2008;26(26):4304-10.

[70] Shin NY, Kim MJ, Lim JS, Park MS, Chung YE, Choi JY, et al. Accuracy of gadoxetic acid-enhanced magnetic resonance imaging for the diagnosis of sinusoidal obstruction syndrome in patients with chemotherapy-treated colorectal liver metastases. Eur Radiol. Apr;22(4):864-71.

[71] Garcea G, Ong SL, Maddern GJ. Predicting liver failure following major hepatectomy. Dig Liver Dis. 2009 Nov;41(11):798-806.

[72] Imamura H, Sano K, Sugawara Y, Kokudo N, Makuuchi M. Assessment of hepatic reserve for indication of hepatic resection: decision tree incorporating indocyanine green test. J Hepatobiliary Pancreat Surg. 2005;12(1):16-22.

[73] Fan ST, Lai EC, Lo CM, Ng IO, Wong J. Hospital mortality of major hepatectomy for hepatocellular carcinoma associated with cirrhosis. Arch Surg. 1995 Feb;130(2): 198-203.

[74] Seifalian AM, El-Desoky A, Davidson BR. Hepatic indocyanine green uptake and excretion in a rabbit model of steatosis. Eur Surg Res. 2001 May-Jun;33(3):193-201.

[75] Krieger PM, Tamandl D, Herberger B, Faybik P, Fleischmann E, Maresch J, et al. Evaluation of chemotherapy-associated liver injury in patients with colorectal cancer liver metastases using indocyanine green clearance testing. Ann Surg Oncol. Jun; 18(6):1644-50.

[76] Stockmann M, Lock JF, Riecke B, Heyne K, Martus P, Fricke M, et al. Prediction of postoperative outcome after hepatectomy with a new bedside test for maximal liver function capacity. Ann Surg. 2009 Jul;250(1):119-25.

[77] Stockmann M, Lock JF, Malinowski M, Niehues SM, Seehofer D, Neuhaus P. The LiMAx test: a new liver function test for predicting postoperative outcome in liver surgery. HPB (Oxford). Mar;12(2):139-46.

[78] de Graaf W, van Lienden KP, van Gulik TM, Bennink RJ. (99m)Tc-mebrofenin hepatobiliary scintigraphy with SPECT for the assessment of hepatic function and liver functional volume before partial hepatectomy. J Nucl Med. Feb;51(2):229-36.

[79] de Graaf W, van Lienden KP, Dinant S, Roelofs JJ, Busch OR, Gouma DJ, et al. Assessment of future remnant liver function using hepatobiliary scintigraphy in patients undergoing major liver resection. J Gastrointest Surg. Feb;14(2):369-78.

[80] Rous P, Larimore LD. Relation of the Portal Blood to Liver Maintenance : A Demonstration of Liver Atrophy Conditional on Compensation. J Exp Med. 1920 Apr 30;31(5):609-32.

[81] Kinoshita H, Sakai K, Hirohashi K, Igawa S, Yamasaki O, Kubo S. Preoperative portal vein embolization for hepatocellular carcinoma. World J Surg. 1986 Oct;10(5): 803-8.

[82] Makuuchi M, Thai BL, Takayasu K, Takayama T, Kosuge T, Gunven P, et al. Preoperative portal embolization to increase safety of major hepatectomy for hilar bile duct carcinoma: a preliminary report. Surgery. 1990 May;107(5):521-7.

[83] Farges O, Jagot P, Kirstetter P, Marty J, Belghiti J. Prospective assessment of the safety and benefit of laparoscopic liver resections. J Hepatobiliary Pancreat Surg. 2002;9(2):242-8.

[84] Wicherts DA, de Haas RJ, Andreani P, Sotirov D, Salloum C, Castaing D, et al. Impact of portal vein embolization on long-term survival of patients with primarily unresectable colorectal liver metastases. Br J Surg. 2010 Feb;97(2):240-50.

[85] Pamecha V, Glantzounis G, Davies N, Fusai G, Sharma D, Davidson B. Long-term survival and disease recurrence following portal vein embolisation prior to major hepatectomy for colorectal metastases. Ann Surg Oncol. 2009 May;16(5):1202-7.

[86] Denys AL, Abehsera M, Leloutre B, Sauvanet A, Vilgrain V, O'Toole D, et al. Intrahepatic hemodynamic changes following portal vein embolization: a prospective Doppler study. Eur Radiol. 2000;10(11):1703-7.

[87] Archer SG, Gray BN. Vascularization of small liver metastases. Br J Surg. 1989 Jun; 76(6):545-8.

[88] Uemura T, Miyazaki M, Hirai R, Matsumoto H, Ota T, Ohashi R, et al. Different expression of positive and negative regulators of hepatocyte growth in growing and shrinking hepatic lobes after portal vein branch ligation in rats. Int J Mol Med. 2000 Feb;5(2):173-9.

[89] Yokoyama Y, Nagino M, Nimura Y. Mechanisms of hepatic regeneration following portal vein embolization and partial hepatectomy: a review. World J Surg. 2007 Feb; 31(2):367-74.

[90] Jaeck D, Oussoultzoglou E, Rosso E, Greget M, Weber JC, Bachellier P. A two-stage hepatectomy procedure combined with portal vein embolization to achieve curative resection for initially unresectable multiple and bilobar colorectal liver metastases. Ann Surg. 2004 Dec;240(6):1037-49; discussion 49-51.

[91] Wicherts DA, Miller R, de Haas RJ, Bitsakou G, Vibert E, Veilhan LA, et al. Long-term results of two-stage hepatectomy for irresectable colorectal cancer liver metastases. Ann Surg. 2008 Dec;248(6):994-1005.

[92] Narita M, Oussoultzoglou E, Bachellier P, Rosso E, Pessaux P, Jaeck D. Two-stage hepatectomy procedure to treat initially unresectable multiple bilobar colorectal liver metastases: technical aspects. Dig Surg. 2011;28(2):121-6.

[93] Vreuls CP, Van Den Broek MA, Winstanley A, Koek GH, Wisse E, Dejong CH, et al. Hepatic sinusoidal obstruction syndrome (SOS) reduces the effect of oxaliplatin in colorectal liver metastases. Histopathology. May 9.

[94] Rubbia-Brandt L, Tauzin S, Brezault C, Delucinge-Vivier C, Descombes P, Dousset B, et al. Gene expression Profiling Provides Insights into Pathways of Oxaliplatin Related Sinusoidal Obstruction Syndrome in Humans. Mol Cancer Ther. 2011 Feb 17;10(4):687-96.

[95] Rubie C, Frick VO, Ghadjar P, Wagner M, Justinger C, Graeber S, et al. Effect of preoperative FOLFOX chemotherapy on CCL20/CCR6 expression in colorectal liver metastases. World J Gastroenterol. Jul 14;17(26):3109-16.

[96] Brand S, Olszak T, Beigel F, Diebold J, Otte JM, Eichhorst ST, et al. Cell differentiation dependent expressed CCR6 mediates ERK-1/2, SAPK/JNK, and Akt signaling resulting in proliferation and migration of colorectal cancer cells. J Cell Biochem. 2006 Mar 1;97(4):709-23.

[97] Robinson SM, White SA. Hepatic Sinusoidal Obstruction Syndrome (SOS) reduces the effect of Oxaliplatin in colorectal liver metastases. Histopathology. 2012;In Press.

Chapter 18

Liver Tumors in Infancy

Julio C. Wiederkehr, Izabel M. Coelho,
Sylvio G. Avilla, Barbara A. Wiederkehr and
Henrique A. Wiederkehr

Additional information is available at the end of the chapter

http://dx.doi.org/10.5772/51764

1. Introduction

Hepatic tumors in children are relatively rare, accounting for 1 to 4% of all pediatric solid tumors. [1] Primary liver masses constitute the third most common group of solid abdominal tumors of childhood [2] with an incidence of 0.4 to 1.9 per million children each year. [3,4]

Liver masses in children can be malignant, benign, or indeterminate and they are a diverse group of epithelial and mesenchymal tumors whose incidence can vary considerably with patient age. [5] Two thirds of liver tumors in children are malignant. [6] Unlike liver tumors in adults, in which the predominant histology is hepatocellular carcinoma, hepatoblastoma accounts for two thirds of liver tumors in children. [7] Other liver malignancies in children include sarcomas, germ cell tumors, and rhabdoid tumors, as well as the more familiar hepatocellular carcinoma. Benign tumors of the liver in children include vascular tumors, hamartomas, adenomas, and focal nodular hyperplasia. The histology and anatomy of a pediatric liver tumor guides the treatment and prognosis. [8]

In this chapter we outline the epidemiology, etiology, pathology, clinical presentation, diagnosis and management of each of the most important types of liver tumor. Also aspects of the surgical anatomy and resection techniques and other ways to improve ressecability in liver tumors in childhood will be described such as portal vein thrombosis, chemotherapy and transarterial chemoembolization (TACE).

2. Epidemiology

The incidence of hepatic tumors in childhood is consistently quoted from many series as being in the region of 0.5-2.5 per million population [9] and approximately 100–150 new cases of liver tumors are diagnosed in the U.S. annually. [7] Two thirds of liver tumors in children are malignant. [6] acounting for slightly more than 1% of all pediatric malignancies and among those there is a male preponderance of 1.8 : 1. [7,10]

Hepatoblastoma presents in a younger age group, being a uncommon diagnosis over the age of 4 years. Hepatocellular carcinoma has its peak onset in early adolescence, although the range is wide. The older age at onset for hepatocarcinoma may well reflect its close association with other underlying disease processes. [10]

There are several suggestions that the incidence of malignant liver tumors is increasing in the U.S. Surveillance, Epidemiology, and End Results data from 1972–1992 showed a 5% annual increase. [7] Liver cancer represented 2% of all malignancies in infants in the early 1980s with the incidence doubling to 4% 10 years later. [11]

At a population level, there has been a dramatic increase in survival in countries in which a modern health system has been implemented, although the increased survival is lower for hepatocarcinoma in comparison with hepatoblastomas. [10] According to Litten & Tomlinson [8], it has been suggested that the improvements in technology, care, and outcomes for premature infants have been driving forces in the increase of the incidence in hepatic tumors. Hepatoblastoma is more commonly diagnosed in children with a history of prematurity than in full-term infants. Interestingly, those tumors that arise in ex-premature infants do not present at a younger age than those of term infants. [8]

3. Hepatoblastoma

Hepatoblastoma is the most common malignant tumor of the liver in children and is an embryonal tumor in the classic sense of incomplete differentiation; [12] accounts for 1% of all pediatric malignancies and for 79% of all liver cancers in children under age. [13] Its overall incidence is 0.5–1.5 per million, however the incidence in children under the age of 18 months is 11.2 cases per million. [14]

Hepatoblastoma is diagnosed in very young children with a peak in the newborn period reflecting those tumors that developed prenatally, and an overall median age at diagnosis of 18 months; 90 percent of cases are manifest by the fourth birthday, several have been present at birth, and there is an hypothesized association with prematurity. [15] Only 5% of new hepatoblastoma cases are diagnosed in children >4 years of age. [8]

The increased incidence of HB in children born before 28 weeks gestation (with birth weight <1500 g) compared with term gestations, may be explained by the exposure of rapidly dividing hepatoblasts to endogenous metabolites and hormones as well as exogenous chemicals that would normally be eliminated via the placenta. Inefficiency and compromise of the immature detoxification mechanisms could produce multiple somatic mutations and epigenetic (ie, methylation) modifications of the genome. [16, 17]

For poorly understood reasons, hepatoblastoma occurs in males significantly more frequently than it does in females with a male:female ratio that ranges from 1.2 to 3.6:1. [14] Most commonly, these tumors present in the right lobe of the liver. [18] There is an increased incidence of hepatoblastoma in Beckwith-Wiedemann Syndrome, which has a relative risk of 2280 suggesting a role for genetic aberrations of chromosome 11 in the pathogenesis of hepatoblastoma,[19, 20] hemihypertrophy, and familial adenomatous polyposis (FAP) witch has a relative risk of 1220 suggesting a role for aberrations of chromosome 5 in the pathogenesis. [21] Screening for cases in FAP kindred families is recommended by testing for germline mutations in the APC tumor suppressor gene. [22, 23] Inactivation of the APC tumor-suppressor gene (found on chromosome 5) is found in 67–89% of sporadic hepatoblastoma [24, 25] This gene is known to regulate B-catenin and modulate the wnt signaling pathway, suggesting a role for this signaling pathway in the development of hepatoblastoma. [26] Additional biologic markers may include Trisomy 2, 8, and 20 and translocation of the NOTCH2 gene on chromosome 1. [27]

Many etiological factors have been linked with the development of malignant hepatic tumors in childhood (Table 1). Broadly speaking, genetic influences are particularly important in the development of hepatoblastoma, whereas environmental factors and coexisting liver disease are strongly associated with hepatocellular carcinoma. [10]

Hepatoblastoma	Hepatocellular carcinoma
Beckwith-Wiedemann Syndrome	Hepatitis B
Hemihypertrophy	Hepatitis C
Familial adenomatous polyposis (FAP)	Hereditary tyrosinemia
	α_1-Antitrypsin deficiency
Gardner syndrome	Cirrhosis secondary to biliary atresia
Glycogen storage disease type I	Glycogen storage disease type I
Trisomy 18	Neurofibromatosis
Fetal alcohol syndrome	
Prematurity and low birth weight	Familial adenomatous polyposis
Maternal exposure to:	Drug/toxin exposure:
Oral contraceptives	Androgens
Gonadotropins	Oral contraceptives
Metals	Methotrexate
Petroleum products	Aflatoxins
Paints and pigments	
Paternal exposure to:	Fanconi anemia
Metals	
Meckel diverticulum	

Table 1. Conditions associated with hepatoblastoma and hepatocellular carcinoma.

Hepatoblastomas are composed of cells resembling the developing fetal and embryonic liver, hence the classification as an embryonal tumor. Indeed, the cells comprising hepatoblastoma mark similarly to hepatic stem cells, defined as pluripotent hepatoblasts capable of differentiating into hepatocytes or cholangiocytes. [28, 29]

According to the Childhood Epithelial Liver Tumors – International Criteria (CELTIC) group, the pathology of hepatoblastoma is classified into four groups based on the work of Weinberg and Finegold: fetal, embryonal, macrotrabecular and small-cell undifferentiated. [10]

Histologically, these tumors can be divided into epithelial (56%) or mixed epithelial/ mesenchymal tissue. The epithelial group is further subdivided into fetal (31%), embryonal (19%), macrotrabecular (3%) and small-cell undifferentiated subtypes (3%). Themajority of hepatoblastomas is epithelial and consist of a mixture of embryonal and fetal cell types (Fig. 1). [8, 30]

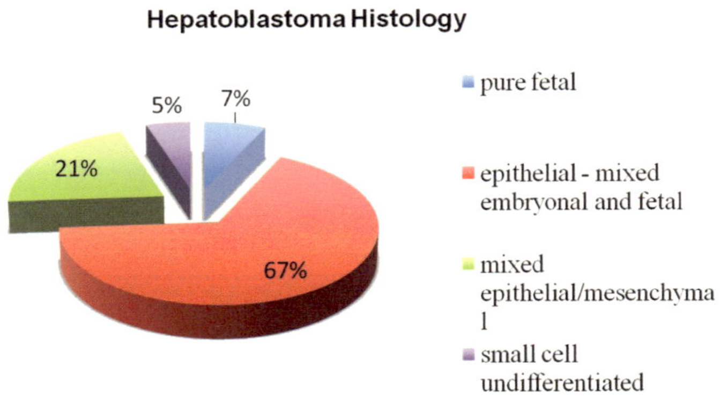

Figure 1. Distribution of histologic subtypes of hepatoblastoma. The majority are epithelial and consist of embryonal and fetal cell types. Pure fetal histology accounts for approximately 7% of hepatoblastomas and is associated with a favorable prognosis. Small cell undifferentiated hepatoblastoma accounts for 5% of hepatoblastoma cases and is associated with a poor prognosis. [8]

Of the five histologic subtypes—pure fetal, embryonal, mixed epithelial, mesenchymal/ macrotrabecular, and small cell undifferentiated—fetal carries the most favorable prognosis. [31] Approximately 5% of hepatoblastomas are of the small cell undifferentiated subtype. This subtype is associated with a worse prognosis. [32] In the mixed epithelial/ mesenchymal type, the presence of mesenchymal elements is associated with improved prognosis and the most common mesenchymal elements are cartilage and osteoid. [33]

Hepatoblastomas usually presents as a palpable asymptomatic mass with abdominal distension. [10] Less common presentations include weight loss, anorexia, emesis and abdominal pain and usually indicate advanced disease. [34] One of the more unusual presenting features of hepatoblastoma is its association with sexual precocity due to the release of human chorionic gonadotropic hormone (β-HCG) by the tumor. Osteoporosis is said to occur in up to 20% of the cases and when severe can lead to bone fractures and vertebral compression. [35] The tumor may rupture spontaneously, producing an acute abdomen and hemoperitoneum. [10]

Approximately 90% of patients demonstrate elevated serum AFP levels and there is a correlation between AFP levels and extent of disease. [36]

The right lobe of the liver is most commonly involved with disease but in 35% of patients there is bilateral disease. [37] Distant metastasis are present in 20% of patients at the time of diagnosis with the lung being the most common site of metastasis; other common sites are the brain and bone and metastasis occur more commonly with disease relapse. [38]

	Hepatoblastoma (%)	Hepatocellular carcinoma (%)
Abdominal mass	71	58
Weight loss	24	21
Anorexia	22	22
Pain	18	16
Vomiting	13	10
Jaundice	7	10

Table 2. Signs and symptoms of liver tumors in children. [10]

Overall, the diagnosis is based on laboratory tests (such as full blood count, liver function tests, α-Fetoprotein – AFP and other markers), imaging (abdominal radiography, ultrasonography, computer tomography, magnetic resonance imaging, hepatic angiography, chest radiography and positron-emission tomography – PET) and biopsy.

The full blood count can reveal anemia (usually normocytic, normochromic) in at least 50% of children with hepatoblastoma. [13, 39] The platelet count is also often abnormal with up to one-third of patients demonstrating thrombocytosis and fewer patients having thrombocytopenia. Thrombocytosis is thought to be related to increased levels of circulating thrombopoietin. [40]

Liver function tests are commonly normal in hepatoblastoma. [10] The serum alpha-fetoprotein (AFP) level is elevated in 90% of children with hepatoblastoma and tumors that fail to express AFP at diagnosis are felt to be biologically more aggressive. [41, 42] AFP levels must be interpreted with caution because AFP is commonly elevated in normal neonates up to 6 months of age and may be slightly elevated in other tumors, as well as after hepatic damage or during regeneration of liver parenchyma.

The imaging study is important in evaluation liver neoplasms. CT, MRI and ultrasound are the most commonly used modalities for pediatric doctors in their medical researches as well as their clinical practice. Ultrasound is accepted as a first-line imaging method because of its less irradiation, greater convenience and better real-time. [43] Ultrasound is extremely valuable in detecting much smaller lesions, especially in detecting fluid and blood-flow in a lesion, and it also can evaluate the hepatic vascular anatomy.[44] As a rule, the initial diagnosis of live tumor is usually made by the abdominal ultrasound examination, which will identify the liver as the organ of origin. Hepatoblastoma are seen as a hyperechoic, solid, intrahepatic mass on US. [45]

Both CT and MRI define the extent of tumor involvement showing its segmental extension and its proximity to the portal vein, to help determine the resectability. Evaluation with CT demonstrates a delineated hypoattentuated mass compared with the surrounding normal tissue and allows identification of calcifications. [46] The use of contrast allows assessment of vascular involvement by the tumor. Combined MRI and contrast enhanced MR-angiography gives the best evaluation of the vascular structures and the tumor blood supply, and this best enables the planning of a resection. A diagnostic biopsy is recommended in all children with a suspected hepatoblastoma. Given the potential side effects of chemotherapy, it is not a good clinical practice to start therapy in a patient in the absence of a tissue diagnosis. Additionally, it is necessary to rule out HCC. Although it is rare, HCC have been reported in children under the age of three and they carry a worse prognosis. [47]

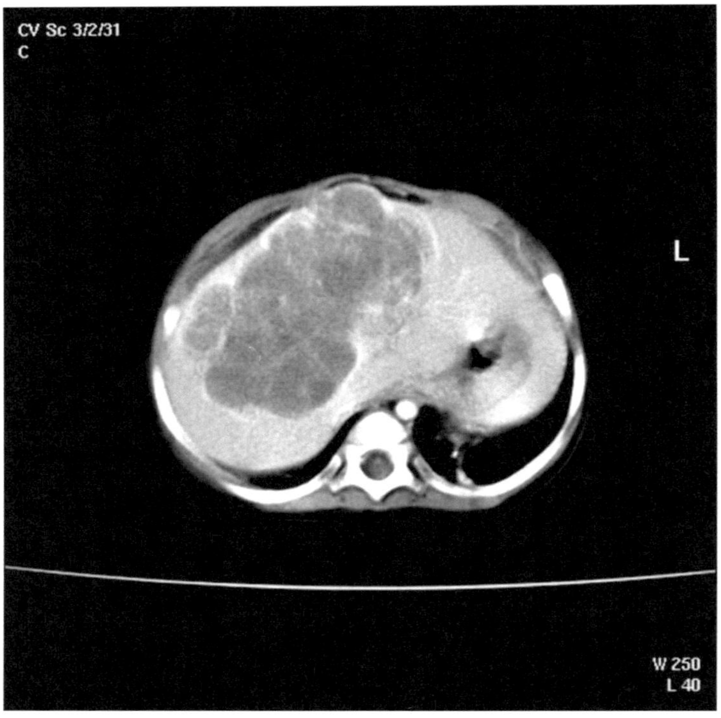

Figure 2. CT scan of an infant with a large central hepatoblastoma.

Large multinodular expansile masses, hepatoblastomas radiographically appear well demarcated from the normal liver but are not encapsulated. They may invade hepatic veins, disseminate to the lungs, or penetrate the liver capsule to reach contiguous tissues. [12]

Historically, North Americans have staged liver tumors similar to other solid tumors, staging system continues to be used by the children's oncology group (COG) and depends upon extent of surgery at the time of initial diagnosis.

http://dx.doi.org/10.5772/51764

Relative number of patients presenting in each stage in the COG trial 9645 (1999–2003) is as follows: Stage I (22%) indicates complete resection at diagnosis, Stage II (0.5%) microscopic residual after attempted complete resection at diagnosis, Stage III (53%) biopsy at diagnosis with gross residual tumor, and Stage IV (23%) metastatic disease at diagnosis.[48, 49] The traditional COG staging system has been criticized for being rather subjective, depending to a large extent on the surgeon rather than the tumor.[12, 50] To address this concern specific surgical guidelines have been proposed by the COG liver tumor committee which define the anatomic and biologic characteristics of a tumor for which resection at diagnosis is recommended. In addition the upcoming COG hepatoblastoma (AHEP 0731) protocol will add a risk-based stratification of treatment as follows: low risk (Stage I/II lacking any unfavorable biologic feature); intermediate risk (Stage III or Stage I/II with small cell undifferentiated histology); and high risk (Stage IV or Stage I/II/III with AFP <100 at diagnosis). [12]

3.1. Stage Information

There are two standard surgical staging systems for pediatric liver tumors. The Childhood Liver Tumour Strategy Group (SIOPEL) uses a presurgical-based staging system, while the Children's Oncology Group (COG) uses a postsurgical-based staging system. The staging systems support different treatment strategies. The presurgical staging system is used with neoadjuvant chemotherapy followed by definitive surgery (with the exception of Pretreatment Extent of Disease [PRETEXT] stage 1), while the postsurgical staging system has surgery as the initial strategy.

Both systems are used in the United States. In a retrospective comparison of the two staging systems at diagnosis using data from patients entered on a North American randomized trial, both staging systems predicted outcome. The presurgical PRETEXT staging system may add prognostic information for patients staged postsurgically at stage 3. [51] The COG is investigating the use of PRETEXT stage before and after chemotherapy to determine the optimal surgical approach. [52]

3.2. Presurgical Staging for Hepatoblastoma and Hepatocellular Carcinoma

The PRETEXT staging system for hepatoblastoma categorizes the primary tumor based on extent of liver involvement at diagnosis. The staging system was devised for use in an international hepatoblastoma treatment program in which only children with PRETEXT stage 1 hepatoblastoma undergo initial resection of tumor. All others are treated with chemotherapy prior to attempted resection of the primary tumor. The liver tumors are staged by interpretation of computerized tomography or ultrasound with or without additional imaging by magnetic resonance. The presence or absence of metastases is noted in addition to the PRETEXT stage, but does not alter the PRETEXT stage. Tumor involvement of the vena cava, hepatic veins, and portal vein, and extrahepatic extension are also noted.

The imaged liver is divided into four quadrants and involvement of each quadrant with tumor is determined. Stage increases and prognosis decreases as the number of quadrants radiologically involved with tumor increases from one to four. [53, 50] Experienced radiologist review is important because it may be difficult to discriminate between real invasion beyond the anatomic border of a given sector and displacement of the anatomic border. [50, 43]

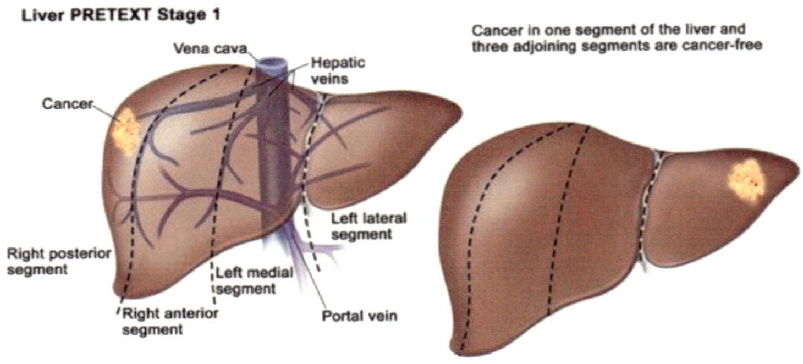

Figure 3. Pretext stage 1 - Tumor involves only one quadrant; three adjoining liver quadrants are free of tumor. [http://www.cancer.gov/PublishedContent/MediaLinks/308970.html]

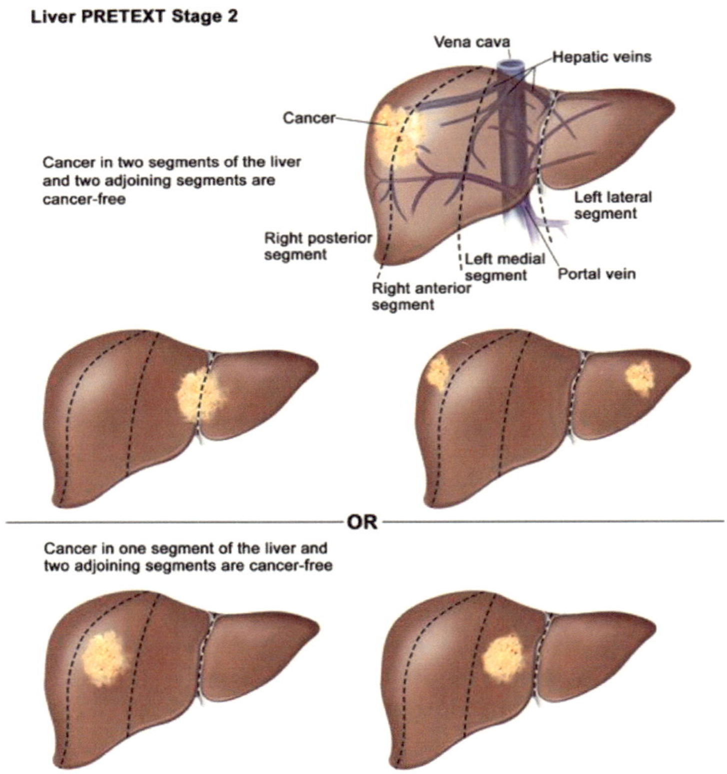

Figure 4. Pretext stage 2 - Tumor involves one or two quadrants; two adjoining quadrants are free of tumor. [http://www.cancer.gov/PublishedContent/MediaLinks/308970.html]

http://dx.doi.org/10.5772/51764

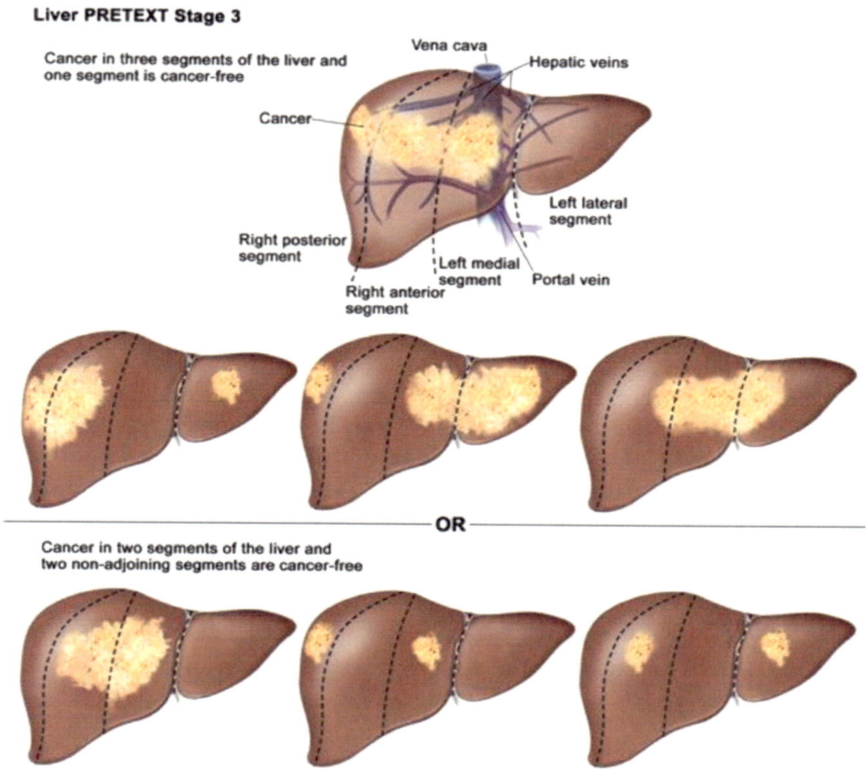

Figure 5. Pretext stage 3 - Tumor involves three quadrants and one quadrant is free of tumor or tumor involves two quadrants and two nonadjoining quadrants are free of tumor. [http://www.cancer.gov/PublishedContent/MediaLinks/308970.html]

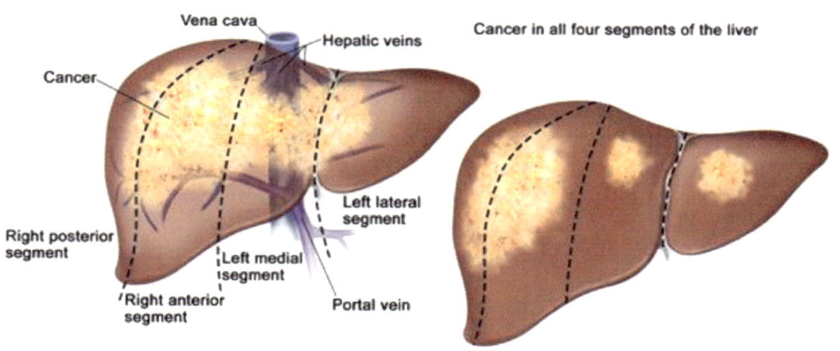

Figure 6. Pretext stage 4 - Tumor involves all four quadrants; there is no quadrant free of tumor. [http://www.cancer.gov/PublishedContent/MediaLinks/308970.html]

3.3. Treatment - Chemotherapy

During the past 30 years, there has been an improved survival for patients with HB based on refinements in surgical techniques, a better understanding of the hepatic segmental anatomy, advances in chemotherapy, and the advent of liver transplantation as a therapeutic modality for patients with unresectable disease. HB is a surgical neoplasm and only complete tumor resection results in a realistic hope for cure. Long-term disappearance of tumor with complete remission with chemotherapy alone has been anecdotally observed. However, chemotherapy is a cornerstone in the management of HB. [55]

Although chemosensitivity varies between patients, it is an essential component of the management and complementary to radical surgical resection to affect a cure. In general, surgeons agree that preoperative chemotherapy helps to reduce the size of most tumors and obtains better demarcation between the tumor and surrounding liver tissue. [56, 57, 58] Consequently, tumors are more likely to be completely resected without increasing perioperative morbidity or mortality. It is also speculated that residual microscopic disease may behave more aggressively under the influence of hepatotrophic factors stimulating liver regeneration if preoperative chemotherapy has not been used. [58] On the other hand, von Schweinitz et al. [59] have shown that there is little to be gained from prolonging chemotherapy beyond the planned treatment regimen, which incurs the risk of developing chemoresistance. [55]

Even if unresectable at diagnosis, most hepatoblastomas are unifocal and chemosensitive, especially to "platinum" derivative chemotherapeutic agents. With the routine addition of cisplatin to the chemotherapy in the late 1980s, overall survival in hepatoblastoma increased from 30% to 70%. [60, 61] Twenty years later, cisplatin remains the backbone of the chemotherapy regimen. In current trials by COG (America), SIOPEL (Europe, South America), GPOH (German), and JPLT (Japan) chemotherapeutic agents used in combination with cisplatin have differed slightly. Although most use some form of doxorubicin, COG currently recommends Cisplatin/5FU/Vincristin (C5V) for low-risk tumors, C5V+Doxorubicin for intermediate risk, and hopes to investigate new agents with up-front window therapy in high-risk tumors. [48, 49] Irinotectan, with or without doxorubicin, has been used in both America and Europe for patients with relapse. [62] Because tumor cells may become resistant to chemotherapy over prolonged exposure [63] and because cumulative chemotherapy toxicity may be unwarranted, prolonged (44 cycles) courses of neoadjuvant chemotherapy are discouraged by all study groups. Early referral for complex surgical planning may be indicated for large invasive tumors potentially requiring transplantation. [12]

Two principle strategies exist. In the United States, tumor resection at diagnosis, whenever prudently possible, has been advocated with the argument that toxicity of chemotherapy can be reduced by avoidance of unnecessary neoadjuvant chemotherapy, that some tumors may become resistant to prolonged courses of chemotherapy [64] and the highest survival rates have historically been observed in patients with initially resected tumors—although these tumors also tend to be the smaller more favorable tumors. Proposed COG Surgical guidelines advocate definitive surgical resection at diagnosis for localized, unifocal PRETEXT I and II tumors followed by chemotherapy. When the tumor is large (PRETEXT III or IV), multicentric, shows radiographic evidence of portal or hepatic venous invasion, or pulmonary metastatic lesions the chance of curative resection may be improved neoadjuvant chemotherapy and delayed primary resection. Alternatively, the SIOPEL study group discourages resection of hepatoblastoma at diagnosis favoring neoadjuvant chemotherapy in all patients with the argument that the chemotherapy renders most tumors smaller, better demarcated, and more likely to be completely resected, and that the toxicity of neoadjuvant chemotherapy is offset by the increased rates of surgical resectability. Both COG and SIOPEL have invested considerable effort in attempts to decrease the significant ototoxiciy attendant to the use of cisplatin based chemotherapy in young infants and toddlers. [12]

In the Intergroup Hepatoblastoma/ Hepatocellular Carcinoma Study, 28% of HB tumors were completely resected at diagnosis (Stage I) and 4% (Stage II) were incompletely excised. These patients had a 91% and 100% 5-year survival, respectively. However, the surgical guidelines of the protocol lacked clear recommendations regarding which tumor should or should not be resected at diagnosis. The study compared the use of cisplatin and doxorubicin in one treatment arm to cisplatin, vincristine, and 5-fluorouracil (5-FU) in the other arm. The overall 3- year survival rates were 63% and 71%, respectively. [65] Although the difference between the groups was not significant, the cisplatin/ doxorubicin group had a higher toxicity rate. A significant response to preoperative chemotherapy was observed in Stage III patients allowing complete tumor resection in 70–80% of these cases. Pre-operative chemotherapy had no effect on operative mortality; however, increased transfusion requirement and a higher operative morbidity was observed in patients that received chemotherapy preoperatively. [55]

The studies coordinated by the SIOPEL group have concentrated on using preoperative chemotherapy. [56, 66] In SIOPEL-1, all patients were treated preoperatively with four courses of cisplatin and doxorubicin (PLADO); surgical resection was followed by two more courses of chemotherapy. If the tumor was judged unresectable by imaging after four courses of chemotherapy, attempting surgical resection was delayed until after the sixth course. If the tumor remained localized to the liver but was still unresectable, liver transplantation was recommended as the primary operative procedure if some response to chemotherapy had been obtained in the absence of extrahepatic tumor extent or metastatic disease. The SIOPEL-2 pilot study [67]was designed to test the efficacy and toxicity of two chemotherapy regimens, one for patients with HB confined to the liver and involving no more then three hepatic sections "standard-risk (SR) HB", and one for instances of HB extending into all four sections and/or with lung metastases or intra-abdominal extrahepatic spread or tumor rupture at presentation or with serum AFP < 100 units at presentation "high-risk (HR) HB". Those with SR-HB were treated with four courses of cisplatin monotherapy, delayed surgery, and then two more courses of cisplatin. Patients with HR-HB were given cisplatin alternating with carboplatin and doxorubicin, pre- and postoperatively. For SR-HB patients (n = 77), and HR-HB patients (n = 58), the 3-year progression-free survival rates were 89% and 48%, respectively. For SR-HB patients, the efficacy of cisplatin monotherapy and the cisplatin/doxorubicin combination are now being compared in a prospective randomized trial (SIOPEL-3 study). For HR-HB patients, intensified chemotherapy with cisplatin, doxorubicin, and carboplatin is being investigated in a SIOPEL-4 study. [55]

In unifocal HB, PRETEXT grouping based on imaging studies at diagnosis in some cases may lead to overstaging the tumor from PRETEXT III to PRETEXT IV when the anatomic border separating a lateral section from the sections of the liver harboring the bulging mass is simply displaced (due to compression) but not invaded. [56, 68] Indeed, repeat imaging studies after chemotherapy, when the tumor has shrunken, can demonstrate that the anatomic border is free from invasion and allow for correct staging and performance of a partial hepatectomy (right or left trisegmentectomy). In multifocal HB with lesions scattered in the different sections of the liver, clearance of one section, (e.g. the left lateral section) [69] can apparently be achieved by chemotherapy in some cases, tempting the surgeon to perform a partial rather than a total hepatectomy. However, this strategy is not recommended because of the high-risk of leaving viable malignant tumor cells in the remaining section. Therefore, in multifocal hepatoblastoma, liver transplantation is the best treatment option, whatever the apparent result of chemotherapy. Further intensification of chemotherapy when the response to completion of full courses of chemotherapy according to protocol is considered unsatisfactory, and hazardous attempts at partial liver resection in order to avoid liver transplantation "at any cost" are no longer justified since the efficacy of primary liver transplantation for unresectable HB has been validated during the last decade. [55]

Even patients presenting with metastatic disease are potentially curable with a combination of chemotherapy, complete tumor resection by partial hepatectomy or transplantation, and pulmonary metastasectomy. The role of pulmonary metastasectomy has yet to be clearly defined, although it appears that surgical resection of lung deposits may be more likely to cure patients with disease present at diagnosis but persistent after neoadjuvant therapy rather than patients with pulmonary relapse. [12] Data from the most recent COG study, 9645, show 3-year event-free survival of 90% for Stage I–II, 50% for Stage III, and only 20% for Stage IV (Malogolowkin et al., 2007). In the European SIOPEL II 3-year survival for standard risk tumors was 90% and for high-risk tumors was 50%. Cure from hepatoblastoma mandates a complete gross resection of the primary tumor at some point during the treatment regimen. [12]

3.4. Surgical resection

The objective of the surgical procedure is to obtain a complete resection of the tumor, both macro- and microscopically, which is paramount for cure of HB (and other liver cancers). The surgical strategy should be based on a sound knowledge of segmental liver anatomy as described by Couinaud, [70] vascular occlusion techniques and expertise in performing the different types of liver resections, including the most extensive procedures (left or right trisegmentectomies). Intraoperative ultrasound is useful in confirming the location of major vessels and other structures. Nonanatomical, atypical resections are best avoided, except in rare cases (i.e., pedunculated tumor), because of an increased risk of incomplete tumor removal and a higher incidence of postoperative complications. [58] Very extensive liver resections (up to 80% of the liver mass) can be tolerated by young children with HB and hepatic regeneration can be complete within 3 months, despite the administration of toxic agents since they usually have no underlying liver disease and excellent hepatic reserve. [71] Liver function rapidly returns to normal without long-term sequelae. Complete tumor resection can be easily achieved with a partial hepatectomy when the intrahepatic extent is limited to one or two sections (PRETEXT I and II). When the tumor involves three sections (PRETEXT III), preoperative neoadjuvant chemotherapy can make lesions initially considered "unresectable" become resectable with a trisegmentectomy. [55]

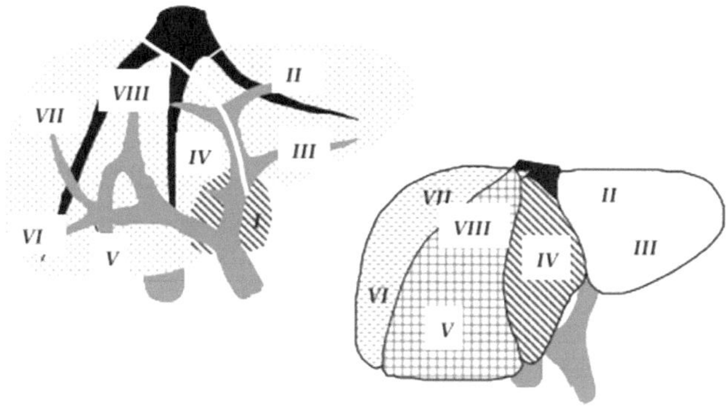

Figure 7. Couinaud's liver segmentation.

In centrally located HB, resection of Couinaud's segments 4, 5 and 8 ("central hepatectomy") can occasionally be performed by expert hands. When an accessory right hepatic vein of appropriate size is present to drain remaining segments 5–7, subtotal hepatectomy removing segments 1–4 and 8 can be successfully performed. [55]

3.5. Liver transplantation

A growing experience with liver transplantation has shown that liver transplant is a good treatment option in children with unresectable primary tumors and without demonstrable metastatic disease after neoadjuvant chemotherapy and pulmonary metastasectomy if necessary. In large solitary, and especially multifocal, hepatoblastomas invading all four sectors of the liver, transplantation has resulted in long-term disease free survival in up to 80% of children. [73] While most agree that "extreme" resection of tumors without liver transplant will avoid the need for long-term immunosuppressive therapy, hazardous attempts at partial hepatectomy in children with major venous involvement or with extensive multifocal tumors should be discouraged. [56, 69, 74, 75, 76] Extensive hepatic surgery in children should be carried out in centers that have a facility for liver transplant, where surgical expertise, as well as willingness to embark on more radical surgery with a transplant "safety net" is likely to be greater. [76]

Previous studies have validated the concept of total hepatectomy and primary orthotopic liver transplantation (OLT) for unresectable HB. In SIOPEL-1, [77] 12 patients (8% of all patients enrolled from 1990 to 1994) underwent liver transplantation as the primary surgical option (after appropriate preoperative chemotherapy) in seven children, and as a rescue procedure in five children because of incomplete partial resection or tumor relapse after partial hepatectomy. The long-term, disease-free patient survival was 66% for the entire series and 85% and 40% for primary transplants and rescue transplants, respectively. Current follow up is >10 years for all patients. All eight patients with PRETEXT IV tumors and all six patients with multifocal HB were cured of their disease. Of the seven patients with macroscopic extension into the portal vein and/or the hepatic veins/vena cava, 71% became long-term, disease-free survivors, as well as four of five (80%) children who had lung metastases at presentation with complete clearance of lung lesions after chemotherapy. [55]

An extensive review of the world experience collected 147 cases of liver transplantation for HB. [77] Data were contributed by 24 centers (12 in North America, 10 in Europe, 1 in Japan and Australia each). Twenty-eight (19% of the total) patients presented with macroscopic venous extension and 12 (8%) with lung metastases. A total of 106 patients (72%) underwent a primary transplant and 41 (28%) received a rescue transplant, either for incomplete resection with partial hepatectomy or for tumor relapse after previous partial hepatectomy. Twenty-eight (19%) received a live, donor-related liver transplant, and 119 (81%) received a deceased donor liver graft. Median follow up since diagnosis for surviving patients was 38 months (range 1– 121 months). Overall disease-free survival at 6 years post-transplant was 82% and 30% for primary transplants and for rescue transplants, respectively. Multivariate statistical analysis showed no difference in regard to gender, age, and lung metastases at presentation or type of transplant. For primary transplants, the only parameter significantly related to overall survival was macroscopic venous invasion ($P = 0.045$). Remarkably, the 6-year, disease-free survival (82%) for the 106 patients who received a primary transplant was similar to the 3-year, progression-free survival (89%) for the 77 HB patients with standard-risk hepatoblastoma confined to the liver and involving no more than 3 hepatic sections that were enrolled in the SIOPEL-2 study. [67] In a recent review of the UNOS database in the USA concerning liver transplantation in 135 children transplanted for unresectable or recurrent HB (1987–2004), the one, five, and 10-year survival was 79%, 69%, and 66% respectively. [78] The median age at transplantation was 2.9 ± 2.5 years. Sixteen percent received a graft from a live donor. Fifty-five percent of the deaths were due to metastases or recurrent disease. The latest ELTR report, including 129 patients transplanted for HB has shown a 1- and 5-year survival of 100% and 74%, respectively. [55, 79]

3.6. Timing of transplantation

Timing of liver transplantation should not be delayed in excess of a few weeks after the last course of chemotherapy (as per protocol). An expeditious access to organ donors is required to meet this requirement. If this is not possible with deceased donors (including split liver grafts), a live-related donor is a valuable option. [55]

According to the results of published studies, the following guidelines have been developed for early consultation with a transplant surgeon: [55]

1. Multifocal PRETEXT IV HB is a clear and undisputed indication for primary liver transplantation, whatever the result of chemotherapy. Apparent clearance of one liver lobe should not distract from this guideline because of the high probability of persistent microscopic viable neoplastic cells. Pediatric oncologists should resist the temptation to in-

tensify chemotherapy in a vain effort to avoid transplantation. These patients should be treated within the same protocol as patients with localized tumors amenable to partial hepatectomy, with as many cycles of chemotherapy before and after transplantation as patients submitted to partial hepatectomy for a localized HB.

2. Primary liver transplantation may be the best option for large, solitary PRETEXT IV HB, involving all four sections of the liver, unless tumor downstaging is clearly demonstrated after initial chemotherapy. If this is the case, a clear retraction of the tumor from the anatomic border of one lateral sector would allow performance of a radical trisegmentectomy.

3. Unifocal, centrally located PRETEXT II and III tumors involving main hilar structures or all three main hepatic veins should be considered for primary liver transplantation because these venous structures would presumably not become free of tumor after chemotherapy. Heroic attempts at partial hepatectomy would be best avoided because of the risk of incomplete resection of malignant tissue.

3.7. Contraindications

Persistence of viable extrahepatic tumor deposit after chemotherapy, not amenable to surgical resection, is the only absolute contraindication for liver transplantation. Macroscopic venous invasion (portal vein, hepatic veins, vena cava) is not a contraindication if complete resection of the invaded venous structures can be accomplished. When there is evidence or suspicion of invasion of the retrohepatic vena cava, it should be resected "en-bloc" and reconstructed. Review of the world experience showed that venous extent was associated with a significantly shorter survival (P = 0.045). [77] Of the nine TNM IV A/IVB patients (eight with major intrahepatic venous invasion) reported by Reyes and associates, seven were alive and disease-free 21–146 months after transplantation. [80]

Patients with lung metastases at presentation should not be excluded from liver transplantation if the metastases clear completely after chemotherapy and/or surgical resection. Long-term, disease-free survival was obtained in 80% of such patients in the SIOPEL-l study and 58% in the world experience. Complete eradication of metastatic lesions by chemotherapy and surgical resection of any suspicious remnant after chemotherapy is a paramount pre-requisite for transplantation. [81] When tumor resection by partial hepatectomy is incomplete or when intrahepatic relapse is observed after a previous partial hepatectomy, performing a rescue liver transplantation may be a relative contraindication because of the disappointing results observed in the SIOPEL-l study and in the reported world experience. [55]

3.8. Outcomes

In experienced surgical units, major intraoperative complications of liver resection for HB such as severe bleeding, air embolism, and unrecognized bile duct injury are infrequent and operative mortality is very low, even after extended hepatectomies, since children with HB have no underlying liver disease. As an example, summarizes the 25 years (1978–2003) of experience gained at Cliniques Saint-Luc, Brussels [82] with 53 children treated for HB.

There were 39 partial hepatectomies, including 23 right or left trisegmentectomies, and 13 primary liver transplants (two from deceased donors and 11 from living related donors). Only one child died from surgical complications (extensive portal vein thrombosis present at diagnosis). Postoperative bleeding requiring reoperation was encountered in 2 patients (3.5%). The incidence of biliary complications was 7.6% after partial hepatectomy and 23% following liver transplantation. Actuarial disease-free survival was 89% and 79% in transplant patients and in children treated with partial hepatectomy, respectively. [55]

Although individual centers treat relatively small numbers of patients with liver cancer, the best overall survival rates are obtained in experienced units that include liver transplantation in their surgical armamentarium. [55, 83, 84, 85]

The most recent report from King's college, London [86] confirms that the modern strategy of combining chemotherapy and radical tumor resection enables the majority of children with HB to be cured. From October 1993 to February 2007, 25 liver transplantations were performed for HB: 18 from deceased donors and 7 from living donors. Fifteen and ten patients were PRETEXT IV and III, respectively. All patients received preoperative chemotherapy following the successive SIOPEL protocols. Patient and graft survival after cadaveric transplantation was 91%, 77.6% and 77.6% after 1, 5 and 10 years, respectively, without retransplantation. Patient and graft survival after living related liver transplantation was 100%, 83.3% and 83.3%, respectively. All surviving children but one remain disease-free, with a median follow up of 6.8 years (range: 0.9–14.9). There were five deaths at a median of 13 months post-OLT, secondary to tumor recurrence in 4 and respiratoryfailure in one. [55]

A remote data entry system is accessible online, worldwide, and free of charge. Registration is open for patients transplanted since January 1st, 2006 (http://www.pluto.cineca.org). PLUTO stands for Pediatric Liver Unresectable Tumor Observatory and was developed by the SIOPEL strategy group. This will allow online registration of children undergoing liver transplantation for a malignant liver tumor. The aim is to establish an international multicenter database with prospective registration of children (<18 years) presenting with unresectable tumor (HB, HCC, epithelioid hemangioendothelioma and other rare malignant tumors) undergoing primary orrescue liver transplantation.

4. Hepatocellular carcinoma

Hepatocellular carcinoma (HCC) in childhood is rare and accounts for less than 0.5% of all pediatric malignancies, [87, 88] is the second most common malignant hepatic neoplasm in children. HCC presents at an older age than does hepatoblastoma, with most HCC cases diagnosed in children older than 5 years. [89] Its relative frequency is 0.5 to 1.0 cases per million children. It is more frequently encountered in older children and teenagers than in infants. [88,90] HCC is more often encountered in males and older children between age 10 and 14 yr and the median age of onset is 12 year. [88]

Previous reports from Southeast Asia cite an annual incidence of pediatric hepatic tumors that is roughly four times higher than western reports in children with less than 15 years of age. [91] This finding is largely based on the high hepatitis carrier rate, with a Taiwanese report stating that 80% of primary liver tumors in children were hepatocellular carcinoma. With the introduction of hepatitis B vaccine in Southeast Asia, however, there has been a marked reduction in the incidence of hepatocellular carcinoma, although the impact of the hepatitis B vaccine has mainly reduced the incidence of liver tumors in males. [92] Occasionally, malignant tumors in children are seen with features of both hepatocellular carcinoma and hepatoblastoma. These tumors are more common in children with a diagnosis at later ages than that typical of hepatoblastoma.

There is an association with pediatric HCC and pre-existing liver cirrhosis, most often because of biliary atresia, Fanconi's syndrome, and hepatitis B. However, most pediatric HCC are de novo tumors and are not necessarily related to cirrhosis. [75] In certain metabolic diseases such as hereditary tyrosinemia and glycogen storage disease type IA, there is an increased incidence of HCC. Hereditary tyrosinemia, caused by a deficiency in fumarylacetoacetate hydrolase, results in a greatly increased susceptibility to HCC. This is because of the accumulation of toxic metabolites in the liver, and the incidence of HCC is 50% by age two. Current medical therapies for tyrosinemia markedly reduce but do not eliminate the risk of development of HCC. Glycogen storage disease type IA is caused by a deficiency in glucose- 6-phosphatase. This results in the development of hepatic adenomas in 50% of patients, and about 11% of patients with adenomas because of glycogen storage disease type IA will undergo malignant transformation into HCC. [93] Other risk factors for HCC include previous treatment with androgenic steroids, oral contraceptives and methotrexate. [94] Unlike adult HCC, pediatric HCC often demonstrate reduced levels of cyclin D1 expression. [95] Whether this is involved in the pathogenesis of pediatric HCC is still unclear. [96]

HCC is a malignancy of hepatocyte origin. The tumor is noted to have a fibrous capsule and is also predisposed to vascular invasion. [97] There are two distinct groups of HCC patients in childhood: those developing HCC in the context of advanced chronic liver disease (CLD), and children who develop sporadic HCC without preceding liver disease. The latter group typically affects older children. Their clinical behavior and biologic behavior are similar to HCC in adults. Approximately 26% of cases are histologically of a fibrolamellar type, [98] which does not appear to make a prognostic difference. Sporadic HCC in children has a relatively poor outcome, [75] while the several small series that report on HCC developing in CLD do so in the context of liver transplantation (LT) [82, 99, 100, 101, 102] The fibrolamellar subtype of HCC (FLHCC) accounts for 3% of HCCs and is not associated with underlying liver disease. FLHCC lesions are solitary, encapsulated, and well defined. Up to 75% of patients will have elevated serum AFP levels. [89, 97].

As for the pathology, HCC macroscopically are usually multifocal and invasive, commonly involving both lobes and frequently associated with vascular invasion, extrahepatic extension, or both at the time of diagnosis. Areas of hemorrhage and necrosis are common, and the lesions themselves vary in consistency from soft to firm. This significantly reduces the resectability rate. Czauderna et al report only a 36% complete tumor resection rate in a series of 39 children recorded by the International Society of Pediatric Oncology over a 4-year time period. [75] The microscopic features distinguishing hepatocellular carcinoma from hepatoblastoma are the presence of tumor cells larger than normal hepatocytes, broad cellular trabeculae, considerable nuclear pleomorphism, nucleolar predominance, frequent tumor giant cells, and absence of hemopoiesis. [33,94] The fibrolamellar variant of HCC is probably a separate clinical entity. Histologically, the tumor cells are plump, with deeply eosinophilic cytoplasm and a marked fibrous stroma separating epithelial cells into trabeculae. [103]

HCC often present as abdominal swelling associated with dull aching pain and discomfort. Other frequent complaints are of rapid weight loss and weakness. [75] The most common clinical sign is hepatomegaly. HCC frequently presents at the time of diagnosis with metastatic spread, most commonly to the regional lymph nodes, lungs and bones. [96]

4.1. Laboratory findings

Although most children with HB have an elevated serum AFP level, this marker is elevated in 50–70% of patients with HCC and less markedly than in HB. Approximately 60–80% of HCC present with significantly elevated AFP levels. [96] All children with HCC should be screened for exposure to viral hepatitis B and C. Similar to HB, some children with HCC may be anemic and others may demonstrate thrombocytosis. Children with cirrhosis-associated HCC may present with elevated serum liver enzyme levels (AST) and those with splenomegaly may show pancytopenia. Careful assessment of hepatic functional reserve in children with cirrhosis is important prior to embarking on major hepatic resection. However, no specific data are available for children regarding tests used in adults (Iodocyanine-green (ICG) dye clearance, galactose elimination capacity). Therefore, the evaluation of the hepatic functional reserve in children is based on standard liver tests including total bilirubin, prothrombine time and INR. [55]

4.2. Imaging

The diagnostic imaging in children with HCC is not different from HB. HCC is often multifocal and may present with a variable number and distribution of tumor nodules. While identifying larger nodules is not difficult, recognizing lesions less than 1.0 cm is still a challenge. Positron emission tomography (PET) using 18- fluorodeoxyglucose may be useful in identifying unsuspected extrahepatic disease. [104]

Three-dimensional CT image analysis techniques are now available to estimate tumor volume and provide detailed intrahepatic anatomy that resembles the actual intraoperative findings. CT volumetry may permit calculation of resected tumor volume and anticipated size of the remnant liver in planning resection. [105] Diagnostic laparoscopy is useful to determine if extra- hepatic disease is present and may avoid unnecessary attempts at resection. Plain radiograph and CT of the chest should be obtained to rule out lung metastases. Hepatic arteriography is currently limited to instances of HCC managed by hepatic artery infusion or transcatheter chemoembolization which can be performed in older children. [55]

On US imaging, HCC may appear as a solitary or multicentric mass most commonly involving the right lobe of the liver, or as a diffusely infiltrating lesion. At diagnosis, these masses appear solid, rarely contain calcification, and have variable echogenicity. Small lesions appear homogeneous and are most often hypoechoic. The capsule can be seen as a hypoechoic halo. Larger lesions become necrotic, and therefore demonstrate a more heterogeneous appearance. Doppler US may detect the high-velocity flow that is related to neovascularity, but Doppler US is most useful for identifying venous invasion. Portal venous invasion is identified in up to 60% of cases, [106] with hepatic venous invasion identified less commonly. Doppler US may differentiate neoplastic thrombus from bland (benign) thrombus by detecting internal neovascularity in the former. [97]

Potentially curative therapies can treat the very early and early stages of the disease. However, less than 30% of HCC patients are detected with the disease in those stages. [107] Another 20% of patients with terminal stage HCC receive recommendations for the best supportive treatment. Since HCC is unresectable in the majority of patients at the time of the first diagnosis, patients are often directed to nonsurgical treatments. Physicians have long overlooked radiotherapy (RT) for HCC as radiation might induce fatal hepatic toxicity at doses lower than the therapeutic doses. [108] However, such limitation has been overcome by recent developments in RT technology involving precise delivery of focused high-dose on partial volume of the liver. [109, 110, 111, 112, 113, 114] According to the Korean Liver Cancer Study Group (KLCSG) practice guidelines, RT is considered appropriate for unresectable, locally advanced HCC without extrahepatic metastasis, Child-Pugh class A or B, and tumors occupying less than two-thirds of the liver. [115]

4.3. Results of resection

Based on recent experience, the optimal treatment should have been total hepatectomy and liver transplantation. Katzenstein et al. reported on 46 children enrolled in the POG and CCG studies - 8 with stage I, 25 with stage III, 13 with stage IV. [49] The overall event-free survival at 5 years was 17%. The outcome was not more favorable in 10 children with FL-HCC. No difference in survival was observed whatever the chemotherapy regimen was given. 369 The German Cooperative Liver Study Group [116] reported the results of two prospective trials. The survival rate of HCC was 33% and 25% in HB-89 (12 patients – 1989–1993) and 25% in HB-94 (25 patients – 1994–1998), respectively. The SIOPEL-1 study (1990–1994) enrolled 39 patients with HCC who were treated with neoadjuvant chemotherapy (PLADO). Thirty-one percent had metastases, 39% had extrahepatic extension/vascular invasion, 56% had multifocal HCC while 31% had pre-existing liver disease. A partial response to PLADO was observed in 49%, a complete tumor resection was possible in 36% (2 with liver transplantation). The 5-year event-free survival was 17%. Adverse prognostic factors included multifocality, metastases and vascular invasion. In SIOPEL-2 pilot study (1994–1998), 21 patients were treated with "super-PLADO" (carboplatin, cisplatin and doxorubicine). Eighteen percent had metastases, 35% had extrahepatic extension/vascular invasion and 53% had multifocal HCC. Partial response to SUPER-PLADO was observed in 46%; complete tumor resection was performed in 47% (one with liver transplantation). The 3-year overall survival was 22%. In SIOPEL-3 (1999–2004), 65 patients were treated with SUPER-PLADO with a partial response in 40%. Thirteen underwent primary surgery. Forty-four percent were never resectable. The 3-year event-free survival was 10%. Currently, the new

SIOPEL-5 study is evaluating non-cirrhotic HCC patients staged according to the PRETEXT system and receiving neoadjuvant PLADO chemotherapy and thalidomide (an anti-angiogenic agent) followed by surgery and postoperative metronomic chemotherapy.

4.4. Liver transplantation for hepatocellular carcinoma

Experience with liver transplantation in children with unresectable HCC is somewhat limited but results have significantly improved over the recent years. Beaunoyer et al. reported on 10 children with underlying liver disease in 5 and cirrhosis in 5. Six had one nodule >5 cm and 7 had >3 nodules. The 5-year actuarial survival was 83%; two died, one of recurrence, while 2 with macrovascular invasion survived. Number and size of lesions or gross vascular invasion did not significantly impact survival. [82] Reyes et al. reported on 19 children with HCC who underwent total hepatectomy and liver transplantation in 1989–1998; two thirds had underlying liver disease. [80] The 5-year disease-free survival was 63% (3/6 died of recurrent HCC). In their experience, risk factors for recurrence were tumor size, vascular invasion and lymphnode involvement. [80] Austin et al. analyzed the aggregated outcome for OLT in HCC in 41 children <18 years (UNOS data). Patient survival was 63% at 5 year and 58% at 10 year. Recurrence was the primary cause of death in 86%. [78]

The most conventional criteria for transplantation are the so-called Milan criteria: [117] no more than three tumors, each not more than 3 cm in size, or a single tumor, not more than 5 cm in diameter, and no evidence of extrahepatic disease or vascular invasion. Recent studies suggest that, in an otherwise normal liver, the present cut-off for tumor size might be expanded to 6.5 cm or 7 cm. [118, 119] The evidence supports the moderate expansion of the Milan criteria although findings from different studies lack consistency and prospective validation by pretransplant imaging. [79] There are no hard data implying that Milan criteria can appropriately select children with a low risk of recurrence of HCC after transplantation. Indeed, Milan criteria are derived from experience in adults with cirrhosis, whereas the majority of children with HCC have no underlying cirrhosis. There is no prospective trial in children while the role of OLT in non-cirrhotic liver is unknown. Moreover, there are differences in biology [120] between adult and pediatric HCC with different molecular findings: mutation of c- met gene in children with HCC, not in adults, level of glycin D1 (regulatory protein of G1 phase cycle) expression is lower in children, loss of heterozygosity on chromosomal arm, 13q, higher in children. There is evidence that childhood HCC might be less chemoresistant than adult HCC; a partial response was observed in 49% enrolled in SIOPEL-1 study. [75] The SIOPEL group has launched in 2005 a new SIOPEL-5 trial directed to non-cirrhotic hepatocellular carcinoma in children and adolescents. It is based on the hypothesis that the addition of an antiangiogenic drug (Thalidomide) to PLADO will result in an improvement of survival with acceptable toxicity. Most likely, Sorafenib will be substituted for Thalidomide on the basis of data obtained in adults with advanced HCC. [121]

Patients with unresectable disease restricted to the liver will be submitted to liver transplantation. Since the majority of children with HCC in western countries have no underlying liver disease, recent data suggest that liver transplantation may be quite useful treatment in carefully selected unresectable cases. [78, 80, 82] Unlike the adult population, the frequency

http://dx.doi.org/10.5772/51764

of HCC in the pediatric population is low; therefore, the experience in the application of liver transplantation in the pediatric population for HCC is limited. [122, 123, 124, 125] In patients whose disease is confined to the liver, the use of liver transplantation is indicated. Because chemotherapy is not beneficial at present in this group, results in patients with more extensive disease are poor. [126]

5. Benign tumors

In general, benign tumors of the liver may arise from hepatocytes, bile duct epithelium, the supporting mesenchymal tissue, or a combination of two or more of these. In addition to true neoplastic conditions of the liver, a variety of nodular diseases may occur that resemble, and must therefore be differentiated from, tumours. Although most patients with benign hepatic tumors are asymptomatic, a minority may present with symptoms that may be local or systemic. In these patients, the relationship between the symptoms and the hepatic lesions may be difficult to correlate, and additional evaluation is necessary to rule out other causes for the patients complaints. In most cases patients with benign hepatic lesions have no preexisting liver disease, and the finding of a coexisting chronic liver disease such as cirrhosis, chronic hepatitis B or C, or hemochromatosis should raise a suspicion for a malignant tumor. A conclusive diagnosis of a focal hepatic lesion is essential because it may represent a primary or secondary malignancy, which may require immediate treatment. In addition, some benign lesions carry specific risks such as rupture, bleeding, malignant transformation, consumptive coagulopathy, and disseminated intravascular coagulation. [127]

Primary liver masses constitute the third most common group of solid abdominal tumors of childhood, [2, 128, 129] with an incidence of 0.4 to 1.9 per million children each year. [129, 130] Benign primary liver masses described in children include hemangioma/infantile hepatic hemangioendothelioma, focal nodular hyperplasia, simple hepatic cysts, mesenchymal hamartomas, adenomas, nodular regenerative hyperplasia, hematomas, arterial venous malformations, granulomas, and lymphangiomas. [2, 12, 128, 129, 130, 131, 132, 133]

Infantile hepatic hemangioendothelioma is a tumor derived from vascular endothelial cells, which is the most diagnosed benign hepatic tumor in children. Hence it accounts for approximately 12% of all childhood hepatic tumors,the most common benign vascular tumor of the liver in infancy, and the most common symptomatic liver tumor during the first 6 months of life. [134, 135, 136, 137]

While the majority of benign masses may be of little consequence, morbidity and mortality can occur from benign masses, mass effect from a tumor can cause pain, biliary obstruction and inferior vena cava obstruction, limit lung capacity, or cause feeding difficulty. [2, 12, 129, 138] Most of the recent radiology literature concerning the liver has focused on lesions detection or identification of specific features (enhancement patterns) that may help distinguish benign from malignant hepatic tumours. Except for hemangioma and focal nodular hyperplasia (FNH), little is know about imaging characteristics that can help identify and distinguish among the many less common bening liver masses. [139]

5.1. Infantile hepatic hemangioendothelioma

More than 90% are diagnosed before the age of 6 years. The typical presentation is of hepatomegaly, hemangiomas of the skin, and heart failure resulting from massive arteriovenous shunting. [127, 140] In addition to heart failure, this tumor may cause consumption coagulopathy (Kasabach–Merritt syndrome) and obstructive jaundice. [127, 141] Although well circumscribed, this tumor is not encapsulated and often has scattered calcifications. Microscopically, this tumor consists of multiple small vessels lined by plump endothelial cells and surrounded by fibrous stroma.

Ultrasonography usually shows hepatomegaly and solitary or multiple hepatic lesions, which may vary from anechoic to hyperechoic. The unenhanced CT scan demonstrates the lesion as a well-defined hypo-attenuating mass, occasionally with calcifications. After contrast injection, the lesion may show enhancement resembling hemangioma and may become isodense on delayed images. Angiography shows dilated, irregular vascular lakes that commonly persist beyond the venous phase. 99mTc-sulfur colloid scintigraphy shows the lesion as a cold spot because of a lack of Kupffer cells within the tumor. [127]

The prognosis of this lesion is dependent on its size and its effect on the heart function. Spontaneous regression is frequent but death may occur within the first 6 months of life because of cardiac failure or replacement of the normal hepatic parenchyma. [127, 142] The prognosis is usually good if heart failure is managed successfully.

Treatment is dictated by tumor-related symptoms produced by tumor size. Management of congestive heart failure may be sufficient in some cases. If symptoms are not relieved, treatment should be aimed at decreasing the tumor size. [127]

Other treatments include hepatic artery ligation, transcatheter endovascular embolization, and radiation therapy. [127, 143, 144] Liver transplant is increasingly recognized as a viable treatment modality for infantile hemangioendothelioma when other treatments fail. [127, 145]

5.2. Focal Nodular Hyperplasia (FNH)

FNH is very rare in pediatric population with an age prevalence in children 7-8 years old, although some cases are diagnosed in early childhood or even in the prenatal period. [146, 147] The female sex is predominant with a M/F ratio of less than 1/10 in one of the largest series. [147, 148]

The majority (70-90%) of FNH at presentation is asymptomatic and the most common way that the disease is discovered is when, during an occasional physical examination, hepatomegaly or a palpatory abdominal mass are detected. The lesion is more often unique, but about 8% of cases may show multiple nodules, up to 30. The diameter of lesions is extremely variable, from less than 1 cm to more than 15 cm but usually is less than 5 cm. [147]

The diagnosis in the majority of cases could be by Ultrasound, CT Scan and MRI. Needle biopsy or open air biopsy are necessary when the radiological investigations are doubtful, above all in case of absence of the central scar, and not rarely the differential diagnosis from

http://dx.doi.org/10.5772/51764

other nodular lesions of liver may be difficult. The differential diagnosis includes different nodular lesions of the liver. [147]

The natural evolution of FNH is unpredictable. In about 2/3 of cases, remain stable and in about 1/3-1/4 of cases show a gradual spontaneous improvement as far as a complete remission. In rare instances an increase in number as well as in size may occur [9]. The recent studies in molecular biology have confirmed that FNH is not a pre-neoplastic lesion: the tissue parenchymal organization is pretty the same of usual liver tissue and, moreover, even though in some cases a clonal origin of FNH nodules have been demonstrated, until now no somatic mutation in the β-catenin gene or in the other genes implicated in the hepatocellular adenoma (where a malignant transformation is possible) have been discovered. [147, 149, 150]

About the management the first step is, of course, the stop of oral contraceptive. Considering the body of evidence that FNH doesn't undergo malignant transformation and that there are only sporadic cases followed by spontaneous rupture and consequent abdominal bleeding, we agree with the opinion that in asymptomatic cases it is opportune a careful follow-up with an ultrasound scan every 6-12 months, and that elective surgery has probably to be limited to the patients suffering of abdominal pain or with a voluminous or growing mass. [147, 149]

5.3. Nodular regenerative Hyperplasia (NRH)

Nodular regenerative hyperplasia (NRH) is a disease characterized by multiple nodules composed by hepatocytes, without a fibrous tissue or central scar. The rare pediatric cases are mostly in association with the congenital absence of portal vein (sometimes complicated by heart disease or multi-cystic kidney dysplasia). Indeed, only about 200 cases have been reported. Symptoms, when present, are mainly associated with the complication of portal hypertension. [151, 152, 153, 154]

CT presentation is really different from FNH, as there are multiple hypodense lesions with poor or absent enhancement after contrast administration. [147, 155] The typical imaging showing anechoic and regular profile of the mass at ultrasound, easily recognize cystic lesions: however CT and MRI may be necessary in selected cases. [147]

5.4. Hamartomas

Mesenchymal hamartoma is a rare, benign, developmental tumor of the liver, with occasional risk of malignancy. Histologically, it appears as a disordered arrangement of the mesenchyme, bile ducts, and hepatic parenchyma. Cords of normal appearing hepatocytes are separated by zones of loose, poorly cellular mesenchyme. The porous nature of the mesenchyme permits accumulation of fluid. [156, 157] Grossly, it has stromal and cystic components with no capsules, and can grow to large sizes. [157, 158] The typical presentation is one of asymptomatic, rapid abdominal distention with a palpable mass on physical examination. The rapid expansion of the tumor is believed to be due to degeneration of the mesenchyme and fluid accumulation. Other uncommon associated symptoms are vomiting, fever, constipation, diarrhea, and weight loss. [156, 157] Laboratory investigations usually reveal normal liver function with elevated alpha-fetoprotein, which is believed to be secreted by the proliferating hepatocytes within the tumor. [157, 159] The radiological appearance is one of a large, uni or multi-cystic, avascular mass occupying part of the liver. [157, 158] Surgical resection has been the standard treatment for this tumor.

6. Sarcoma

The third most common hepatic malignancy, after hepatoblastoma and hepatocellular carcinoma, is undifferentiated embryonal sarcoma. [8, 160, 161] It is believed to be a primitive mesenchymal neoplasm, which usually behaves in a highly malignant fashion. [162] It was first recognized as a clinicopathologic entity by Stocker and Ishak in 1978. [156] Before their report, this tumor had been described under different names such as embryonal sarcoma [163] mesenchymoma, [164] primary sarcoma [165] or fibromyxosarcoma. [166]

These tumors occur in children 5–10 years of age and are mesenchymal in appearance. [8, 167] Diagnosis of primary hepatic sarcoma is challenging due to the lack of specific presenting symptoms, lack of serological markers, non-specific findings on radiological imaging and the rarity of the disease. [86] However, leukocytosis and elevated aspartate aminotransferase and alkaline phosphatase are not uncommon laboratory findings. [156, 161, 162, 168, 169] The serum α-fetoprotein level is always normal. [156, 161, 162, 169] There is no correlation with hepatitis B or C virus infection. Most tumors have prominent areas of cystic degeneration. [161, 162] Multinucleated giant tumor cells with eosinophilic cytoplasm and frequent mitosis are usually present. (Stocker and Ishak,1978 and [162] et al.,2001) PAS-positive, diastase-resistant hyaline globules, which are believed to be lysosomes or apoptotic bodies, are frequently seen within tumor cells as well as in extracellular stromata. [156, 162, 168, 170, 171]

Regarding the radiological imaging, undifferentiated embryonal sarcoma often show a misleading cystic appearance on CT and magnetic resonance imaging (MRI) in contrast to a predominantly solid appearance on ultrasound. [86, 172]

Undifferentiated embryonal sarcoma of the liver behaves in a highly malignant fashion, [162, 173] and the median survival has been less than a year. [156, 162] Complete surgical resection is the key to a favorable outcome. However, despite apparent complete resectability in somecases, local recurrence and distant metastases have been major impediments to achieving long-term disease-free survival. [162, 173] Multidisciplinary treatment (chemotherapy and radiotherapy) has been used to achieve superior and local control and disease-free survival in patients with Undifferentiated embryonal sarcoma of the liver. [160, 167, 173]

Author details

Julio C. Wiederkehr[1,2*], Izabel M. Coelho[1,2], Sylvio G. Avilla[1,2], Barbara A. Wiederkehr[2] and Henrique A. Wiederkehr[2]

*Address all correspondence to: julio.wieder@uol.com.br

1 Federal University of Paraná, Curitiba, Brazil

2 Hospital Pequeno Príncipe, Curitiba, Brazil

References

[1] Kim, E. H., Koh, K. N, Park, M, Kim, B. E, Im, H. J, & Seo, J. J. (2011). Clinical features of infantile hepatic hemangioendothelioma. *Korean Journal of Pediatrics*, 54(6), 260, doi:10.3345/kjp.2011.54.6.260.

[2] Luks, F. I., Yazbeck, S., Brandt, M. L., et al. (1991). Benign liver tumors in children: a 25- year experience. *J Pediatr Surg*, 26, 1326-30.

[3] Reymond, D., Plaschkes, J., Luthy, A. R., et al. (1995). Focal nodular hyperplasia of the liver in children: review of follow-up and outcome. *J Pediatr Surg*, 30, 1590-3.

[4] Ehren, H., Mahour, G. H., & Isaacs, H., Jr. (1983). Benign liver tumors in infancy and childhood. Report of 48 cases. *Am J Surg*, 145, 325-9.

[5] Emre, S., & Mc Kenna, G. J. (2004). Liver tumors in children. *Pediatric transplantation*, 8(6), 632-8.

[6] Weinberg, AG, & Finegold, MJ. (1983). Primary hepatic tumors of childhood. *Hum Pathology*, 14, 512-537.

[7] Multerys, M., Goodman, M. T., Smith, MA, et al. (1999). Hepatic Tumors. In Ries LAG, SmithMA,GurneyJGet al. (eds). Cancer Incidence, SurvivalamongChildren, Adolescents: United States SEER Program 1975-1995. *SEER Program, NIH Pub.* [99-4649], Bethesda, MD, National Cancer Institute, 91-97.

[8] Litten, J. B., & Tomlinson, G. E. (2008). Liver tumors in children. *The oncologist*, 13(7), 812-20.

[9] Dimmick, J. E., Rogers, P. C. J., & Blair, G. (1994). Hepatic Tumors. *In: Pochedly C, ed. Neoplastic Siseases of Childhood*, Chur, Switzerland, Harwood Academic, 973-1010.

[10] Kelly, D. (2008). *Diseases of the Liver and Biliary System in Children ed.*, Wiley-Blackwell, Oxford.

[11] Kenney, LB, Miller, B. A., Ries, L. A., et al. (1998). Incidence of cancer in infants in the U.S.: 1980-1990. *Cancer*, 82, 1396-1400.

[12] Meyers, R. L. (2007). Tumors of the liver in children. *Surgical oncology*, 16(3), 195-203.

[13] Mann, J. R., Kasthuri, N., Raafat, F., et al. (1990). Malignant hepatic tumours in children: incidence, clinical features and aetiology. *Paediatr Perinat Epidemiol*, 4, 276-289.

[14] Bulterys, M., Goodman, M. T., Smith, M. A., et al. (1999). Cancer Inci- dence and Survival Among Children and Adolescents: United States SEER Program1975-1995. *National Cancer Institute SEER Program. NIHPublication* [99-4649], 91-97.

[15] Owe, T., Kubota, A., Okuyama, H., et al. (2003). Hepatoblastoma in children of extremely low birth weight: a report from a single prenatal center. *Journal of Pediatric Surgery*, 38, 134-7.

[16] Honda, S., Haruta, M., Sugawara, W., et al. (2008). The methylation status of RASSF1A promoter predicts responsiveness to chemotherapy and eventual cure in hepatoblastoma patients. *Int J Cancer*, 5, 1117-25.

[17] Sakamoto, L. H., De Camargo, B., Cajaiba, M., et al. (2010). MT1G hypermethylation: a potential prognostic marker for hepatoblastoma. *Pediatr Res*, 67, 387-93.

[18] Exelby, P. R., Filler, R. M., & Grosfeld, J. L. (1975). Liver tumors in children in the particular reference to hepatoblastoma and hepatocellular carcinoma: American Academy of pediatrics surgical section survey- 1974. *Journal of pediatric surgery*, Saunders, Retrieved from, http://linkinghub.elsevier.com/retrieve/pii/0022346875900950?showall=true.

[19] DeBaun, M. R., & Tucker, M. A. (1998). Risk of cancer during the first four years of life in children from the Beckwith-Wiedemann Syndrome Registry. *J Pediatr*, 132, 398-400.

[20] Steenman, M., Westerfeld, A., & Mannens, M. (2000). Genetics of Beckwith-Weidemann Syndrome associated tumours: common genetic pathways. *Genes Chromosomes Cancer*, 28, 1-13.

[21] Giardello, F. M., Offerhaus, G. J., Krush, A. J., et al. (1991). Risk of hepatoblastoma in familial adenomatous polyposis. *J Pediatr*, 119, 766-768.

[22] Aretz, S., Koch, A., Uhlhaas, S., et al. (2006). *Pediatric Blood Cancer*, 47, 811-8.

[23] Hirschman, B. A., Pollock, B. H., & Tomlinson, G. E. (2005). The spectrum of APC mutations in children with hepatoblastoma from familial adenomatous polyposis kindreds. *Journal of Pediatrics*, 147, 263-6.

[24] Wei, Y., Fabre, H., Branchereau, S., et al. (2000). Activation of B-catenin in epithelial and mesenchymal hepatoblastomas. *Oncogene*, 19, 498-506.

[25] Jeng, Y. M., Wu, M. Z., Chang, M. H., et al. (2000). Somatic mutations of B-catenin play a crucial role in the tumorigenesis of sporadic hepatoblastoma. *Cancer*, 152, 45-5.

[26] Udatsu, Y., Kusafuka, T., Kuroda, S., et al. (2001). High frequency of beta catenin mutations in hepatoblastoma. *Pediatr Surg Int*, 17, 508-512.

[27] Tomlinson, G. E., Douglass, E. C., Pollock, B. H., et al. (2006). Cytogenetic analysis of a large series of hepatoblastoma: numerical aberrations with recurring translocations involving 1q12-21. *Genes Chromosomes Cancer*, 44, 177-84.

[28] Ruck, P., Xiao, J. C., Pietsch, T., et al. (1997). Hepatic stem-like cells in hepatoblastoma: Expression of cytokeratin 7, albumin and oval cell associated antigens detected by OV-1 and OV-. *Histopathology*, 31, 324-329.

[29] Ruck, P., & Xiao, J. C. (2002). Stem-like cells in hepatoblastoma. *Med Pediatr Oncol*, 39, 504-507.

[30] Stocken, J. T. (1994). Hepatoblastoma. *Semin Diagn Pathol*, 11, 136-143.

[31] Malogolowkin, M. H., Katzenstein, H. M., Krailo, M., et al. (2006). Intensified platinum therapy is an ineffective strategy for improving outcome in pediatric patients with advanced hepatoblastoma. *Journal of Clinical Oncology*, 24, 2879-84.

[32] Haas, J. E., Feusner, J. H., & Finegold, M. J. (2001). Small cell undifferentiated histology in hepatoblastoma may be unfavorable. *Cancer*, 92, 3130-4.

[33] Hass, J. E., Mczynski, K. A., Krailo, M., et al. (1989). Histopathology and prognosis in childhood hepatoblastoma and hepatocellular carcinoma. *Cancer*, 64, 1082-1095.

[34] Perilongo, G., & Shafford, E. A. (1999). Liver tumours. *Eur J Cancer*, 19, 953-958.

[35] Teng, C. T., Daeschner, C. W., Jr., Singleton, E. B., Rosenberg, H. S., Cole, V. W., Hill, L. L., & Brennan, J. C. (1961). Liver disease and osteoporosis in children. I. Clinical observations. *Journal of Pediatrics*, 59, 684-702.

[36] Van Tornout, J. M., Buckley, J. D., Quinn, J. J., et al. (1997). Timing and magnitude of decline in alpha-fetoprotein levels in tested children with unresectable or metastatic hepatoblastoma are predictors of outcome: a report from the Children's Cancer Group. *J Clin Oncol*, 15, 1190-1197.

[37] Hartley, A. L., Birch, J. M., Kelsey, A. M., et al. (1990). Epidemiological and familial aspects of hepatoblastoma. *Med Pediatr Oncol*, 18, 103-119.

[38] Feusner, J. R., Krailo, M. A., Hass, J. E., et al. (1993). Treatment of pulmonary metastasis of initial stage I hepatoblastoma in child- hood: report from the children's cancer group. *Cancer*, 71, 859-864.

[39] Lack, E. E., Neave, C., & Vawter, G. F. (1982). Hepatoblastoma- A clinical and pathologic study of 54 cases. *Am J Suj Pathol*, 6, 693-705.

[40] Nickerson, H. J., Silberman, T. L., & McDonald, T. P. (1980). Hepatoblastoma, thrombocytosis and increased thrombopoetin. *Cancer*, 315-7.

[41] Meyers, R. L., Katzenstein, H. M., Rowland, J. H., et al. (2008). PRETEXT and other prognostic factors in hepatoblastoma. *Pediatric Blood Cancer*.

[42] Perilongo, G. (2006). State of the art: Treatment of childhood liver tumors. Geneva, Switzerland. *In: 38th annual meeting of SIOP*.

[43] Roebuck, D. J., Olsen, O., & Pariente, D. (2006). Radiological staging in children with hepatoblastoma. *Pediatr Radiol*, 36, 176-82.

[44] Roebuck, D. (2008). Focal liver lesion in children. *Pediatr Radiol*, 38(3), 518-22.

[45] De Campo, M., & De Campo, J. F. (1988). Ultrasound of primary hepatic tumors in childhood. *Pediatric Radiol*, 19, 19-24.

[46] Helmberger, J. R., Ros, P. R., Medgo, P. J., et al. (1999). Pediatric liver neoplasms: a radiology-pathological correlation. *Eur Radiol*, 9, 1339-1347.

[47] Von Schweiniz, D., Burger, D., Weiner, P., et al. (1992). Therapy of malignant liver tumors in childhood. An intermittent report of the HB-89 multicenter. *Clin Pediatr*, 204, 214-220.

[48] Katzenstein, H. M., Krailo, M., Malogolowkin, M. H., et al. (2007, February). Biology and treatment of children with all stages of hepatoblastoma: COG proposal AHEP-0731. *submitted to CTEP and NCI.*

[49] Katzenstein, H. M., Krailo, M., Malogolowkin, M. H., et al. (2002). Hepatocellular carcinoma in children and adolescents: results from the Pediatric Oncology Group and the Children's Cancer Group intergroup study. *J Clin Oncol*, 20(12), 2789-97.

[50] Aronson, D. C., Schnater, J. M., Staalman, C. R., et al. (2005). Predictive value of pre-treat- ment extent of disease system in hepatoblastoma: Results from the International Society of Pediatric Oncology Liver Tumor Study Group SIOPEL-1 study. *J Clin Oncol*, 23, 1245-1262.

[51] Meyers, R. L., Rowland, J. R., Krailo, M., et al. (2009). Predictive power of pretreatment prognostic factors in children with hepatoblastoma: a report from the Children's Oncology Group. *Pediatr Blood Cancer*, 53(6), 1016-22.

[52] Douglass, E. C., Reynolds, M., Finegold, M., et al. (1993). Cisplatin, vincristine, and fluorouracil therapy for hepatoblastoma: a Pediatric Oncology Group study. *J Clin Oncol*, 11(1), 96-9.

[53] Brown, J., Perilongo, G., Shafford, E., et al. (2000). Pretreatment prognostic factors for children with hepatoblastoma-- results from the International Society of Paediatric Oncology (SIOP) study SIOPEL 1. *Eur J Cancer*, 36(11), 1418-25.

[54] http://www.cancer.gov/PublishedContent/MediaLinks/308970.html.

[55] Otte, J. B. (2010). Progress in the surgical treatment of malignant liver tumors in children. *Cancer treatment reviews*, 36(4), 360-71, Elsevier Ltd.

[56] Czauderna, P., Otte, J. B., Aronson, D. C., et al. (2005). Guidelines for surgical treatment of hepatoblastoma in the modern era : recommendations from the childhood liver tumour strategy group of the international society of paediatric oncology (SIOPEL). *European Journal of Cancer*, 41, 1031-6.

[57] Stringer, M. (2006). Liver tumors. *Semin Pediatr Surg*, 9, 196-208.

[58] Fuchs, J., Rydzynski, J., Hecker, H., et al. (2002). The influence of preoperative chemotherapy and surgical technique in the treatment of hepatoblastoma-a report from

http://dx.doi.org/10.5772/51764

the German cooperative liver tumours studies HB-89 and HB-94. *Eur J Pediatr Surg*, 12, 255-61.

[59] Von Schweinitz, D., Faundez, A., Teichmann, B., et al. (2000). Hepatocyte growth-factor- scatter-factor can stimulate postoperative tumor-cell proliferation in childhood hepatoblastoma. *Int J Cancer*, 85, 151-9.

[60] Ortega, J. A., Douglass, E. C., Feusner, J. H., et al. (2000). Randomized comparison of cisplatin/vincristin/5-fluorouracil and cisplatin/doxorubicin for the treatment of pediatric hepatoblastoma (HB): a report from the Children's cancer group and the pediatric oncology group. *Journal of Clinical Oncology*, 18, 2665-75.

[61] Schnater, J. M., Aronson, D. C., Plaschkes, J., et al. (2002). Surgical view of the treatment of patients with hepatoblastoma. *Cancer*, 94, 1111-20.

[62] Malogolowkin, M. H., Katzenstein, H. M., Krailo, M., et al. Redefining the role of doxorubicin for the treatment of children with hepatoblastoma. *Journal of Clinical Oncology*.

[63] Von Schweinitz, D., & Haberle, B. (2007, March). German liver tumor study: HB 99. Poland, Gdansk. *In: First international symposium childhood hepatoblastoma.*

[64] Von Schweinitz, D., Hecker, H., Harms, D., et al. (1995). Complete resection before development of drug resistance is essential for survival from advanced hepatoblastoma-a report fro the German cooperative pediatric liver tumor study HB-89. *Journal of Pediatric Surgery*, 30, 845-52.

[65] Ortega, J. A., Douglass, E., Feusner, J., et al. (1994). A randomized trial of cisplatin/ vincristine/5-fluorouracil vs. CCP/doxorubicin continuous infusion for the treatment of hepatoblastoma: results from the pediatric inter-group hepatoma study (abstr). *Proc Am Soc Clin Oncol (ASCO)*, 13, 416.

[66] Pritchard, J., Brown, J., Shafford, E., et al. (2000). Cisplatin, doxorubicin and delayed surgery for childhood hepatoblastoma: a successful approach-results of the first prospective study of the International Society of Pediatric Oncology. *J Clin Oncol*, 18, 3819-28.

[67] Perilongo, G., Shafford, E., Maibach, R., et al. (2004). Risk-adapted treatment for childhood hepatoblastoma Final report of the second study of the International Society of Pediatric Oncology- SIOPEL 2. *Eur J Cancer*, 40, 411-21.

[68] Meyers, R. L., Malogolowkin, M. H., Rowland, J. M., & Krailo, M. (2006, May 27). Predictive value of the PRETEXT staging system in children with hepatoblastoma. *In: Presented at the 37th annual meeting American Pediatric Surgical Association, Hilton Head, SC.*

[69] Dall'Igna, P., Cecchetto, G., Toffolutti, T., et al. (2003). Multifocal hepatoblastoma is there a place for partial hepatectomy? *Med Pediatr Oncol*, 40, 113-6.

[70] Couinaud, C. (1992). The anatomy of the liver. *Ann Ital Chir*, 63, 693-7.

[71] Wheatley, J. M., Rosenfield, N. S., Berger, L., & La Quaglia, M. P. (1996). Liver regeneration in children after major hepatectomy for malignancy-evaluation using a computer-aided technique of volume measurement. *J Surg Res*, 61, 183-9.

[72] Von Schweinitz, D. (2006). Management of liver tumors in childhood. *Semin Pediatr Surg*, 15, 17-24.

[73] Otte, J. B., & De Ville de Goyet, J. (2005). The contribution of transplantation to the treatment of liver tumors in children. *Semin Pediatr Surg*, 14, 233-8.

[74] Chardot, C., Sant Martin, C., Gilles, A., et al. (2002). Living related liver transplantation and vena cava reconstruction after total hepatectomy including the vena cava for hepatoblastoma. *Transplantation*, 73, 90-2.

[75] Czauderna, P., Mac Kinley, G., Perilongo, G., et al. (2002). Hepatocellular carcinoma in children: results of the first prospective study of the international society of pediatric oncology group. *Journal of Clinical Oncology*, 20, 2798-804.

[76] Millar, A. J. W., Hartley, P., Khan, D., et al. (2001). Extended hepatic resection with transplantation back-up for an unresectable tumor. *Pediatric Surgery International*, 17, 378-81.

[77] Otte, J. B., Pritchard, J., Aronson, D. C., et al. (2004). Liver transplantation for hepatoblastoma: Results from the International Society of Pediatric Oncology (SIOP) study SIOPEL-1 and review of the world experience. *Pediatr Blood Cancer*, 42, 74-83.

[78] Austin, M. T., Leys, C. M., Feurer, I. D., et al. (2006). Liver transplantation for childhood hepatic malignancy: a review of the United Network for Organ Sharing (UNOS) database. *J Pediatr Surg*, 41, 182-6.

[79] Hoti, E., & Adam, R. (2008). Liver transplantation for primary and metastatic liver cancers. *Transplant Int*, 21, 1107-17.

[80] Reyes, J. D., Carr, B., Dvorchik, I., et al. (2000). Liver transplantation and chemotherapy for hepatoblastoma and hepatocellular cancer in childhood and adolescence. *J Pediatr*, 136(6), 795-804.

[81] Perilongo, G., Brown, J., Shafford, E., et al. (2000). Hepatoblastoma presenting with lung metastases: treatment results of the first cooperative, prospective study of the International Society of Pediatric Oncology on childhood liver tumors. *Cancer*, 89, 1845-53.

[82] Beaunoyer, M., Vanatta, J. M., Ogihara, M., et al. (2007). Outcomes of transplantation in children with primary hepatic malignancy. *Pediatr Transplant*, 11(6), 655-60.

[83] Pimpalwar, A. P., Sharif, K., Ramani, P., et al. (2002). Strategy for hepatoblastoma management: transplant versus nontransplant surgery. *J Pediatr Surg*, 37, 240-5.

[84] Tiao, G. M., Bobey, N., Allen, S., et al. (2005). The current management of hepatoblastoma: a combination of chemotherapy, conventional resection, and liver transplantation. *J Pediatr*, 146, 204-11.

[85] Molmenti, E. P., Wilkinson, K., Molmenti, H., et al. (2002). Treatment of unresectable hepatoblastoma with liver transplantation in the pediatric population. *Am J Transplant*, 6, 535-8.

[86] Faraj, W., Mukherji, D., El Majzoub, N., Shamseddine, A., Shamseddine, A., & Khalife, M. (2010). Primary undifferentiated embryonal sarcoma of the liver mistaken for hydatid disease. *World journal of surgical oncology*, 8(58).

[87] Moore, S. W., Hesseling, P. B., Wessels, G., et al. (1997). Hepatocellular carcinoma in children. *Pediatr Surg Int*, 12, 266-70 .

[88] Bellani, F. F., & Massimino, M. (1993). Liver tumors in childhood: Epidemiology and clinics. *J Surg Oncol*, 3, 119-121.

[89] Dubois, J., Garel, L., Russo, P., et al. (1993). Pediatric case of the day. *Radiographics*, 13, 691-2.

[90] Parkin, D. M., Stiller, C. A., Draper, G. J., et al. (1988). The international incidence of childhood cancer. *Int J Cancer*, 42, 511-520.

[91] Chen, J. C., Chang, M. L., Lin, J. N., et al. (2005). Comparison of childhood hepatic malignancies in a hepatitisBhyper-endemic area. *World J Gastroenterol*, 11, 5289-5294.

[92] Chang, M. L., Chen, J. C., Lai, M. S., et al. (1997). Universal hepatitis B vaccination in Taiwan and the incidence of hepatocellular carcinoma in children. Taiwan Childhood Hepatoma Study Group. *N Engl J Med*, 336, 1855-1859.

[93] Howell, R. R., Stevenson, R. E., Ben-Menachem, Y., et al. (1976). Hepatic adenoma in type I glycogen storage disease. *JAMA*, 236, 1481-1489.

[94] Weinberg, A. G., & Finegold, M. J. (1983). Primary Hepatic Tumor of Childhood. *Hum Pathol*, 14, 512-537.

[95] Kim, H., Lee, M. J., Kim, M. R., et al. (2000). Expression of cyclin D1, cyclin E, cdk4 and loss of heterozygosity of 8p13q 17p in hepatocellular carcinoma. *Comparison study of childhood and adult hepatocellular carcinoma. Liver*, 20, 173-178.

[96] Emre, S., & Mc Kenna, G. J. (2004). Liver tumors in children. *Pediatric transplantation*, 8(6), 632-8.

[97] Varich, L. (2010). Ultrasound of Pediatric Liver Masses. *Ultrasound Clinics*, 5(1), 137-152, Elsevier Ltd.

[98] Katzenstein, H. M., Krailo, M. D., Malogolowkin, M. H., et al. (2003). Fibrolamellar hepatocellular carcinoma in children and adolescents. *Cancer*.

[99] Arikan, C., Kilic, M., Nart, D., et al. (2006). Hepatocellular carcinoma in children and effect of living-donor liver transplantation on outcome. *Pediatr Transplant*, 10, 42-7.

[100] Sevmis, S., & Karakayali, H. (2008). Ozc carcinoma in children. *Pediatr Transplant*, 12, 52-6.

[101] Hadzic, N., Quaglia, A., Portmann, B., et al. (2011). Hepatocellular carcinoma in children with biliary atresia; King's College Hospital Experience. *J Pediatr.*

[102] Hadzic, N., & Finegold, M. J. (2011). Liver neoplasia in children. *Clinics in liver disease,* 15(2), 443-62, vii-x., Elsevier Ltd.

[103] Craig, J. R., Peters, R., Edmondson, H. A., & Omata, M. (1980). Fibrolamellar carcinoma of the liver: a tumor of adolescentes and Young adults with distinctive clinicopathologic features. *Cancer,* 46, 372-9.

[104] Hain, S. F., & Fogelman, I. (2004). Recent advances in imaging hepatocellular carcinoma: diagnosis, staging and response assessment functional imaging. *Cancer J,* 10, 121-7.

[105] Shoup, M., Gonen, M., D'Angelica, M., et al. (2003). Volumetric analysis predicts hepatic dysfunction in patients undergoing major liver resection. *J Gastrointest Surg,* 7, 325-30.

[106] Rumack, C. M., Wilson, S. R., & Charboneau, J. W. (2005). *Diagnostic ultrasound* (3rd edition), St Louis (MO), Mosby.

[107] Bruix, J., & Sherman, M. (2005). Practice Guidelines Committee, American Association for the Study of Liver Diseases. Management of hepatocellular carcinoma. *Hepatology,* 42, 1208-1236.

[108] Cochrane, A. M., Murray-Lyon, I. M., Brinkley, D. M., & Williams, R. (1977). Quadruple chemotherapy versus radiotherapy in treatment of primary hepatocellular carcinoma. *Cancer,* 40, 609-6.

[109] Lawrence, T. S., Tesser, R. J., & ten Haken, R. K. (1990). An application of dose volume histograms to the treatment of intrahepatic malignancies with radiation therapy. *Int J Radiat Oncol Biol Phys,* 19, 1041-1047.

[110] Lawrence, T. S., Ten Haken, R. K., Kessler, M. L., et al. (1992). The use of 3-D dose volume analysis to predict radiation hepatitis. *Int J Radiat Oncol Biol Phys,* 23, 781-788.

[111] Robertson, J. M., Mc Ginn, C. J., Walker, S., et al. (1997). A phase I trial of hepatic arterial bromodeoxyuridine and conformal radiation therapy for patients with primary hepatobiliary cancers or colorectal liver metastases. *Int J Radiat Oncol Biol Phys,* 39, 1087-1092.

[112] Seong, J., Keum, K. C., Han, K. H., et al. (1999). Combined transcatheter arterial chemoembolization and local radiotherapy of unresectable hepatocellular carcinoma. *Int J Radiat Oncol Biol Phys,* 43, 393-397.

[113] Shim, S. J., Seong, J., Han, K. H., et al. (2005). Local radiotherapy as a complement to incomplete transcatheter arterial chemoembolization in locally advanced hepatocellular carcinoma. *Liver Int,* 25, 1189-1196.

[114] Park, W., Lim, D. H., Paik, S. W., et al. (2005). Local radiotherapy for patients with unresectable hepatocellular carcinoma. Int J Radiat Oncol Biol Phys , 61, 1143-1150.

[115] Park, JW. (2004). Korean Liver Cancer Study Group and National Cancer Center. Practice guideline for diagnosis and treatment of hepato- cellular carcinoma. *Korean J Hepatol*, 10, 88-98.

[116] Von Schweinitz, D. (2004). Treatment of liver tumors in children. *In: Clavian PA, Fong Y, Lyerly H, et al. editors. Liver tumors: current and emerging therapies*, Boston, Jones and Bartlett.

[117] Mazzaferro, V., Regalia, E., Doci, R., et al. (1996). Liver transplantation for the treatment of small hepatocellular carcinoma in patients with cirrhosis. *New Engl J Med*, 334, 693-9.

[118] Yao, F. Y., Ferrell, L., Bass, N. M., et al. (2001). Liver transplantation for hepatocellular carcinoma: expansion of the tumor size limits does not adversely impact survival. *Hepatology*, 33, 1394-403.

[119] Roayaie, S., Frischer, J. S., Emre, S. H., et al. (2002). Long-term results with multimodal adjuvant therapy and liver transplantation for the treatment of hepatocellular carcinoma larger than 5 centimetres. *Ann Surg*, 235, 533-9.

[120] Terracciano, L., & Tornillo, L. (2003). Cytogenetic alteration in liver cell tumors as detected by comparative genomic hybridization. *Pathologica*, 95, 71-82.

[121] Llovet, J. M., Ricci, S., Mazzaferro, V., et al. (2008). Sorafenib in advanced hepatocellular carcinoma. *New Engl J Med*, 359, 420-2.

[122] Srinivasan, P., Mc Call, J., Pritchard, J., et al. (2002). Orthotopic liver transplantation for unresectable hepatoblastoma. *Transplantation*, 74, 652-5.

[123] Tagge, E. P., Tagge, D. U., Reyes, J., et al. (1992). Resection, including transplan- tation, for hepatoblastoma and hepatocellular carcinoma: impact on survival. *J Pediatr Surg*, 27, 292-6, discussion 297.

[124] Freeman, R. B., Jr., & Edwards, E. B. (2000). Liver transplant waiting time does not correlate with waiting list mortality: implications for liver allocation policy. *Liver Transplant*, 6, 543-52.

[125] Organ Procurement and Transplantation Network-HRSA. (1998). Final rule with comment period. *Fed Regist*, 63, 16296-338.

[126] Tiao, G. M., Alonso, M. H., & Ryckman, F. C. (2006). Pediatric liver transplantation. *Seminars in pediatric surgery*, 15(3), 218-27.

[127] Schiff, E. R., Maddrey, W. C., & Sorrel, M. F. (2011). *Schiff's Disease of the Liver* (11th ed.), Wiley-Blackwell.

[128] Ehren, H., Mahour, G. H., & Isaacs, H., Jr. (1983). Benign liver tumors in infancy and childhood. *Report of 48 cases. Am J Surg*, 145, 325-9.

[129] Kochin, M. D., Tamir, A., Miloh, M. D., Ronen Arnon, M. D., Kishore, R., Iyer, M. D., Frederick, J., Suchy, M. D., Nanda Kerkar, M., Zenge, J. P., Fenton, L., Lovell, M. A.,

Grover, T. R., et al. (2002). Case report: infantile hemangioendothelioma. *Curr Opin Pediatr*, 14, 99-102.

[130] Reymond, D., Plaschkes, J., Luthy, A. R., et al. (1995). Focal nodular hyperplasia of the liver in children: review of follow-up and outcome. *J Pediatr Surg*, 30, 1590-3.

[131] Bakshi, P., Srinivasan, R., Rao, K. L., et al. (2006). Fine needle aspiration biopsy in pediatric space- occupying lesions of liver: a retrospective study evaluating its role and diagnostic efficacy. *J Pediatr Surg*, 41, 1903-8.

[132] Schwartz, M. E., Konstadoulakis, M. M., Roayaie, S., et al. (2008). The Mount Sinai experience with orthotopic liver transplantation for benign tumors: brief report and literature review: case reports. *Transplant Proc*, 40, 1759-62.

[133] Finegold, M. J., Egler, R. A., Goss, J. A., et al. (2008). Liver tumors: pediatric population. *Liver Transpl*, 14, 1545-56.

[134] Zenge, J. P., Fenton, L., Lovell, M. A., & Grover, T. R. (2002). Case report: infantile hemangioendothelioma. *Curr Opin Pediatr*, 14, 99-102.

[135] Mortelé, K. J., Vanzieleghem, B., Mortelé, B., Benoit, Y., & Ros, P. R. (2002). Solitary hepatic infantile hemangioendothelioma: dynamic gadolinium-enhanced MR imaging findings. *Eur Radiol*, 12, 862-865.

[136] Ingram, J. D., Yerushalmi, B., Connell, J., Karrer, F. M., Tyson, R. W., & Sokol, R. J. (2000). Hepatoblastoma in a neonate: a hypervascular presentation mimicking hemangioendothelioma. *Pediatr Radiol*, 30, 794-797.

[137] Roos, J. E., Pfiffner, R., Stallmach, T., Stuckmann, G., Marincek, B., & Willi, U. (2003). Infantile hemangioendothelioma. *Radiographics : a review publication of the Radiological Society of North America*, 23(6), 1649-55.

[138] Stringer, M. D., & Alizai, N. K. (2005). Mesenchymal hamartoma of the liver: a systematic review. *J Pediatr Surg*, 40, 1681-90.

[139] Horton, K. M., Bluemke, D. A., Ralph, H., Soyer, P., & Fishman, E. K. (1999). *CT and MR Imaging of Benign Hepatic*, 431-451.

[140] Zafrani, E. S. (1989). Update on vascular tumours of the liver. *J Hepatology*, 8(1), 125-30.

[141] Linderkamp, O., Hopner, F., Klose, H., et al. (1976). Solitary hepatic hemangioma in a newborn infant complicated by cardiac failure, consumption coagulopathy, microangiopathic hemolytic anemia, and obstructive jaundice. Case report and review of the literature. *Eur J Pediatr*, 125(1), 239.

[142] Hobbs, K. E. (1990). Hepatic hemangiomas. *World J Surg*, 14(4), 468-71.

[143] DeLorimier, A. A., Simpson, E. B., Baum, R. S., et al. (1967). Hepatic-artery ligation for hepatic hemangiomatosis. *N Engl J Med*, 277(7), 333-7.

[144] Warmann, S., Bertram, H., Kardorff, R., et al. (2003). Interventional treat- ment of infantile hepatic hemangioendothelioma. *J Pediatr Surg*, 38(8), 1177-81.

[145] Walsh, R., Harrington, J., Beneck, D., et al. (2004). Congenital infantile hepatic hemangioendothelioma type II treated with orthotopic liver transplantation. *J Pediatr Hematol Oncol*, 26(2), 121-3.

[146] Lack, E. E., & Ornvold, K. (1986). Focal nodular hyperplasia and hepatic adenoma: a review of eight cases in the pediatric age group. *J Surg Oncol*, 33, 129-35.

[147] Farruggia, P., Alaggio, R., Cardella, F., Tropia, S., Trizzino, A., Ferrara, F., & D'Angelo, P. (2010). Focal nodular hyperplasia of the liver: an unusual association with diabetes mellitus in a child and review of literature. *Italian journal of pediatrics*, 36, 41, doi: 10.1186/1824-7288-36-41.

[148] Luciani, A., Kobeiter, H., Maison, P., Cherqui, D., Zafrani, E. S., Dhumeaux, D., & Mathieu, D. (2002). Focal nodular hyperplasia of the liver in men: is presentation the same in men and women? *Gut*, 50, 877-80.

[149] Rebouissou, S., Bioulac-Sage, P., & Zucman-Rossi, J. (2008). Molecular pathogenesis of focal nodular hyperplasia and hepatocellular adenoma. *J Hepatol*, 48, 163-170.

[150] Raidl, M., Pirker, C., Schulte-Hermann, R., Aubele, M., Kandioler-Eckersberger, D., Wrba, F., Micksche, M., Berger, W., & Grasl-Kraupp, B. (2004). Multiple chromosomal abnormalities in human liver (pre)neoplasia. *J Hepatol*, 40, 660-668.

[151] Vernier-Massouille, G., Cosnes, J., Lemann, M., Marteau, P., Reinisch, W., Laharie, D., & Cadiot, G. (2007). Nodular regenerative hyperplasia in patients with inflammatory bowel disease treated with azathioprine. *Gut*, 56(10), 1404-9.

[152] Stromeyer, F. W., & Ishak, K. G. (1981). Nodular transformation (nodular "regenerative" hyperplasia) of the liver.A clinicopathologic study of 30 cases. *Hum Pathol*, 12, 60-71.

[153] Wanless, I. R., Godwin, T. A., Allen, F., et al. (1980). Nodular regenerative hyperplasia of the liver in hematologic disorders: a possible response to obliterative portal venopathy. A morphometric study of nine cases with an hypothesis on the pathogenesis. *Medicine*, 59, 367-79.

[154] Naber, A. H., Van Haelst, U., & Yap, S. H. (1991). Nodular regenerative hyperplasia of the liver: an important cause of portal hypertension in non-cirrhotic patients. *J Hepatol*, 12, 94-9.

[155] Reshamwala, P. A., Kleiner, D. E., & Heller, T. (2006). Nodular regenerative hyperplasia: not all nodules are created equal. *Hepatology*, 44, 7-14.

[156] Stocker, J. T., & Ishak, K. G. (1983). Mesenchymal hamartoma of the liver: Report of 30 cases and review of the literature. *Pediatr Pathol*, 1, 245-67.

[157] Gupta, R., Parelkar, S. V., & Sanghvi, B. (2009). Mesenchymal hamartoma of the liver. *Indian J Med Paediatr Oncol*, 30, 141-143, doi:.

[158] Kirks, D. R., & Griscom, N. T. (1990). Practical pediatric imaging. Lippincott Williams and Wilkins, 3rd ed, Boston, Little, Brown, *Diagnostic radiology of infants and children*, 808-815.

[159] Ito, H., Kishikawa, T., Toda, T., Arai, M., & Muro, H. (1984). Hepatic mesenchymal hamartoma of an infant. *J Pediatr Surg*, 19, 315-7.

[160] Bisogno, G., Pilz, T., Perilongo, G., et al. (2002). Undifferentiated sarcoma of the liver in childhood: A curable disease. *Cancer*, 94, 252-257.

[161] Lack, E. E., Schloo, B. L., Azumi, Net, et al. (1991). Undifferentiated (embryonal) sarcoma of the liver.Clinical and pathological study of 16 cases with emphasis on immunohistochemical features. *Am J Surg Pathol*, 15, 1-16.

[162] Chuang, W.-yu., Lin, J.-nan., Hung, I.-jih., & Hsueh, C. (2001). *Undifferentiated Sarcoma of the Liver*, 399-404.

[163] Foster, J. H., & Berman, M. M. (1977). *Solid Liver Tumors*, Philadelphia, W. B. Saunders, 198-202.

[164] Donovan, E. J., & Santulli, T. V. (1946). Resection of the left lobe of the liver for mesenchymoma- Report of case. *Ann Surg*, 124, 90-3.

[165] Willeford, G., & Stembridge, V. A. (1950). Primary sarcoma of liver- Report of a case. *Am J Dis Child*, 80, 404-7.

[166] Dintzman, M., Reiss, R., & Haimoff, H. (1966). Right hepatectomy. *Isr J Med Sci*, 2, 743-9.

[167] Noguchi, K., Yokoo, H., Nakanishi, K., Kakisaka, T., Tsuruga, Y., Kamachi, H., Matsushita, M., et al. (2012). A long-term survival case of adult undifferentiated embryonal sarcoma of liver. *World journal of surgical oncology*, 10(1), 65.

[168] Walker, N. I., Horn, M. J., Strong, R. W., Lynch, S. V., Cohen, J., Ong, T. H., & Harris, O. D. (1992). Undifferentiated (embryonal) sarcoma of the liver: Pathologic findings and long-term survival after complete surgical resection. *Cancer*, 69(1), 52-59.

[169] Aoyama, C., Hachitanda, Y., Sato, J. K., Said, J. W., & Shimada, H. (1991). Undifferentiated (embryonal) sarcoma of the liver. A tumor of uncertain histogenesis showing divergent differentiation. *Am J Surg Pathol*, 15, 615-24.

[170] Chou, P., Mangkornkanok, M., & Gonzalez-Crussi, F. (1990). Undifferentiated (embryonal) sarcoma of the liver: ultrastructure, immunohistochemistry, and DNA ploidy analysis of two cases. *Pediatr Pathol*, 10, 549-62.

[171] Keating, S., & Taylor, G. P. (1985). Undifferentiated (embryonal) sarcoma of the liver: ultrastructural and immunohistochemical similarities with malignant fibrous histiocytoma. *Hum Pathol*, 16, 693-9.

[172] Buetow, P. C., Buck, J. L., Pantongrag-Brown, L., Marshall, W. H., Ros, P. R., Levine, M. S., & Goodman, Z. D. (1997). Undifferentiated embryonal sarcoma of the liver: pathological basis of imaging findings in 28 cases. *Radiology*, 203, 779-783.

[173] Urban, C. E., Mache, C. J., Schwinger, W., Pakisch, B., Ranner, G., Riccabona, M., Schimpl, G., Brandesky, G., Messner, H., Pobegen, W., Becker, H., & Grienberger, H. (1993). Undifferentiated (embryonal) sarcoma of the liver in childhood. Successful combined-modality therapy in four patients. *Cancer*, 72, 2511-6.

[174] Newman, K. D., Schisgall, R., Reaman, G., & Guzzetta, P. C. (1989). Malignant mesenchymoma of the liver in cildren. *J Pediatr Surg*, 24, 781-3.

[175] Kirks, D. R., & Griscom, N. T. (1990). Practical pediatric imaging. editors. Lippincott Williams and Wilkins, 3rd ed., Boston, Little, Brown, *Diagnostic radiology of infants and children*, 808-815.

Chapter 19

Liver Tumors in Infancy and Children

Chunbao Guo and Mingman Zhang

Additional information is available at the end of the chapter

http://dx.doi.org/10.5772/51500

1. Introduction

The liver is the third-most-common site for intra-abdominal malignancy in children, following adrenal neuroblastoma and wilms tumor. Although the overall incidence of childhood cancer has been slowly increasing since 1975, cancer in children and adolescents is still rare, the incidence of primary malignant liver tumors per year is 1-1.5 per million children in the United States [1, 2, 3, 4]. This yields a relative low rate for hepatic tumors (1.3% of all pediatric malignancies). Tumors of the liver may be either malignant or benign. Two thirds of liver tumors in children are malignant. Of these malignant tumors, hepatoblastoma (HB) and hepatocellular carcinoma (HCC) are the most common and account for 70 persent of all hepatic neoplasms. Unlike liver tumors in adults, in which the predominant histology is hepatocellular carcinoma, hepatoblastoma accounts for two thirds of liver tumors in children. Other liver malignancies in children include sarcomas, germ cell tumors, as well as rhabdoid tumors. Benign tumors of the liver in children include vascular tumors, hamartomas, adenomas, and focal nodular hyperplasia (FNH). The histology and anatomy of a pediatric liver tumor guides the treatment and prognosis [5, 6, 7, 8].

Recently, dramatic improvements in survival have been achieved for children and adolescents with liver cancer. Children and adolescents with liver cancer should be referred to multidisciplinary team incorporates the skills of the primary care physician, pediatric surgical subspecialists, radiation therapists, pediatric oncologists/hematologists, rehabilitation specialists, pediatric nurse specialists, social workers, and others to ensure that children receive treatment, supportive care, and rehabilitation that will achieve optimal survival and quality of life. Almost all liver masses in children are surgically treated, either primarily or following systemic chemotherapy [9, 10]. The conditions that eventuate in this choice of therapy, when and how to accomplish it, and the medical and surgical consequences for children of transplantation for tumors are described in guidelines for pediatric cancer centers and their role in the treatment of pediatric patients with cancer by the American Academy of Pediatrics [11, 12, 13]. Clinical trials for children and adolescents with cancer are generally designed to compare potentially better therapy with therapy that is currently accepted as standard. Clinical trials are available in many clinical institutes for liver cancer that occur in children and adolescents, and the opportunity to participate in these trials is offered to most patients/families [14].

2. Epidemiology of pediatric hepatic tumors

Benign lesions in children represent 30% of hepatic tumors and are most commonly vascular in origin (eg, hemangiomas, hemangioendotheliomas). Two-thirds of hepatic neoplasms in children are malignant. Liver cancer is also rare malignancy in children and adolescents and account for approximately 1% of all pediatric malignancies. The malignant liver tumor is divided into two major histologic subgroups: hepatoblastoma, affecting around 80% of children, and hepatocellular carcinoma (HCC) [15, 16]. The age of onset of liver cancer in children is related to tumor histology. Hepatoblastoma usually occur before the age of 3 years, and approximately 90% of malignant liver tumors in children aged 4 years and younger are hepatoblastomas. There are 2 distinct groups of HCC patients in childhood: children who develop sporadic HCC without preceding liver disease, and those developing HCC in the context of advanced chronic liver disease (CLD). Sporadic HCC in children has a relatively poor outcome, while the several small series that report on HCC developing in CLD do so in the context of liver transplantation (LT). Some biologic differences may exist between HCCs developing in adults and children. One study reported an high radiological response (49%) in pediatric HCC, higher than adult HCC [17].

The incidence of hepatocellular carcinoma is negligible in children aged 14 years and younger. In china, the incidence of hepatic tumors in children 14 years and younger is 2.6 per 100,000, of which 81 persent are hepatoblastoma. The incidence of hepatoblastoma in the United States increased in the last 25 years, whereas the incidence of hepatocellular carcinoma in the United States has not changed appreciably over time. The cause for the increase in incidence of hepatoblastoma is unknown, but the increasing survival of very low birth weight premature infants, which is known to be associated with hepatoblastoma, may contribute. In Japan, the risk of hepatoblastoma in children who weighed less than 1,000 g at birth are 15 times the risk in normal birth weight children. Other data has confirmed the high incidence of hepatoblastoma in very low birth weight premature infants. In several asian countries, the incidence of hepatocellular carcinoma in children is 10 times more than that in North America. The high incidence appears to be related to the incidence of perinatally acquired hepatitis B, which can be prevented in most cases by vaccination and administration of hepatitis B immune globulin to the newborn [18, 19].

Additional rare malignant liver tumors in children are sarcoma, including its 3 variants rhabdomyosarcoma, embryonal or undifferentiated sarcoma, and angiosarcoma predominantly presenting in early childhood. Also included is the exceedingly uncommon cholangiocarcinoma, which can present at any age, often in the context of chronic biliary disease.The overall survival rate for children with hepatoblastoma is 70%, but is only 25% for those with hepatocellular carcinoma.

3. Clinical presentation and diagnosis

Most children with liver tumors commonly present insidiously with nonspecific abdominal discomfort, a palpable abdominal mass, feeding difficulties, and abdominal distension. Chronic fatigue secondary to anemia thrombocytopenia, and leukocytosis and lack of appetite are often reported. Jaundice and biochemical derangement are signs of advanced neoplastic change. Children with both HB and HCC may also present with weight loss, fever, and anorexia [20, 21, 22].

Fetal and neonatal presentations include hydramnios, fetal hydrops, congestive heart failure, and respiratory distress. Occasionally, the child may present acutely with vomiting, fever and clinical signs of abdominal irritation, often suggestive of tumor rupture with intraperitoneal spread. Patients with congestive heart failure have been shown to have lower survival rates. Very rarely HB can present with signs of precocious puberty/virilization due to b-HCG secretion by the tumor. Laboratory studies are performed to assess baseline CBC count, electrolyte levels, liver enzyme levels, liver synthetic function, and α -fetoprotein (AFP) levels Serum AFP remains the key clinical marker of malignant neoplastic change, response to the treatment, and relapse. AFP levels are elevated in 50%-70% of children with hepatic neoplasms, and multiple studies confirm that AFP is a valuable surveillance marker in children who have previously undergone hepatic resection for malignancy. However, there are some variants of both HB and HCC that have low or normal AFP. These variants may have distinct histologic features and poorer prognoses [23, 24]. The initial workup for hepatic masses includes radiographic assessment using ultrasonography.

All children with a palpable abdominal mass usually undergo an initial ultrasound to confirm the location and to characterize the consistency as cystic or solid. Cystic or vascular lesions may not require any further imaging. However, definitive characterization of the mass requires a computed tomography (CT) or magnetic resonance imaging (MRI) scan. Calcifications can be seen in a minority of liver tumors. Hypervascularized hepatic lesions with delayed contrast excretion are highly suspicious of a malignant tumor.

Abdominal ultrasonography usually demonstrates a large mass, possibly with some satellite lesions and areas of hemorrhage within the tumor. CT scanning of the abdomen and chest are used for indeterminate or solid lesions to further delineate the location and to assess resectability (Fig. 1) and evaluate for the presence of pulmonary metastasis. MRI angiography is frequently helpful preoperatively to determine resectability because it delineates the vascular anatomy more precisely. Local radiological availability, expertise extent, and multiplicity of the lesions and to detect metastases may facilitate surgical planning and may determine resectability, however, definitive diagnosis can be proven only through biopsy findings [25, 26, 27].

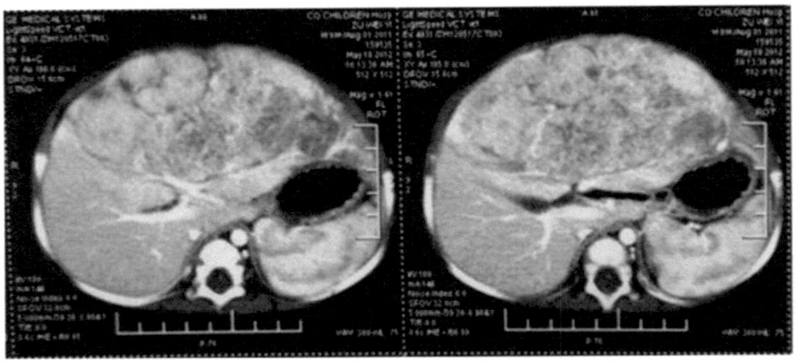

Figure 1. CT scan of a hepatoblastoma amenable to surgical resection.

Any child with a suspected liver tumor should also have AFP and ß-HCG serum assays. The alpha-fetoprotein (AFP) and beta-hCG tumor markers are very helpful in diagnosis and management of liver tumors. Alttough elevation of AFP levels is not diagnostic of hepatic malignancy. AFP is markedly elevated in90% of hepatoblastoma cases and in many cases of hepatocellular carcinoma, and it returns to normal with effective therapy. The level of AFP at diagnosis and rate of decrease in AFP during treatment should be compared to the age-adjusted normal range. Caution should be taken in normal term infants who can have AFP levels in excess of 100,000 ng/ml, however, with a half-life of approximately 1 week, the AFP level normalizes to 10 ng/ml over the first few months of life. Absence of elevated AFP levels at diagnosis occurs in a few percentage of children with hepatoblastoma and appears to be associated with poor prognosis, as well as with the small cell undifferentiated variant of hepatoblastoma. Lack of a significant decrease of AFP levels with treatment may predict a poor response to therapy.

Beta-hCG is a hormone commonly produced by liver tumors and, in excess, can result in precocious puberty. It's levels may also be elevated in children with hepatoblastoma or hepatocellular carcinoma, which may result in isosexual precocity in boys. Extremely high levels of beta-hCG are associated with infantile choriocarcinoma of the liver [28, 29].

Because of the association between familial adenomatous polyposis and hepatoblastoma, obtaining a thorough family history is an important aspect of the management of a child with a liver tumor and his family, with particular attention to any family history of colon cancer or colonic polyps.

A chest CT is an important aspect of the workup because the lung parenchyma is the most common distant site for metastasis. A CBC typically displays mild normocytic and normochromic anemia with thrombocytosis.

Tissue diagnosis of the tumor is essential, although some advocate that in the presence of very high AFP in a young child (6 months to 3 years). The practice in the United States is not to treat without a tissue sample except under the most urgent life-threatening circumstances, such as tumor growth into the right atrium. But this may not be necessary, as avoiding the biopsy theoretically reduces the risks of the tumor seeding. In Europe, The Childhood

Liver Tumor Study Group of the Inter-national Society of Pediatric Oncology (SIOPEL) has developed a preoperative evaluation of the tumor extent (PRETEXT) grading system. The rationale for this recommendation is provided in the section on pathology. Segmental assessment of the extent of the tumor and its relation with the main hepatic vessels is of foremost importance for planning the intensity of chemotherapy and eventual surgery., which could provide a valuable tool for the risk stratification. Formal staging of the tumor should include chest and brain CT and bone scanning [30, 31].

Benign hepatic tumors are usually diagnosed incidentally. Some children may develop the Kasabach-Merritt phenomenon, a triad of coagulopathy, hemolytic anemia and thrombocytopenia due to intralesional pooling of the blood. IHE can have an acute presentation, typically within the first couple of weeks or months of life. Dramatic abdominal distension can lead to major respiratory distress, prompting the need for assisted ventilation and intensive care support. Nowadays some IHEs may be detected on routine antenatal ultrasonography, due to their characteristic vascular multichannel appearance. A proportion of children develop a bizarre secondary hypothyroidism that is thought to be secondary to tumor production of the enzyme iodothyronine deiodinase, which stimulates the conversion of thyroxine to reverse triiodothyronine and of triiodothyronine to 3,3'-diio-dothyronine, leading to a biochemical picture of hypothyroidism, requiring thyroxin supplementation. This phenomenon resolves once the tumor is removed or significantly decreases in size, usually within the first 2 years of life.

3.1. Risk factors

Similar to other embryonal tumors, altered imprinting at the 11–15 locus has been observed in hepatoblastoma. Rearrangements involving the pericentric region of chromosome 1 also appear to be important in hepatoblastoma, with roughly 18% of hepatoblastomas displaying an imbalanced translocation involving this region. Hepatoblastoma is associated with several genetic syndromes and familial cancer predisposition conditions, such as familial adenomatous polyposis and Beckwith-Wiedemann syndrome in addition to several other rare syndromes. Other compelling evidence suggests that acquired aberrations in the ß-catenin/Wnt pathways are important in the pathogenesis of hepatoblastoma. Acquired chromosomal changes in tumors include numerical chromosomal changes, most commonly trisomies of chromosomes 2, 8, and 20. Finally, epigenetic changes in methylation patterns of DNA may be altered in hepatoblastoma.

There is limited but compelling evidence that parental exposures are associated with a higher incidence of liver tumors and, more specifically, hepatoblastoma. Children from parents who have been exposed to metals used in soldering and welding, petroleum, or paints are at a higher risk for hepatoblastoma. Recent reports have also implicated parental smoking as a risk factor for hepatoblastoma [32, 33].

3.2. Beckwith-Wiedemann syndrome

The incidence of hepatoblastoma is increased 1,000 to 10,000-fold in infants and children with Beckwith-Wiedemann syndrome (BWS). BWS can be caused by either genetic mutations and be familial, or much more commonly, by epigenetic changes and be sporadic. Hepatoblastoma is also increased in hemihypertrophy, an overgrowth syndrome caused by the same epigenetic changes in chromosome 11p15.5 that cause many cases of BWS, but in a genetically mosaic fashion. Either mechanism can be associated with an increased incidence of embryonal tumors including Wilms tumor and hepatoblastoma. The gene dosage and ensuing increase in expression of insulin-like growth factor 2 (IGF 2) has been implicated in the macrosomia and embryonal tumors in BWS and hemihypertrophy. When sporadic, the types of embryonal tumors associated with BWS have frequently also undergone somatic changes in the BWS locus and IGF 2. All children with BWS or isolated hemihypertrophy should be screened regularly by ultrasound to detect abdominal malignancies at an early stage. Screening using AFP levels has helped in the early detection of hepatoblastoma in children with BWS or hemihypertrophy. Other somatic overgrowth syndromes, such as Simpson-Golabi-Behmel syndrome, may also be associated with hepatoblastoma.

3.3. Familial adenomatous polyposis

There is an association between hepatoblastoma and familial adenomatous polyposis (FAP); children in families that carry the APC gene are at an 800-fold increased risk for hepatoblastoma. However, hepatoblastoma occurs in less than 1% of FAP family members, so ultrasound and AFP screening for hepatoblastoma in members of families with FAP is controversial. The predisposition to hepatoblastoma may be limited to a specific subset of APC mutations. It has been recommended that all children with hepatoblastoma be examined for congenital hypertrophy of the retinal pigment epithelium, a marker of APC mutation carriers in 70% of polyposis families. In the absence of APC germline mutations, childhood hepatoblastomas do not have somatic mutations in the APC gene; however, they frequently have mutations in the beta-catenin gene, the function of which is closely related to APC.

3.4. Hepatitis B and hepatitis C infection

Hepatocellular carcinoma is associated with hepatitis B and hepatitis C infection, especially in children with perinatally acquired hepatitis B virus [33]. Compared with adults, the incubation period from hepatitis virus infection to the genesis of hepatocellular carcinoma is extremely short in a small subset of children with perinatally acquired virus. Widespread hepatitis B immunization has decreased the incidence of hepatocellular carcinoma in Asia. Mutations in the met/hepatocyte growth factor receptor gene occur in childhood hepatocellular carcinoma, and this could be the mechanism that results in a shortened incubation period.Hepatocellular carcinoma may also arise in very young children with mutations in the bile salt export pump ABCB11, which causes progressive familial hepatic cholestasis. Several specific types of nonviral liver injury and cirrhosis are associated with hepatocellular carcinoma in children including tyrosinemia and biliary cirrhosis.

http://dx.doi.org/10.5772/51500

3.5. Undifferentiated Embryonal Sarcoma of the Liver

Undifferentiated embryonal sarcoma of the liver (UESL) is the third most common liver malignancy in children and adolescents, comprising 9% to 13% of liver tumors. Widespread infiltration throughout the liver and pulmonary metastasis are common, usually between the ages of 5 and 10 years. It could also presents as an abdominal mass, often with pain or malaise. It may appear solid or cystic on imaging, frequently with central necrosis. Distinctive features are characteristic intracellular hyaline globules and marked anaplasia on a mesenchymal background. Many UESL contain diverse elements of mesenchymal cell maturation, such as smooth muscle and fat.

Strong clinical and histological evidence suggest that some UESLs arise from mesenchymal hamartomas of the liver (MHL), which are large benign multicystic masses that present in the first 2 years of life. Many MHLs have a characteristic translocation with a breakpoint at 19q13.4 and several UESLs have the same translocation. In a report of 11 cases of UESL, five arose in association with MHL, and transition zones between the histologies were noted. Some UESLs arising from MHLs may have complex karyotypes not involving 19q13.4.

3.6. Infantile Choriocarcinoma of the Liver

Choriocarcinoma of the liver is a very rare tumor that appears to originate in the placenta and presents with a liver mass in the first few months of life. Infants are often unstable due to hemorrhage from the tumor. Clinical diagnosis may be made without biopsy based on extremely high serum beta-hCG levels and normal AFP levels for age.

3.7. Epithelioid Hemangioendothelioma

Epithelioid hemangioendothelioma (EHE) is a rare vascular cancer that occurs in the liver and other organs.

Generally, children with liver masses display normal growth and development unless they show the phenotypes associated with Beckwith-Wiedemann syndrome or the other genetic cancer predisposition syndromes associated with liver tumors.

4. Screening

Hepatic neoplasms develop in a myriad of chronic liver disorders of childhood, often without or with minimal symptoms. Therefore, regular screening with abdominal ultrasound and serum AFP measurement should be in place for all children with CLD at least annually. Therefore, awareness of antecedent conditions that permit screening is essential. Detection of a liver tumor prior to dissemination and/or massive growth is the single most important management tool for all tumor types at all ages. Children with chronic hepatitis B should be also regularly checked, but because communities in which immunization has yet to be provided are typically impoverished and medically underserved, recommendations for screening have not yet been implemented. Some of the conditions with known increased propensity to develop malignancies such as tyrosinemia type 1 (even on nitizinone treatment) or bile salt export pump (BSEP) deficiency should be assessed every 6 months. However, there is no formal guideline for the frequency and manner of screening at this time [34, 35].

Extraordinary advances in neonatal care in the past 25 years have led to a wholly new population of children, the long-term survivors of birth as early as 22 to 23 weeks of gestation with a weight less than 1000 g. In addition to many other chronic problems, they have extraordinary susceptibility to HB. HB is dramatically more common in expremature babies but arranging effective screening programs could prove to be difficult because of their increasing numbers and fact that their long term care is typically provided outside hepatological clinics. Monitoring much smaller cohorts of children with Beckwith-Wiedemann Syndrome for HB is more feasible, and one study has suggested abdominal ultrasonography and serum AFP every 3 months until 4 years of age.

There are several conditions for which screening of children for primary liver cancer is recommended by virtue of the attendant risk. Hepatitis B virus can cause HCC as early as age 4 following perinatal transmission from infected carrier mothers. Vaccination and perinatal administration of hepatitis B immunoglobulin have already reduced the incidence dramatically. A relative risk for such prematures versus term babies of 16- to 52-fold is recognized around the world. HB occurs at the same age as HB in term babies or later. Screening of infants with hemihypertrophy or hemiaplasia, as part of the Beckwith-Wiedemann over-growth syndrome, has been carried out for many years via ultrasound to detect intraabdominal malignancies. These include Wilms' tumor and adreno cortical carcinoma, in addition to the less common HB, which has a relative risk of 2280. HB is not the only proliferative lesion of the Beckwith-Wiedemann syndrome liver, as hemangioendothelioma and mesenchymal hamartoma have also been observed, either con-currently or sequentially [37, 38].

In familial adenomatous polyposis (FAP), the first manifestation of an autosomal dominant mutation in a family may be HB in a baby, with the colonic polyps detected only afterwards in a parent. The relative risk for children in such cohorts is 800-fold, but many examples are due to new germ-line mutations at 5q21,22 or only in the tumor.

A series from the Children's Oncology Group focused primarily on known FAP families but raised the issue of de novo cases or the potential for infants of parents too young to be aware of the symptoms of FAP themselves.

The largest report of sporadic cases looked at 50 patients and found 5 germline antigen-presenting cell (APC) mutations. This led the authors to recommend routine screening for APC mutations in all cases of sporadic HB, including both a screen for APC deletion or duplication and sequencing through the gene itself. In the only prospective screening study to date, 20 children with confirmed or suspected FAP were followed for 10 years by ultrasonography, and no tumors were detected. In FAP, other forms of hepatocellular neoplasia are also observed, including adenoma and HCC, as well as biliary adenomas.

The timelines of the development of these various cancers in distinct tissues are not linked, and therefore, surveillance for these cancers needs to continue throughout the patient's life

[39]. Chronic cholestatic syndromes may be the substrate for liver cancers, with HB, cholangiocarcinoma, and in the Alagille syndrome of a paucity of intrahepatic bile ducts due to Jagged 1 or NOTCH mutations. Also, we have observed HB in three 2-year olds with congenital hepatic fibrosis and autosomal recessive polycystic disease. HB and HCC have been seen in the explants of infants with cirrhosis due to biliary atresia as early as 1 year. On the basis of the growth rate of HCC and with the aim of detecting tumors when they are 3 cm in diameter, the American Association for the Study of Liver Disease and the European Association for the Study of the Liver recommend screening ultrasound examinations at 6-month intervals, and some institutions shorten this interval to 3 months when the patient is on a transplant waiting list. These organizations have also published diagnostic criteria for liver nodules detected during the screening process.

HCC can be diagnosed noninvasively by computed tomography (CT) or magnetic resonance imaging (MRI) if a lesion 2cm in diameter within a cirrhotic liver demonstrates rapid contrast enhancement during the arterial phase and washout on the delayed venous phase. These guidelines were developed for cirrhotic adults, and there are no validated evidence-based guidelines for screening for tumors in children and adolescents with chronic liver disease.

According to adult data, ultrasound is insensitive for the diagnosis of HCC in the cirrhotic liver and should not be used for the detection of focal liver lesions in this setting. MRI is more sensitive than multidetector 3-phase CT for the diagnosis of regenerative and dysplastic nodules and is comparable to CT for the detection of HCC. There is a lower false-positive rate with MRI. Interval growth is probably the best indicator of malignancy, and there is a definite need for the establishment of protocols for follow-up imaging in centers that care for children with diffuse liver disease.

In the case of hereditary tyrosinemia type 1 due to fumaryl acetoacetate hydrolase deficiency, prompt medical management, by blocking an enzyme upstream in the tyrosine catabolic pathway, can avert the injury that otherwise leads to HCC more often than any other metabolic defect. However, a low risk of developing HCC remains even with adequate medical management, so these children require life-long surveillance. Therefore, for the conditions listed, periodic abdominal ultrasonography and serum alpha fetoprotein measurements, at 3-month intervals in the case of Beck-with-Wiedemann syndrome and similarly for the first 3 years of life for others and then every 6 months thereafter, are advocated [40, 41]. In addition, recognition of the rare sequential occurrences of mesenchymal hamartoma and sarcoma and of hemangioendothelioma with angiosarcoma indicates the need for surveillance ultrasonography whenever a complete resection or transplant has not taken place [42, 43].

5. Staging

The process used to find out if cancer has spread within the liver or to other parts of the body is called staging. The staging system would be useful in determining treatment plans and offers good prognostic value for overall and disease-free survival outcome. Historically, north Americans have staged liver tumors similar to other solid tumors, with surgical resectability and the presence of metastases as the primary criteria. The European staging system considers only the pretreatment extent of disease, and was developed by the Childhood Liver Tumor Strategy Group. After childhood liver cancer has been diagnosed, tests are done to find out if cancer cells have spread within the liver or to other parts of the body. The PRETEXT staging system divides the liver into four sectors, and the number of segments involved by tumor indicates stage. A lettering system further indicates extrahepatic involvement.The information gathered from the staging process determines the stage of the disease [44, 45].

The following tests and procedures may be used in the staging process: -CT scan (CAT scan): This procedure is also called computed tomography, computerized tomography, or computerized axial tomography. The pictures are made by a computer linked to an x-ray machine. A procedure that makes a series of detailed pictures of areas inside the body, taken from different angles. A dye may be injected into a vein or swallowed to help the organs or tissues show up more clearly.

-MRI (magnetic resonance imaging): Also called nuclear magnetic resonance imaging (NMRI), a procedure that uses a magnet, radio waves, and a computer to make a series of detailed pictures of areas inside the body.

-Ultrasound exam: A procedure in which high-energy sound waves (ultrasound) are bounced off internal tissues or organs and make echoes. The echoes form a picture of body tissues called a sonogram. The picture can be printed to be looked at later.

-Surgery: An operation will be done to look at or remove the tumor. Tissues removed during surgery will be checked by a pathologist.

There are 2 staging systems for childhood liver cancer.

-Presurgical (before surgery) staging: This staging system is called PRETEXT, based on imaging procedures such as MRI or CT, where the tumor has shown within the four parts (sections) of the liver.

The liver is divided into 4 vertical sections.

In PRETEXT stage 1(Fig. 2A), the cancer is found in one section of the liver. Three sections of the liver that are next to each other do not have cancer in them.

In PRETEXT stage 2 (Fig. 2B), cancer is found in one or two sections of the liver. Two sections of the liver that are next to each other do not have cancer in them.

In PRETEXT stage 3(Fig. 2C), the cancer is found in three sections of the liver and one section does not have cancer. OR, cancer is found in two sections of the liver and two sections that are not next to each other do not have cancer in them.

http://dx.doi.org/10.5772/51500

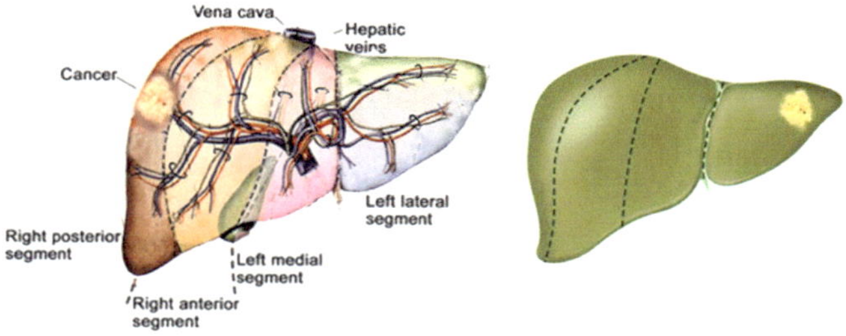

Figure 2.

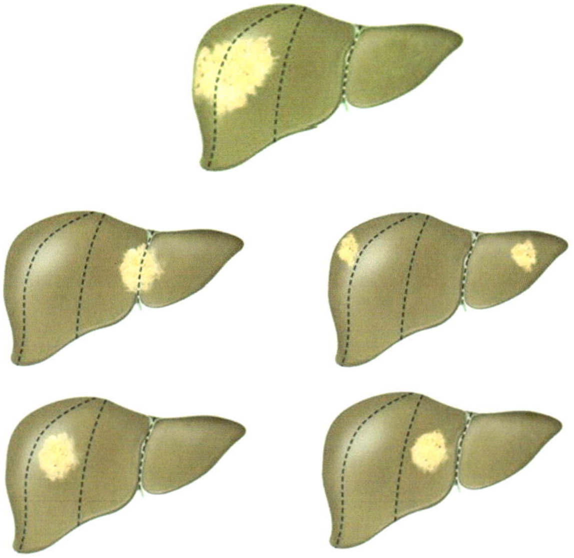

Figure 3.

Postsurgical (after surgery) staging: The stage is based on the amount of tumor that remains after the patient has had surgery to look at or remove the tumor.

Stage I

In stage I, all of the cancer was removed by surgery in the liver.

Stage II

In stage II, a small amount of cancer remains in the liver, but it can be seen only with a microscope, or the tumor cells may have spilled into the abdomen before surgery or during surgery.

Stage III

In stage III:

In stage III, the tumor cannot be removed by surgery; orcancer that can be seen without a microscope remains after surgery; or the cancer has spread to nearby lymph nodes.

Stage IV

In stage IV, the cancer has spread to other parts of the body. Cancer invades the surrounding normal tissue. Cancer invades the lymph system and travels through the lymph vessels to other places in the body. Cancer invades the veins and capillaries and travels through the blood to other places in the body.

The metastasis is described as when cancer cells break away from the primary (original) tumor and travel through the lymph or blood to other places in the body, another (secondary) tumor may form [46]. The secondary (metastatic) tumor is the same type of cancer as the primary tumor. For example, if breast cancer spreads to the bones, the cancer cells in the bones are actually breast cancer cells. The disease is metastatic breast cancer, not bone cancer.

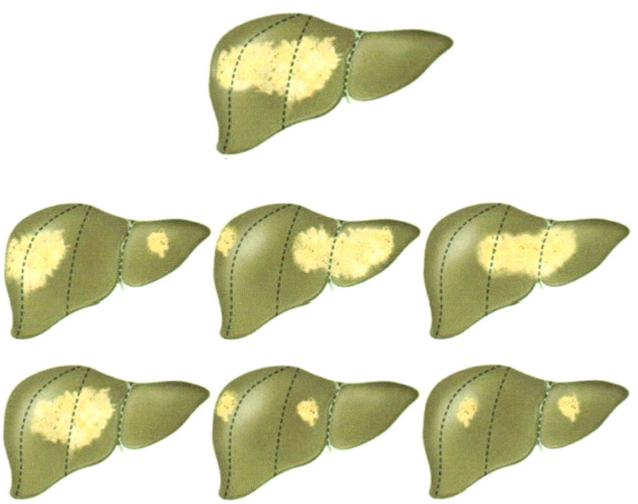

Figure 4.

In PRETEXT stage 4(Fig. 2D), cancer is found in all four sections of the liver.

http://dx.doi.org/10.5772/51500

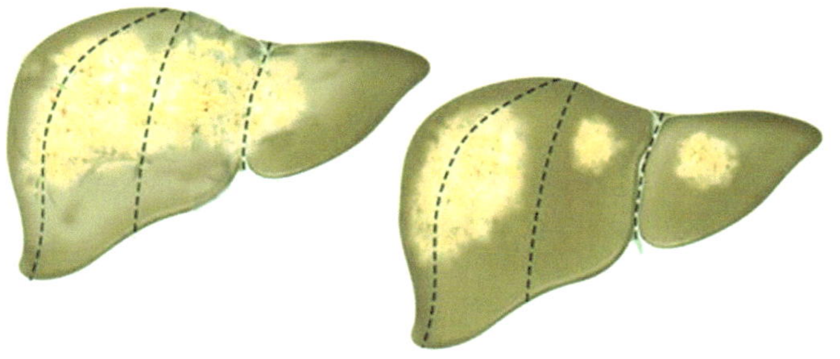

Figure 5.

6. Management

The key to successful treatment of malignant liver tumors in children is surgical removal, either by tumor resection/partial hepatectomy or Live Transplantation. Historically, complete surgical resection of the primary tumor has been required to cure malignant liver tumors in children. Complete surgical resection of the primary tumor continues to be the goal of definitive surgical procedures, but surgical resection is often combined with other treatment modalities (e.g., chemotherapy) to achieve this goal. SIOPEL recommends initial chemotherapy, while the American guidelines from COG require primary resection if possible, followed by chemotherapy, unless the tumor is pure fetal type HB stage 1, when the chemotherapy is not given. Both strategies have been successful in increasing the 5-year survival rates in HB to approximately 80% due to effective chemotherapy (cisplatinum in combination with doxorubicin or vincristine). Moreover, the timing and nature of surgical interventions are better defined for HB, and they are well-placed within the management protocols. For HCC, however, complete surgical excision or transplantation are essential for cure, and chemotherapy is not effective. On the whole, treatment planning by a multidisciplinary team of cancer specialists with experience treating tumors of childhood is required to determine and implement optimum treatment [47, 48].

The most important step in the management of benign tumors in children is confirmation of their genuine benign nature. Multiphase contrast CT imaging and, less frequently, direct angiography are required for the radiological diagnosis. Some of the benign tumors, including IHE, mesenchymal hamartoma, and FNH, would have characteristic radiological features, not always requiring a tissue diagnosis.

Many of the improvements in survival in childhood cancer have been made using new therapies that have attempted to improve on the best available, accepted therapy. Clinical trials in pediatrics are designed to compare potentially better therapy with therapy that is currently accepted as standard.Because of the relative rarity of cancer in children, all children with liver cancer should be considered for entry into a clinical trial. This comparison may be done in a randomized study of two treatment arms or by evaluating a single new treatment, comparing the results with those previously obtained with standard therapy [49].

6.1. Surgical approaches

The timing of the surgical approach is critical. For this reason, surgeons with experience in pediatric liver resection and transplantation should be involved early in the decision-making process for determining optimal timing and extent of resection.There are three ways in which surgery is used to treat primary pediatric liver cancer, including initial surgical resection (alone or followed by chemotherapy), delayed surgical resection (chemotherapy followed by surgery) and orthotopic liver transplantation [50].

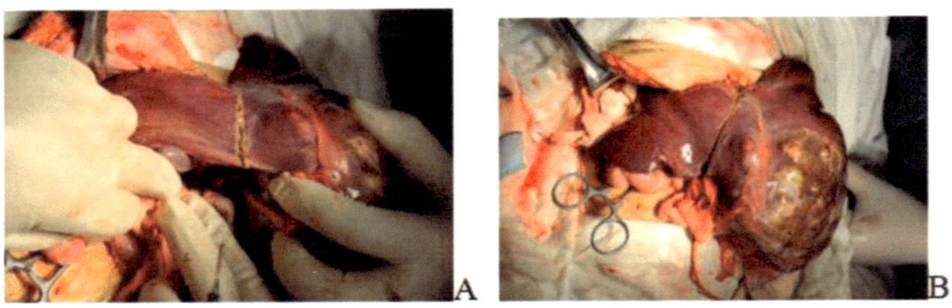

Figure 6. The lesion to resect is marked out.

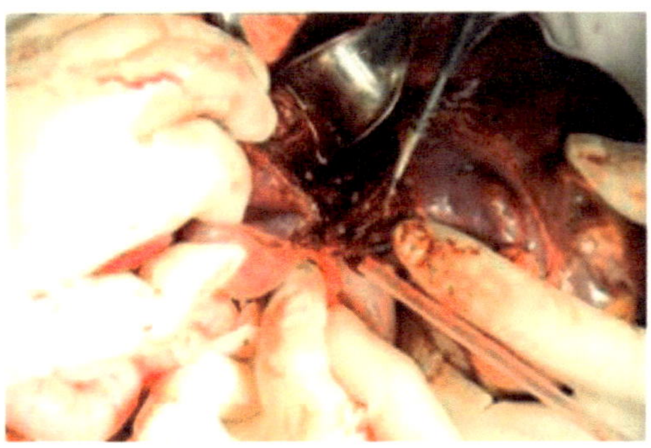

Figure 7. Electrocautery is useful for dissecting through the liver capsule and parenchyma.

Resection is typically performed through a bilateral subcostal incision, and, occasionally, a right thoracoabdominal approach is necessary for large lesions arising high in the right lobe. Surgical resection has seen applications of newer technology. Intraoperative ultrasonography has been widely applied to determine the exact location of the tumor relative to the vessels. Once deemed resectable, the resection is marked out (Fig. 3, 4), and various tools may then be used to perform the resection; electrocautery, bipolar devices such as LigaSure, and argon beam coagulation for hemostasis have been used.

The most frequently performed procedure is a right hepatectomy (60%) because hepatoblastomas (HBs) occur 3 times more often in the right lobe than in the left. The hilar plate is divided, exposing the bifurcation of the hepatic artery and portal vein. These structures are ligated (Fig. 5).

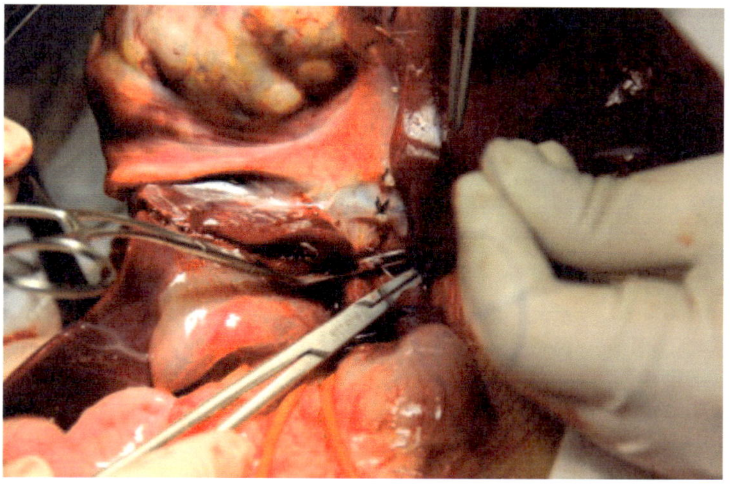

Figure 8. Suture and ligation may be useful in sealing blood vessels and hepatic ducts.

In an extended right hepatectomy, the middle hepatic vein is ligated and segment 4 is resected. The right hepatic vein is identified and ligated before any division of the hepatic parenchyma. At completion, only segments 2 and 3 and the caudate lobe remain.

Left hepatic lobectomy begins the same way right hepatectomy, with division of the left hepatic artery and left branch of the portal vein. The left and middle hepatic veins are identified after dissection through the sinus venosus. The liver is then transected after vascular isolation of the resected segments. An extended left hepatectomy includes removal of all or most of segments 5 and 8. Unresectability is usually determined by involvement of hilar structures or all hepatic veins, multicentricity, and invasion of inferior vena cava (IVC) or portal vein. Centrally located tumors are, by definition, more likely unresectable.

Laparoscopic and robotic resections of both benign and malignant liver tumors have been described. Their role in standard practice is still being defined.

If preoperative chemotherapy is to be administered, it is very important to consult frequently with the surgical team concerning the timing of resection, as prolonged chemotherapy can lead to unnecessary delays and in rare cases, tumor progression. If the tumor can be completely excised by an experienced surgical team, less postoperative chemotherapy may be needed.

In PRETEXT stage 3 or 4 disease patients with involvement of major liver vessels, early involvement with an experienced pediatric liver surgeon is especially important, patients with. Although initially thought to be a contraindication to resection, experienced liver surgeons could also perform aggressive approaches avoiding transplantation for vascular involvement patients. Accomplishing a complete resection is imperative since rescue transplant of incompletely resected patients has an inferior outcome compared to patients who are transplanted as the primary surgical therapy.

Surgical resection of distant disease has also contributed to the cure of children with hepatoblastoma and is often performed at the same time as resection of the primary tumor. Resection of pulmonary metastases is recommended when the number of metastases is limited. When possible, resection of areas of locally invasive disease, such as in the diaphragm, and of isolated brain metastasis is recommended. Second resection of positive margins and/or radiation therapy may not be necessary in patients with incompletely resected hepatoblastoma whose residual tumor is microscopic and who receive subsequent chemotherapy.

Major intraoperative complications include hemorrhage, air embolism, tumor embolus, and bile duct injury. Only 20% of the liver is necessary to maintain hepatic function; thus, postoperative insufficiency is rare. Postoperative complications include hemorrhage, bile leak, abscess formation, pulmonary complications, and wound problems. Postoperative care consists of adequate fluid replacement, intravenous albumin supplementation, vitamin K, and clotting factors for the first 3-4 days. The liver function test results generally normalize within the first 2 weeks, and hepatic insufficiency is reasonably rare. Postoperative monitoring consists of frequent ultrasonography, chest radiography, and serial α -fetoprotein (AFP) level measurements, generally at 3-month to 6-month intervals.

Tumor rupture at presentation, resulting in major hemorrhage that can be controlled by transcatheter arterial embolization or partial resection to stabilize the patient, does not preclude a favorable outcome when followed by chemotherapy and definitive surgery. The decision as to which surgical approach to use depends on many factors including: PRETEXT stage, size of the primary tumor, presence of multifocal hepatic disease, AFP levels, Vascular involvement, preoperative chemotherapy as well as orthotopic liver transplantation criteria.

In North American clinical trials, the Children's Oncology Group (COG) has recommended that surgery be performed initially if a complete resection can be accomplished. COG is investigating the use of PRETEXT stage at diagnosis and after chemotherapy to determine the optimal surgical approach and its timing. In European clinical trials, only patients with PRETEXT stage 1 receive resection surgery and all other patients are biopsied [51, 52, 53].

It is difficult to compare the North American and European approaches. Somewhat comparable results for children with PRETEXT stage 1 and 2 tumors were obtained in two international studies. The 5-year survival of PRETEXT stage 1 and 2 patients(chemotherapy prior to attempted surgical resection of the primary liver tumor) is 90% to 100% on the European studies and seems to be similar to that of children treated on North American studies where surgery was performed before chemotherapy. In comparison, a survey of children with liver tumors who were treated prior to the consistent use of combination chemotherapy found that 45 of 78 patients (57%) with hepatoblastoma who had complete excision of the tumor survived while no children with positive margins or gross disease following resection survived.

6.2. Orthotopic liver transplantation

Orthotopic liver transplantation was first described in 1968 by Starzl. Liver transplantation has recently been associated with significant success in the treatment of children with unresectable hepatic tumors. The criteria currently used to evaluate adult transplant candidates may not be applicable for pediatric patients. The main indication for transplantation is non-metastatic, unresectable lesions. Extrahepatic disease and lymph node involvement did not prove to be contraindications. Hepatoblastoma (HB) now constitutes an indication for 3% of all pediatric liver transplantations, whereas the role of liver transplantation for HCC is more controversial. In hepatocellular carcinoma, vascular invasion, distant metastases, lymph node involvement, tumor size, and male gender were significant risk factors for recurrence. Because of the poor prognosis in patients with hepatocellular carcinoma, liver transplant should be considered for disorders such as tyrosinemia and familial intrahepatic cholestasis early in the course, prior to the development of liver failure and malignancy. Because no good medical therapy for pediatric HCC has been identified, liver transplantation should be carefully evaluated as front-line therapy. Additionally, successful transplantation has been used benign lesions such as diffuse hepatic hemangiomas. In addition, liver transplantation may be an option in children with unresectable primary tumors, without metastatic disease, after neoadjuvant chemotherapy and pulmonary metastasectomy, if necessary. It has been suggested that adjuvant chemotherapy following transplant may decrease the risk of tumor recurrence. Generally, preoperative and postoperative chemotherapy are recommended, in addition to postoperative immunosuppression [54, 55, 56].

Transplantation may also be used in selected cases of tumor recurrence but is much less successful when used for salvage therapy. There are discrepant results on the outcomes for patients with lung metastases at diagnosis who undergo orthotopic liver transplantation following complete resolution of lung disease in response to pretransplant chemotherapy. Some studies have reported favorable outcomes for this group of patients, while others have noted high rates of hepatoblastoma recurrence. All of these studies are limited by small patient numbers; further study is needed to better define outcomes for this subset of patients [57, 58].

A review of the world experience has documented a posttransplant survival rate of 70% to 80% for children with hepatoblastomas. Intravenous invasion, positive lymph nodes, and contiguous spread did not have a significant adverse effect on outcome.

The primary cause of death for both HB and HCC was metastatic disease. Generally, the 5-year survival rate for patients transplanted for HB is 70%.

A study of the United Network for Organ Sharing (UNOS) database reported 135 patients undergoing 135 transplants for HB and 43 transplants for HCC with 1-year, 5-year, and 10-year survival of 79%, 69%, and 66% for HB, respectively, and 86%, 63%, and 58% for HCC, respectively [59, 60]. Liver transplantation for hepatic hemangioma has been studied in 59 patients in Europe with 1-year, 5-year, and 10-year patient survival rates of 93%, 83%, and 72%, respectively.

The availability of donor organs has increased with the use of split-liver grafting and other "technical variant" techniques, along with living-related liver transplant techniques. Prognosis in terms of graft and patient survival appear to be the same between full-size liver and technical variant liver transplants; however, morbidity following transplant appears to be higher in those patients who receive technical variant grafts [61, 62, 63, 64].

Early failure of liver transplant (< 30 d) is usually due to vascular complications or primary nonfunction. Late failure is usually more a result of infection, posttransplant lymphoproliferative disease, chronic rejection, biliary complications, or recurrence of malignant disease. These failures may warrant retransplantation. The predictors of success after retransplantation remain unknown. The United Network for Organ Sharing (UNOS) Standard Transplant and Research Files registry reported all children younger than 18 years listed for a liver transplant in the United that the 5-year survival rates of 69% for hepatoblastoma and 63% for hepatocellular carcinoma and the 10-year survival rates were similar to the 5-year rates. Application of the Milan criteria for UNOS selection of recipients of deceased donor livers is controversial. However, living donor liver transplants are more common with children and the outcome is similar [65, 66, 67, 68, 69].

6.3. Chemotherapy

In recent years, virtually all children with hepatoblastoma have been treated with chemotherapy, which may reduce the incidence of surgical complications at the time of resection, and in some centers, even children with resectable hepatoblastoma are treated with preoperative chemotherapy. For PRETEXT stage 1 hepatoblastoma, it was resected and treated with doxorubicin and cisplatin chemotherapy. The pre-resection neoadjuvant chemotherapy (doxorubicin and cisplatin) was given to all children with PRETEXT stage 2, 3, or 4 hepatoblastoma with or without metastases. The chemotherapy was well tolerated. This strategy resulted in an OS of 75% at 5 years after diagnosis. Identical overall results were seen in a follow-up international study. Following chemotherapy, and excluding those who received liver transplant (less than 5% of patients), complete resection was obtained in 87% of children. In contrast, an American Intergroup protocol for treatment of children with hepatoblastoma, encouraged resection at the time of diagnosis for all tumors amenable to resection without undue risk. The protocol did not treat children with stage I tumors of purely fetal histology with preoperative or postoperative chemotherapy unless they developed progressive disease. Further study will be needed to determine whether presurgical chemotherapy is preferable to resection followed by chemotherapy for children with PRETEXT stage 2, 3, and 4 hepatoblastoma [70, 71].

Routine assessment of hearing, renal, and cardiac function is standard during treatment for pediatric malignancies. Post-chemotherapy neutropenia rarely represents additional concerns during the surgical treatment. Platinum compounds (cisplatin and carboplatin), which have been a backbone of the successful treatment for pediatric liver tumors, are also quite ototoxic. Around 40% of children develop significant hearing loss, which typically affects

http://dx.doi.org/10.5772/51500

high-register tones, and could be delayed. Chronic dose-related nephrotoxicity remains a significant long-term issue for both chemotherapy for malignant liver tumors and calcineurin inhibitor-based immunosuppression. Therefore, early use of calcineurin inhibitor-sparing agents, such as mycophenolate mofetil or sirolimus, is recommended for children after LT for liver tumors. Nevertheless, it is prudent not to give chemotherapy 2 weeks before or after resection or LT.

In rare cases, intensive platinum- and doxorubicin-based multidrug chemotherapy can induce complete regressions in approximately 50% of patients, with subsequent 3-year event-free survival of 56% for pulmonary metastases and eliminated multinodular tumor foci in the liver. Chemotherapy has been much more successful in the treatment of hepatoblastoma than in hepatocellular carcinoma.

6.4. Other Treatment Approaches

Other treatment approaches such as transarterial chemoembolization, have been used for patients with postsurgically-staged stage III hepatoblastoma. Transarterial chemoembolization has been used in a few children to successfully shrink tumor size to permit resection.Cryosurgery, intratumoral injection of alcohol, and radiofrequency ablation can successfully treat small (<5 cm) tumors in adults with cirrhotic livers. Some local approaches such as cryosurgery, radiofrequency ablation, and transarterial chemoembolization that suppress hepatocellular carcinoma tumor progression are used as bridging therapy in adults to delay tumor growth while on a waiting list for cadaveric liver transplant [72].

7. Medical issues related to current chemotherapy

It is no surprise that most of the toxicity data stem from HB treatment survivors, while information from the HCC setting is lacking.

7.1. Recurrent hepatic tumors

The prognosis for a patient with recurrent or progressive hepatoblastoma depends on many factors, including the site of recurrence, prior treatment, and individual patient considerations. If possible, isolated metastases should be resected completely in patients whose primary tumor is controlled. For example, in patients with stage I hepatoblastoma at initial diagnosis, aggressive surgical treatment of isolated pulmonary metastases that develop in the course of the disease may make extended disease-free survival possible. Liver transplant should be considered for patients with isolated recurrence in the liver. Combined vincristine/irinotecan has been used with some success. Some patients treated with cisplatin/vincristine/fluorouracil could be salvaged with doxorubicin-containing regimens, but patients treated with doxorubicin/cisplatin could not be salvaged with vincristine/fluorouracil. Treatment in a clinical trial should be considered if all of the recurrent disease cannot be surgically removed. Phase I and phase II clinical trials may be appropriate and should be considered [73, 74].

The prognosis for a patient with recurrent or progressive hepatocellular carcinoma is poor. Chemoembolization or liver transplant should be considered for those with isolated recurrence in the liver. Phase I and phase II clinical trials may be appropriate and should be considered [75, 76].

8. Summary and future issues

Management of pediatric liver tumors has significantly improved over the last 2 decades. The principal reasons are that efficient chemotherapy and established medico-surgical treatment algorithms for HB have now integrated LT as a very valuable complementary treatment option. The management options for HCC are less effective and not well defined, broadly mirroring the therapeutic guidelines in adults except for a more cautionary approach to neoadjuvant and loco-regional methods. In the pediatric context the main clinical aims are to reduce chemotherapy toxicity (predominantly ototoxicity and nephrotoxicity) in children treated for HB and to investigate additional modes of treatment for HCC.

Improved understanding of HB and HCC biology may improve risk stratification a presentation and direct the treatment at specific molecular targets in the future. Management of less common benign and malignant tumors should benefit from establishing international collaborative pediatric networks such as the Pediatric Liver Unresectable Tumor Observatory (PLUTO).

Author details

Chunbao Guo* and Mingman Zhang*

*Address all correspondence to:

*Address all correspondence to:

Dept. of hepatobiliary Surgery, Children's Hospital, Chongqing Medical University, ChongqingP.R. China, P.R. China

References

[1] Smith, N. L., Altekruse, S. F., Ries, L. A., Melbert, D. L., O'Leary, M., Smith, F. O., & Reaman, G. H. (2010). Outcomes for children and adolescents with cancer: challenges for the twenty-first century. *J Clin Oncol.*, 28(15), 2625-34.

[2] Guidelines for the pediatric cancer center and role of such centers in diagnosis and treatment. (1997). *American Academy of Pediatrics Section Statement Section on Hematology/Oncology. Pediatrics*, 99(1), 139-41.

[3] Eheman, C., Henley, S. J., Ballard-Barbash, R., Jacobs, E. J., Schymura, Noone. A. M., Pan, L., Anderson, Fulton. J. E., Kohler, J. A., Ward, E., Plescia, M., Ries, L. A., & Edwards, B. K. (2012). Annual Report to the Nation on the status of cancer, 1975-2008, featuring cancers associated with excess weight and lack of sufficient physical activity. *Cancer.*, 118(9), 2338-66.

[4] Darbari, A., Sabin, K. M., Shapiro, C. N., & Schwarz, K. B. (2003). Epidemiology of primary hepatic malignancies in U.S. children. *Hepatology*, 38(3), 560-6.

[5] Czauderna, P., Otte, J. B., Aronson, D. C., Gauthier, F., Mackinlay, G., Roebuck, D., Plaschkes, J., & Perilongo, G. (2005). Childhood Liver Tumour Strategy Group of the International Society of Paediatric Oncology (SIOPEL). Guidelines for surgical treatment of hepatoblastoma in the modern era--recommendations from the Childhood Liver Tumour Strategy Group of the International Society of Paediatric Oncology (SIOPEL). *Eur J Cancer*, 41(7), 1031-6.

[6] Exelby, P. R., Filler, R. M., & Grosfeld, J. L. (1975). Liver tumors in children in the particular reference to hepatoblastoma and hepatocellular carcinoma: American Academy of Pediatrics Surgical Section Survey--1974. *J Pediatr Surg.*, 10(3), 329-37.

[7] Katzenstein, H. M., Krailo, Malogolowkin. M. H., Ortega, J. A., Liu-Mares, W., Douglass, E. C., Feusner, J. H., Reynolds, M., Quinn, J. J., Newman, K., Finegold, Haas. J. E., Sensel, M. G., Castleberry, R. P., & Bowman, L. C. (2002). Hepatocellular carcinoma in children and adolescents: results from the Pediatric Oncology Group and the Children's Cancer Group intergroup study. *J Clin Oncol.*, 20(12), 2789-97.

[8] Czauderna, P., Mackinlay, G., Perilongo, G., Brown, J., Shafford, E., Aronson, D., Pritchard, J., Chapchap, P., Keeling, J., Plaschkes, J., & Otte, J. B. (2002). Liver Tumors Study Group of the International Society of Pediatric Oncology. Hepatocellular carcinoma in children: results of the first prospective study of the International Society of Pediatric Oncology group. *J Clin Oncol.*, 20(12), 2798-804.

[9] Ortega, J. A., Douglass, E. C., Feusner, J. H., Reynolds, M., Quinn, J. J., King, D. R., Liu-Mares, W., & Sensel, M. G. (2000). Randomized comparison of cisplatin/vincristine/fluorouracil and cisplatin/continuous infusion doxorubicin for treatment of pediatric hepatoblastoma: A report from the Children's Cancer Group and the Pediatric Oncology Group. *J Clin Oncol.*, 18(14), 2665-75.

[10] Katzenstein, H. M., Krailo, Malogolowkin. M. H., Ortega, J. A., Liu-Mares, W., Douglass, E. C., Feusner, J. H., Reynolds, M., Quinn, J. J., Newman, K., Sensel, M. G., Castleberry, R. P., & Bowman, L. C. (2002). Hepatocellular carcinoma in children and adolescents: results from the Pediatric Oncology Group and the Children's Cancer Group intergroup study. *J Clin Oncol.*, 20(12), 2789-97.

[11] Andres, A. M., Hernandez, F., Lopez-Santamaría, M., Gámez, M., Murcia, J., Leal, N., López, Gutierrez. J. C., Frauca, E., Sastre, A., & Tovar, J. A. (2007). Surgery of liver tumors in children in the last 15 years. *Eur J Pediatr Surg.*, 17(6), 387-92.

[12] D'Antiga, L., Vallortigara, F., Cillo, U., Talenti, E., Rugge, M., Zancan, L., Dall'Igna, P., De Salvo, G. L., & Perilongo, G. (2007). Features predicting unresectability in hepatoblastoma. *Cancer.*, 110(5), 1050-8.

[13] Hemming, A. W., Reed, A. I., Fujita, S., Zendejas, I., Howard, R. J., & Kim, R. D. (2008). Role for extending hepatic resection using an aggressive approach to liver surgery. *J Am Coll Surg.*, 206(5), 870-5.

[14] Czauderna, P., Mackinlay, G., Perilongo, G., Brown, J., Shafford, E., Aronson, D., Pritchard, J., Chapchap, P., Keeling, J., Plaschkes, J., Otte, J. B., Liver, Tumors., Study, Group., of, the., International, Society., & of, Pediatric. (2002). Hepatocellular carcinoma in children: results of the first prospective study of the International Society of Pediatric Oncology group. *J Clin Oncol.*, 20(12), 2798-804.

[15] Otte, J. B., Pritchard, J., Aronson, D. C., Brown, J., Czauderna, P., Maibach, R., Perilongo, G., Shafford, E., Plaschkes, J., International, Society., of, Pediatric., & Oncology, . S. I. O. P. (2004). Liver transplantation for hepatoblastoma: results from the International Society of Pediatric Oncology (SIOP) study SIOPEL-1 and review of the world experience. *Pediatr Blood Cancer.*, 42(1), 74-83.

[16] Austin, M. T., Leys, C. M., Feurer, I. D., Lovvorn, H. N., O'Neill, J. A., Pinson, C. W., & Pietsch, J. B. (2006). Liver transplantation for childhood hepatic malignancy: a review of the United Network for Organ Sharing (UNOS) database. *J Pediatr Surg.*, 41(1), 182-6.

[17] Czauderna, P., Otte, J. B., Aronson, D. C., Gauthier, F., Mackinlay, G., Roebuck, D., Plaschkes, J., & Perilongo, G. (2005). Childhood Liver Tumour Strategy Group of the International Society of Paediatric Oncology (SIOPEL).Guidelines for surgical treatment of hepatoblastoma in the modern era--recommendations from the Childhood Liver Tumour Strategy Group of the International Society of Paediatric Oncology (SIOPEL). *Eur J Cancer.*, 41(7), 1031-6.

[18] Tsukuma, H., Hiyama, T., Tanaka, S., Nakao, M., Yabuuchi, T., Kitamura, T., Nakanishi, K., Fujimoto, I., Inoue, A., Yamazaki, H., et al. (1993). Risk factors for hepatocellular carcinoma among patients with chronic liver disease. *N Engl J Med.*, 328(25), 1797-801.

[19] González-Peralta, R. P., Langham, M. R., Jr Andres, J. M., Mohan, P., Colombani, P. M., Alford, M. K., & Schwarz, K. B. (2009). Hepatocellular carcinoma in 2 young adolescents with chronic hepatitis C. *J Pediatr Gastroenterol Nutr.*, 48(5), 630-5.

[20] Ni, Y. H., Chang, M. H., Hsu, H. Y., Hsu, H. C., Chen, C. C., Chen, W. J., & Lee, C. Y. (1991). Hepatocellular carcinoma in childhood. Clinical manifestations and prognosis. *Cancer*, 68(8), 1737-41.

[21] Stocker JT.Hepatic tumors in children. Clin Liver Dis. (2001). , 5(1), 259-81.

[22] De Ioris, M., Brugieres, L., Zimmermann, A., Keeling, J., Brock, P., Maibach, R., Pritchard, J., Shafford, L., Zsiros, J., Czaudzerna, P., & Perilongo, G. (2008). Hepatoblastoma with a low serum alpha-fetoprotein level at diagnosis: the SIOPEL group experience. *Eur J Cancer.*, 44(4), 545-50.

[23] Meyers, R. L., Rowland, J. R., Krailo, M., Chen, Z., Katzenstein, H. M., & Malogolowkin, M. H. (2009). Predictive power of pretreatment prognostic factors in children with hepatoblastoma: a report from the Children's Oncology Group. *Pediatr Blood Cancer*, 53(6), 1016-22.

[24] Schneider, D. T., Calaminus, G., & Göbel, U. (2001). Diagnostic value of alpha 1-fetoprotein and beta-human chorionic gonadotropin in infancy and childhood. *Pediatr Hematol Oncol.*, 18(1), 11-26.

[25] Nicol, K., Savell, V., Moore, J., Teot, L., Spunt, S. L., Qualman, S., Children's, Oncology., Group, Soft., & Tissue, Sarcoma. (2007). Distinguishing undifferentiated embryonal sarcoma of the liver from biliary tract rhabdomyosarcoma: a Children's Oncology Group study. *Pediatr Dev Pathol.*, 10(2), 89-97.

[26] Katzenstein, H. M., Steelman, C. K., Wulkan, M. L., Gow, K. W., Bridge, J. A., Kenney, Thompson. K., de Chadarévian, J. P., & Abramowsky, C. R. (2011). Undifferentiated embryonal sarcoma of the liver is associated with mesenchymal hamartoma and multiple chromosomal abnormalities: a review of eleven cases. *Pediatr Dev Pathol.*, 14(2), 111-6.

[27] Stringer, M. D., & Alizai, N. K. (2005). Mesenchymal hamartoma of the liver: a systematic review. *J Pediatr Surg.*, 40(11), 1681-90.

[28] Malogolowkin, M. H., Stanley, P., Steele, D. A., & Ortega, J. A. (2000). Feasibility and toxicity of chemoembolization for children with liver tumors. *J Clin Oncol.*, 18(6), 1279-84.

[29] Zsíros, J., Maibach, R., Shafford, E., Brugieres, L., Brock, P., Czauderna, P., Roebuck, D., Childs, M., Zimmermann, A., Laithier, V., Otte, J. B., de Camargo, B., Mac, Kinlay. G., Scopinaro, M., Aronson, D., Plaschkes, J., & Perilongo, G. (2010). Successful treatment of childhood high-risk hepatoblastoma with dose-intensive multiagent chemotherapy and surgery: final results of the SIOPEL-3HR study. *J Clin Oncol.*, 28(15), 2584-90.

[30] Clericuzio, C. L., Chen, E., Mc Neil, D. E., O'Connor, T., Zackai, E. H., Medne, L., Tomlinson, G., & De Baun, M. (2003). Serum alpha-fetoprotein screening for hepatoblastoma in children with Beckwith-Wiedemann syndrome or isolated hemihyperplasia. *J Pediatr.*, 143(2), 270-2.

[31] Malogolowkin, M. H., Stanley, P., Steele, D. A., & Ortega, J. A. (2000). Feasibility and toxicity of chemoembolization for children with liver tumors. *J Clin Oncol.*, 18(6), 1279-84.

[32] Tanimura, M., Matsui, I., Abe, J., Ikeda, H., Kobayashi, N., Ohira, M., Yokoyama, M., & Kaneko, M. (1998). Increased risk of hepatoblastoma among immature children with a lower birth weight. *Cancer Res.*, 58(14), 3032-5.

[33] Mc Laughlin, C. C., Baptiste, M. S., Schymura, M. J., Nasca, P. C., & Zdeb, M. S. (2006). Maternal and infant birth characteristics and hepatoblastoma. *Am J Epidemiol.*, 163(9), 818-28.

[34] Chang, M. H., Chen, T. H., Hsu, H. M., Wu, T. C., Kong, M. S., Liang, D. C., Ni, Y. H., Chen, C. J., & Chen, D. S. (2005). Taiwan Childhood HCC Study Group. Prevention of hepatocellular carcinoma by universal vaccination against hepatitis B virus: the effect and problems. *Clin Cancer Res.*, 11(21), 7953-7.

[35] Zsíros, J., Maibach, R., Shafford, E., Brugieres, L., Brock, P., Czauderna, P., Roebuck, D., Childs, M., Zimmermann, A., Laithier, V., Otte, J. B., de Camargo, B., Mac, Kinlay. G., Scopinaro, M., Aronson, D., Plaschkes, J., & Perilongo, G. (2010). Successful treatment of childhood high-risk hepatoblastoma with dose-intensive multiagent chemotherapy and surgery: final results of the SIOPEL-3HR study. *J Clin Oncol.*, 28(15), 2584-90.

[36] Schnater, J. M., Aronson, D. C., Plaschkes, J., Perilongo, G., Brown, J., Otte, J. B., Brugieres, L., Czauderna, P., Mac, Kinlay. G., & Vos, A. (2002). Surgical view of the treatment of patients with hepatoblastoma: results from the first prospective trial of the International Society of Pediatric Oncology Liver Tumor Study Group. *Cancer*, 94(4), 1111-20.

[37] Yoon, J. M., Burns, R. C., Malogolowkin, M. H., & Mascarenhas, L. (2007). Treatment of infantile choriocarcinoma of the liver. *Pediatr Blood Cancer.*, 49(1), 99-102.

[38] Brown, J., Perilongo, G., Shafford, E., Keeling, J., Pritchard, J., Brock, P., Dicks-Mireaux, C., Phillips, A., Vos, A., & Plaschkes, J. (2000). Pretreatment prognostic factors for children with hepatoblastoma-- results from the International Society of Paediatric Oncology (SIOP) study SIOPEL 1. *Eur J Cancer*, 36(11), 1418-25.

[39] Perilongo, G., Shafford, E., Maibach, R., Aronson, D., Brugières, L., Brock, P., Childs, M., Czauderna, P., Mac, Kinlay. G., Otte, J. B., Pritchard, J., Rondelli, R., Scopinaro, M., Staalman, C., Plaschkes, J., International, Society., of, Paediatric., & Oncology-S, I. O. P. E. L. . (2004). Risk-adapted treatment for childhood hepatoblastoma. final report of the second study of the International Society of Paediatric Oncology--SIOPEL 2. *Eur J Cancer.*, 40(3), 411-21.

[40] DeBaun, M.R., & Tucker, M.A. (1998). Risk of cancer during the first four years of life in children from The Beckwith-Wiedemann Syndrome Registry. *J Pediatr.*, 132, (3 Pt 1):398-400.

[41] Sparago, A., Russo, S., Cerrato, F., Ferraiuolo, S., Castorina, P., Selicorni, A., Schwienbacher, C., Negrini, M., Ferrero, G. B., Silengo, M. C., Anichini, C., Larizza, L., & Riccio, A. (2007). Mechanisms causing imprinting defects in familial Beckwith-Wiedemann syndrome with Wilms' tumour. *Hum Mol Genet*, 16(3), 254-64.

[42] Algar, E. M., St, Heaps. L., Darmanian, A., Dagar, V., Prawitt, D., Peters, G. B., & Collins, F. (2007). Paternally inherited submicroscopic duplication at 1115 implicates insulin-like growth factor II in overgrowth and Wilms' tumorigenesis. *Cancer Res.*

[43] Steenman, M., Westerveld, A., & Mannens, M. (2000). Genetics of Beckwith-Wiedemann syndrome-associated tumors: common genetic pathways. *Genes Chromosomes Cancer.*, 28(1), 1-13.

[44] Roebuck, D. J., Olsen, Ø., & Pariente, D. (2006). Radiological staging in children with hepatoblastoma. *Pediatr Radiol.*, 36(3), 176-82.

[45] Tiao, G. M., Bobey, N., Allen, S., Nieves, N., Alonso, M., Bucuvalas, J., Wells, R., & Ryckman, F. (2005). The current management of hepatoblastoma: a combination of chemotherapy, conventional resection, and liver transplantation. *J Pediatr.*, 146(2), 204-11.

[46] Atri, P., Paredes, J. L., Di Cicco, L. A., Sindhi, R., Soltys, K. A., Mazariegos, G. V., & Kane, T. D. (2010). Review of outcomes of primary liver cancers in children: our institutional experience with resection and transplantation. *Surgery*, 148(4), 778-82.

[47] Otte, J. B., Pritchard, J., Aronson, D. C., Brown, J., Czauderna, P., Maibach, R., Perilongo, G., Shafford, E., & Plaschkes, J. (2004). International Society of Pediatric Oncology (SIOP). Liver transplantation for hepatoblastoma: results from the International Society of Pediatric Oncology (SIOP) study SIOPEL-1 and review of the world experience. *Pediatr Blood Cancer*, 42(1), 74-83.

[48] Douglass, E. C., Reynolds, M., Finegold, M., Cantor, A. B., & Glicksman, A. (1993). Cisplatin, vincristine, and fluorouracil therapy for hepatoblastoma: a Pediatric Oncology Group study. *J Clin Oncol.*, 11(1), 96-9.

[49] Pritchard, J., Brown, J., Shafford, E., Perilongo, G., Brock, P., Dicks-Mireaux, C., Keeling, J., Phillips, A., Vos, A., & Plaschkes, J. (2000). Cisplatin, doxorubicin, and delayed surgery for childhood hepatoblastoma: a successful approach--results of the first prospective study of the International Society of Pediatric Oncology. *J Clin Oncol.*, 18(22), 3819-28.

[50] Perilongo, G., Shafford, E., Maibach, R., Aronson, D., Brugières, L., Brock, P., Childs, M., Czauderna, P., Mac, Kinlay. G., Otte, J. B., Pritchard, J., Rondelli, R., Scopinaro, M., Staalman, C., & Plaschkes, J. (2004). International Society of Paediatric Oncology-SIOPEL 2.Risk-adapted treatment for childhood hepatoblastoma. final report of the second study of the International Society of Paediatric Oncology--SIOPEL 2. *Eur J Cancer*, 40(3), 411-21.

[51] Feusner, J. H., Krailo, M. D., Haas, J. E., Campbell, J. R., Lloyd, D. A., & Ablin, A. R. (1993). Treatment of pulmonary metastases of initial stage I hepatoblastoma in childhood. *Report from the Childrens Cancer Group. Cancer*, 71(3), 859-64.

[52] Perilongo, G., Brown, J., Shafford, E., Brock, P., De Camargo, B., Keeling, J. W., Vos, A., Philips, A., Pritchard, J., & Plaschkes, J. (2000). Hepatoblastoma presenting with

lung metastases: treatment results of the first cooperative, prospective study of the International Society of Paediatric Oncology on childhood liver tumors. *Cancer*, 89(8), 1845-53.

[53] Malogolowkin, M. H., Katzenstein, H. M., Krailo, M., Chen, Z., Quinn, J. J., Reynolds, M., & Ortega, J. A. (2008). Redefining the role of doxorubicin for the treatment of children with hepatoblastoma. *J Clin Oncol.*, 26(14), 2379-83.

[54] Lubienski, A. Hepatocellular carcinoma: interventional bridging to liver transplantation. *Transplantation*, 2005. 80(1 Suppl):S113-9.

[55] Otte, J. B., Pritchard, J., Aronson, D. C., Brown, J., Czauderna, P., Maibach, R., Perilongo, G., Shafford, E., Plaschkes, J., International, Society., of, Pediatric., & Oncology, . S. I. O. P. (2004). Liver transplantation for hepatoblastoma: results from the International Society of Pediatric Oncology (SIOP) study SIOPEL-1 and review of the world experience. *Pediatr Blood Cancer*, 42(1), 74-83.

[56] Reyes, Carr. B., Dvorchik, I., Kocoshis, S., Jaffe, R., Gerber, D., Mazariegos, G. V., Bueno, J., & Selby, R. (2000). Liver transplantation and chemotherapy for hepatoblastoma and hepatocellular cancer in childhood and adolescence. *J Pediatr.*, 136(6), 795-804.

[57] Austin, M. T., Leys, C. M., Feurer, I. D., Lovvorn, H. N., O'Neill, J. A., Pinson, C. W., & Pietsch, J. B. (2006). Liver transplantation for childhood hepatic malignancy: a review of the United Network for Organ Sharing (UNOS) database. *J Pediatr Surg.*, 41(1), 182-6.

[58] Beaunoyer, M., Vanatta, J. M., Ogihara, M., Strichartz, D., Dahl, G., Berquist, W. E., Castillo, R. O., Cox, K. L., & Esquivel, C. O. (2007). Outcomes of transplantation in children with primary hepatic malignancy. *Pediatr Transplant.*, 11(6), 655-60.

[59] Guiteau, J. J., Cotton, R. T., Karpen, S. J., O'Mahony, C. A., & Goss, J. A. (2010). Pediatric liver transplantation for primary malignant liver tumors with a focus on hepatic epithelioid hemangioendothelioma: the UNOS experience. *Pediatr Transplant.*, 14(3), 326-31.

[60] Suh, M. Y., Wang, K., Gutweiler, J. R., Misra, M. V., Krawczuk, L. E., Jenkins, R. L., & Lillehei, C. W. (2008). Safety of minimal immunosuppression in liver transplantation for hepatoblastoma. *J Pediatr Surg.*, 43(6), 1148-52.

[61] Browne, M., Sher, D., Grant, D., Deluca, E., Alonso, E., Whitington, P. F., & Superina, R. A. (2008). Survival after liver transplantation for hepatoblastoma: a 2-center experience. *J Pediatr Surg.*, 43(11), 1973-81.

[62] Faraj, W., Dar, F., Marangoni, G., Bartlett, A., Melendez, H. V., Hadzic, D., Dhawan, A., Mieli-Vergani, G., Rela, M., & Heaton, N. (2008). Liver transplantation for hepatoblastoma. *Liver Transpl.*, 14(11), 1614-9.

[63] Austin, M. T., Leys, C. M., Feurer, I. D., Lovvorn, H. N., 3rd O'Neill, J. A., Pinson, C. W., & Pietsch, J. B. (2006). Liver transplantation for childhood hepatic malignancy: a

review of the United Network for Organ Sharing (UNOS) database. *J Pediatr Surg.*, 41(1), 182-6.

[64] Heaton, N., Faraj, W., Melendez, H. V., Jassem, W., Muiesan, P., Mieli-Vergani, G., Dhawan, A., & Rela, M. (2008). Living related liver transplantation in children. *Br J Surg.*, 95(7), 919-24.

[65] Reyes, Carr. B., Dvorchik, I., Kocoshis, S., Jaffe, R., Gerber, D., Mazariegos, G. V., Bueno, J., & Selby, R. (2000). Liver transplantation and chemotherapy for hepatoblastoma and hepatocellular cancer in childhood and adolescence. *J Pediatr.*, 136(6), 795-804.

[66] Sevmis, S., Karakayali, H., Ozçay, F., Canan, O., Bilezikci, B., Torgay, A., & Haberal, M. (2008). Liver transplantation for hepatocellular carcinoma in children. *Pediatr Transplant.*, 12(1), 52-6.

[67] Madanur, Battula. N., Davenport, M., Dhawan, A., & Rela, M. (2007). Staged resection for a ruptured hepatoblastoma: a 6-year follow-up. *Pediatr Surg Int.*, 23(6), 609-11.

[68] Schnater, J. M., Aronson, D. C., Plaschkes, J., Perilongo, G., Brown, J., Otte, J. B., Brugieres, L., Czauderna, P., Mac, Kinlay. G., & Vos, A. (2002). Surgical view of the treatment of patients with hepatoblastoma: results from the first prospective trial of the International Society of Pediatric Oncology Liver Tumor Study Group. *Cancer*, 94(4), 1111-20.

[69] Otte, J.B. (2008). Should the selection of children with hepatocellular carcinoma be based on Milan criteria? *Pediatr Transplant.*, 12(1), 1-3.

[70] Douglass, E. C., Reynolds, M., Finegold, M., Cantor, A. B., & Glicksman, A. (1993). Cisplatin, vincristine, and fluorouracil therapy for hepatoblastoma: a Pediatric Oncology Group study. *J Clin Oncol.*, 11(1), 96-9.

[71] Ortega, J. A., Douglass, E. C., Feusner, J. H., Reynolds, M., Quinn, J. J., Finegold, Haas. J. E., King, D. R., Liu-Mares, W., Sensel, M. G., & Krailo, M.D. (2000). Randomized comparison of cisplatin/vincristine/fluorouracil and cisplatin/continuous infusion doxorubicin for treatment of pediatric hepatoblastoma: A report from the Children's Cancer Group and the Pediatric Oncology Group. *J Clin Oncol.*, 18(14), 2665-75.

[72] Habrand, J. L., Nehme, D., Kalifa, C., Gauthier, F., Gruner, M., Sarrazin, D., & Terrier-Lacombe, Lemerle. J. (1992). Is there a place for radiation therapy in the management of hepatoblastomas and hepatocellular carcinomas in children? *Int J Radiat Oncol Biol Phys.*, 23(3), 525-31.

[73] Feusner, J. H., Krailo, M. D., Haas, J. E., Campbell, J. R., Lloyd, D. A., & Ablin, A. R. (1993). Treatment of pulmonary metastases of initial stage I hepatoblastoma in childhood. *Report from the Childrens Cancer Group. Cancer*, 71(3), 859-64.

[74] Perilongo, G., Brown, J., Shafford, E., Brock, P., De Camargo, B., Keeling, J. W., Vos, A., Philips, A., Pritchard, J., & Plaschkes, J. (2000). Hepatoblastoma presenting with lung metastases: treatment results of the first cooperative, prospective study of the International Society of Paediatric Oncology on childhood liver tumors. *Cancer.*, 89(8), 1845-53.

[75] Robertson, P. L., Muraszko, K. M., & Axtell, R. A. (1997). Hepatoblastoma metastatic to brain: prolonged survival after multiple surgical resections of a solitary brain lesion. *J Pediatr Hematol Oncol.*, 19(2), 168-71.

[76] Perilongo, G., Maibach, R., Shafford, E., Brugieres, L., Brock, P., Morland, B., de Camargo, B., Zsiros, J., Roebuck, D., Zimmermann, A., Aronson, D., Childs, M., Widing, E., Laithier, V., Plaschkes, J., Pritchard, J., Scopinaro, M., Mac, Kinlay. G., & Czauderna, P. (2009). Cisplatin versus cisplatin plus doxorubicin for standard-risk hepatoblastoma. *N Engl J Med.*, 361(17), 1662-70.

Chapter 20

Laparoscopic Radiofrequency Ablation of Liver Tumors

Mirela Patricia Sîrb Boeti, Răzvan Grigorie and
Irinel Popescu

Additional information is available at the end of the chapter

http://dx.doi.org/10.5772/52830

1. Introduction

The biological effects of radiofrequency (RF) waves were first reported on liver lesions by McGahan et al. in 1990 [1].

The early reports on the efficacy and safety of radiofrequency ablation (RFA) for liver tumors have encouraged rapid spreading of the technique for the treatment of unresectable or even resectable tumors. Nowadays RFA constitutes a wide-range therapeutical option for a variety of tumors. The vast majority of the reports about RFA refer to malignant liver tumors. There are only few authors who attest the efficiency of this in situ ablative method for benign liver tumors (e.g. hepatic cavernous hemangioma, hepatic adenoma). RFA must be integrated in a complex multimodal treatment for patient with liver tumors. Selected patients may also benefit of simultaneous and/or consecutive association of RFA with other treatments like surgery, chemotherapy, and other in situ ablation procedures.

All the authors concur to the fact that RFA is a technology-based treatment. However, the importance of operator experience in this treatment must not be alluded. Not only the complete knowledge of the RF armamentarium but also patient and approach selection for RFA are mandatory to certify this method as an effective and safe technique for treatment of the liver tumors [2].

It must be underscore that RFA is not just a simple technique of inserting a needle to "cook" the tumors but is a new technology in the treatment of liver tumors with a steep learning curve which may offer these patients a 50-95% chance of destroying these lesions [3].

While RFA is most commonly performed in the radiology departments through a percutaneous approach, our experience over 5 years determines us to advocate for the laparoscopic ablation of liver tumor using RF. Even if it is still a debate on the correlation of the different

RFA approaches with the results in terms of recurrence and survival, our recommendation is to use laparoscopic RFA (LRFA) whenever possible.

With this paper we intend to offer a review regarding the laparoscopic ablations with RF for patients suffering from liver tumors. We aim to describe the RF and ultrasound equipment, define the selection criteria of the patients for this kind of approach, present the ablation procedure, and the follow-up criteria, and discuss the LRFA outcomes in terms of procedural-related morbidity and mortality, tumor recurrence, and patient survival.

2. Methods

A review of relevant articles was undertaken based on a Medline search from January 1998 till January 2012.

2.1. Mechanism of RFA

When high-frequency (350-500 kHz) alternating current passes the tissues, polar molecules (e.g. water molecules) are orientated in conformity with the field polarity [4]. With every change of the polarity of the alternating current polar molecules are moving in attempt to follow its direction. Their ionic vibration results in dielectrical losses into tissues because of molecular friction. The dielectric losses generate heat (frictional heating) which causes thermal tissues injuries. The extension and type of the thermal lesions depend on the temperature and duration of current applications. These lesions begin at 42^{0}C. Above this level the time of lethal exposion drops progressively: 8 min at 46^{0}C, 4-5 min at 50ºC. At 60ºC the cellular death is inevitable due to irreversible lesions of mitochondrial and cytoplasmatic enzymes secondary to thermal protein denaturation [5]. Tissue desiccation occurs at 100ºC. But quick tissue heating over 100ºC has the disadvantage of fast increasing thetissue impedance due to charring, which consecutively restricts the heat propagation and eventually coagulation necrosis [5]. Malignant cells are more prone to damages due to hyperthermia than normal cells [6].

2.2. Indications of RFA

RFA is now gaining popularity as the preferred modality of local ablation for patients with malignant liver tumors who are not surgical candidates (table 1).

RFA is used to treat liver lesions considered unresectable due to their bulky volume, position near key vessels, multiplicity or insufficiency of remnant liver parenchyma.

In terms of the extend of hepatic disease we consider safe to perform LRFA on patients with total tumor volume less than 20% contrary with opinion of other authors who reported good results in patients with up to 50% total liver replacement [3].

RFA has an important role in converting nonresectable in resectable tumors and also in increasing resectability of multiple liver tumors. Resections of such tumors are feasible d'emblee or in two-stage procedure. RFA of the small and deeply situated tumor(s) in one hepatic lobe can be associated with resection of a large tumor or multiple tumors located in the controlateral lobe or with controlateral portal vein ligation. The procedure can also be performed before liver resection for tumors located in the section plane in order to obtain disease-free margins.

Patients with liver tumor but with general contraindications for hepatic resection or those who refuse the operation are also candidates for RFA.

Moreover, the application of RFA has now expanded to patients as a bridge to liver transplantation. RFA proved benefits for patients with cirrhotic and HCC who are within Milano criteria on the waiting list for liver transplantation. It also have been shown to result in down staging the HCC in cirrhotic patients beyound the Milano criteria and thus in listing these patients for liver transplantation.

Patient with primary or metastatic hepatic tumor(s) which are not candidates for hepatic resection
Tumor characteristics
multiple diffuse bilobar
in association with hepatic resection
in association with transarterial chemoembolization of hepatic artery
deeply situated
near the portal pedicles, hepatic veins, inferior vena cava
recurrence after major hepatectomies
small HCC on cirrhosis in patients (in Milan criteria) on waiting list for LTx
large HCC on cirrhosis in patients (out of Milan criteria) to be included on the waiting list after downstaging
large unresectable tumor for downstaging followed by hepatectomy
number ≤ 5 (14)
maximum diameter ≤ 5 (7, 8) cm
Poor liver parenchyma function
Patient with benign hepatic tumor
Co-morbidities which increase the anesthesia-surgical risk
Patient refusal of hepatic resection
Patient expectation survival ≥ 3 months
Other tumor localizations which can be treated
Written informed consent of the patient

Table 1. Indications of RFA.

Based on some studies there are authors who plead for RFA even as a substitute to hepatic resection for small liver tumors.

Patients with hepatic malignancies, except those with neuroendocrine tumors, should be approached with curative intent and the goal of extending survival. Curative intent means that similar to liver resection the ablation has to completely destroy not only the tumor but also at least 0.5-1 cm zone of normal liver parenchyma.

RFA was successfully used to treat patients with symptomatic and rapid-growth hepatic cavernous hemangioma [7]. Application of LRFA for the treatment of benign tumor proved to be safe and indicated also in patients with liver adenoma [8].

2.2.1. LRFA advantages

We advocate the laparoscopic approach to ablate the liver tumors with RF due to its advantages over the other two methods: percutaneous and open.

Laparoscopy represents a reliable diagnostic tool. Some authors consider that every liver resection must be preceded by abdominal laparoscopic assessment of the disease [9]. By identifying extrahepatic lesions, laparoscopy can up-stage the patients with cancer and can deem these as unresectable or untreatable with in situ ablation procedures (except those with neuroendocrine tumors).

Two third of the patients with advanced liver insufficiency being evaluated for orthotopic liver transplantation are restaged after exploratory laparoscopy, laparoscopic ultrasound (LUS) and Ultrasound-guided biopsy, half being downstaged and half upstaged [10]. This finding determines some authors to indicate laparoscopic staging followed by LRFA for patients with adenocirrhosis evaluated for liver transplantation unless there are unequivocal clinical data supporting the stage of hepatocellular carcinoma [10].

Unsuspected intra-abdominal extrahepatic metastases can be noted in up to 26% of patients with colorectal liver metastases [11].

Moreove laparoscopy either alone or in association with intraoperative ultrasound examination can diagnose other liver lesions missed by the preoperative imaging examinations in up to 38% cases [12]. LUS can detect lesions less than 2 cm in diameter.

The laparoscopic approach proved to be safe for the treatment of subcapsular tumors due to the possibility of direct visualization and active protection of the surrounding structures (gallbladder, stomach, duodenum, colon, diaphragm) and possibility to control the potential bleeding from these lesions.

The pneumoperitoneum creates a working camera which not only removes the surrounding structures from the liver but also reduces the respiratory movements of the liver and thus facilitates the placement of the RF needle.

LRFA is also able to ablate deep-sited lesions difficult or impossible to be visualized by percutaneous US or to be punctured percutaneously. Some authors consider that for lesions located beneath the diaphragm laparoscopic approach can be associated [13] or even replaced with the thoracoscopic one [14, 15].

For treating patients with large or multiple liver tumors LRFA seems to be the first choice. Nevertheless, for tumors larger than 60 mm in diameter, tumors more than 5, and tumors close to the hepatic vein or inferior vena cava, some author consider RFA via laparotomy to be safer than LRFA [16].

During LRFA the Pringle maneuver can be used if it is necessary. Pneumoperitoneum per se has the advantage to decrease the blood flow and increase the area of ablation [17].

In patients with multiple hepatic lesions surgeons with high expertise can performed LRFA in association with laparoscopic hepatic resection.

Comparing with the open technique, LRFA determines less intra-operative blood loss and fewer postoperative complications [16].

Due to its minimal surgical trauma, LRFA determines a fast recovery time and short hospital stay. It is our practice to discharge the patient 24-48 hours after the operation.

The benefits of LRFA in cirrhotic patients are certain when comparing with the open approach. First, preservation of the abdominal wall and lack of the need to mobilize the liver avoid interruption of large collateral veins and perihepatic ligaments, thus decreasing postoperative ascitic syndrome. Second, nonexposure of the viscera restricts the electrolytic and protein losses and hence the fluids requirements which secondary improves absorption of ascitis. Third, the laparoscopic approach is associated with lower intraoperative blood loss due to the haemostatic effect of the positive pressure of peritoneum, meticulous intraoperative manipulations of the tissue under magnification, and smaller abdominal incisions. It was reported that intraoperative blood loss is a major risk factor of postoperative morbidity and death [18].

For liver tumor recurrences, LRFA can be repeated as needed.

It is still not finally settled which is the best RFA approach in terms of recurrence and survival but we favor the laparoscopic one based on literature data and our experience.

2.2.2. Hepatocellular carcinoma (HCC)

Hepatocellular carcinoma (HCC) is the fifth most common malignancy and fourth in annual mortality. Its incidence continues to grow up secondary to the increasing prevalence of viral hepatitis [19]. Hepatic resection and liver transplantation are considered the mainstay of treatment of HCC being proven as the most effective treatments in means of disease-free interval and survival. However, less than 20% of HCC can be treated surgically because of multifocal diseases, proximity of the tumor to key vascular or biliary structures precluding a margin-negative resection, and inadequate functional hepatic reserve with cirrhosis. Usually, noncirrhotic or Child A cirrhotic patients with single small HCC (≤5 cm) or up to three lesions ≤3 cm are indicated for surgery.

2.2.2.1. Bridge to transplantation

The efficacy of RFA in wait-listed transplant candidates has been studied. Johnson et al. reported eight pretransplant patients treated solely by RFA and matched to a similar group by age, sex, Child-Turcotte-Pugh class, and Model for End-Stage Liver Disease (MELD) score who did not undergo treatment prior to transplant.[20] Patients pretreated with RFA were able to remain on the transplant list for longer periods of time than their matched counterparts. Dropout rates without RFA have been shown to be as high as 40%; however, the use of RFA has decreased them to as low as 20%. The use of RFA as a bridge to transplantation has proven to be an effective strategy. Control of tumor size and the theoretical prevention of metastatic disease formation allow patients to remain on the waiting list for longer periods, increasing their likelihood of obtaining a donor organ. RFA remains limited in its ability to provide complete necrosis of large tumors and should not be expected to do so in patients who are near the upper limits of transplant candidacy because of size criteria.

The need for an accurate intrahepatic staging is crucial for patients with HCC candidates to an aggressive surgical or ablative treatment. Combinations of resection and ablation may be required in certain cases, extending the indications for the laparoscopic approach to hepatocellular carcinoma in liver cirrhosis. Laparoscopy with LUS seems to be useful to identify unsuspected new nodules and to help in choosing the most suitable treatment. Laparoscopy with LUS could represent a sound preliminary examination in patients who are candidates to liver transplantation in order to both improve the staging and guide an interstitial therapy as a bridge to the transplantation itself [21].

2.2.2.2. Resection versus RFA

Surgical resection is the gold standard of treatment for HCC in noncirrhotic and cirrhotic patients who can tolerate hepatic resection. Noncirrhotic patients with HCC can usually undergo resection. However, patients with underlying cirrhosis are rarely candidates for resection and often face a dismal prognosis. As a result, prospective studies comparing patients who are surgical candidates and underwent RFA with those who underwent resection are fairly limited.

2.2.2.3. The use of RFA in nonsurgical candidates

The reported rate of resectable HCC is low and ranges from 9% to 27%. It is limited by the proximity of the tumor to major vascular and biliary structures that would preclude negative resection margins, but more importantly by the degree of underlying liver disease and Ability of the patient to tolerate hepatectomy. Small tumors are generally best suited for RFA and provide the best results. However, larger lesions have also been ablated with mixed success, occasionally even providing overall long-term survival of some patients with HCC. Small lesions are generally considered those that are <3–3.5 cm in diameter.

Larger lesions are known to be more difficult to treat using RFA. Tumors >3 cm may require repositioning of the electrode or multiple treatment sessions in order to obtain clear margins. However, even using a more aggressive approach, the efficacy of RFA has been proven to be limited by tumor size. Lesions measuring >5 cm have at best only a 50% chance of being completely ablated.

Therefore, most authors do not recommend the use of RFA for tumors >5–6 cm because of the technical limitations of the current used equipment and their inability to provide complete coagulative necrosis.

Despite the tumor size limitations of RFA, its use in unresectable HCC is significant. Those who are not transplant candidates or are unable to undergo resection face a dismal prognosis, and RFA provides a chance for survival, especially for patients with smaller lesions. However, the use of RFA should be discouraged in patients with large lesions or those who have evidence of metastatic disease, because these groups have such a poor outcome that RFA is unlikely to provide any tangible benefit.

2.2.2.4. Surgical resection in combination with LRFA

Patients with multifocal disease may be treated by a combined approach using both surgical resection and RFA. The bulk of the tumor burden is initially resected, and RFA is then performed on any remaining unresectable lesions. However, there are few data to support this approach, especially in the setting of HCC. Most agree that if HCC has progressed so extensively, the patient is unlikely to be cured even by aggressive combined modalities of this nature. Additionally, although well tolerated intraoperatively, RFA combined with hepatic resection does place the patient at a higher risk for postoperative liver failure and death. This is especially true in the cirrhotic patient with poor hepatic reserve prior to intervention. Therefore, the role of LRFA in conjunction with resection must be used judiciously and mandates further reviews before it can be recommended in the treatment of HCC.

2.2.3. Metastatic colorectal cancer

The liver is the most common site of distant metastases second only to lymph nodes [22]. Initially considered to be a terminal diagnosis, treatment of these lesions has provided significantly better outcomes for many of these patients, in comparision to those untreated.

Akin with the primary liver masses, surgical resection remains the gold standard therapy for liver metastases from colorectal cancer.

Colorectal cancer is the leading cause of cancer death in US. At the time of exploration for their primary tumor 16-25% of patients have liver metastases and about 25% will develop such lesions in the disease course.

Colorectal cancer is responsible for up to 75% of liver metastases that undergo surgical treatment. For those who undergo resection of isolated liver metastases, the 5-year survival rate has recently been shown to be as high as 58% [23]. Prospective studies that compare RFA with Resection in operative candidates are extremely limited.

Unfortunately, up to 80% of the patients diagnosed with stage IV disease are not candidates for resection. For unresectable liver metastases, alternative options, such as RFA alone or in conjunction with other therapeutic modalities, are being explored to further improve survival [24]. Criteria for unresectable metastases include bilobar disease that cannot be completely excised, proximity to major vasculature structures precluding margin-negative resection, and comorbid conditions that preclude surgery [25]. For these untreated patients, survival is <5%–10% at 5 years [26].

Large trials evaluating the combination of RFA and resection are limited, and therefore it is difficult to draw definitive conclusions regarding its efficacy and safety. As larger portions of hepatic parenchyma are resected or ablated, the risk for liver failure increases, making it difficult to support the use of a combined approach without achieving a survival benefit. At this time, there are few data to support combining RFA with surgical resection.

2.2.4. Liver metastasis from neuroendocrine tumors

Liver metastases occur in 5-90% of patients with neuroendocrine tumors and the specific pattern of these is an indolent course, which may be dominated by symptoms related to hormonal secretion.

The goal of surgical resection and RFA in most cases of both primary and metastatic liver disease is curative. However, neuroendocrine tumors represent a unique group of slowly growing, often highly symptomatic tumors that are unlikely to be cured by resection. The untreated patients with unresectable neuroendocrine liver metastases have a 5-year survival rate of 25-38%.[27] In patients with metastatic neuroendocrine tumors who are unlikely to be cured by surgery or unable to tolerate an invasive form of treatment, RFA has been shown to ameliorate the symptoms (95%), significantly or completely control the symptoms (80%), and partially or significantly decrease the circulating hormone levels (65%) [28, 29]. LRFA seems appealing for these patients because the recurrence rate after resection is >80% at 5 years. Moreover, in case of liver recurrence, LRFA can be repeated for maintaining tumor control in the liver without increasing morbidity.

2.2.5. Liver metastasis from nonneuroendocrine and noncolorectal tumors

Regarding the nonneuroendocrine and noncolorectal liver metastases there are few reports on the utility of RFA to treat them. Patients with liver metastases from sarcoma, breast cancer, gastric cancer, pancreatic adenocarcinoma, or malignant melanoma are predicted to have a short survival due to the rapid diffusely disseminated disease. The overall median survival for these patients is 33 months. The aim for these patients is to prolong life with treatments which have low side effects and offer a good quality of life. Notwithstanding the curative intention of the treatments, most of them are ultimately proven to be palliative due to the progression of the disease. For these patients LRFA has not only curative but also debulking target. For the patients with nonresectable liver metastases, LRFA offers an overall median survival of more than 51 months [30].

2.3. Contraindications of LRFA

These contraindication are:

- Patients ≤ 18 years-old or ≥ 80 years-old,
- Sever coagulopathy (PLT <50.000/mm3, PT, APTT >1,5N),
- Renal failure (serum creatinin > 2,5 mg/dl),
- Jaundice (bilirubinemia > 3 mg/dl, bile duct dilatation),
- Acute infection,
- Tumor vascular or organ invasion,

- Patients with cardiac pacemaker, implanted metallic pieces,
- Sever mental disturbances,
- Pregnancy and breast feeding.

2.4. Patient preparation for LRFA

For all patients admitted for LRFA a baseline evaluation has to be done within one week before the procedure. Besides history and clinical examinations, there are some mandatory laboratory tests and imaging examinations.

Laboratory tests consist of complete blood cell counts, coagulation profile, renal and liver panel, and appropriate serum tumor markers.

Imaging examinations include percutaneous abdominal ultrasound, computer tomography, magnetic resonance imaging (MRI), chest Rx, and, in selected cases, positron emission tomography using ^{18}FDG [12].

The patients known with cardiac problems should have a pretreatment cardiologic assessment in order to prevent the possible arrhythmia due to RFA. Without being an absolute contraindication, patients with implanted cardiac pacemakers need special attention before, during and after the procedure.

Due to the great risk of biliary injury during RFA of the central liver tumors, some authors place preoperative prophylactic biliary stents in patients with such lesions [12].

A dose of intravenous antibiotics is given just before RFA. The duration of administration depends on the various protocol used, being up to 5 days [2].

Informed consent of the patient is obtained before the procedure.

For LRFA the most used is the supine position of the patient. Only when there is a predominance of the disease in the posterior segments of the liver the patient is put on the operating table in left lateral position [31].

The LRFA is performed under general anesthesia.

2.5. The RF-equipment

2.5.1. The RF-equipment

Historically, the major impediment on RFA has been the size of the area to be ablated which could be the explanation of the Achilles' heel of this procedure: local tumor recurrence. In order to improve the results, RF equipments have been continuously perfected.

The rapid increase of temperature (above 100°C) during RFA, leading to charring of the tissue and increase of impedance, was shown to be the main cause of the small coagulation volumes. Many electrodes have been designed to improve energy deposition on tissue and further increase coagulation volume. Nowadays there are various single or combined type of electrodes. The main types are: single, cluster, multitined expandable, spiral expandable, cooled, wet (perfused), monopolar or bipolar electrodes (table 2).[32]

RF system	Rita Model 1500x	**Cool –tip**	Boston RF 3000	**Berchtold**	**Surtron**	Celon Power-Olympus
Power	250 W	200 W	200 W	60 W	200W	250 W
Frequency	460 kHz	480 kHz	480 kHz	375 kHz	480kHz	470 kHz
Ablation control	Impedance and temperature	Impedance	Impedance	Impedance	Impedance	Impedance
Energy delivery	Monopolar bipolar	Monopolar	Monopolar	Monopolar	Monopolar	Bipolar multipolar
Electrode diameter	2.2 mm	1.6mm/ 3x1.6mm	2.5 mm	1.7 mm		1.8 mm
Electrode geometry	"Christmas tree"	Single, Cluster	"Umbrella"	Single, Cluster	Single	Single
Active part of the electrode	5cm/7cm	Single/ Cluster 3cm/2,5cm	4 cm	1.5 cm		4 cm
Electrode	Expended± wet ±flexible	Cooled single/cluster	Expended	Wet		Cooled
MRI	Yes (XL)	Yes (single or cluster)	Yes (3.5cm)	Yes	Yes	Yes (mono/ multipolar)

Table 2. Different characteristics of RF equipments and probes.

2.5.2. The ultrasound equipment

The ultrasound equipment used for ablation must have either a fixed or flexible linear laparoscopic ultrasound probe (figure 1A) or a fixed forward-viewing convex-array transducer (figure 2B) and the possibility of Doppler imaging.

For improvement of tumor visualization and targeting for RFA, a prototype tracked ultrasound-guided laparoscopic surgery system was design and used in clinical practice by some authors [33]. By tracking two-dimensional ultrasound images in physical space, the system generates three-dimensional ultrasound volumes. Once the tumor is manually identified in this volume, a targeting system is used to guide the tip of the RFA probe inside the tumor [33].

A picture-in-picture box with the quarter-size laparoscopic image superimposed over the full-sized ultrasound image is of paramount importance for the coordination of the movement of the instruments.

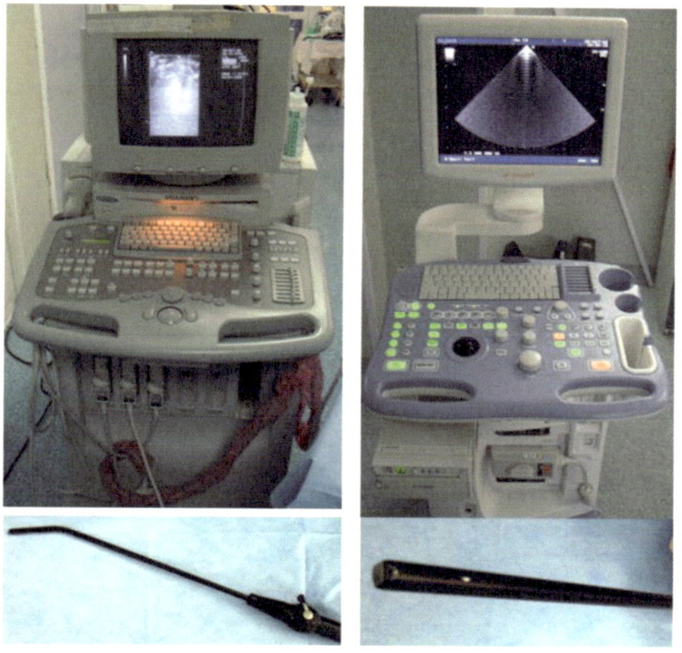

Figure 1. Ultrasound equipment. A. Ultrasound machine with flexible liniar transductor for laparoscopy. B. Ultrasound machine with fixed convex transductor for laparoscopy

2.6. LRFA technique

2.6.1. Pneumoperitoneum induction

In many centers the Veress technique remains the most widespread method of induction of peritoneum. Because the most common complications of laparoscopic surgery are related to insertion of the Veress needle and the first trocar, alternatives such Hasson's open method or optical access trocar-insertion emerged. These alternative methods are especially useful in patients with previous operations and intraabdominal adhesions.

The Hasson's open method implies the transversing of the tissue planes under direct view and carries the disadvantages of continuous air leaks and prolonged operating time. Besides it can be cumbersome in obese patients.

The optical access trocars have been developed as an alternative means of transversing the tissue planes under direct view. We advocate the use of optical access trocar which in our department is the standard device for obtaining abdominal access in laparoscopic practice since 1995 [34]. The method consists in introduction into abdomen of a 12-mm disposable Optiview® trocar (Ethicon Endo-surgery Cincinnati, OH) or a 5-12 mm Visiport™ Plus Optical trocar (Covidien)with an inserted 0^0 laparoscope.

2.6.2. *Trocar insertion*

Most of the patients submitted for LRFA can be treated with placement of two right subcostal ports. The umbilical placement of one trocar represents an impediment to reach the dome of the liver from such a location.

Selected patients need insertion of the third or fourth trocar (figure 2). The additional trocars may be needed for dissection of the intra-abdominal adhesions, performing cholecystectomy, retraction of the adjacent organs, or multiple needle insertion for treating multiple tumors.

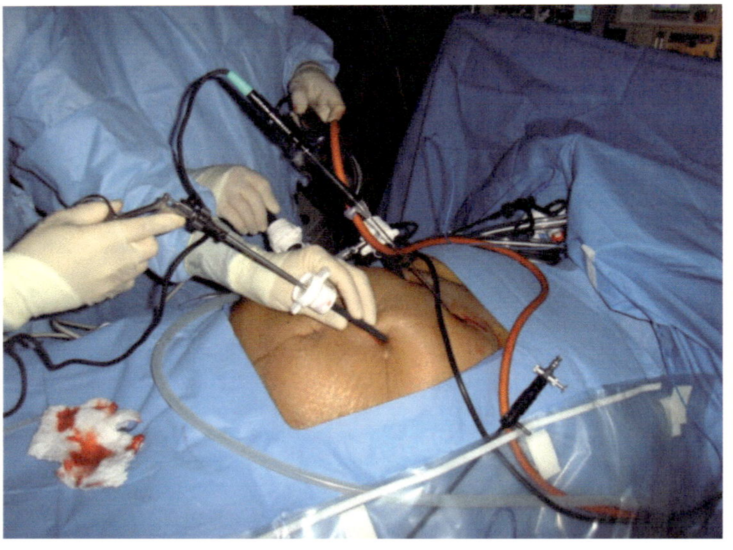

Figure 2. Patient with previous laparotomy, placed in supine position for LRFA of bilateral liver metastases. Three trocars are inserted: one for video, one for ultrasound transductor, and one aditional trocar for forceps. The RF probe is percutaneously introduced.

2.6.3. *Abdominal exploration*

All adhesions that interfere with proper exploration of the abdomen are taken down. A systematic and thorough visual exploration of the abdominal cavity is performed, and all peritoneal surfaces are carefully examined for possible deposits, paying special attention to the undersurface of the diaphragm, the hepatic round ligament, and the omentum. Lymph nodes in the hepatoduodenal ligament are examined for enlargement. The quality of the liver parenchyma with regard to the degree of cirrhosis or steatosis is also assessed.

Laparoscopic ultrasound is performed systematically in a longitudinal fashion, different from the transverse orientation in intraoperative ultrasound. For laparoscopic ultrasound liver scanning, most authors use the linear probe. For a better visualization of the upper segments or caudate lobe some authors favor the use of others probes. In some cases for a better contact between the convex liver surface and the probe, instillation of normal saline solution

http://dx.doi.org/10.5772/52830

into peritoneum can be very helpful to provide an acoustic window. Sometimes the abdomen need to be desufflated to improve contact with the liver. The laparoscope and LUS probe can be interchanged between the ports to provide different views of the liver and to enable varying placements of the probe on the liver surface. Generally it is not needed to take down the falciform ligament but the creation of a window in the falciform ligament allows the exploration of the liver in patients with dense midline adhesions. Maintaining visual guidance of the probe's position on the liver with the laparoscope aids in orientation. Scanning is started with visualization of the point at which the three liver veins drain into the inferior caval vein. The number and size of hepatic lesions and their segmental locations are carefully documented. The exact location of the liver masses relative to the central vascular structures is aided by color Doppler, and the distance to the vessels is measured in centimeters, considering a safe margin for ablation of 1 cm. Color Doppler is also used to assess the vascularity of the hepatic lesions. The distance between hepatic lesion and surrounding viscera is evaluated in order to plan the ablation process.

2.6.4. Tumor biopsy

Once the lesions are mapped in the liver, a core biopsy is performed under ultrasound guidance using an 18-gauge spring-loaded biopsy gun (Microinvasive) and sent for frozen section to confirm malignancy. In some HHC, obtaining of proper amount of tumoral tissue is difficult due to its inconsistency and repeated biopsy are needed. The tumor biopsy can also be Obtained after the RFA having the advantage of harvesting a more consistent tissue fragment and avoiding the possible bleeding from liver puncture site. Tissue samples are taken only from representative tumors and not from all.

2.6.5. RF needle insertion

Laparoscopic introduction of the RF electrodes into the liver tumors are ultrasound guided and the operator has to plan very carefully the insertions. This represents the most difficult part of the procedure, and most beginners under treat due to this.

Introduction of the electrodes especially to ablate large tumors, tumors near great vessels or poor visualized tumor is very demanding using the fix or flexible linear-type ultrasound probe (figure 1A). Often small and deep-seated tumors necessitate repeated trial-and-error insertions of the RF electrode. The safety and the complete necrosis of ablation is very much dependent on the RF electrode positioning.

For ablation of liver tumors under the guidance of a linear-type probe, the RF electrode must be inserted from the abdominal wall cranially and parallel to the ultrasound probe. For accurate tumoral insertion of the RF probe operator has to mentally establish in three dimensions the insertion site and angle on the abdominal wall and also on the surface of the liver. For small and deep-seated tumors, insertion of the electrode can be very difficult due to the impossibility to observe the needle on a single image. Therefore, the ultrasound probe has to be moved according to the position of the needle tip.

Continuous monitorization of the position of the needle tip on the ultrasound image immediately after puncturing the liver is possible using the laparoscopic system with a fixed forward-viewing convex-array transducer, with a guide groove on the back of the shaft (figure 1B) [35]. Perpendicular direction of scanning of this transducer enable the easy and accurate puncture of the deep-seated tumors. Unlike with other conventional linear-type, it is not necessary to consider the insertion site on the abdominal wall and surface of the liver. This transducer facilitates the needle insertion in tumors situated in segment VII, VIII, for which scanning by linear-type probes is more difficult [35]. Some authors advocate the use of the forward-viewing convex-array probe for lesions situated in segment I arguing that this US-probe makes not only the imaging of the caudate lobe easily but also avoid the insertion of the needle through segment IV which has the risk to damage major vessels and biliary ducts [36].

Positioning the needle tip depends on the type of the electrode used. If a straight (nonexpendable) electrode is used then it is advanced under US-guidance until its tip reaches and passes the deep margin of the lesion in order to obtain a safe oncological rim of normal parenchyma. Depending on the tumor size and noninsulated distance of the electrode it might take more than one application to complete the lesion ablation. Repositioning the electrode is performed to obtain overlapping spherical or cylindrical ablations.

If the electrode has Christmas tree-type deployment then the tip of the electrode is positioned also in correlation with the tumor diameter and the active size of the electrode. If only one ablation is planned the tip of the electrode is advanced till it reaches the superficial margin and the prongs are progressively deployed. If more than one ablation is intended then the tip of the electrode is positioned into the tumor considering the dimension of the prongs. After completing the first ablation, the prongs are undeployed, the electrode is retracted by 2-2.5 cm, the prongs are again deployed, and ablation reinitiated.

If one considers the use of an umbrella-type expandable electrode, the tip of the electrode usually targets the center of the tumor. In case of a large tumor, the positioning of the electrode is similar with the previous expandable type.

Using the first-generation RITA Medical System model 30 (4 arrays) or model 70 (7 arrays), a single ablation cycle is enough to destroy a tumor <3 cm. For tumors >3 cm overlapping ablations are necessary using these probes. Using the second-generation of probes - RITA Medical System Starbust XL (9 arrays, 5 cm) - the tumors <3 cm are ablated with a single 3 cm ablation, those of 3-4 cm with a single 4 cm ablation, those of 4-5 cm with one cycle of a 5 cm ablation and those of >5 cm with application of 2-4 cycles of ablation to obtain adequate margins [29]. The new RITA System Starbust XLi enhanced permits ablation of the 5-7 cm sized tumors with a single ablation cycle.

In patients with multiple lesions the duration of the ablation process can be shorten using simultaneously two RF needles. However these simultaneous ablations are very demanding due to real-time monitorization. In case of performing these, care must be taken to place the needles apart otherwise much larger ablation area can result.

Withdrawal of the RF needle after the ablation needs some consideration to discuss. RFA of the needle track is needed not only to control the bleeding but also to avoid recurrences along it. Bleeding from the needle track is seldom a problem but it might be cumbersome in cirrhotic patients. Generally RF ablation with application of a 20-30W power suffices. If not, laparoscopy permits us to control the bleeding by other means: electrocautery, haemostatics, argon application.

2.6.6. Real-time monitoring of the ablation process

The ablation process is assessed in three ways:

1. monitoring the thermocouples temperatures,
2. observing the ablation effect by ultrasound,
3. checking the absence of the Doppler signal into the previously vascularized tumors.

Except of RITA generators all the others deliver energy to tissues automatically based on impedance feed-back control. Because the damages of the tissues are well established at certain temperatures, we favor the use of RITA generators which control the ablation process using the thermocouple temperature. The device can be manually preset to the target temperature. We use for ablation a preset 105^{0}C temperature at thermocouples. During the ablation procedure the temperatures of the thermocouples are monitorized and visualized on the display of the device. The process can also be registered on a notebook connected to the system.

Aiming the enlargement of the ablation area, many authors have developed their own protocol of ablation [37]. Due to animal experimental studies and our clinical experience, LRFA has become a standardized operation. The time of ablation process depends on the tumor volume. The mainstay is to achieve the target temperature progressively till the full deployment appropriate to the tumor diameter. Our protocol is to deploy progressively the prongs of the RF needle. The prongs are deployed at 2 cm and subsequently to 3 cm until target temperature of 105^{0}C is reached at all thermocouples. Then the catheter is advanced to 4 cm and consecutively to 5 cm and maintain for 7 min at each deployment [37]. If the target temperatures cannot be achieved the prongs are completely retracted and the catheter rotated with 45^0 and then the prongs redeployed. While advancing the deployment of the prongs, the temperature of the thermocouples decreases and then progressively increases. Sometimes the reposition of the needle is needed to avoid the vicinity of the great vessels or to maintain the prongs inside the liver parenchyma. Even when one to three prongs cannot reach the highest temperature, the ablation procedure is continued taking them out of equation.

After the ablation is ceased, the monitoring of the thermocouples temperature is observed and it should be noticed that it drops rapidly over the 10-20 s and slower after. The temperatures higher then 60-70^{0}C at 1 min after ablation are considered relevant to a successful ablation. In case of uncertain ablation, the needle is 45^0 rotated and the tines are again fully deployed. If the temperatures are above 60^{0}C the ablation is well done. If not, the ablation is repeated.

The ultrasound visualization of the tumor ablation is possible due to the microbubbles formation into the tissue. These are caused by out gassing of dissolved nitrogen. The area of the tumor becomes progressively hypoechoic and due to the gas shadow the deep edge of the tumor is obscured (figure 3). This justify the planning of the ablation process from the deepest tumor area to the superficial one. In about 10 min the gas is reabsorbed and the tumor regains the initial aspect with the exception of some amount of gas and the needle track.

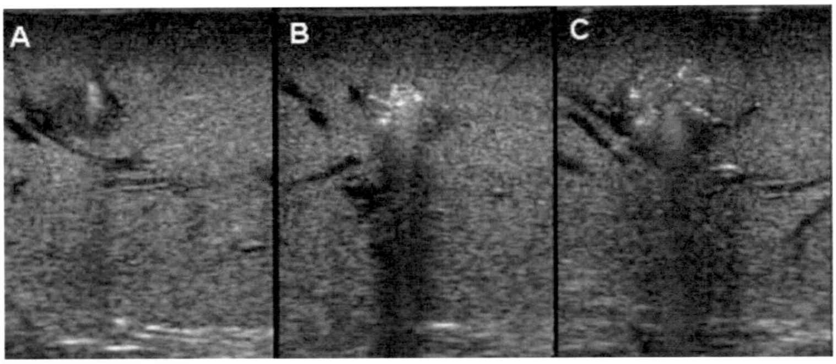

Figure 3. RFA ablation of HCC. A. Positioning the tip of the electrode in the hepatic tumor. B. RFA is started and microbubbles of gas determine appearance of hyperechoic images in the tumor. C. The extension of ablated tissue obscures the deep edge of the tumor. From image collection of Dr. Boros Mirela.

Doppler control of the ablation process is useful in case of vascularized tumors to certify the disappearance of the flow. Usage of the micro bubble contrast agents (e.g. SonoVue ® Bracco International B.V., Holland) can add more help in assessment of the liver blood flow.

Fluorescence spectroscopy was tried in porcine models aiming to detect hepatocellular thermal damage in real time and hence ensure adequate tumor ablation [38].

Due to the skin burn complications reported after RFA, the monitorization of the skin temperature under the grounding pads needs to be mentioned. Especially in patients with large or multiple tumors the position of the grounding pads is essential. The common position is at the same distance on the anterior surface of the tights. These neutral electrodes are needed only when RF monopolar electrodes are used. The bipolar electrodes do not necessitate these pads. It was showed that placing the ground pad over the patient's back resulted in delivering an increased power to the tumor itself and decreasing the time to reach the target temperature [31]. When planning to use two needles two pair of grounding pad are mounted on the patient's back and tight. After completing the ablation the peripheral small tumors become volcanic crater-like and the larger ones appear as a depressed mass.

2.2.7. Useful intraoperative maneuvers

2.6.7.1. Saline-enhanced LRFA

Hypertonic saline injected through a side port on the shaft of the electrode prior to ablation can be uniformly distributed within an encapsulated HCC and thus increase ionicity and conduction within the tumor. The result is an increased volume of ablation up to 6-7 cm diameter. On the contrary, this method is not safe for patients with scirrhous colorectal liver metastases due to the unpredictability distribution of hypertonic saline.

2.6.7.2. Saline infusion systems

The electrodes designed with tiny channels can be used to infuse small volumes of saline into tumor during ablation process in order to prevent desiccation and charring of the tumor that would otherwise prevent conductivity and limit the ablation volume.

2.6.7.3. Vascular occlusion

The application of the Pringle maneuver for limited amounts of time has been shown by some authors [39] to increase ablation volumes but was found inefficient by others [40]. The vascular pedicle occlusion might be justified due to reduction of the heat-sink effect [41]. Total vascular exclusion of the liver was shown to result in the greatest increase in necrosis volume when compared to no occlusion or Pringle maneuver [42].

The possibility of vessel damage or thrombosis secondary to RFA with vascular inflow occlusion was pointed out by some authors [43]. These vascular side effects could be increased in such cases when one or more of electrode prongs are placed in the lumen of a vessel [44]. Moreover, increased ablation secondary to Pringle maneuver carries with it an associated risk of biliary, portal, or parenchymal injury [45].

We consider reasonable not to perform Pringle maneuver also because laparoscopy results in a 30-40% reduction of the blood flow as it was stated by other authors [46].

2.6.7.4. Cooling of the biliary tract

Despite the major vessels, major biliary ducts are deemed to be vulnerable to hyperthermia. Damage of these ducts were reported to occur when the RF needle was located less than 5 mm apart from these [36]. As with the biliary ducts, gallbladder is submitted to damages during and after the ablation process. For tumors situated in segment I, IV, V, in the proximity of the gallbladder cholecystectomy may be recommended before starting the ablation in order to avoid organ perforation or inflammation. The method to prevent the occurrence of biliary system damages is cooling it by pouring cold saline solution onto the surface of the bile duct and gallbladder [36] or by infusing a 4^0 C saline solution quickly through a catheter placed in the bile duct via choledochotomy [47].

3. Results

3.1. Follow-up

Postablation syndrome is a self-limited flu-like syndrome. This systemic inflammatory reaction occurs in one third of patients after RFA and usually depends on the extension of the ablated lesion(s) and ablation time. Its clinical manifestations are milder compared with cryotherapy and consist in transient fever, pain, malaise, myalgia, nausea, and vomiting [48]. The laboratory tests which attest the inflammation are leukocytosis, elevation of serum transaminases, and bilirubin level. The laboratory analysis are performed in the first day after ablation. The WBC count increases more in patients with normal livers and less in patients with previous chemotherapy and cirrhosis [49]. The most dramatic elevations are noticed with AST (14-fold) and ALT (10-fold) but with a fast return to baseline within a week. Serum bilirubin, alkaline phosphatase, and GGT also increase immediately after ablation but with a slower return to baseline up to 3 months. The degree of these elevations is more pronounced in patients with normal hepatic parenchyma than in patients with hepatic steatosis, fibrosis, or cirrhosis [49]. Despite what it would be expected because of the cell death, serum potassium and lactate dehydrogenase levels remain stable after RFA.

To test the tumor markers, blood sample is obtained 1 week after ablation, every 3 months for 2 years, and every 6 months thereafter.

Grayscale ultrasonography of LRFA ablated liver tumor may show hypoechoic, hyperechoic, or mixed appearance. It can be used to early diagnose the hepatic abscess as complication of RFA.

The triphasic (noncontrast, arterial, portal-venous) CT scan is performed to establish a baseline at 1 week postablation and on regular basis every 3 months for 2 years, 6 months for 2 years and yearly thereafter (figure 4).

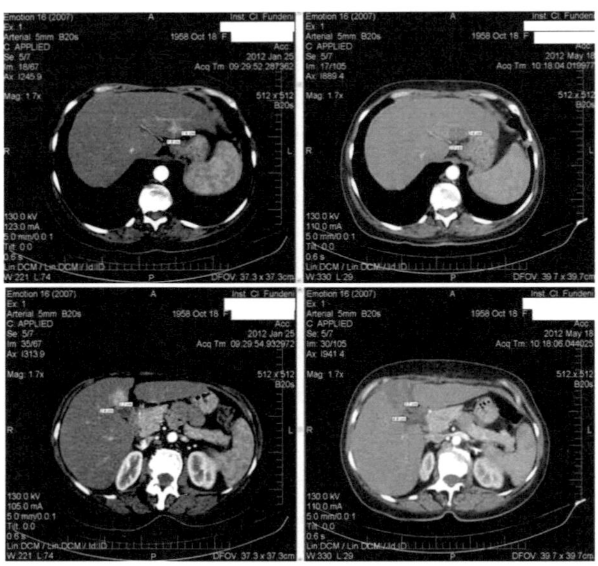

Figure 4. LRFA of a multicentric HCC on cirrhotic liver. The upper images show a hepatic tumor in segment II pre and postablation. The lower images show a hepatic tumor in segment IV pre and postablation. Tactic cholecystectomy was performed during the same operation. There is no tumor recurrence after 3 months postablation.

http://dx.doi.org/10.5772/52830

In the first week postablation, the destroyed tumors appear on contrast-enhanced CT (CECT) with low attenuation when comparing to the normal liver tissue. CECT scan performed in the first 2 weeks postablation may underestimate the actual result due to the presence of granulomatous hypervascularized healing around necrosis which can be misinterpreted as residual viable tumor.

The small ablated lesions have a spherical, "punched out" shape contrary to the large ablated lesions which have a more irregular shape. The success of ablation is announced by CT demonstration of a larger lesion due to the ablation of a rim of nontumoral hepatic parenchyma (figure 5). On further CT scanning the lesion will decrease in size. Any increase in lesion size, irregularity of the edges, or contrast enhancement diagnoses either the incomplete necrosis or local recurrence. Sometimes the appreciation of the contrast enhancement of the lesion might be very difficult especially when comparing the pre- and postablation hypodense liver masses. The assessment of CT Hounsfield unit of the preablated liver lesion was shown to be very reliable in assessment of its evolution. The quantitative measurement of tissue density expressed in Hounsfield unit scale is reproducible over time and is machine independent. In successfully ablated lesions there is a measurable decrease in contrast uptake, which is indicated by the minimal increase in Hounsfield unit density following the administration of contrast in postablation scans [50].

Contrast-enhanced ultrasonography (CEUS) is also useful to provide information regarding ablated lesion but has low sensitivity in identifying the safety margin and incomplete coverage of the liver in patients at high risk of developing new hepatic tumors.

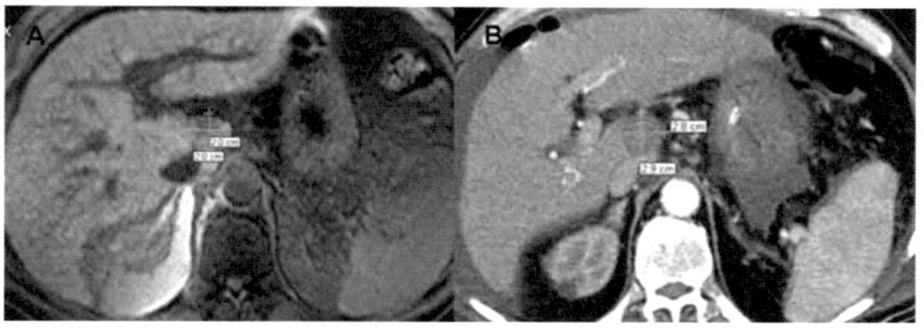

Figure 5. Follow-up of HCC with LFRA. A. RMI is diagnostic for a 2 cm sized tumor situated in caudate lobe. B. Two months after LRFA the tumor is hypodense on CECT and a little larger than prior ablation with a diameter of 2.8 cm. The ablation was successfully completed.

If the CT imaging is doubtful, MRI or PET is indicated. Unenhanced or contrast-enhanced MRI can be used post-LRFA. MRI has a higher sensitivity than CT for detection of recurrences at 2 months (89% vs. 44%) [51] but at 4 months there is no difference between them.

Despite its higher sensitivity for local recurrence comparing with multidetector CT (MDCT), radiolabeled deoxyglucose ([18F]FDG) PET/CT is limited to few centers.

In case of further uncertain imaging results for tumor recurrence, percutaneous biopsy or exploratory laparoscopy with LUS examination and biopsy may be needed [52]. In case of positive malignant fresh sections, the tumor recurrence must be reablated including the whole previous lesion due to the 23% risk of viable tumoral cells in the core of the lesion and respecting 0.5-1 cm edge of oncological safety.[52]

Quality of life is assessed pre- and postablation using different questionnaires.

3.2. Morbidity and mortality

The type of complications after LRFA are mainly the same with those encountered after percutaneous or open approach but with an intermediate rate. The specific complications for the laparoscopic approach are those linked to the introduction of Veress needle and trocars. In LRFA there have not been reported thermal damages of the neighboring organs. The rate of complications seems to be non-related with the histological pattern of the tumor. It has also been proven on large cohort of patients that the rates of complications are comparable if it is the first RFA (5%), repeated RFA (1%), or RFA combined with other procedures (3%) [49].

Hepatic abscess represents the most common complication registered after RFA and is related mostly to large area of necrotic tissue. One explanation for development of hepatic abscess is the retrograde enteric bacterial contamination of the biliary tract from bilioenteric anastomosis or Oddi sphincterectomy. In patients with previous Whipple procedure the incidence of the liver abscess is 40% much more higher than in patients without bilioenteric anastomosis (0.4%) [49]. Considering these, some authors avoid performance of RFA on such patients [2]. In case of performing LRFA for the patients with bilioenteric anastomosis, there should be a close follow-up aiming the early diagnosis and treatment of this complication and a longer antibioprofilaxy. The hepatic abscess can be treated with antibiotics and percutaneous drainage.

Other possible complications are ascitis, liver failure, and respiratory complications.

Thrombocytopenia (excluding patients with preexisting thrombocytemia) and gross mioglobinuria are seldom encountered, being related to the extensive procedure for large or multiple tumors. Acute renal failure due to mioglobinuria is much less encountered as a complication of RFA than cryotherapy and it can be prevented with high hydration of the patient during and after the procedure.

Skin burns are a rare complication with LRFA.

Overall, LRFA is safe and well tolerated, with a per procedure mortality of less than 1%.

3.3. Parietal seeding

Parietal seeding is less a problem in laparoscopic than in percutaneous RFA and can be coped with the aid of a 14 G venous needle or a 2 mm trocar placed through the abdominal wall. The RF electrode is introduced through these large sheaths [53]. For cluster needle such a precaution is not feasible.

3.4. Local recurrence

Local recurrence is defined if the lesion is within 2 cm of the ablated tumor. Remote or distal recurrence is defined when the lesion is at least 2 cm far from the ablated tumor. [53]. Local recurrence is the best measure to assess the technical success of RFA.

Theoretically, the recurrent lesions are due to viable malignant cells that escaped thermal injury during the ablative procedure. This could be the explanation of the recurrences which mainly occur at the periphery of the lesions [50].

The wide range of local recurrence after RFA between 1.8% and 60% reflects difference in tumor type, size, number, liver segmental location, approach, ablation margin, blood vessel proximity, operator experience, and - last but not least - type of RF probe and generator used [54, 55].

The higher rates of recurrence seen within certain tumor histology types are likely a reflection of tumor biology (e.g. density, vascularity, heat conduction) but also of parenchymal milieu (e.g. cirrhosis) [55]. Patients with metastases from colorectal cancer, hepatocellular carcinoma, and melanoma have higher rates of local recurrence comparing with other malignant liver tumors [56].

LRFA results In a tumoral recurrence of 5.8% which is similar with 4.4% obtained in open approach but significant lesser comparing with 16.4% reported with the percutaneous approach [55].

In case of limited hepatic recurrences after other ablative procedures or in selected cases after liver resection, it is our believe that LRFA deserves to be the first-choice treatment. In case of multiple hepatic recurrences, transarterial chemoembolization (TACE) is needed in association with LRFA performed for the larger lesions [57].

3.5. Association of LRFA with other therapeutic methods

In patients with multiple liver masses, LRFA can be performed in association with laparoscopic liver resections [58]. LRFA is indicated for deep-situated (<3 cm) tumors while resection is feasible and safety for exophitic/subcapsular tumors. The association of resection with RFA was found to be a safe procedure with long term outcomes better than the ablation but poorer than resection alone [59].

Due to the progression of the malignant disease most of the patients will develop recurrences after LRFA [53, 60]. Because better survival rates have been obtained with the association of regional chemotherapy, some authors recommend the placement of hepatic arterial infusion pump (HAIP) in all patients who undergo RFA [61]. Concomitant LRFA and HAIP are safe and feasible [62].

LRFA is a therapeutic option for the patients with primary digestive cancer and synchronic liver metastases. A rule of thumb is to perform surgery for the primary indication that brings the patient to the operation (i.e. colorectal, pancreas resection, ileostomy reversal). The surgery for digestive tract can be performed either by laparoscopy or laparotomy and is followed by LRFA. A laparotomy should be converted for LRFA because laparoscopic approach facilitates accurate needle placement [63]. Moreover, LRFA avoids the need of large incision for liver access. For selected cases with colorectal tumors and liver dissemination in which liver resection might increase the operative risk, the ablation of the hepatic lesions is recommended to be performed laparoscopically in the same operative session. The tumor ablation combined with other operative procedures was shown to be safe and not to increase the risk of morbidity and hospital stay [63].

4. Conclusion

Laparoscopic exploration and intraoperative ultrasound permit an accurate staging of malignant disease. In unresectable malignant liver tumors, LRFA represents a safe and effective treatment especially when percutaneus approach to the lesions is deemed difficult. LRFA can also be a substitute for hepatic resection in patients with small malignant tumors or benign liver tumors. LRFA proved to be safe for the treatment of subcapsular tumors due to the possibility of direct visualization, active protection of the surrounding structures, and control of the potential bleeding from these lesions. Deep-situated lesions difficult or impossible to be visualized by percutaneous US and/or punctured percutaneously can be successfully ablated by laparoscopy. Laparoscopic approach is the first choice for ablation of large or multiple liver tumors with possible association of surgical resection or portal vein ligation. LRFA represents a good bridge therapy for prevention of tumor progression and downstaging of multiple lesions for patients with HCC and cirrhosis on the waiting list for liver transplantation. LRFA is associated with less intraoperative blood loss and fewer postoperative complications when compared with open procedure. Due to its minimal surgical trauma, this procedure determines a fast recovery time and short hospital stay. Tumoral recurrence after LRFA is similar to the open approach but significant lesser comparing with percutaneous one. In case of incomplete thermal ablation or tumor recurrence, LRFA can be repeated or followed by transarterial chemoembolization.

Acknowledgements

This chapter was supported by the Sectorial Operational Program Human Resources Development 2007-2013 through the project "Molecular and cellular biotechnologies with medical applications", FSE POSDRU/89/1.5/S/60746.

Author details

Mirela Patricia Sîrb Boeti[1,2*], Răzvan Grigorie[2] and Irinel Popescu[1,2]

*Address all correspondence to: paboet@yahoo.com

1 University of Medicine and Pharmacy "Carol Davila", Bucharest, Romania

2 Fundeni Clinical Institute, Department of General Surgery and Liver Transplantation, Bu-chares, Romania

References

[1] Mc Gahan, J. P., Browning, P. D., Brock, J. M., & Tesluk, H. (1990). Hepatic ablation using radiofrequency electrocautery. *Invest Radiol*, 25(3), 267-70.

[2] Poon, R. T., Ng, K. K., Lam, C. M., Ai, V., Yuen, J., Fan, S. T., et al. (2004). Learning curve for radiofrequency ablation of liver tumors: prospective analysis of initial 100 patients in a tertiary institution. *Ann Surg*, Apr, 239(4), 441-9.

[3] Hildebrand, P., Leibecke, T., Kleemann, M., Mirow, L., Birth, M., Bruch, H. P., et al. (2006). Influence of operator experience in radiofrequency ablation of malignant liver tumours on treatment outcome. *Eur J Surg Oncol*, May, 32(4), 430-4.

[4] Garcea, G., & Berry, D. P. (2007). Focal liver ablation techniques in primary and secondary liver tumors. *In: P.M.Schlag USS, editor. Regional Cancer Therapy (Cancer Drug Discovery and Development). Humana Press Inc., Totowa, NJ.*

[5] Giovannini, M., Moutardier, V., Danisi, C., Bories, E., Pesenti, C., & Delpero, J. R. (2003). Treatment of hepatocellular carcinoma using percutaneous radiofrequency thermoablation: results and outcomes in 56 patients. *J Gastrointest Surg*, Sep, 7(6), 791-6.

[6] Curley, S. A. (2001). Radiofrequency ablation of malignant liver tumors. *Oncologist*, 6(1), 14-23.

[7] Fan, R. F., Chai, F. L., He, G. X., Wei, L. X., Li, R. Z., Wan, W. X., et al. (2006). Laparoscopic radiofrequency ablation of hepatic cavernous hemangioma. *A preliminary experience with 27 patients. Surg Endosc*, Feb, 20(2), 281-5.

[8] Buscarini, L., Rossi, S., Fornari, F., Di Stasi, M., & Buscarini, E. (1995). Laparoscopic ablation of liver adenoma by radiofrequency electrocauthery. *Gastrointest Endosc*, Jan, 41(1), 68-70.

[9] Rahusen, F. D., Cuesta, Borgstein. P. J., Bleichrodt, R. P., Barkhof, F., Doesburg, T., et al. (1999). Selection of patients for resection of colorectal metastases of the liver using diagnostic laparoscopy and laparoscopic ultrasonography. *Ann Surg*, 230(1), 31-7.

[10] Kim, R. D., Nazarey, P., Katz, E., & Chari, R. S. (2004). Laparoscopic staging and tumor ablation for hepatocellular carcinoma in Child C cirrhotics evaluated for orthotopic liver transplantation. *Surg Endosc*, Jan, 18(1), 39-44.

[11] Lefor, A. T., Hughes, K. S., Shiloni, E., Steinberg, S. M., Vetto, J. P., Papa, M. Z., et al. (1998). Intra-abdominal extrahepatic disease in patients with colorectal hepatic metastases. *Dis Colon Rectum*, 31(2), 100-3.

[12] Bilchik, A. J., Wood, T. F., & Allegra, D. P. (2001). Radiofrequency ablation of unresectable hepatic malignancies: lessons learned. *Oncologist*, 6(1), 24-33.

[13] Kang, C. M., Ko, H. K., Song, S. Y., Kim, K. S., Choi, J. S., Lee, W. J., et al. (2007). Dual-scope guided (simultaneous thoraco-laparoscopic) transthoracic transdiaphragmatic intraoperative radiofrequency ablation for hepatocellular carcinoma located beneath the diaphragm. *Surg Endosc*, Jun 26.

[14] Ishikawa, T., Kohno, T., Shibayama, T., Fukushima, Y., Obi, S., Teratani, T., et al. (2001). Thoracoscopic thermal ablation therapy for hepatocellular carcinoma located beneath the diaphragm. *Endoscopy*, Aug, 33(8), 697-702.

[15] Ishikawa, T., Kohno, T., Teratani, T., & Omata, M. (2002). Thoracoscopic radiofrequency ablation therapy for hepatocellular carcinoma above the diaphragm associated with intractable hemothorax. *Endoscopy*, Oct, 34(10), 843.

[16] Topal, B., Aerts, R., & Penninckx, F. (2003). Laparoscopic radiofrequency ablation of unresectable liver malignancies: feasibility and clinical outcome. *Surg Laparosc Endosc Percutan Tech*, Feb, 13(1), 11-5.

[17] Smith, M. K., Mutter, D., Forbes, L. E., Mulier, S., & Marescaux, J. (2004). The physiologic effect of the pneumoperitoneum on radiofrequency ablation. *Surg Endosc*, Jan, 18(1), 35-8.

[18] Shimata, M., Takenaka, K., Fujiwara, Y., Giot, T., Shirabe, K., Yanaga, K., et al. (1998). Risk factors linked to postoperative morbidity in patients with hepatocellular carcinoma. *Br J Surg*, 85(2), 195-8.

[19] Kew, M. C. (2002). Epidemiology of hepatocellular carcinoma. *Toxicology*, 181-182, 35-8.

[20] Johnson, E. W., Holck, P. S., Levy, A. E., Yeh, M. M., & Yeung, R. S. (2004). The role of tumor ablation in bridging patients to liver transplantation. *Arch Surg*, Aug, 139(8), 825-9.

[21] Montorsi, M., Santambrogio, R., Bianchi, P., Dapri, G., Spinelli, A., & Podda, M. (2002). Perspectives and drawbacks of minimally invasive surgery for hepatocellular carcinoma. *Hepatogastroenterology*, Jan, 49(43), 56-61.

[22] Liu, L. X., Zhang, W. H., & Jiang, H. C. (2003). Current treatment for liver metastases from colorectal cancer. *World J Gastroenterol*, Feb, 9(2), 193-200.

[23] Abdalla, E. K., Vauthey, J. N., Ellis, L. M., Ellis, V., Pollock, R., Broglio, K. R., et al. (2004). Recurrence and outcomes following hepatic resection, radiofrequency ablation, and combined resection/ablation for colorectal liver metastases. *Ann Surg*, Jun, 239(6), 818-25.

[24] Fahy, B. N., & Jarnagin, W. R. (2006). Evolving techniques in the treatment of liver colorectal metastases: role of laparoscopy, radiofrequency ablation, microwave coagulation, hepatic arterial chemotherapy, indications and contraindications for resection, role of transplantation, and timing of chemotherapy. *Surg Clin North Am*, Aug, 86(4), 1005-22.

[25] Curley, S. A., Izzo, F., Delrio, P., Ellis, L. M., Granchi, J., Vallone, P., et al. (1999). Radiofrequency ablation of unresectable primary and metastatic hepatic malignancies: results in 123 patients. *Ann Surg*, Jul, 230(1), 1-8.

[26] Bentrem, D. J., Dematteo, R. P., & Blumgart, L. H. (2005). Surgical therapy for metastatic disease to the liver. *Annu Rev Med*, 56, 139-56.

[27] Touzios, J. G., Kiely, J. M., Pitt, S. C., Rilling, W. S., Quebbeman, E. J., Wilson, S. D., et al. (2005). Neuroendocrine hepatic metastases: does aggressive management improve survival? *Ann Surg*, 241, 776-85.

[28] Mazzaglia, P. J., Berber, E., Milas, M., & Siperstein, A. E. (2007). Laparoscopic radiofrequency ablation of neuroendocrine liver metastases: a 10-year experience evaluating predictors of survival. *Surgery*, Jul, 142(1), 10-9.

[29] Berber, E., Flesher, N., & Siperstein, A. E. (2002). Laparoscopic radiofrequency ablation of neuroendocrine liver metastases. *World J Surg*, Aug, 26(8), 985-90.

[30] Berber, E., Ari, E., Herceg, N., & Siperstein, A. (2005). Laparoscopic radiofrequency thermal ablation for unusual hepatic tumors: operative indications and outcomes. *Surg Endosc*, Dec, 19(12), 1613-7.

[31] Siperstein, A., Garland, A., Engle, K., Rogers, S., Berber, E., String, A., et al. (2000). Laparoscopic radiofrequency ablation of primary and metastatic liver tumors. Technical considerations. *Surg Endosc*, Apr, 14(4), 400-5.

[32] Salmi, A., & Metelli, F. (2003). Laparoscopic ultrasound-guided radiofrequency thermal ablation of hepatic tumors: a new coaxial approach. *Endoscopy*, Sep, 35(9), 802.

[33] Bao, P., Sinha, T. K., Chen, C. C., Warmath, J. R., Galloway, R. L., & Herline, A. J. (2007). A prototype ultrasound-guided laparoscopic radiofrequency ablation system. *Surg Endosc*, Jan, 21(1), 74-9.

[34] String, A., Berber, E., Foroutani, A., Matcho, J. R., Pearl, J. M., & Siperstein, A. (2001). Use of the optical access trocar for safe and rapid entry in various laparoscopic procedures. *Surg Endosc*, 15, 570-3.

[35] Hozumi, M., Ido, K., Hiki, S., Isoda, N., Nagamine, N., Ono, K., et al. (2003). Easy and accurate targeting of deep-seated hepatic tumors under laparoscopy with a forward-viewing convex-array transducer. *Surg Endosc*, Aug, 17(8), 1256-60.

[36] Inamori, H., Ido, K., Isoda, N., Hozumi, M., Onobuchi, Y., Nagae, G., et al. (2004). Laparoscopic radiofrequency ablation of hepatocellular carcinoma in the caudate

lobe by using a new laparoscopic US probe with a forward-viewing convex-array transducer. *Gastrointest Endosc*, Oct, 60(4), 628-31.

[37] Berber, E., Herceg, N. L., Casto, K. J., & Siperstein, A. E. (2004). Laparoscopic radiofrequency ablation of hepatic tumors: prospective clinical evaluation of ablation size comparing two treatment algorithms. *Surg Endosc*, Mar, 18(3), 390-6.

[38] Zhou, X., Strobel, D., Haensler, J., & Bernatik, T. (2005). Hepatic transit time: indicator of the therapeutic response to radiofrequency ablation of liver tumours. *Br J Radiol*, May, 78(929), 433-6.

[39] Rossi, S., Garbagnati, F., De Accocella, F. I., Leonardi, F., Quaretti, L., et, P., et al. (1999). Relationship between the shape and size of radiofrequency induced thermal lesions and hepatic vascularization. *Tumori*, Mar, 85(2), 128-32.

[40] Scott, D. J., Fleming, J. B., Watumull, L. M., Lindberg, G., Tesfay, S. T., & Jones, D. B. (2002). The effect of hepatic inflow occlusion on laparoscopic radiofrequency ablation using simulated tumors. *Surg Endosc*, Sep, 16(9), 1286-91.

[41] Patterson, E. J., Scudamore, C. H., Owen, D. A., Nagy, A. G., & Buczkowski, A. K. (1998). Radiofrequency ablation of porcine liver in vivo: Effects of blood flow and treatment on lesion size. *Surg Oncol*, 227(4), 559-65.

[42] Chang, C. K., Hendy, M. P., Smith, J. M., Recht, M. H., & Welling, R. E. (2002). Radiofrequency ablation of the porcine liver with complete hepatic vascular occlusion. *Ann Surg Oncol*, Jul, 9(6), 594-8.

[43] Goldberg, S. N., Gazelle, G. S., Compton, C. C., Mueller, P. R., & Tanabe, K. K. (2000). Treatment of intrahepatic malignancy with radiofrequency ablation: radiologic-pathologic correlation. *Cancer*, Jun 1, 88(11), 2452-63.

[44] Shen, P., Fleming, S., Westcott, C., & Challa, V. (2003). Laparoscopic radiofrequency ablation of the liver in proximity to major vasculature: effect of the Pringle maneuver. *J Surg Oncol*, May, 83(1), 36-41.

[45] Denys, A., Doenz, F., Qanadli, S. D., & Chevallier, P. (2005). Radiofrequency tumor ablation: from the liver to the lung passing by the kidney]. *Rev Med Suisse*, Jul 13, 1(27), 1774-8.

[46] Jakimowicz, J., Stultines, G., & Smulders, F. (1998). Laparoscopic insufflation in the abdomen reduces portal venous flow. *Surg Endosc*, 12, 129-32.

[47] Elias, D., Sideris, L., Pocard, M., Dromain, C., & de Baere, T. (2004). Intraductal cooling of the main bile ducts during radiofrequency ablation prevents biliary stenosis. *J Am Coll Surg*, May, 198(5), 717-21.

[48] Chapman, W. C., Debelak, J. P., Wright, P. C., Washington, M. K., Atkinson, J. B., Venkatakrishnan, A., et al. (2000). Hepatic cryoablation, but not radiofrequency ablation, results in lung inflammation. *Ann Surg*, May, 231(5), 752-61.

[49] Berber, E., & Siperstein, A. E. (2007). Perioperative outcome after laparoscopic radiofrequency ablation of liver tumors: an analysis of 521 cases. *Surg Endosc*, Apr, 21(4), 613-8.

[50] Berber, E., Foroutani, A., Garland, A. M., Rogers, S. J., Engle, K. L., Ryan, T. L., et al. (2000). Use of CT Hounsfield unit density to identify ablated tumor after laparoscopic radiofrequency ablation of hepatic tumors. *Surg Endosc*, Sep, 14(9), 799-804.

[51] Dromain, C., de Baere, T., Elias, D., Kuoch, V., Ducreux, M., Boige, V., et al. (2002). Hepatic tumors treated with percutaneous radio-frequency ablation: CT and MR imaging follow up. *Radiology*, 223(1), 255-62.

[52] Mason, T., Berber, E., Graybill, J. C., & Siperstein, A. (2007). Histological, CT, and Intraoperative Ultrasound Appearance of Hepatic Tumors Previously Treated by Laparoscopic Radiofrequency Ablation. *J Gastrointest Surg*, Oct, 11(10), 1333-8.

[53] Santambrogio, R., Opocher, E., Costa, M., Cappellani, A., & Montorsi, M. (2005). Survival and intra-hepatic recurrences after laparoscopic radiofrequency of hepatocellular carcinoma in patients with liver cirrhosis. *J Surg Oncol*, Mar 15, 89(4), 218-25.

[54] Ahmad, A., Chen, S. L., Kavanagh, M. A., Allegra, D. P., & Bilchik, A. J. (2006). Radiofrequency ablation of hepatic metastases from colorectal cancer: are newer generation probes better? *Am Surg*, Oct, 72(10), 875-9.

[55] Mulier, S., Ni, Y., Jamart, J., Ruers, T., Marchal, G., & Michel, L. (2005). Local recurrence after hepatic radiofrequency coagulation: multivariate meta-analysis and review of contributing factors. *Ann Surg*, Aug, 242(2), 158-71.

[56] Amersi, F. F., Mc Elrath-Garza, A., Ahmad, A., Zogakis, T., Allegra, D. P., Krasne, R., et al. (2006). Long-term survival after radiofrequency ablation of complex unresectable liver tumors. *Arch Surg*, Jun, 141(6), 581-7.

[57] Nicoli, N., Casaril, A., Marchiori, L., Mangiante, G., & Hasheminia, A. R. (2001). Treatment of recurrent hepatocellular carcinoma by radiofrequency thermal ablation. *J Hepatobiliary Pancreat Surg*, 8(5), 417-21.

[58] Belli, G., D'Agostino, A., Fantini, C., Cioffi, L., Belli, A., Russolillo, N., et al. (2007). Laparoscopic radiofrequency ablation combined with laparoscopic liver resection for more than one HCC on cirrhosis. *Surg Laparosc Endosc Percutan Tech*, Aug, 17(4), 331-4.

[59] Elias, D., Goharin, A., El Otmany, A., Taieb, J., Duvillard, P., Lasser, P., et al. (2000). Usefulness of intraoperative radiofrequency thermoablation of liver tumours associated or not with hepatectomy. *Eur J Surg Oncol*, Dec, 26(8), 763-9.

[60] Santambrogio, R., Podda, M., Zuin, M., Bertolini, E., Bruno, S., Cornalba, G. P., et al. (2003). Safety and efficacy of laparoscopic radiofrequency ablation of hepatocellular carcinoma in patients with liver cirrhosis. *Surg Endosc*, Nov, 17(11), 1826-32.

[61] Bilchik, A. J., Rose, D. M., Allegra, D. P., Bostick, P. J., Hsueh, E., & Morton, D. L. (1999). Radiofrequency ablation: a minimally invasive technique with multiple applications. *Cancer J Sci Am*, Nov, 5(6), 356-61.

[62] Cheng, J., Glasgow, R. E., O'Rourke, R. W., Swanstrom, L. L., & Hansen, P. D. (2003). Laparoscopic radiofrequency ablation and hepatic artery infusion pump placement in the evolving treatment of colorectal hepatic metastases. *Surg Endosc*, Jan, 17(1), 61-7.

[63] Berber, E., Senagore, A., Remzi, F., Rogers, S., Herceg, N., Casto, K., et al. (2004). Laparoscopic radiofrequency ablation of liver tumors combined with colorectal procedures. *Surg Laparosc Endosc Percutan Tech*, Aug, 14(4), 186-90.

Chapter 21

Surgical Management in Portal Hypertension

Hiroshi Yoshida, Yasuhiro Mamada,
Nobuhiko Taniai, Takashi Tajiri and Eiji Uchida

Additional information is available at the end of the chapter

http://dx.doi.org/10.5772/52899

1. Introduction

Bleeding from esophagogastricvarices is a catastrophic complication of chronic liver disease. There are various treatments for esophagogastricvarices, such as endoscopic treatment, interventional radioligy, and surgical procedure [1-3]. Recently, "General Rules for Recording Endoscopic Findings of EsophagogastricVarices [4]" were establised and endoscopic treatment further improved survival rates [5].

Many years ago, operation was the only treatment available. A number of surgical procedures have been developed to manage esophagogastricvarices [6]. Broadly, these can be classified as shunting and nonshunting procedures.

We showed the surgical procedures for the treatment of esophagogastricvarices.

2. Operation technique

2.1. Shunting procedures

There are various shunting procedures for the treatment of esophagogastricvarices [7-25]. There are two types of shunting procedures, nonselective shunt and selective shunt. Nonselective shunts, such as portacaval or mesocaval shunts, reduce portal venous pressure and improve esophagogastricvarices. While nonselective shunt is associated with a high risk of hepatic encephalopathy secondary to the hyperammonemia that is caused by impaired protein metabolism in the liver [26-28].

Selective shunts, such as distal splenorenal shunt (DSRS) or left gastric venous caval shunt (Inokuchi shunt), maintain portal pressure and selectively reduce esophagogastricvariceal pressure. Shunt surgery is the best procedure in terms of preventing recurrent bleeding [20-22], but carries a high risk of postoperative encephalopathy, especially after nonselective shunt [26-28]. Even in selective shunt, loss of shunt selectivity occurs occasionally, leading to postoperative encephalopathy [8, 14].

2.1.1. Nonselective shunt

2.1.1.1. Portacaval and mesocaval shunt

The mesocaval shunt was initially used to control bleeding from esophageal varices in children with congenital abnormalities of the hepatobiliary system. The procedure consisted of transposition of the divided inferior vena cava and the divided superior mesenteric vein, hence its name, mesocaval shunt. This operation was modified, and some reports have described a portacaval or mesocaval interposition shunt with a graft (H-graft mesocaval shunt) [9, 10, 29-33]. Millikan et al. [26] have reported that the incidence of hyperammonemia after nonselective shunt procedures was as high as 75%.

2.1.2. Selective shunt

2.1.2.1. Left gastric venous caval shunt (Inokuchi shunt)

To assure postoperative portal perfusion and to prevent Eck's syndrome, in 1967 Inokuchi designed a selective shunt, called the left gastric venous caval shunt [7, 19, 23-25].

After dilatation, and engorgement of the left gastric vein is confirmed by splenoportography, the gastrohepatic ligament is opened and the left gastric vein is identified, and dissected 2 cm towards its junction with the portal system or splenic vein. The vein dissection must be done carefully to avoid hemorrhage, since the wall of the left gastric vein is weak due to increased portal vein pressure. The anastomosis is then performed between the distal end of the transected left gastric vein and the inferior vena cava. The autograft, the great saphenous vein, is anastomosed to the inferior vena cava in an end-to-side fashion, and opposite end is pulled through the suprapancreatic space. After the anastomosis is completed, a splenectomysi done. If splenectomy is not indicated, short gastric vein ligation is necessary in order to decrease the collateral circulation from the greater curvature of the stomach. The selection of a caval anastomosis procedure depends upon anatomical individuality or operative difficulty or both. The left gastric venous-caval shunt can be modified in three ways, left gastric-spermatic (ovarian) shunt, left gastric-adrenal shunt, or left gastric-renal shunt.

Postoperative mean portal pressure was 335 mm of water, and although it is decreased whe compared to 363 mm water at laparotomy, this may be the result of solenectomy. On the other hand, left gastric venous pressure decreased from 316 mm of water to 211 mm of water postoperatively [7].

2.1.2.2. DSRS

Original DSRS: The DSRS is a selective shunt that was developed by Warren (original DSRS) in 1967 [12] to preserve portal blood flow through the liver while lowering variceal pressure. The hope was that both bleeding and hyperammonemia would be prevented. DSRS effectively prevents rebleeding, but still carries a risk of hyperammonemia [14].

The procedure for DSRS consists of anastomosis of the distal end of the splenic vein to the left renal vein, and devascularization of left gastric artery and vein. The specific objectives of DSRS as stated in the original publication [12] were : 1) selective reduction of pressure and volume of flow through gastroesophageal veins; 2) maintaining portal venous perfusion of the liver; and 3) maintaining continual venous hypertension in the intestinal bed. These three objectives formed a basis for much subsequent work.

Henderson et al. [34]compared hemodynamics between alcoholic and nonalcoholic cirrhotic patients after DSRS. Portal perfusion and liver blood flow are maintained, both quantitatively and qualitatively, in nonalcoholic patients with cirrhosis, resulting in better hepatocyte function and improved survival.

Stenosis of a DSRS shunt may lead to inadequate variceal decompression, accompanied by a risk of rebleeding. Henderson et al. [35]reported that the patients with stenosis of a DSRS were successfully managed by balloon dilation. All of the shunts were patent, but showed a mean pressure gradient of 15 millimeters of mercury, which was reduced to a mean of 7 millimeters of mercury by dilation. Although, repeat angiography should be performed in patients with rebleeding or reappearance of varices after DSRS to determine the cause.

DSRS + splenopancreatic disconnection (SPD): Belghiti et al. [8] reported loss of shunt selectivity during long-term follow-up in patients who underwent original DSRS, confirmed via the pancreatic vein. Warren et al. [36] subsequently improved the DSRS procedure by adding SPD, i.e., skeletonization of the splenic vein from the pancreas to its bifurcation at the splenic hilum. The operation technique is as follows: The pancreas is approached through the lesser sac, with the additional takedown of the splenic flexure to improve access to the retropancreatic plane. The whole pancreas is mobilized along its inferior border from the superior mesenteric vein to the splenic hilus. The pancreatic perforating veins are ligated as they enter the splenic vein. It is imperative to sufficiently dissect the splenic vein from the pancreas and to carefully manipulate the junction between the splenic and superior mesenteric vein to ensure that skeletonization proceeds to the renal vein without kinking. The key to the entire procedure lies in accurate identification and ligation of the pancreatic perforating veins as they enter the splenic vein. The anastomosis should also be performed without tension or kinking of the splenic vein. Typically, the anastomosis lies just in front of the ligated adrenal vein on the left renal vein with continuous suture.

Moon et al. [37] examined the outcomes of DSRS+SPD in children to evaluate the usefulness of this operation. The platelet count and white cell count increased significantly after DSRS +SPD. Spleen size decreased significantly. No patient underwent subsequent transplantation or endoscopic treatment for esophagogastricvarices after DSRS+SPD.

DSRS + SPD + gastric transection (GT): Loss of shunt selectivity was still observed via collateral pathways through the stomach [20]. We therefore modified DSRS by additionally performing SPD and GT to prevent loss of shunt selectivity. GT involved transection and anastomosis of the upper stomach with an autosuture instrument. The short gastric arteries and veins were spared. Katoh et al. [38] performed transection and re-suture of the seromuscular layer of the upper stomach to prevent loss of selectivity after DSRS + SPD. They called this procedure "superselective DSRS." We performed transection of all layers, whereas Katoh et al. transected only the seromuscular layer of the upper stomach.

We compared long-term results for three types of DSRS for the treatment of esophageal varices. Additional treatment for recurrent varices was required in the original DSRS group (9.1%), DSRS with SPD group (18.2%), and DSRS with SPD plus GT group (4.3%). All of the patients with recurrent varices had shunt stenosis within the first year after DSRS. The prevalence of hyperammonemia in the DSRS with SPD plus GT group was significantly lower than that in the original DSRS group and the DSRS with SPD group ($P<0.01$). There were no significant differences in survival among the three groups. DSRS with SPD plus GT may reduce the incidence of postoperative hyperammonemia [14]. Kanaya et al. [39] have reported that the incidence of hyperammonemia after DSRS with SPD plus gastric disconnection (transection of only the seromuscular layer of the upper stomach) was 3.2%. We found that the prevalence of hyperammonemia after DSRS with SPD plus GT was 0% at 1 year, 9.1% at 5 years, and 9.1% at 10 years [14]. The loss of shunt selectivity promotes hyperammonemia and decreases portal blood flow. High serum ammonia concentrations result in encephalopathy. We previously reported that obliteration of portosystemic shunts followed by partial splenic embolization is beneficial in patients with portosystemic encephalopathy. Portal venous pressures were similar before and after treatment in patients who underwent embolization of portosystemic shunts followed by partial splenic embolization [40, 41]. In patients who had portosystemic encephalopathy after DSRS, however, elevated portal venous pressures after embolization of portosystemic shunts can notreduced by partial splenic embolization. Fisher et al. [42] have reported normalization of hyperammonemia after administration of a solution enriched with branched chain amino acids. All patients with hyperammonemia in our study should received branched chain amino acids [14]. However, patients with hyperammonemia require long-term nutritional support, negatively affecting their quality of life. Liver dysfunction was controlled with good nutritional support. We found no significant differences in cumulative survival among the original DSRS group, DSRS with SPD group, and DSRS with SPD plus GT group [14]. Kanaya et al. [39] have reported better 5- and 7-year survival rates after DSRS with SPD plus gastric disconnection than after standard DSRS.

Santambrogio et al. [43] compared endoscopic injection sclerotherapy (EIS) with DSRS for the prevention of recurrent variceal bleeding in cirrhotic patients who underwent long-term follow-up. They concluded that DSRS with a correct portal-azygos disconnection more effectively prevents varicealrebleeding than EIS in a subgroup of patients with good liver function. However, this positive effect did not influence long-term survival because other factors (e.g., hepatocellular carcinoma) were more important determinants of the outcomes of the cirrhotic patients with portal hypertension.

Rikkers et al. (13)performed a prospective, randomized trial to evaluate the effectiveness of DSRS for the treatment of cirrhotic patients who previously had bleeding from esophageal varices. A total of 55 patients were randomly assined to receive a DSRS (26 patients) or a nonselective shunt (29 patients). Three operative deaths occurred in each group. Early post-operative angiography revealed preservation of hepatic portal perfusion in 14 of 16 selective patients (88%), but in only 1 of 20 nonselective patients ($p<0.001$). Quantitative measures of hepatic function (maximal rate of urea synthesis and Child's score) were similar to preoperative values in the selective shunt, but had significantly decreased in the nonselective shunt on the first postoperative evaluation. Encephalopathy has not developed in any patient with continued portal perfusion, as compared with 45% of patients without portal flow ($p<0.05$). No significant differences the between selective and nonselective shunt have been detected with respect to total cumulative mortality (10 selective, 38%; 8 nonselective, 28%), shunt occlusion (2 selective, 10%; 5 nonselective, 18%), or recurrent variceal hemorrhage (1 selective, 4%; 2 nonselective, 8%). Overall, postoperative encephalopathy has developed in significantly fewer selective patients (3 selective, 12%; 15 nonselective, 52%; $p<0.001$). Therefore, they conclude that the DSRS, especially when its objective of maintaining hepatic portal perfusion is achieved, results in significantly less morbidity than nonselective shunt.

Warren et al. (44) reported the metabolic basis of portosystemic encephalopathy and compared the effects of selective vs. nonselective shunts. Metabolic studies were done in the Clinical Research Unit during a 14-day stay under carefully controlled dietary conditions. Maximal rate of urea systhesis did not change in patients with DSRS, but decreased significantly in those with nonselective shunt. Likewise, ammonium chloride tolerance, defined as the smallest dose required to produce a 40-µg/dL rise in the plasma ammonia concentration, was unchanged in the DSRS group, but significantly worsened in the nonselective shunt group.

Galambos et al. [45]compared nonselective shunt with selective shunt for the treatment of bleeding esophageal varices in a randomized controlled trial. A total of 48 patients were randomly assigned to receive a nonselective shunt (24 patients) or a selective shunt (24 patients). Mortality rates, the frequencies of shunt occlusion, and the frequencies of recurrent gastrointestinal bleeding were similar. Encephalopathy developed more often after a nonselective shunt than after a selective shunt. Nonselective shunts consistently diverted the hepatopetal mesenteric-portal flow from the liver. Deterioration of hepatic function was greater after nonselective than selective shunt.

2.2. Nonshunting procedures

Historically, nonshunting procedures were developed in an attempt to decrease the high rates of encephalopathy associated with portosystemic anastomoses. An alternative to total shunt was developed by Sugiura and Futagawa in 1973 [46]. Esophageal transection (ET) disrupts the blood supply to esophagogastricvarices. ET solves the problem of hepatic encephalopathy; unfortunately, however, varices can recur because portal pressure remains high.

Various nonshunting procedures, such as the Hassab operation, ET, splenectomy, or terminal esophago-proximal gastrectomy, have been developed to treat esophagogastricvarices

[46-49]. All nonshunting procedures performesplenectomy. Portal vein thrombosis is not a rare complication of splenectomy and can be fatal in patients with hypersplenism. Kawanaka et al. reported that low antithrombin 3 activity and futher decreases in this activity are associated with portal vein thrombosis after splenectomy in cirrhotic patients, and that treatment with antithrombin 3 concentrates is likely to prevent the development of portal vein thrombosis in thease patients [50].

2.2.1. Splenectomy

Splenectomy was one of the earliest nonshunting procedures. It was found to be generally ineffective for preventing recurrent variceal bleeding [51]. Despite elimination of the splenic component of the portal circulation, portal hypertension is maintained after simple splenectomy, and the risk of continued bleeding via the splenic venous branches is high.

Recently, laparosopicsplenectomy is wadely accepted as a standard treatment for hematologic disorders such as idiopathic thrombocytopenic purpura. Laparoscopic splenectomy is improved safty in liver cirrhosis patients with portal hypertension [52].

2.2.2. Hassab operation

In 1967, Hassab [47] reported a successful technique for gastroesophageal decongestion and splenectomy, developed in Egypt. Most of his patients had schistosomiasis. The operation entailed removal of the spleen as well as devascularization of the cardiac portion of the stomach and abdominal portion of the esophagus, including the supraphrenic veins. By ligating the left gastric artery and splenic artery, portal blood flow was also decreased, thereby decompressing the portal system. Recently, the Hassab operation has been employed in patients with varices limited to the stomach.

2.2.3. Terminal esophago-proximal gastrectomy

Terminal esophago-proximal gastrectomy involves proximal gastric transection and autosuture proximal gastrectomy in association with extensive devascularization and splenectomy [49].

2.2.4. ET

Among non-shunting procedures for the treatment of esophagogastricvarices, ET has been the most popular operation. ET in Japan was first performed in 1967 [53], using a modification of Walker's procedure for transthoracic ET [54]. The procedure was then refined by Sugiura and Futagawa in 1973 [46]. ET consists of paraesophagealdevascularization, esophageal transection and reanastomosis, splenectomy, and pyloroplasty. First, splenectomy with devascularization of the greater curvature was performed. Devascularization of the lesser curvature was done from the angle to the esophagogastric junction, and the left gastric artery was ligated and divided. The esophagus and cardia were devascularized from the lesser to the greater curvature. Then, the vagal nerve and paraesophageal vessels were ligated and divided. The esophagus was completely transected above the esophagogastric junction, and the mucosa was anastomosed with interrupted sutures, performed recently with an autosuture instrument. ET was done using three different approaches, transthoracic, thoracoabdominal, and transabdominal. Devascularization of the esophagus and the stomach is most extensive and complete in the thoracoabdominal approach; however, this is the most drastic procedure.

Sugiura et al. [55] reported on 636 patients with portal hypertension in whom ETs with paraesophagogastricdevascularization were performed to manage esophageal varices. The operative mortality rates were as follows: emergency cases 13.7%, elective cases 3.2%, prophylactic cases 4.3%, and overall 5.2%. There were no deaths among the 233 patients in Child's class A; the 232 patients in class B had a 2% mortality rate, and the 171 patients in class C had a 17% mortality rate. The 10-year actuarial survival rates in patients with cirrhosis were 55% in emergency cases, 72% in prophylactic cases, and 72% in elective cases. In patients without cirrhosis, the corresponding survival rates were 90%, 96%, and 95%, respectively. The recurrence rate of variceal bleeding or varices was less than 5%. They concluded that the Sugiura procedure is safe and effective for controlling esophageal varices and prolongs the long-term survival of patients with portal hypertension.

In our study, however, the recurrence rate of varices after ET was high [21]. We examined hemodynamic changes associated with recurrent esophageal varices after ET and evaluated the effectiveness of EIS for their treatment. Nineteen patients with recurrent esophageal varices after ET were treated by EIS. Endoscopic varicealography during injection sclerotherapy (EVIS), following oral blockage of flow by a balloon, identified three patterns: type 1 (common type), continuous filling by the feeder vessel of the varix; type 2 (retrograde disappearing type), confirmed hepatofugal flow; and type 3 (immediate washout type), immediate washout of contrast medium. Angiography showed that the hepatofugal feeder vessel was the right gastric vein in all cases. Recurrent esophageal varices were classified as type 1 in 14 patients (73.7%), type 2 in 4 (21.1%), and type 3 in 1 (5.3%). Fewer treatment sessions were required in type 1 than in type 2 varices ($p<0.005$). Recurrent varices were completely eradicated in all patients except the patient with type 3 disease. Cumulative re-recurrence rates at 5 and 10 years were higher in type 1 than in type 2 varices without significance (28.6% and 71.4% vs. 25.0% and 25.0%, respectively). Cumulative survival rates after EIS at 5 and 10 years also were similar for type 1 and type 2 varices (77.1% and 66.1% vs. 66.7% and 66.7%). EIS was thus effective for the management of recurrent esophageal varices after ET, excluding type 3 disease [56].

Cleva et al. [57] compared the systemic hemodynamic effects of DSRS with those of esophagogastricdevascularization and splenectomy in patients treated for schistosomal portal hypertension. The hyperdynamic circulatory state observed in Manson's schistosomiasis was corrected by esophagogastricdevascularization and splenectomy, but persisted in patients who underwent DSRS. Similarly, the elevated mean pulmonary artery pressure resolved after esophagogastricdevascularization and splenectomy, but persisted after DSRS. They concluded that esophagogastricdevascularization and splenectomy seems to be the most physiologic operation for patients with schistosomal portal hypertension.

We compared the long-term results of DSRS and ET in cirrhotic patients with complete variceal eradication who were followed up for at least 3 years. There was no recurrent varix in the DSRS group. The cumulative recurrence rates of varices in the ET group were 31.6% and

52.5% at 5 and 10 years, respectively. The cumulative rates of hyperammonemia at 5 and 10 years were significantly higher in the DSRS group (30.4%, 30.4%) than in the ET group (0%, 5.6%) (p=0.009). The cumulative survival rates in the DSRS group vs. the ET group were 90.9% vs. 94.7% at 5 years and 85.2% vs. 81.7% at 10 years (NS). These results suggest that DSRS is more effective than ET in preventing recurrence of esophageal varices, but is associated with a higher incidence of hyperammonemia [21]. In that study, no patient who underwent DSRS with complete eradication had recurrent varices. When collateral pathways to the esophagus develop after DSRS, flow is via the short gastric veins, the splenic vein, and the left renal vein. After ET, collateral pathways to the esophagus develop across the transection site and generate new varices. Most of the recurrent varices in the ET group were supplied by the right gastric vein across the transection site [56]. However, collateral flow in the DSRS group decreased hepatic blood flow and led to the development of postoperative hyperammonemia. Rikkers et al. [58] reported that patients with no hepatic portal perfusion had the worst survival and greatest morbidity after DSRS.

Idiopathic portal hypertension (IPH) is a disease of unknown etiology characterized by splenomegaly, anemia, and portal hypertension. This disorder develops in the absence of liver cirrhosis, extrahepatic portal vein occlusion, schistosomiasis, or any other identifiable cause [59, 60]. We evaluated the results of shunting and nonshunting procedures for the treatment of esophagogastricvarices in patients with IPH. Esophagogastricvarices were completely eradicated in 3 (75.0%) patients in the shunting group and 4 (80.0%) in the nonshunting group. Additional endoscopic treatment (one session) was performed in 2 patients with incompletely eradicated varices. There was no recurrence in the shunting group. In the nonshunting group, esophagogastricvarices recurred in all 4 patients with completely eradicated varices. All recurrent esophageal varices were completely eradicated. Postoperative platelet counts ($\times 10^4/\mu L$) were significantly lower in the shunting group (10.0±2.6) than in the nonshunting group (42.0±14.0) (p=0.0029). The increase in the platelet count after operation was significantly lower in the shunting group (1.7±0.2 times) than in the nonshunting group (5.8±2.9 times) (p=0.0267). No patient received anticoagulants postoperatively. Portal venous thrombus did not develop in the shunting group, but appeared in 4 patients (80.0%) in the nonshunting group. No patient had loss of shunt selectivity or portal-systemic encephalopathy. One patient in the nonshunting group died of cerebral hemorrhage; all others are alive. Shunting procedure, DSRS, was suggested to be useful for the management of esophagogastricvarices in patients with IPH [61].

Author details

Hiroshi Yoshida[1*], Yasuhiro Mamada[2], Nobuhiko Taniai[2], Takashi Tajiri[2] and Eiji Uchida[2]

*Address all correspondence to: hiroshiy@nms.ac.jp

1 Department of Surgery, Nippon Medical School Tama Nagayama Hospital, Japan

2 Department of Surgery, Nippon Medical School, Japan

References

[1] Yoshida H, Mamada Y, Taniai N, Tajiri T. New methods for the management of esophageal varices. World J Gastroenterol. 2007 Mar 21;13(11):1641-5.

[2] Yoshida H, Mamada Y, Taniai N, Tajiri T. New methods for the management of gastric varices. World J Gastroenterol. 2006 Oct 7;12(37):5926-31.

[3] Yoshida H, Mamada Y, Taniai N, Yoshioka M, Hirakata A, Kawano Y, et al. Treatment modalities for bleeding esophagogastricvarices. J Nippon Med Sch. 2012;79(1):19-30.

[4] Tajiri T, Yoshida H, Obara K, Onji M, Kage M, Kitano S, et al. General rules for recording endoscopic findings of esophagogastricvarices (2nd edition). Dig Endosc. 2010 Jan;22(1):1-9.

[5] Yoshida H, Mamada Y, Taniai N, Yamamoto K, Kawano Y, Mizuguchi Y, et al. A randomized control trial of bi-monthly versus bi-weekly endoscopic variceal ligation of esophageal varices. Am J Gastroenterol. 2005 Sep;100(9):2005-9.

[6] Yoshida H, Mamada Y, Taniai N, Tajiri T. New trends in surgical treatment for portal hypertension. Hepatol Res. 2009 Oct;39(10):1044-51.

[7] Inokuchi K, Kobayashi M, Kusaba A, Ogawa Y, Saku M, Shiizaki T. New selective decompression of esophageal varices. By a left gastric venous-caval shunt. Arch Surg. 1970 Feb;100(2):157-62.

[8] Belghiti J, Grenier P, Nouel O, Nahum H, Fekete F. Long-term loss of Warren's shunt selectivity. Angiographic demonstration. Arch Surg. 1981 Sep;116(9):1121-4.

[9] Shields R. Small-diameter PTFE portosystemic shunts: portocavalvsmesocaval. HPB Surg. 1998;10(6):413-4.

[10] Mercado MA, Morales-Linares JC, Granados-Garcia J, Gomez-Mendez TJ, Chan C, Orozco H. Distal splenorenal shunt versus 10-mm low-diameter mesocaval shunt for variceal hemorrhage. Am J Surg. 1996 Jun;171(6):591-5.

[11] Paquet KJ, Lazar A, Koussouris P, Hotzel B, Gad HA, Kuhn R, et al. Mesocaval interposition shunt with small-diameter polytetrafluoroethylene grafts in sclerotherapy failure. Br J Surg. 1995 Feb;82(2):199-203.

[12] Warren WD, Zeppa R, Fomon JJ. Selective trans-splenic decompression of gastroesophagealvarices by distal splenorenal shunt. Ann Surg. 1967 Sep;166(3):437-55.

[13] Rikkers LF, Rudman D, Galambos JT, Fulenwider JT, Millikan WJ, Kutner M, et al. A randomized, controlled trial of the distal splenorenal shunt. Ann Surg. 1978 Sep;188(3):271-82.

[14] Tajiri T, Onda M, Yoshida H, Mamada Y, Taniai N, Umehara M, et al. Long-term results of modified distal splenorenal shunts for the treatment of esophageal varices. Hepatogastroenterology. 2000 May-Jun;47(33):720-3.

[15] Stipa S, Balducci G, Ziparo V, Stipa F, Lucandri G. Total shunting and elective management of variceal bleeding. World J Surg. 1994 Mar-Apr;18(2):200-4.

[16] Klein AS, Fair JH, Cameron JL. Suprarenal mesocaval shunt. SurgGynecol Obstet. 1991 Oct;173(4):319-22.

[17] Sato Y, Hatakeyama K. Left gastric venous caval direct shunt in esophagogastricvarices. Hepatogastroenterology. 2002 Sep-Oct;49(47):1251-2.

[18] Inokuchi K, Beppu K, Koyanagi N, Nagamine K, Hashizume M, Sugimachi K. Exclusion of nonisolated splenic vein in distal splenorenal shunt for prevention of portal malcirculation. Ann Surg. 1984 Dec;200(6):711-7.

[19] Inokuchi K. Selective decompression of esophageal varices by a left gastric venacaval shunt. SurgAnnu. 1978;10:215-36.

[20] Henderson JM, Warren WD, Millikan WJ, Galloway JR, Kawasaki S, Kutner MH. Distal splenorenal shunt with splenopancreatic disconnection. A 4-year assessment. Ann Surg. 1989 Sep;210(3):332-9; discussion 9-41.

[21] Tajiri T, Onda M, Yoshida H, Mamada Y, Taniai N, Yamashita K. Comparison of the long-term results of distal splenorenal shunt and esophageal transection for the treatment of esophageal varices. Hepatogastroenterology. 2000 Nov-Dec;47(36):1619-21.

[22] Rikkers LF. Definitive therapy for variceal bleeding: a personal view. Am J Surg. 1990 Jul;160(1):80-5.

[23] Inokuchi K, Beppu K, Koyanagi N, Nagamine K, Hashizume M, Iwanaga T, et al. Fifteen years' experience with left gastric venous caval shunt for esophageal varices. World J Surg. 1984 Oct;8(5):716-21.

[24] Inokuchi K, Kobayashi M, Ogawa Y, Saku M, Nagasue N. Results of left gastric vena caval shunt for esophageal varices: Analysis of one hundred clinical cases. Surgery. 1975 Nov;78(5):628-36.

[25] Inokuchi K. A selective portacaval shunt. Lancet. 1968 Jul 6;2(7558):51-2.

[26] Millikan WJ, Jr., Warren WD, Henderson JM, Smith RB, 3rd, Salam AA, Galambos JT, et al. The Emory prospective randomized trial: selective versus nonselective shunt to control variceal bleeding. Ten year follow-up. Ann Surg. 1985 Jun;201(6):712-22.

[27] Rikkers LF, Jin G. Variceal hemorrhage: surgical therapy. GastroenterolClin North Am. 1993 Dec;22(4):821-42.

[28] Rikkers LF, Sorrell WT, Jin G. Which portosystemic shunt is best? GastroenterolClin North Am. 1992 Mar;21(1):179-96.

[29] Smith RB, 3rd, Warren WD, Salam AA, Millikan WJ, Ansley JD, Galambos JT, et al. Dacron interposition shunts for portal hypertension. An analysis of morbidity correlates. Ann Surg. 1980 Jul;192(1):9-17.

[30] Sarfeh IJ, Rypins EB. The emergency portacaval H graft in alcoholic cirrhotic patients: influence of shunt diameter on clinical outcome. Am J Surg. 1986 Sep;152(3): 290-3.

[31] Sarfeh IJ, Rypins EB, Fardi M, Conroy RM, Mason GR, Lyons KP. Clinical implications of portal hemodynamics after small-diameter portacaval H graft. Surgery. 1984 Aug;96(2):223-9.

[32] Sarfeh IJ, Rypins EB, Mason GR. A systematic appraisal of portacaval H-graft diameters. Clinical and hemodynamic perspectives. Ann Surg. 1986 Oct;204(4):356-63.

[33] Sarfeh IJ, Rypins EB, Raiszadeh M, Milne N, Conroy RM, Lyons KP. Serial measurement of portal hemodynamics after partial portal decompression. Surgery. 1986 Jul; 100(1):52-8.

[34] Henderson JM, Millikan WJ, Jr., Wright-Bacon L, Kutner MH, Warren WD. Hemodynamic differences between alcoholic and nonalcoholic cirrhotics following distal splenorenal shunt--effect on survival? Ann Surg. 1983 Sep;198(3):325-34.

[35] Henderson JM, El Khishen MA, Millikan WJ, Jr., Sones PJ, Warren WD. Management of stenosis of distal splenorenal shunt by balloon dilation. SurgGynecol Obstet. 1983 Jul;157(1):43-8.

[36] Warren WD, Millikan WJ, Jr., Henderson JM, Abu-Elmagd KM, Galloway JR, Shires GT, 3rd, et al. Splenopancreatic disconnection. Improved selectivity of distal splenorenal shunt. Ann Surg. 1986 Oct;204(4):346-55.

[37] Moon SB, Jung SE, Ha JW, Park KW, Seo JK, Kim WK. The usefulness of distal splenorenal shunt in children with portal hypertension for the treatment of severe thrombocytopenia and leukopenia. World J Surg. 2008 Mar;32(3):483-7.

[38] Katoh H, Shimozawa E, Kojima T, Tanabe T. Modified splenorenal shunt with splenopancreatic disconnection. Surgery. 1989 Nov;106(5):920-4.

[39] Kanaya S, Katoh H. Long-term evaluation of distal splenorenal shunt with splenopancreatic and gastric disconnection. Surgery. 1995 Jul;118(1):29-35.

[40] Yoshida H, Mamada Y, Taniai N, Yamamoto K, Kaneko M, Kawano Y, et al. Long-term results of partial splenic artery embolization as supplemental treatment for portal-systemic encephalopathy. Am J Gastroenterol. 2005 Jan;100(1):43-7.

[41] Yoshida H, Mamada Y, Taniai N, Tajiri T. Partial splenic embolization. Hepatol Res. 2008 Mar;38(3):225-33.

[42] Fischer JE, Rosen HM, Ebeid AM, James JH, Keane JM, Soeters PB. The effect of normalization of plasma amino acids on hepatic encephalopathy in man. Surgery. 1976 Jul;80(1):77-91.

[43] Santambrogio R, Opocher E, Costa M, Bruno S, Ceretti AP, Spina GP. Natural history of a randomized trial comparing distal spleno-renal shunt with endoscopic sclerotherapy in the prevention of varicealrebleeding: a lesson from the past. World J Gastroenterol. 2006 Oct 21;12(39):6331-8.

[44] Warren WD, Rudman D, Millikan W, Galambos JT, Salam AA, Smith RB, 3rd. The metabolic basis of portasystemic encephalopathy and the effect of selective vs nonselective shunts. Ann Surg. 1974 Oct;180(4):573-9.

[45] Galambos JT, Warren WD, Rudman D, Smith RB, 3rd, Salam AA. Selective and total shunts in the treatment of bleeding varices. A randomized controlled trial. N Engl J Med. 1976 Nov 11;295(20):1089-95.

[46] Sugiura M, Futagawa S. A new technique for treating esophageal varices. J Thorac-Cardiovasc Surg. 1973 Nov;66(5):677-85.

[47] Hassab MA. Gastroesophageal decongestion and splenectomy in the treatment of esophageal varices in bilharzial cirrhosis: further studies with a report on 355 operations. Surgery. 1967 Feb;61(2):169-76.

[48] Hassab MA. Gastro-esophageal decongestion and splenectomy GEDS (Hassab), in the management of bleeding varices. Review of literature. Int Surg. 1998 Jan-Mar; 83(1):38-41.

[49] Yamamoto S, Hidemura R, Sawada M, Takeshige K, Iwatsuki S. The late results of terminal esophagoproximalgastrectomy (TEPG) with intensive devascularization and splenectomy for bleeding esophageal varices in cirrhosis. Surgery. 1976 Jul;80(1): 106-14.

[50] Kawanaka H, Akahoshi T, Kinjo N, Konishi K, Yoshida D, Anegawa G, et al. Impact of antithrombin III concentrates on portal vein thrombosis after splenectomy in patients with liver cirrhosis and hypersplenism. Ann Surg. 2010 Jan;251(1):76-83.

[51] Smith GW. Splenectomy and coronary vein ligation for the control of bleeding esophageal varices. Am J Surg. 1970 Feb;119(2):122-31.

[52] Kawanaka H, Akahoshi T, Kinjo N, Konishi K, Yoshida D, Anegawa G, et al. Technical standardization of laparoscopic splenectomy harmonized with hand-assisted laparoscopic surgery for patients with liver cirrhosis and hypersplenism. J HepatobiliaryPancreat Surg. 2009;16(6):749-57.

[53] Idezuki Y, Sugiura M, Sakamoto K, Abe H, Miura T, Hatano S, et al. Rationale for transthoracic esophageal transection for bleeding varices. Dis Chest. 1967 Nov;52(5): 621-31.

[54] Walker RM. Transection operations for portal hypertension. Thorax. 1960 Sep; 15:218-24.

[55] Sugiura M, Futagawa S. Results of six hundred thirty-six esophageal transections with paraesophagogastricdevascularization in the treatment of esophageal varices. J Vasc Surg. 1984 Mar;1(2):254-60.

[56] Yoshida H, Onda M, Tajiri T, Toba M, Umehara M, Mamada Y, et al. Endoscopic injection sclerotherapy for the treatment of reccurent esophageal varices after esophageal transection.. Dig Endosc. [original]. 2002;14:93-8.

[57] de Cleva R, Herman P, D'Albuquerque L A, Pugliese V, Santarem OL, Saad WA. Pre- and postoperative systemic hemodynamic evaluation in patients subjected to esophagogastricdevascularization plus splenectomy and distal splenorenal shunt: a comparative study in schistomomal portal hypertension. World J Gastroenterol. 2007 Nov 7;13(41):5471-5.

[58] Rikkers LF, Cormier RA, Vo NM. Effects of altered portal hemodynamics after distal splenorenal shunts. Am J Surg. 1987 Jan;153(1):80-5.

[59] Boyer JL, Sen Gupta KP, Biswas SK, Pal NC, BasuMallick KC, Iber FL, et al. Idiopathic portal hypertension. Comparison with the portal hypertension of cirrhosis and extrahepatic portal vein obstruction. Ann Intern Med. 1967 Jan;66(1):41-68.

[60] Okuda K, Kono K, Ohnishi K, Kimura K, Omata M, Koen H, et al. Clinical study of eighty-six cases of idiopathic portal hypertension and comparison with cirrhosis with splenomegaly. Gastroenterology. 1984 Apr;86(4):600-10.

[61] Yoshida H, Mamada Y, Taniai N, Mineta S, Kawano Y, Mizuguchi Y, et al. Shunting and nonshunting procedures for the treatment of esophageal varices in patients with idiopathic portal hypertension. Hepatogastroenterology. 2010 Sep-Oct;57(102-103): 1139-44.

Chapter 22

Vasoactive Substances and Inflammatory Factors in Progression of Liver Cirrhosis with Portal Hypertension

Hao Lu, Guoqiang Li, Ling Lu, Ye Fan,
Xiaofeng Qian, Ke Wang and Feng Zhang

Additional information is available at the end of the chapter

http://dx.doi.org/10.5772/52663

1. Introduction

Portal hypertension (PH), a detrimental complication of many diseases, is abnormalities in pre-, intra- or post-hepatic portal venous system. Intrahepatic PH is the most common type, which is mainly cause by liver cirrhosis [1], liver cancer, and sometimes intrahepatic vascular abnormalities [2].

Hepatic venous pressure gradient (HVPG) is the difference between wedged hepatic venous pressure and infra vena cava pressure. PH is defined as an HVPG higher than 5 mmHg [3]. According to absence or presence of complications (splenomegaly and hypersplenism, esophageal varices and ascites), PH can be classified into compensated or decompensated phase. Meanwhile, an HVPG higher than 10 mmHg has been considered as a direct predictor of decompensation and a 10-year-follow-up study showed the significant worse long-term survival when HVPG > 10 mmHg [4-6].

In cirrhotic PH, increased intrahepatic vascular resistance (IHVR) is the primary factor [7, 8] and subsequently increased portal vein inflow (PVI) worsens the situation of PH patients. This review will focus on the physiopathological changes happened in PH.

2. Correlation between vasoactive substances and IHVR/PVI

2.1. Nitric oxide

Nitric oxide (NO) is a potential vasodilator, produced by NO synthase (NOS). In a rat PH model induced by Thioacetamide, contraction of hepatic stellate cells, which resulting the increase of intrahepatic vascular tone, was inhibited by incubated with nitroflurbiprofen *in vitro*, a nitric oxide-releasing cyclooxygenase inhibitor in a dose-dependent manner. In wild-type BDL mice, expression of NOS, especially eNOS was down-regulated [9]. Moreover, the significantly elevated total intrahepatic resistance was reduced significantly *in vivo* by the drug, indicating a potential role of NO on portal pressure [10]. In another rat PH model induced by bile-duct-ligation, intrahepatic vascular resistance increased significantly. Besides, relative level of phos-NOS decreased compared with sham group, leading to an inhibition of intrahepatic NO, although the relative mRNA level was increased [11]. Intrahepatic NO production is largely mediated by endothelial NO synthase (eNOS) and impaired when cirrhosis and secondary endothelial dysfunction existed, leading to the increase of intrahepatic vascular resistance. But the inhibition of NO might be the result of up-regulation of caveolin-1, a down-regulator of eNOS [12].

Contrastingly, extrahepatic NO is increased in PH patients. A clinical trial has shown that serum nitrate level was positively correlated with clinical presentation, (e.g. pulse rate, jaundice, hepatic encephalopathy, lower limb edema) and esophageal varices [13]. It is well established that NO results in dilation of splanchnic and systemic circulation as a powerful vasodilator and blood level of NO is increased as PH progresses [14-16]. Administration of CCl4 to eNOS(-/-) mice also led to an elevated NO production, which is eNOS independent [17]. Another study suggested that iNOS might be involved [18].

2.2. Carbon monoxide

Carbon monoxide (CO), a vasodilator producing by heme oxygenases (HOs) from heme [19], changes as HO-1 expression altered in PH patients [20, 21], which shares the same characters with NO [12]. Expression of intrahepatic HO-1 and -2 decreased in cirrhotic rats than that in normal ones. In situ perfusion with CO-releasing molecule-2, which leads to relaxation of hepatic stellate cells, and HO-1 inducer hemin could attenuated increased IHVR. ZnPP caused a higher IHVR attributing to inhibition of intrahepatic HO-1 in cirrhotic liver[22].

But things are different in splanchnic and systemic circulation. Reportedly, portal vein pressure (PVP) was significantly higher in bile-duct-ligated rats than that in sham group. Meanwhile, mRNA and protein level of HO-1 was also elevated significantly in lung [23].A clinical study has shown an activated HO/CO system in cirrhotic patients while the HO-1 activity and plasma level of CO were related with the severity of PH [20]. Arterial blood gas analysis showed an increase of COHb in bile-duct-ligated rats which could be reversed by ZnPP [23]. HO-1 could promote expression of VEGF and thereafter lead to formation of collateral vessels and higher splanchnic circulation [24].

2.3. Endothelin

Endothelin-1 (ET-1) is the most powerful vasoconstrictor in ETs family [25], which is primarily synthesized and acts in liver mainly in a paracrine fashion via ET A receptor causing vessel constriction [26]. In liver cirrhotic rats induced by carbon tetrachloride, both plasma

ET-1 level and PVP elevated dramatically while the mean hepatic tissue portal inflow reduced. And, perfusion with an antagonist of ET A receptor led to a reduction of plasma ET-1 level and PVP but did not improve the hepatic infusion suggesting that ET-1 was involved in development of PH [26]. It is consistent with a previous study which had demonstrated that liver blood inflow fluctuated in ET A and B receptors antagonist infusion groups and control group [27]. ET A and B receptors play different roles in CCl4-induced portal hypertensive rats. Antagonism of ET A or B receptor led to a reduced or increased of PVP and sinusoidal area in the cirrhotic rats respectively [28]. However, activation of ET B receptor leads to production of other vasoactive molecules, e.g. TXA_2 [29]. Besides, antagonism of ET A receptor alone cannot improve splanchnic circulation indicating ET B receptor plays a role on regulation in PH [30].

2.4. RAAS

It is well established that renin -angiotensin II (Ang II) -aldosterone -system (RAAS) plays an important role on body circulation. Ang II promotes proliferation and contraction of HSC and formation of collagen, leading to liver fibrosis [31]. In hepatorenal syndrome, a severe complication of cirrhotic portal hypertension with hyperdynamic circulation, systemic resistance, circulatory renin activity and plasma aldosterone were significantly increased [32]. Besides, angiotensin converting enzyme (ACE) and Ang II elevated in liver cirrhosis [33, 34]. Role of RAAS on portal pressure provides a new therapeutic alternative [35]. Animal model studies and clinical trials have shown that blockade of Ang II type 1 receptor (AT1R) significantly reduced portal perfusion pressure and HVPG [36-39]. ACE inhibitor also effects to reduce portal pressure in cirrhotic patients [40]. Inhibition of RAAS by losartan could also lead to a reduction of eNOS and ROS level in BDL rats [41].

2.5. Catecholamines

Catecholamines (CA) cause general physiological changes including increases in heart rate, blood pressure, blood glucose levels, and a general reaction of the sympathetic nervous system. In BDL cirrhotic rats, noradrenaline correlated with perfusion pressure dose-dependently, and this constrictive effect might be normalized by phentolamine but not propranolol, indicating that noradrenaline influences PVP through α-receptor on portal-systemic collaterals [42]. In short-term PH induced by partial portal vein ligation (PVL), antagonism of phentolamine on α-receptor was reduced; meanwhile, release of noradrenaline was down-regulated as NO up-regulated, indicating a potential role of CA, together with NO, on hyperhemodynamics and increased PVI [43]. Besides, expressions of tyrosine hydroxylase and dopamine β-hydroxylase were down-regulated in superior mesenteric artery revealing genetic regulation of adrenergic neurotransmitter system participating in the splanchnic vasodilation in PH [44]. Nevertheless, protein level of α-receptor was higher in cirrhotic livers than in normal livers; activation of these α-receptors located on HSC induced calcium spikes and HSC constriction through MAPK, NK-κB and AP-1 pathways, resulting in increased intrahepatic resistance [45]. When response to β-blockers was defined as a reduction $> 10\%$ in HVPG from baseline, the proportion of non-responsers decreased, the rate of first-bleeding among them increased and the diagnostic acuracy improved significantly contrasting with a 20% cut-off value.[46] Also, acute responsers to β-blockers have a better long-term outcome.[47]

2.6. Cannabinoid

Correlation between Cannabinoid and portal hypertension was paid attention in the last decades. Administration of anandamide, an endogenous cannabinoid, resulted in a drop of systemic circulation, mainly mean arterial pressure, although venous pressure changes verified, because of its effect on heart rate. Contrastingly, PVI and PVP increased in a dose-dependent fashion [48]. Treatment with antagonist of cannabinoid CB1 receptor in rats might lead to an elevation of blood pressure and a reduction of PVI and PVP, indicating cannabinoid is responsible for the dilation of systemic circulation [49]. It is in agreement with human. In cirrhotic patients, plasma level of cannabinoid was increased regardless of well-compensated or not [50]. But things are different in liver. Expression of CB1 receptor was dramatically down-regulated in both wild-type and eNOS knock-out group mice [9]. However, more researches are needed.

2.7. Cyclooxygenase, prostanoids and TXA_2

Activation of COX-2/prostanoid pathway promotes production of TXA_2 and PGE_2 [51]. In BDL rats, TXB_2, a stable metabolic of TXA_2 in isolated liver perfusate and PVP were increased in a time-dependent manner. Both inhibition of Kuffer cells and COX attenuate these changes. Further results indicated that COX-2 interact with Kuffer cells-derived TXA_2 was involved and its expression increased significantly [52]. Another group reported that COX-1 and PGI2 were responsible for decreased splanchnic resistance and increased PVI [53, 54]. However, elevated PVP of intrahepatic or pre-hepatic hypertension rats might be reduced by short- or long-term administration of COX inhibitor [18]. It is consistent with Graupera M et. al. [55]. In BDL portal hypertensive rats, elevated ET-1 interacted with Kuffer cells, increasing the responsiveness of p38MAPK through ET B receptor, activating $cPLA_2$ and promoting production of TXA_2, contributing to progression of portal hypertension [29].

2.8. Reactive oxygen species

Reactive oxygen species (ROS) is involved in many pathologic processes. In the case of PH, ROS level increases when circulatory NO decreases [56]. Administration of tempol, a type of superoxide dismutase, normalizes these changes with statistical significance in endothelial cells and cirrhotic liver, reduces intrahepatic vessel resistance and consequently increases PVI [57]. ROS also takes part in oxidative stress [58], lipid peroxidation, apoptosis and dysfunction of endothelial cells [41]. Reportedly, carvedilol, a β-blocker might ameliorate oxidative stress as well as inflammation and fibrosis in a CCl4-induced liver damage model, by reducing depletion of antioxidant enzyme, formation of collagen, and activation of NF-κB pathway, indicating a relationship between ROS and liver damage and fibrosis [59].

http://dx.doi.org/10.5772/52663

3. Cytokines and liver fibrosis

Cytokine is a group of soluble protein or polypeptide, regulating immunologic response and hematopoiesis, participating inflammatory damage and repair. It consists of interleukins (IL), interferons (IFN), tumor necrosis factors (TNF), colony stimulating factors (CSF), chemokines, and growth factors. It has been reported that serum levels IL-6, TNF-α [60, 61], and IL-1β [62] were elevated in hepatoportal sclerosis, and plasma IL-6 level was correlated with the deterioration of liver function [63]. Although IL-6 was increased, expression of IL-6 receptor in cirrhotic liver was decreased, leading to a reduction of hepatocyte response to IL-6, accompanied by an increase of gp130, indicating gp130 might be the potential negative regulator of liver IL-6 signal pathway [64]. In chronic patients with hepatitis C and/or schistosomal, plasma IL-4 level, as well as ROS, was increased and correlated with portal vein diameter, suggesting IL-4 might plays a role on PVI [65]. A clinical trial has shown that administration of probiotic led to a trend to reduction of plasma endotoxin, a mild but significant increase of TNF-α and a significant reduction of aldosterone [66]. Besides, increased PVP induced a up-regulation of α-smooth muscle actin and collagen ◎ and ethanol exposure enhanced expression of TGF-β and production of extracellular matrix via ERK1/2-JNK and p38MAPK pathway respectively, leading to fibrosis of liver [67]. Reportedly, IL-18 gene knock-out mice fed with methionine-choline-deficient diet (MCDD) showed significant exacerbated inflammation, revealing IL-18 was a negative regulator of non-alcoholic fatty liver disease and non-alcoholic steatohepatitis. Tnf mRNA, but not il-6 or il-1b levelm was higher in db/db (Asc-/-) group than db/db (wt) group, indicating TNF-α expression drove the progression of non-alcoholic steatohepatitis [68]. In another type of liver cirrhosis caused by chronic infection of schistosomiasis, inflammation and following tissue repair led to obstruction of intrahepatic vessels and increased intrahepatic resistance. These defenses in liver was mediated by IL-10. But surprisingly, blockade of IL-10R resulted in an elevation of PH and a reduction of parasitic antigen specific B cells, but worsened pulmonary accumulation of eggs without an increase of PVP [69]. Co-infection of bacteria led to production of IL-17 [70]. Consistently, knock-out of IL-10, IL-12p40, and IL-13Rα2 contributed to a progressive and lethal liver fibrosis, showing the anti-fibrosis effects of these Th2-derived interleukins in schistosomiasis mansoni treated mice [71]. As demonstrated by Pinter M et. Al. [72], responders to sorafenib showed a decreased HVPG and VEGF, PDGF, PIGF, RhoA kinase, and TNF-α expression, revealed a potential effect of these growth factors and TNF-α on HVPG. And level of soluble TNF-α receptor in portal vein and hepatic vein was correlated with model for end-stage liver disease score, in accordance with previous studies [73]. However, intrahepatic TNF-α, IL-1β, IL-4, and IL-10 were down-regulated while splanchnic levels were increased [74]. It is shown that IFN is involved in progression of hypertension, especially in viral infection- associated hepatitis [60, 75, 76]. Nowadays, IFN is usually used as antiviral treatment. Combination of 5-fluorouracil and IFN might reduce the portal hypertension related events [77]. Also, combination with IFN enhanced the viral clearance effect of ribavirin [78]. But IFN alone therapy only led to a temporary reduction of viral DNA load [79]. As documented, TGF-β promotes liver fibrosis in rats with biliary cirrhosis, cooperates with IFN-γ, IL-4, and TNF-α, etc [80]. More studies are needed to illustrate the detail effects of cytokines network on portal hypertension and liver fibrosis.

4. Molecules in further physiopathological progression

4.1. Splenomegaly and hypersplenism

Volume of spleen or splenomegaly in cirrhotic hypertension patients is primarily attributed to increased splanchnic circulation and congestion, in which vasoactive substances play important roles. And the main pathologic changes are lower counts of red blood cells, white blood cells, and platelets. Compared to normal spleen, lymphocytes in PH spleen were relatively reduced with a similar distribution; but total number of lymphocytes was increased due to the increase of spleen weight, with an elevated proliferation [81, 82]. MicroRNAome analysis showed that microRNA, expecially miR-615-3p was up-regulated in PH spleen significantly [83, 84]. It targeted on ligand-dependent nuclear receptor corepressor (LCoR), promoted the phagocytic capacity of macrophages through PPARγ pathway [84]. On the other hand, phagocytic capacity of macrophages might be inhibit by Phosphatidylinositol 3-kinase regulatory subunit 1 (PI3KR1) knock-down, accompanied by down-regulation of IL-1β and TNF-α [85]. Similarly, expressions of IL-1β and NALP3, a potential NF-κB activator participating in inflammation and immunologic response were up-regulated significantly in CCl_4-induced cirrhotic PH group compared to control group, together with typical splenomegaly histopathological changes [86]. In cirrhotic spleen, different from extrahepatic portal vein obstruction, thromopoietin (TPO) was reduced and this reduction is positively correlated with exacerbation of liver function, leading to a decrease of platelet counts [87].

4.2. Esophageal varices

Cirrhotic hypertension is characterized by hyperdynamic circulation and increased intrahepatic resistance as discussed before in this review. Splanchnic vasodilation results in increasing in HVPG. When HVPG is higher than 12 mmHg, risk of esophageal varices dramatically increased [88, 89]. Generally speaking, esophageal varices, as well as development of other collateral vessels, occur after HVPG and is followed by variceal bleeding [90]. Angiogenesis is associated with esophageal varices and portal hypertension, and expressions of VEGF are up-regulated, alone or together with TNF-α or PEGF[91-93]. Inhibition of VEGF/VEGF receptor pathway led to a decrease in hyperdynamic splanchnic circulation and collateral vessels [94]. Besides, metabolic disturbances occurred in cirrhotic PH lead to an elevation of glucagon [95]. The ratio of glycated albumin (GA) to glycated hemoglobin (HbA1c) was associated positively with the progression of liver cirrhosis, and patients with elevated GA/HbA1c ratio have severer esophageal variceal and higher risk of bleeding in HCV-related cirrhotic patients. This parameter might become a potential biomarker to predict the prognosis of these patients [96].

4.3. Ascites

Portal hypertension in cirrhotic liver diseases is a main cause of ascites. As discussed before, vasoactive substances lead to an elevation of intrahepatic vessels resistance and a relative decrease of blood back-flow to liver. Besides, mechanisms below are involved: 1) hyperdynamic circulation. Hyperdynamic circulation is associated with disturbance of vasoactive substances. It is characterized by increased cardiac index and plasma volume and decreased systemic and splanchnic resistance [90]. 2) hypoalbuminemia following damage of liver function. One of the hyperalbuminemia occurred in cirrhotic PH is dysfunction of hepatocytes. In is shown that hypertension is a negative regulator to the number and structure of hepatocytes [97]. Poor blood supply induced by liver fibrosis and disturbance of hemodynamics results in intrahepatic hypoxia and damage of hepatocytes. Besides, primary liver diseases also cause inflammation and damage in liver. 3) renal function changes. This part will be discussed below.

4.4. Hepatorenal syndrome

It is well established that main cause of hepatorenal syndrome (HRS) is constriction of vessels in kidney induced by reduction of effective circulating blood volume (ECBV). As discussed previously, ECBV is reduced by systemic and splanchnic vasodilation induced by changes of NO, ET, PGs and TXA_2. Besides, some localized physiopathologic should be paid attention on. Expression of HO-1 in kidney was significantly reduced in BDL-induced cirrhotic rats [98]. Cyctatin C was increased in decompensated liver cirrhosis and HRS, thus it could be used as a predictor of HRS [99, 100]. Additionally, plasma level of ADAMTS13 was decreased and supplemental therapy might improve prognosis of patients with severe liver cirrhosis and HRS [101, 102].

4.5. Hepatic encephalopathy

Hepatic encephalopathy (HE) in portal hypertension is defined as C type HE. In PVL-induced PH rats, chemokine changes in splanchnic system, liver, and central nervous system (CNS) are different [103]. As reported, in CNS, CX3CL1/CX3CR1 and SDF1-α/CXCR4 were increased. The former one promotes inflammation in CNS while the latter one modulates neuron activity through inhibitory neurotransmitters, e.g. gamma-amino butyric acid (GABA) [104]. ROS also participates in pre-hepatic portal hypertension [105, 106]. GABA level is also negatively regulated by dehydroepiandrosterone sulfate (DHEAS), which reduced in cirrhotic HE [107]. Besides, IL-6 has synergistic effect with ammonia in cirrotic HE patients [108]. Ammonia impairs brain eNOS activity, leading to significant abnormality of NO regulation and disturbance of blood supply [109]. Due to liver dysfunction in HE patients, elevated plasma manganese also indicates a bad prognosis [110].

5. Conclusion

Portal hypertension concerns a great number of molecules and complicated physiopathologic mechanisms. It can be classified into pre-, intra-, and post-hepatic PH according to the primary disease, with similar but not same involvement of molecules and mechanisms. However, we can still conclude that: 1) vasoactive substances play an important in systemic, splanchnic, hepatic, and even neurologic circulations which are closely related to blood supply, affecting the development, progression, and outcome of PH; 2) imbalance of pro-/anti-inflammatory cytokines lead to a systemic and/or localized regulation of signal pathways and modulate gene expression and silencing, cell proliferation and apoptosis, tissue damage and repair, and eventually life and death; 3) accumulating research advancements provide us new targets for treatment of PH, but it has a long way to go from bench to bedside.

Acknowledgements

This study was supported by the International Collaboration Foundation of Jiangsu Province (BZ2011041, BK2009439, ZX05 200904, WS2011106), Development of Innovative Research Team in the First Affiliated Hospital of NJMU and the National Nature Science Foundation of China (81210108017, 81100270, 81070380). First Innovation Team Foundation of Jiangsu province Hospital (for Sun BC).

Author details

Hao Lu, Guoqiang Li, Ling Lu, Ye Fan, Xiaofeng Qian, Ke Wang and Feng Zhang*

*Address all correspondence to: zhangf@njmu.edu.cn

Liver Transplantation Center, First Affiliated Hospital of Nanjing Medical Univerisity, Nanjing, China

Hao Lu and Guoqiang Li contribute equally to this work.

References

[1] Bari K,Garcia-Tsao G. Treatment of portal hypertension. World J Gastroenterol 2012;18:1166-1175. PMID: 22468079

[2] Arya A, Kakani N, Hussain N, Chandok N. Massive avascular malformations causing life threatening portal hypertension. Ann Hepatol 2012;11:552-553. PMID: 22700638

[3] Bosch J. Vascular deterioration in cirrhosis: the big picture. J Clin Gastroenterol 2007;41 Suppl 3:S247-253. PMID: 17975472

http://dx.doi.org/10.5772/52663

[4] Bruix J, Castells A, Bosch J, Feu F, Fuster J, Garcia-Pagan JC, et al. Surgical resection of hepatocellular carcinoma in cirrhotic patients: prognostic value of preoperative portal pressure. Gastroenterology 1996;111:1018-1022. PMID: 8831597

[5] Llovet JM, Fuster J, Bruix J. Intention-to-treat analysis of surgical treatment for early hepatocellular carcinoma: resection versus transplantation. Hepatology 1999;30:1434-1440. PMID: 10573522

[6] Zipprich A, Garcia-Tsao G, Rogowski S, Fleig WE, Seufferlein T, Dollinger MM. Prognostic indicators of survival in patients with compensated and decompensated cirrhosis. Liver Int 2012. PMID: 22679906

[7] Bosch J,Garcia-Pagan JC. Complications of cirrhosis. I. Portal hypertension. J Hepatol 2000;32:141-156. PMID: 10728801

[8] Rodriguez-Vilarrupla A, Fernandez M, Bosch J, Garcia-Pagan JC. Current concepts on the pathophysiology of portal hypertension. Ann Hepatol 2007;6:28-36. PMID: 17297426

[9] Biecker E, Sagesser H, Reichen J. Vasodilator mRNA levels are increased in the livers of portal hypertensive NO-synthase 3-deficient mice. Eur J Clin Invest 2004;34:283-289. PMID: 15086360

[10] Laleman W, Van Landeghem L, Van der Elst I, Zeegers M, Fevery J, Nevens F. Nitro-flurbiprofen, a nitric oxide-releasing cyclooxygenase inhibitor, improves cirrhotic portal hypertension in rats. Gastroenterology 2007;132:709-719. PMID: 17258737

[11] Luo W, Meng Y, Ji HL, Pan CQ, Huang S, Yu CH, et al. Spironolactone Lowers Portal Hypertension by Inhibiting Liver Fibrosis, ROCK-2 Activity and Activating NO/PKG Pathway in the Bile-Duct-Ligated Rat. PLoS One 2012;7:e34230. PMID: 22479572

[12] Goh BJ, Tan BT, Hon WM, Lee KH, Khoo HE. Nitric oxide synthase and heme oxygenase expressions in human liver cirrhosis. World J Gastroenterol 2006;12:588-594. PMID: 16489673

[13] El-Sherif AM, Abou-Shady MA, Al-Bahrawy AM, Bakr RM, Hosny AM. Nitric oxide levels in chronic liver disease patients with and without oesophageal varices. Hepatol Int 2008;2:341-345. PMID: 19669263

[14] Bories PN, Campillo B, Azaou L, Scherman E. Long-lasting NO overproduction in cirrhotic patients with spontaneous bacterial peritonitis. Hepatology 1997;25:1328-1333. PMID: 9185747

[15] Arkenau HT, Stichtenoth DO, Frolich JC, Manns MP, Boker KH. Elevated nitric oxide levels in patients with chronic liver disease and cirrhosis correlate with disease stage and parameters of hyperdynamic circulation. Z Gastroenterol 2002;40:907-913. PMID: 12436367

[16] Moriyama A, Masumoto A, Nanri H, Tabaru A, Unoki H, Imoto I, et al. High plasma concentrations of nitrite/nitrate in patients with hepatocellular carcinoma. Am J Gastroenterol 1997;92:1520-1523. PMID: 9317076

[17] Theodorakis NG, Wang YN, Wu JM, Maluccio MA, Sitzmann JV, Skill NJ. Role of endothelial nitric oxide synthase in the development of portal hypertension in the carbon tetrachloride-induced liver fibrosis model. Am J Physiol Gastrointest Liver Physiol 2009;297:G792-799. PMID: 19628654

[18] Xu J, Cao H, Liu H, Wu ZY. Role of nitric oxide synthase and cyclooxygenase in hyperdynamic splanchnic circulation of portal hypertension. Hepatobiliary Pancreat Dis Int 2008;7:503-508. PMID: 18842497

[19] Pannen BH, Kohler N, Hole B, Bauer M, Clemens MG, Geiger KK. Protective role of endogenous carbon monoxide in hepatic microcirculatory dysfunction after hemorrhagic shock in rats. J Clin Invest 1998;102:1220-1228. PMID: 9739056

[20] Tarquini R, Masini E, La Villa G, Barletta G, Novelli M, Mastroianni R, et al. Increased plasma carbon monoxide in patients with viral cirrhosis and hyperdynamic circulation. Am J Gastroenterol 2009;104:891-897. PMID: 19277027

[21] Makino N, Suematsu M, Sugiura Y, Morikawa H, Shiomi S, Goda N, et al. Altered expression of heme oxygenase-1 in the livers of patients with portal hypertensive diseases. Hepatology 2001;33:32-42. PMID: 11124818

[22] Van Landeghem L, Laleman W, Vander Elst I, Zeegers M, van Pelt J, Cassiman D, et al. Carbon monoxide produced by intrasinusoidally located haem-oxygenase-1 regulates the vascular tone in cirrhotic rat liver. Liver Int 2009;29:650-660. PMID: 18795901

[23] Guo SB, Duan ZJ, Li Q, Sun XY. Effects of heme oxygenase-1 on pulmonary function and structure in rats with liver cirrhosis. Chin Med J (Engl) 2011;124:918-922. PMID: 21518603

[24] Angermayr B, Mejias M, Gracia-Sancho J, Garcia-Pagan JC, Bosch J, Fernandez M. Heme oxygenase attenuates oxidative stress and inflammation, and increases VEGF expression in portal hypertensive rats. J Hepatol 2006;44:1033-1039. PMID: 16458992

[25] Giaid A. Nitric oxide and endothelin-1 in pulmonary hypertension. Chest 1998;114:208S-212S. PMID: 9741571

[26] Takashimizu S, Kojima S, Nishizaki Y, Kagawa T, Shiraishi K, Mine T, et al. Effect of endothelin A receptor antagonist on hepatic hemodynamics in cirrhotic rats. Implications for endothelin-1 in portal hypertension. Tokai J Exp Clin Med 2011;36:37-43. PMID: 21769771

[27] Watanabe N, Takashimizu S, Nishizaki Y, Kojima S, Kagawa T, Matsuzaki S. An endothelin A receptor antagonist induces dilatation of sinusoidal endothelial fenestrae: implications for endothelin-1 in hepatic microcirculation. J Gastroenterol 2007;42:775-782. PMID: 17876548

[28] Feng HQ, Weymouth ND, Rockey DC. Endothelin antagonism in portal hypertensive mice: implications for endothelin receptor-specific signaling in liver disease. Am J Physiol Gastrointest Liver Physiol 2009;297:G27-33. PMID: 19299580

[29] Miller AM,Zhang JX. Altered endothelin-1 signaling in production of thromboxane A2 in kupffer cells from bile duct ligated rats. Cell Mol Immunol 2009;6:441-452. PMID: 20003820

[30] Andersson A, Fenhammar J, Weitzberg E, Sollevi A, Hjelmqvist H, Frithiof R. Endothelin-mediated gut microcirculatory dysfunction during porcine endotoxaemia. Br J Anaesth 2010;105:640-647. PMID: 20710019

[31] Liu J, Gong H, Zhang ZT, Wang Y. Effect of angiotensin II and angiotensin II type 1 receptor antagonist on the proliferation, contraction and collagen synthesis in rat hepatic stellate cells. Chin Med J (Engl) 2008;121:161-165. PMID: 18272044

[32] Umgelter A, Wagner KS, Reindl W, Luppa PB, Geisler F, Huber W, et al. Renal and circulatory effects of large volume plasma expansion in patients with hepatorenal syndrome type 1. Ann Hepatol 2012;11:232-239. PMID: 22345341

[33] Lotfy M, El-Kenawy Ael M, Abdel-Aziz MM, El-Kady I, Talaat A. Elevated renin levels in patients with liver cirrhosis and hepatocellular carcinoma. Asian Pac J Cancer Prev 2010;11:1263-1266. PMID: 21198274

[34] Beyazit Y, Ibis M, Purnak T, Turhan T, Kekilli M, Kurt M, et al. Elevated levels of circulating angiotensin converting enzyme in patients with hepatoportal sclerosis. Dig Dis Sci 2011;56:2160-2165. PMID: 21290180

[35] Hidaka H, Kokubu S, Nakazawa T, Okuwaki Y, Ono K, Watanabe M, et al. New angiotensin II type 1 receptor blocker olmesartan improves portal hypertension in patients with cirrhosis. Hepatol Res 2007;37:1011-1017. PMID: 17608670

[36] Huang HC, Chang CC, Wang SS, Lee FY, Teng TH, Lee JY, et al. The roles of angiotensin II receptors in the portosystemic collaterals of portal hypertensive and cirrhotic rats. J Vasc Res 2012;49:160-168. PMID: 22285953

[37] Loiola RA, Fernandes L, Eichler R, Passaglia Rde C, Fortes ZB, de Carvalho MH. Vascular mechanisms involved in angiotensin II-induced venoconstriction in hypertensive rats. Peptides 2011;32:2116-2121. PMID: 21945423

[38] Hidaka H, Nakazawa T, Shibuya A, Minamino T, Takada J, Tanaka Y, et al. Effects of 1-year administration of olmesartan on portal pressure and TGF-beta1 in selected patients with cirrhosis: a randomized controlled trial. J Gastroenterol 2011;46:1316-1323. PMID: 21850387

[39] Debernardi-Venon W, Martini S, Biasi F, Vizio B, Termine A, Poli G, et al. AT1 receptor antagonist Candesartan in selected cirrhotic patients: effect on portal pressure and liver fibrosis markers. J Hepatol 2007;46:1026-1033. PMID: 17336417

[40] Tandon P, Abraldes JG, Berzigotti A, Garcia-Pagan JC, Bosch J. Renin-angiotensin-aldosterone inhibitors in the reduction of portal pressure: a systematic review and meta-analysis. J Hepatol 2010;53:273-282. PMID: 20570385

[41] Dal-Ros S, Oswald-Mammosser M, Pestrikova T, Schott C, Boehm N, Bronner C, et al. Losartan prevents portal hypertension-induced, redox-mediated endothelial dysfunction in the mesenteric artery in rats. Gastroenterology 2010;138:1574-1584. PMID: 19879274

[42] Chan CC, Chang CC, Huang HC, Wang SS, Lee FY, Chang FY, et al. Effects of norepinephrine and acetylcholine on portal-systemic collaterals of common bile duct-ligated cirrhotic rat. J Gastroenterol Hepatol 2005;20:1867-1872. PMID: 16336446

[43] Sastre E, Balfagon G, Revuelta-Lopez E, Aller MA, Nava MP, Arias J, et al. Effect of short- and long-term portal hypertension on adrenergic, nitrergic and sensory functioning in rat mesenteric artery. Clin Sci (Lond) 2012;122:337-348. PMID: 21999248

[44] Coll M, Genesca J, Raurell I, Rodriguez-Vilarrupla A, Mejias M, Otero T, et al. Down-regulation of genes related to the adrenergic system may contribute to splanchnic vasodilation in rat portal hypertension. J Hepatol 2008;49:43-51. PMID: 18457899

[45] Sancho-Bru P, Bataller R, Colmenero J, Gasull X, Moreno M, Arroyo V, et al. Norepinephrine induces calcium spikes and proinflammatory actions in human hepatic stellate cells. Am J Physiol Gastrointest Liver Physiol 2006;291:G877-884. PMID: 16782692

[46] Villanueva C, Aracil C, Colomo A, Hernandez-Gea V, Lopez-Balaguer JM, Alvarez-Urturi C, et al. Acute hemodynamic response to beta-blockers and prediction of long-term outcome in primary prophylaxis of variceal bleeding. Gastroenterology 2009;137:119-128. PMID: 19344721

[47] La Mura V, Abraldes JG, Raffa S, Retto O, Berzigotti A, Garcia-Pagan JC, et al. Prognostic value of acute hemodynamic response to i.v. propranolol in patients with cirrhosis and portal hypertension. J Hepatol 2009;51:279-287. PMID: 19501930

[48] Garcia N, Jr., Jarai Z, Mirshahi F, Kunos G, Sanyal AJ. Systemic and portal hemodynamic effects of anandamide. Am J Physiol Gastrointest Liver Physiol 2001;280:G14-20. PMID: 11123193

[49] Shah V. Portal hypertension and the hyperdynamic circulation: nitric oxide in a haze of cannabinoid smoke. Hepatology 2001;34:1060-1061. PMID: 11679979

[50] Fernandez-Rodriguez CM, Romero J, Petros TJ, Bradshaw H, Gasalla JM, Gutierrez ML, et al. Circulating endogenous cannabinoid anandamide and portal, systemic and renal hemodynamics in cirrhosis. Liver Int 2004;24:477-483. PMID: 15482346

[51] Piston D, Wang S, Feng Y, Ye YJ, Zhou J, Jiang KW, et al. The role of cyclooxygenase-2/prostanoid pathway in visceral pain induced liver stress response in rats. Chin Med J (Engl) 2007;120:1813-1819. PMID: 18028778

[52] Yokoyama Y, Xu H, Kresge N, Keller S, Sarmadi AH, Baveja R, et al. Role of thromboxane A2 in early BDL-induced portal hypertension. Am J Physiol Gastrointest Liver Physiol 2003;284:G453-460. PMID: 12431905

[53] Cao H, Xu J, Liu H, Meng FB, Qiu JF, Wu ZY. Influence of nitric oxide synthase and cyclooxygenase blockade on expression of cyclooxygenase and hemodynamics in rats with portal hypertension. Hepatobiliary Pancreat Dis Int 2006;5:564-569. PMID: 17085343

[54] Cao H, Xu J, Hua R, Meng FB, Qiu JF, Wu ZY. Expression of cyclooxygenase in hyperdynamic portal hypertensive rats. Hepatobiliary Pancreat Dis Int 2006;5:252-256. PMID: 16698586

[55] Graupera M, Garcia-Pagan JC, Abraldes JG, Peralta C, Bragulat M, Corominola H, et al. Cyclooxygenase-derived products modulate the increased intrahepatic resistance of cirrhotic rat livers. Hepatology 2003;37:172-181. PMID: 12500202

[56] Vujanac A, Jakovljevic V, Djordjevic D, Zivkovic V, Stojkovic M, Celikovic D, et al. Nitroglycerine effects on portal vein mechanics and oxidative stress in portal hypertension. World J Gastroenterol 2012;18:331-339. PMID: 22294839

[57] Garcia-Caldero H, Rodriguez-Vilarrupla A, Gracia-Sancho J, Divi M, Lavina B, Bosch J, et al. Tempol administration, a superoxide dismutase mimetic, reduces hepatic vascular resistance and portal pressure in cirrhotic rats. J Hepatol 2011;54:660-665. PMID: 21159403

[58] Huang YT, Hsu YC, Chen CJ, Liu CT, Wei YH. Oxidative-stress-related changes in the livers of bile-duct-ligated rats. J Biomed Sci 2003;10:170-178. PMID: 12595753

[59] Hamdy N,El-Demerdash E. New therapeutic aspect for carvedilol: Antifibrotic effects of carvedilol in chronic carbon tetrachloride-induced liver damage. Toxicol Appl Pharmacol 2012. PMID: 22543095

[60] Koksal AS, Koklu S, Ibis M, Balci M, Cicek B, Sasmaz N, et al. Clinical features, serum interleukin-6, and interferon-gamma levels of 34 turkish patients with hepatoportal sclerosis. Dig Dis Sci 2007;52:3493-3498. PMID: 17404864

[61] Cariello R, Federico A, Sapone A, Tuccillo C, Scialdone VR, Tiso A, et al. Intestinal permeability in patients with chronic liver diseases: Its relationship with the aetiology and the entity of liver damage. Dig Liver Dis 2010;42:200-204. PMID: 19502117

[62] Tan G, Pan S, Li J, Dong X, Kang K, Zhao M, et al. Hydrogen sulfide attenuates carbon tetrachloride-induced hepatotoxicity, liver cirrhosis and portal hypertension in rats. PLoS One 2011;6:e25943. PMID: 22022478

[63] [The role of interleukin-6 and nitric oxide in pathogenesis of portal hypertension and decompensation of liver cirrhosis]. Klin Med (Mosk) 2012;90:47-49. PMID: 22567940

[64] Lemmers A, Gustot T, Durnez A, Evrard S, Moreno C, Quertinmont E, et al. An inhibitor of interleukin-6 trans-signalling, sgp130, contributes to impaired acute phase

response in human chronic liver disease. Clin Exp Immunol 2009;156:518-527. PMID: 19438606

[65] Elsammak MY, Al-Sharkaweey RM, Ragab MS, Amin GA, Kandil MH. IL-4 and reactive oxygen species are elevated in Egyptian patients affected with schistosomal liver disease. Parasite Immunol 2008;30:603-609. PMID: 19067841

[66] Tandon P, Moncrief K, Madsen K, Arrieta MC, Owen RJ, Bain VG, et al. Effects of probiotic therapy on portal pressure in patients with cirrhosis: a pilot study. Liver Int 2009;29:1110-1115. PMID: 19490420

[67] Okada Y, Tsuzuki Y, Hokari R, Miyazaki J, Matsuzaki K, Mataki N, et al. Pressure loading and ethanol exposure differentially modulate rat hepatic stellate cell activation. J Cell Physiol 2008;215:472-480. PMID: 18064666

[68] Henao-Mejia J, Elinav E, Jin C, Hao L, Mehal WZ, Strowig T, et al. Inflammasome-mediated dysbiosis regulates progression of NAFLD and obesity. Nature 2012;482:179-185. PMID: 22297845

[69] Fairfax KC, Amiel E, King IL, Freitas TC, Mohrs M, Pearce EJ. IL-10R blockade during chronic schistosomiasis mansoni results in the loss of B cells from the liver and the development of severe pulmonary disease. PLoS Pathog 2012;8:e1002490. PMID: 22291593

[70] Perona-Wright G, Lundie RJ, Jenkins SJ, Webb LM, Grencis RK, MacDonald AS. Concurrent bacterial stimulation alters the function of helminth-activated dendritic cells, resulting in IL-17 induction. J Immunol 2012;188:2350-2358. PMID: 22287718

[71] Mentink-Kane MM, Cheever AW, Wilson MS, Madala SK, Beers LM, Ramalingam TR, et al. Accelerated and progressive and lethal liver fibrosis in mice that lack interleukin (IL)-10, IL-12p40, and IL-13Ralpha2. Gastroenterology 2011;141:2200-2209. PMID: 21864478

[72] Pinter M, Sieghart W, Reiberger T, Rohr-Udilova N, Ferlitsch A, Peck-Radosavljevic M. The effects of sorafenib on the portal hypertensive syndrome in patients with liver cirrhosis and hepatocellular carcinoma--a pilot study. Aliment Pharmacol Ther 2012;35:83-91. PMID: 22032637

[73] Trebicka J, Krag A, Gansweid S, Appenrodt B, Schiedermaier P, Sauerbruch T, et al. Endotoxin and tumor necrosis factor-receptor levels in portal and hepatic vein of patients with alcoholic liver cirrhosis receiving elective transjugular intrahepatic portosystemic shunt. Eur J Gastroenterol Hepatol 2011;23:1218-1225. PMID: 21971377

[74] Garcia-Dominguez J, Aller MA, Garcia C, de Vicente F, Corcuera MT, Gomez-Aguado F, et al. Splanchnic Th(2) and Th(1) cytokine redistribution in microsurgical cholestatic rats. J Surg Res 2010;162:203-212. PMID: 20031157

[75] Dragoteanu M, Balea IA, Dina LA, Piglesan CD, Grigorescu I, Tamas S, et al. Staging of portal hypertension and portosystemic shunts using dynamic nuclear medicine investigations. World J Gastroenterol 2008;14:3841-3848. PMID: 18609707

[76] Di Marco V, Almasio PL, Ferraro D, Calvaruso V, Alaimo G, Peralta S, et al. Peg-interferon alone or combined with ribavirin in HCV cirrhosis with portal hypertension: a randomized controlled trial. J Hepatol 2007;47:484-491. PMID: 17692985

[77] Katamura Y, Aikata H, Takaki S, Azakami T, Kawaoka T, Waki K, et al. Intra-arterial 5-fluorouracil/interferon combination therapy for advanced hepatocellular carcinoma with or without three-dimensional conformal radiotherapy for portal vein tumor thrombosis. J Gastroenterol 2009;44:492-502. PMID: 19330281

[78] Iacobellis A, Ippolito A, Andriulli A. Antiviral therapy in hepatitis C virus cirrhotic patients in compensated and decompensated condition. World J Gastroenterol 2008;14:6467-6472. PMID: 19030197

[79] Pozzi M, Pizzala DP, Maldini FF, Doretti A, Ratti L. Portal pressure reduction after entecavir treatment in compensated HBV cirrhosis. Hepatogastroenterology 2009;56:231-235. PMID: 19453064

[80] Albillos A, Nieto M, Ubeda M, Munoz L, Fraile B, Reyes E, et al. The biological response modifier AM3 attenuates the inflammatory cell response and hepatic fibrosis in rats with biliary cirrhosis. Gut 2010;59:943-952. PMID: 20442198

[81] Li ZF, Zhang S, Huang Y, Xia XM, Li AM, Pan D, et al. Morphological changes of blood spleen barrier in portal hypertensive spleen. Chin Med J (Engl) 2008;121:561-565. PMID: 18364147

[82] Li ZF, Zhang S, Lv GB, Huang Y, Zhang W, Ren S, et al. Changes in count and function of splenic lymphocytes from patients with portal hypertension. World J Gastroenterol 2008;14:2377-2382. PMID: 18416465

[83] Li Z, Zhang S, Huang C, Zhang W, Hu Y, Wei B. MicroRNAome of splenic macrophages in hypersplenism due to portal hypertension in hepatitis B virus-related cirrhosis. Exp Biol Med (Maywood) 2008;233:1454-1461. PMID: 18791127

[84] Jiang A, Zhang S, Li Z, Liang R, Ren S, Li J, et al. miR-615-3p promotes the phagocytic capacity of splenic macrophages by targeting ligand-dependent nuclear receptor corepressor in cirrhosis-related portal hypertension. Exp Biol Med (Maywood) 2011;236:672-680. PMID: 21565892

[85] Zhang W, Zhang S, Li ZF, Huang C, Ren S, Zhou R, et al. Knockdown of PIK3R1 by shRNA inhibits the activity of the splenic macrophages associated with hypersplenism due to portal hypertension. Pathol Res Pract 2010;206:760-767. PMID: 20846792

[86] Xia Z, Wang G, Wan C, Liu T, Wang S, Wang B, et al. Expression of NALP3 in the spleen of mice with portal hypertension. J Huazhong Univ Sci Technolog Med Sci 2010;30:170-172. PMID: 20407867

[87] El-Sayed R, El-Ela MA, El-Raziky MS, Helmy H, El-Ghaffar AA, El-Karaksy H. Relation of serum levels of thrombopoietin to thrombocytopenia in extrahepatic portal vein obstruction versus cirrhotic children. J Pediatr Hematol Oncol 2011;33:e267-270. PMID: 21941130

[88] Boleslawski E, Petrovai G, Truant S, Dharancy S, Duhamel A, Salleron J, et al. Hepatic venous pressure gradient in the assessment of portal hypertension before liver resection in patients with cirrhosis. Br J Surg 2012;99:855-863. PMID: 22508371

[89] Garcia-Tsao G, Groszmann RJ, Fisher RL, Conn HO, Atterbury CE, Glickman M. Portal pressure, presence of gastroesophageal varices and variceal bleeding. Hepatology 1985;5:419-424. PMID: 3873388

[90] Maruyama H,Yokosuka O. Pathophysiology of portal hypertension and esophageal varices. Int J Hepatol 2012;2012:895787. PMID: 22666604

[91] Yin ZH, Liu XY, Huang RL, Ren SP. Expression of TNF-alpha and VEGF in the esophagus of portal hypertensive rats. World J Gastroenterol 2005;11:1232-1236. PMID: 15754412

[92] Huang HC, Haq O, Utsumi T, Sethasine S, Abraldes JG, Groszmann RJ, et al. Intestinal and plasma VEGF levels in cirrhosis: the role of portal pressure. J Cell Mol Med 2012;16:1125-1133. PMID: 21801303

[93] Pan WD, Liu Y, Lin N, Xu R. The expression of PEDF and VEGF in the gastric wall of prehepatic portal hypertensive rats. Hepatogastroenterology 2011;58:2152-2155. PMID: 22024088

[94] Fernandez M, Mejias M, Angermayr B, Garcia-Pagan JC, Rodes J, Bosch J. Inhibition of VEGF receptor-2 decreases the development of hyperdynamic splanchnic circulation and portal-systemic collateral vessels in portal hypertensive rats. J Hepatol 2005;43:98-103. PMID: 15893841

[95] Tsui CP, Sung JJ, Leung FW. Role of acute elevation of portal venous pressure by exogenous glucagon on gastric mucosal injury in rats with portal hypertension. Life Sci 2003;73:1115-1129. PMID: 12818720

[96] Sakai Y, Enomoto H, Aizawa N, Iwata Y, Tanaka H, Ikeda N, et al. Relationship between Elevation of Glycated Albumin to Glycated Hemoglobin Ratio in Patients with a High Bleeding Risk of Esophageal Varices. Hepatogastroenterology 2012;59. PMID: 22440250

[97] Dursun H, Albayrak F, Uyanik A, Keles NO, Beyzagul P, Bayram E, et al. Effects of hypertension and ovariectomy on rat hepatocytes. Are amlodipine and lacidipine protective? (A stereological and histological study). Turk J Gastroenterol 2010;21:387-395. PMID: 21331992

[98] Guo SB, Duan ZJ, Li Q, Sun XY. Effect of heme oxygenase-1 on renal function in rats with liver cirrhosis. World J Gastroenterol 2011;17:322-328. PMID: 21253390

[99] Sharawey MA, Shawky EM, Ali LH, Mohammed AA, Hassan HA, Fouad YM. Cystatin C: a predictor of hepatorenal syndrome in patients with liver cirrhosis. Hepatol Int 2011. PMID: 21484118

[100] Barakat M,Khalil M. Serum cystatin C in advanced liver cirrhosis and different stages of the hepatorenal syndrome. Arab J Gastroenterol 2011;12:131-135. PMID: 22055590

[101] Uemura M, Fujimura Y, Ko S, Matsumoto M, Nakajima Y, Fukui H. Determination of ADAMTS13 and Its Clinical Significance for ADAMTS13 Supplementation Therapy to Improve the Survival of Patients with Decompensated Liver Cirrhosis. Int J Hepatol 2011;2011:759047. PMID: 21994870

[102] Takaya H, Uemura M, Fujimura Y, Matsumoto M, Matsuyama T, Kato S, et al. ADAMTS13 activity may predict the cumulative survival of patients with liver cirrhosis in comparison with the Child-Turcotte-Pugh score and the Model for End-Stage Liver Disease score. Hepatol Res 2012;42:459-472. PMID: 22292786

[103] Merino J, Aller MA, Rubio S, Arias N, Nava MP, Loscertales M, et al. Gut-brain chemokine changes in portal hypertensive rats. Dig Dis Sci 2011;56:2309-2317. PMID: 21347560

[104] Guyon A,Nahon JL. Multiple actions of the chemokine stromal cell-derived factor-1alpha on neuronal activity. J Mol Endocrinol 2007;38:365-376. PMID: 17339399

[105] Rosello DM, Balestrasse K, Coll C, Coll S, Tallis S, Gurni A, et al. Oxidative stress and hippocampus in a low-grade hepatic encephalopathy model: protective effects of curcumin. Hepatol Res 2008;38:1148-1153. PMID: 19000058

[106] Nikonenko AG, Radenovic L, Andjus PR, Skibo GG. Structural features of ischemic damage in the hippocampus. Anat Rec (Hoboken) 2009;292:1914-1921. PMID: 19943345

[107] Ahboucha S, Talani G, Fanutza T, Sanna E, Biggio G, Gamrani H, et al. Reduced brain levels of DHEAS in hepatic coma patients: Significance for increased GABAergic tone in hepatic encephalopathy. Neurochem Int 2012;61:48-53. PMID: 22490610

[108] Luo M, Li L, Yang EN, Cao WK. Relationship between interleukin-6 and ammonia in patients with minimal hepatic encephalopathy due to liver cirrhosis. Hepatol Res 2012. PMID: 22646055

[109] Balasubramaniyan V, Wright G, Sharma V, Davies NA, Sharifi Y, Habtesion A, et al. Ammonia reduction with ornithine phenylacetate restores brain eNOS activity via the DDAH-ADMA pathway in bile duct-ligated cirrhotic rats. Am J Physiol Gastrointest Liver Physiol 2012;302:G145-152. PMID: 21903766

[110] Zeron HM, Rodriguez MR, Montes S, Castaneda CR. Blood manganese levels in patients with hepatic encephalopathy. J Trace Elem Med Biol 2011;25:225-229. PMID: 21975221

Chapter 23

Egyptian Hepatic Veno-Occlusive Disease: Surgical Point of View

Elsayed Ibrahim Salama

Additional information is available at the end of the chapter

http://dx.doi.org/10.5772/50685

1. Introduction

Hepatic veno-occlusive disease (HVOD): was described as a non portal cirrhosis occurring frequently in children and occasionally in adults. Now it is considered an important cause of non cirrhotic portal hypertension particularly in children [1].

Rollins 1989 [2], stated that HVOD is a non-thrombotic obliteration of small intrahepatic veins by loose connective tissues. The venous occlusion may be progressive and lead to massive hepatocellular necrosis. However the precise pathogenesis is still obscure but also most likely relates to venous endothelial injury.

Originally the syndrome was described in South Africa at 1920, but at present it is endemic in Jamaica, encountered in Afghanistan and India. The syndrome was described under different names, from Jamaica the disease was described under the term Jamaican veno-occlusive disease, in India the disease was given the term Indian childhood Cirrhosis (ICC), in Europe HVOD has been called endophlebitis obliterans of which sporadic cases were described, as in Germany. Hepatic veno- occlusive disease was examined by scanning electron microscopy (SEM). SEM correlated its histology and postmortem examination and disclosed microscopic occlusion of the centrilobular and sublobular veins in the liver, these veins were occluded partially or completely by intimal and medial thickening of their walls due to proliferation of collagen and reticulin fibers. In addition to venous obliteration, which had not been demonstrated by other techniques, frequent occlusion of the sinusoidal opening into the central veins was observed by SEM. [4], [5], [6].

Causes of non cirrhotic portal hypertension	
Intrahepatic	**Extrahepatic**
Schistosomiasis	Extrahepatic portal vein thrombosis
Extrahepatic portal vein thrombosis	Splenic vein thrombosis
Biliary cirrhosis, primary and secondary	
Chronic veno-occlusive disease	
Chronic active hepatitis	
Congenital hepatic fibrosis	
Haemochromatosis	
Alcoholic fibrosis	
Sarcoidosis	
Nodular regenerative hyperplasia	
Idiopathic portal hypertension	
Non-cirrhotic portal fibrosis	

Hepatic veno-occlusive disease has been recognized as being due to the toxic effects of some remedies, recently pyrrolizidine alkaloids mostly involved, as in senecio (bush teas) and crotalaria (comfrey trees). It is also now seen as complication of high dose of anti-neoplastic chemotherapy, especially in the setting of bone marrow transplantation. HVOD may be familial, so the term *"veno occlusive familial hepatic disease"* [7], [8], [9].

2. Hepatic veno-occlusive disease (HVOD) in Egypt: Overview

In Egypt Hashem 1939 [7], gave the first reference to this syndrome, in his study of portal cirrhosis among Egyptian children. Since 1939 several reports pointed out the occurrence of a specific syndrome among Egyptian children who rapidly developed abdominal distention with ascites and hepatomegaly. In 1965, Safouh et al [11]; reported that 54 Egyptian children were studied and the term "Hepatic vein occlusion disease in Egyptian children" was applied. At the same year, El Gholmy 1956 [10], studied a group of patients and introduced the term "Infantile cirrhosis of Egypt"

The different reports from Egypt, thereafter, describing the syndrome, the clinical picture, the pathology and the etiology revealed that HVOD is not uncommon among Egyptian infants and young children. They also have shown clearly for the first time that hepatic vein occlusion should be considered in the diagnosis of Egyptian children presenting with hepatosplenomegaly [11].

Safouh 1965 [11], reported that the Egyptian hepatic vein occlusion is the result of enhanced thrombotic activity of the blood with the formation of fibrinous thrombi followed by organization and thickening or closure of the vessels, a finding which seems peculiar to the Egyptian cases and thus differs from the classical HVOD.

3. Clinical Picture of HVOD

Clinical diagnosis is based on; hepatomegaly and/or right upper quadrant pain, ascites or unexplained weight gain and also jaundice may or may not present [7].

The acute stage starts abruptly with abdominal discomfort or pain accompanied by hepatomegaly and ascites, nausea and vomiting are common. Histologically the liver shows an edematous endophlebitis of the central veins associated with centrilobular congestion, hemorrhage and necrosis. Mclean 1969 [12], has shown experimentally that the block occurs first at the outlets of the sinusoids. Patients surviving the acute stage may progress to the subacute stage with persistent hepatomegaly and ascites which then diminish if an adequate collateral circulation becomes established. The chronic stage is a centrilobular type of septal cirrhosis [7].

Clinical picture:
Non febrile onset
Mild continuous dragging pain in right hypochondrium
Anorexia, nausea and vomiting
Rapidly filling ascites
Distended veins over the abdomin
Oliguria and pedal edema
Hepatomegaly
Splenomegaly in some cases

Tandon 1977

4. Diagnosis of HVOD

In the acute phase the diagnosis is usually readily made from the history and the characteristic clinical picture. In the sub-acute and chronic stages the diagnosis may be more difficult. In all stages the diagnosis is confirmed by the characteristic histopathological findings of liver biopsy in the absence of extrahepatic venous obstruction.

4.1. Laboratory Studies:

1. Safouh et al; 1965 [11] reported the following results:

Most of the cases showed some degree of anemia.

Total and differential leukocytic counts did not show any constant deviation from normal.

Liver function tests showed that : * Serum bilirubin was always below 3 mg/dl, * Serum AST varied between 20 and 60 units, * Serum ALT and alkaline phosphatase were found to be normal.

Erythrocyte sedimentation rate (ESR) was low in spite of advanced state of the disease.

The pattern of serum total proteins showed a state of hypoproteinemia ranging from 4-5 gm/dl and the albumen fraction is usually is decreased but globulin fraction may be increased.

2. Millis and Bale 1976 [13], stated that a feature of their cases is the partial immune deficiency. However, such a state of hypogammaglobulinemia reported by them goes parallel with findings in the acute cases only, that their cases were quite a different group of patients suffering from genetic immunodeficiency as observed from the very early appearance of the syndrome in some of them being as early as days.

3. Serum procollagen type III is an early and sensitive marker in VOD after BM transplantation, usually above 100 ng /ml.

4. Serum protein S,C, liedin factor

4.2. Ultrasonographic scaning of the liver:

It is of *definite help* in the diagnosis of this syndrome, it showed that the liver is enlarged especially the caudate lobe, splenic enlargement is usually of mild degree and ascites is always found in acute cases. Narrowing of inferior vena cava could be detected in 40% of cases. Examination of the terminal parts of the hepatic veins demonstrated their occlusion or attenuation, a finding which is considered a new and significant contribution to the early diagnosis of this syndrome [14].

4.3. Inferior vena cava angiogram:

Presented as narrow or closed intra-hepatic portion of the inferior vena cava with marked collaterals [14].

4.4. Liver biopsy:

In the acute stage it shows centrilobular hemorrhage, necrosis and sinusoidal dilatation. In the chronic stage it presents picture of micronodular cirrhosis with normal portal tracts [7].

4.5. Other tools of investigations [14]

- The ascitic fluid is a main laboratory field of investigations. It usually shows protein values ranging between 1-3.5 gms/dl with occasional lymphocytes.
- Other sophisticated modules of investigations might be carried out : liver isotopic scanning, splenoportal venogram and arterio-venography of the portal system.

5. Management of Hepatic veno-occlusive disease:

No effective therapy until now especially in this type of Egyptian children. The target of available line is, may be, to reduce the complications, to reduce the stress of the patients and keep the patients in nearly comfortable life, but the following measures could be used safely [14].

5.1. Preventive measures:

- More investigation for the etiology of the disease especially pyrrolizidine alkaloids.
- Encouraging the breast feeding for two years as Glorious Qura'n says. (Sorra El bakara), regulation and careful inspection of diet after weaning [11].
- Good nutrition of the mother
- What about copper utensils ?? it suspected to play a role in indian cirrhosis !

5.2. Conservative measures :

- Follow up, because a grossly abnormal scan of liver and spleen in a patient with HVOD has been normalized completely without any interference.
- Colonic lavage to wash out the toxic metabolites.

5.3. Medical treatment:

- Low doses of *heparin or anticoagulants*, adapted dose of *prostacyclin.*
- *Anti inflammatory* or *steroids.*
- Use of *Vit C,* use of *Vit. E* and Glutamine (source of glutathione) as antioxidants [15].
- Use of *recombinant tissue plasminogen activator* (rtPA), especially in patients after BM transplantation, *Urokinase* especially in cases with bleeding diathesis leading to thrombotic HVOD [15], [16], [17].
- *Diuretics* for ascites.
- *Large doses of glucose* together with *insulin* to aid glycogen deposition in the liver and so help its nutrition.
- Cupper chelation treatment (Di-penecillamine)

5.4. Surgical treatment [18].

5.4.1. Treatment of ascites :

- Frequent aspiration (partial or full)
- TIPS (transjagular intrahepatic portosystemic shunt)
- Hepatic and portal decompression for interactable ascites.
- LeVeen, peritoneojagular shunt.

5.4.2. Treatment of portal hypertension:

- Porto-systemic shunt as porto-caval, spleno-renal or meso-atrial.
- Acute venous obstruction could be treated by hepatofugal portal flow via veno-venous bypass to drain arterial blood flow.

5.4.3. Liver transplantation:

- It is now a part of the therapeutic armamentarium for this condition.

6. Therapeutic paracentesis [21].

The first study re-evaluating paracentesis as a treatment of cirrhotic patients with ascites consisted of a randomized controlled trial comparing repeated large-volume paracentesis (4-6 l/day until the disappearance of ascites) plus intravenous albumin infusion (40g after each tap) with standard diuretic therapy (frusemide plus spironolactone) in I17 patients with tense ascites and avid sodium retention who were admitted to several hospitals in the Barcelona area. This study, later confirmed by two more trials performed in Milan and Barcelona, showed the following results:

1. paracentesis was more effective than diuretics in eliminating ascites (96.5 versus 72.8%);

2. paracentesis plus albumin infusion did not induce significant changes in hepatic and renal function, serum electrolytes, cardiac output, plasma volume, plasma renin activity and plasma concentration of noradrenaline and antidiuretic hormone.

3. the incidence of hyponatremia, hepatic encephalopathy and renal impairment was much lower in patients treated with paracentesis.

4. the duration of hospital stay was lower in patients treated with paracentesis.

5. there were no significant probability of re-admission, probability of survival and causes of death between the two groups of patients.

Tito et al., later investigated whether ascites can be safely mobilized by total paracentesis (complete removal of ascites by a single paracentesis) plus intravenous albumin infusion

(6-8 g/l removed) in a one day hospitalization regime. The incidence of complications and the clinical course of the disease, as estimated by the probability of readmission to hospital, causes of re-admission, probability of survival and causes of death, were comparable to those reported by the same group of investigators in patients treated with repeated large-volume paracentesis.

In conclusion, these studies demonstrate that mobilization of ascites by paracentesis associated with intravenous albumin infusion does not impair systemic haemodynamics and renal function in patients with cirrhosis and tense ascites. Therapeutic paracentesis should be the treatment of choice for cirrhotic patients admitted to hospital with tense ascites, because it is more effective in mobilizing associated with a lower incidence of complications and reduce the duration of hospitalization. To avoid re-accumulation of ascites, patients treated with paracentesis require dietary sodium restriction and administration of diuretics after the procedures.

Subsequently, a trial was performed to establish whether intravenous albumin infusion is necessary in cirrhotic patients with tense ascites treated with repeated large-volume paracentesis. It was observed that paracentesis plus intravenous albumin does not induce significant changes in standard renal function testes, plasma renin activity and plasma aldosterone concentration. In contrast, paracentesis without albumin was associated with a significant increase in blood urea nitrogen, a marked elevation in plasma renin activity and plasma aldosterone concentration, and a significant reduction in serum sodium concentration. The number of patients developing hyponatremia and renal impairment was remarkably higher in patients treated with repeated large-volume paracentesis without intravenous albumin infusion. There are two detailed investigations assessing the effects of large-volume paracentesis without albumin infusion on systemic haemodynamics vasoactive hormones and renal function. A significant increase in cardiac output was observed 1 hour after treatment in both studies. Some hours later, however, a significant drop below baseline values was observed in cardiac output, pulmonary wedge capillary pressure and central venous pressure. Plasma renin activity increased and plasma atrial natriuretic peptide concentration decreased. The adverse effects observed after complete mobilization of ascites by paracentesis without albumin expansion did not occur in patients in whom ascites was only partially mobilized by paracentesis without colloid replacement. In conclusion, these studies demonstrate that complete mobilization of ascites by paracentesis without plasma volume expansion is followed by a reduction in effective intravascular volume, which leads to activation of the renin-aldosterone system and may impair renal function. The infusion of intravenous albumin is an important measure to prevent these abnormalities in cirrhotic patients with tense ascites treated with large-volume or total paracentesis.

Five randomized controlled trials and one prospective study aimed at investigating whether albumin can be substituted by less expensive plasma expanders (dextran-70, dextran-40, Haemaccel 5% and isotonic saline) have recently been reported. It has been observed that total or repeated large-volume paracentesis associated with intravenous administration of dextran-70 or Haemaccel is not associated with significant changes in renal and hepatic function. The incidence of hyponatremia, renal impairment and hepatic encephalopathy in patients receiving dextran-70 or Haemaccel was comparable with that in patients receiving albumin.

In one study, patients treated with dextran-70 showed a significant increase in plasma renin activity and aldosterone concentration. In a more recent study, however, therapeutic paracentesis plus intravenous dextran-70 administration was not associated with significant changes in plasma renin activity, which was measured 24 and 96 hours after the treatment. Cabrera et al., in one study including 14 patients, have suggested that intravenous isotonic saline infusion can also be a safe and cost effective alternative plasma expander in cirrhotics with tense ascites treated with paracentesis. Further studies are obviously needed to confirm their findings. It seems that dextran-40 is not as effective as albumin in preventing renal and electrolyte complications after therapeutic paracentesis, as renal impairment and/or hyponatremia developed after treatment in a relatively high proportion of patients.

Recently, a multicenter randomized trial comparing therapeutic paracentesis with PVS in cirrhotic patients with refractory or recurrent ascites has been published. More than 40 patients were included in each group. Both treatments were equally effective in mobilizing the ascites during the first hospital stay, although the duration of hospitalization was significantly longer in the shunt group. There were also no significant differences between both groups in the number of patients who developed complications or died. The number of readmissions for any reason or for ascites, was significantly higher, and the time to first readmission for any reason and for ascites significantly shorter in the paracentesis group than in the shunt group. The total time in hospital during follow-up, however, was similar in the two groups. The probability of shunt obstruction was 40 % at 1 -year follow-up. The probability of survival was similar in both groups. In conclusion, this trial shows that, although the LeVeen shunt was better than paracentesis in the long-term control of ascites, it did not reduce the total time in hospital nor prolong survival. On the other hand, patients treated with PVS required frequent re-operations due to obstruction of the prosthesis. Therapeutic paracentesis is therefore an alternative treatment to LeVeen shunt in cirrhotic patients with refractory ascites.

7. Peritoneovenous Shunting

In 1974 LeVeen [19], and colleagues developed a pressure-activated one-way valve for use in a peritoneovenous shunt (PVS). This device consists of a perforated intra-abdominal tube connected through a one-way pressure sensitive valve to a silicone tube that traverses the subcutaneous tissue up to the neck, where it enters one of the jugular veins (usually the internal jugular vein). The tip of the intravenous tube is located in the superior vena cava, near the right atrium or in the right atrium itself. The shunt produces a sustained circulating blood volume expansion by continuous passage of ascitic fluid to the general circulation. Flow in the shunt is maintained if there is a 3-5 cm H2O pressure gradient between the abdominal cavity and the superior vena cava. A loss of this gradient causes the valve to close, preventing blood from flowing back into the tubing. Two additional shunts have been introduced Denver and Cordis-Hakim. These latter shunts include a pumping mechanism that allows flow to be increased or a partially occluded shunt to be cleared.

The intravenous infusion of ascitic fluid through the shunt is associated with an increase in circulating blood volume and cardiac output. Since arterial pressure does not rise, there is a concomitant reduction in peripheral vascular resistance. These hemodynamic changes are associated with an increase in the plasma concentration of atrial natriuretic factor and a suppression of plasma levels of renin, aldosterone, noradrenaline and antidiuretic hormone. Urine volume and free water clearance increase in most patients. However, there is significant natriuresis in less than half of the patients, demonstrating that the PVS does not completely correct the abnormal sodium-retaining state associated with cirrhosis. Finally, in cirrhotic patients with moderate FRF, the PVS may improve renal blood flow and glomerular filtration rate. These hemodynamic and hormonal changes persist in most cases and a significant proportion of patients remains with minimal or no ascites despite a moderate sodium restriction and low diuretic dosage. There are also two studies that suggest that PVS has a positive effect on the nutritional status of patients in whom the shunt functions for a prolonged period of time. Despite these positive effects of PVS, there are a large number of complications, which may occur early in the postoperative period or at any time during follow-up [19], [20].

The role of PVS in the management of cirrhotic patients with ascitcs is still not well established. Only one prospective study showed that PVS is superior to conventional medical therapy in the management of ascites and in improving survival. By contrast, four randomized studies have failed to demonstrate a longer survival time in cirrhotic patients with ascites treated with PVS compared with medical therapy. Of these studies, that which was performed by Stanley et al., 1989 [22], is worth mentioning. They compared PVS with medical treatment (diuretics and occasional paracentesis) in 299 patients with cirrhosis and refractory or recurrent ascites. Although early mortality and probability of survival after randomization were similar in both therapeutic groups, PVS was more effective in the management of ascites than was conventional medical therapy, as indicated by shorter duration of first hospitalization, longer time to recurrence of ascites, and lower diuretic requirements during follow-up. However, these results are not surprising, because PVS was compared with a treatment that by definition was known to be ineffective.

The effect of PVS on survival in patients with FRF has also been studied in a randomized controlled trial. The treated patients had some improvement in renal function, but their survival was unaffected. Several studies have shown that morbidity and survival of cirrhotic patients treated with PVS correlate with the degree of impairment of liver and renal function. Therefore, the best results with this procedure should be expected to occur in those few patients with diuretic-resistant ascites and preserved hepatic function [23].

7.1. Early complications of peritoneovenous shunting

Acute bacterial infection is the most serious early complication. Staphylococcus aureus is a frequent isolate and represents the operative contamination of the shunt in some cases. The prosthesis is usually colonized and the infection cannot be eradicated in most cases unless the shunt is removed a high mortality can be expected. The prophylactic administration of anti-staphylococcal antibiotics 24 hours before and 48 hours after surgery reduces the incidence of early postoperative infection. Biochemical disseminated intravascular coagulation (DIC) is seen in practically every cirrhotic patient treated with PVS in the early postoperative period. Bleeding caused by DIC develops most commonly in those patients with severe liver disease, but is now very uncommon, because many surgeons remove the ascitic fluid before inserting the shunt and replace it with normal saline. DIC is thought to develop because of infusion of factors present in ascitic fluid that activate coagulation (thromboplastin, activated clotting factors, endotoxin, collagen, plasminogen activator and fibrin split products). Postoperative fever, probably related to the passage of endotoxin contained in the ascitic fluid to the general circulation, is almost a constant and disappears spontaneously within the second postoperative week. Rapid expansion of the plasma volume is associated with a rise in portal pressure and may increase the risk of variceal haemorrhage. This complication can also be prevented by removing most ascitic fluid before the insertion of the shunt [24].

7.2. Long-term complications of peritoneovenous shunting

Obstruction of the shunt is the most common complication during follow-up. It occurs in more than 30% of patients and is usually due to deposition of fibrin within the valve or the intravenous catheter, thrombotic obstruction of the venous limb of the prosthesis, or thrombosis of the superior vena cava or right atrium initiated at the venous end of the shunt or damaged endothelium. Shunt obstruction is generally associated with ascites re-accumulation. Shunt patency can be assessed by Doppler ultrasound or by technetium 99m scintigraphy using intraperitoneal radioisotope injection. If the obstruction is confirmed, a shuntogram after the injection of contrast into the proximal limb of the shunt may identify the site of obstruction. Venography or digital angiography is necessary in the case of obstruction of the venous tip of the shunt. Superior vena cava syndrome secondary to total obstruction of the vein and pulmonary embolism are much less common. It is not clear that the insertion of a titanium tip into the venous end of the LeVeen shunt prevents thrombotic obstruction and the development of superior vena cava thrombosis. Finally, another long-term complication of PVS is small-bowel obstruction, which occurs in approximately 10% of patients and is due to intraperitoneal fibrosis [25].

8. Transjugular intrahepatic portosystemic shunt (TIPS)

The feasibility of intrahepatic portosystemic shunting was first demonstrated by Rosch and colleagues 1969 in pigs. Colapinto et al; 1982 [27] reported the first application of this technique to humans. This was attempted following transhepatic obliteration of varices in 20 severely ill patients with variceal hemorrhage. The authors inflated a balloon catheter in the intrahepatic track and left it there for 12 hours. In an initial report all six shunts studied were patent 12 hours after the procedure and one was still patent at autopsy 6 weeks late.

Many demonstrated prolonged patency of the shunt for up to 10 months and ease of recanalizing the radiopaque shunt when occlusion occurred. This expandable stent was then used successfully in patients with portal hypertension. Similar good results were soon reported with the self-expanding Wall stent. Percutaneous portography was used in the early cases to facilitate transjugular portal vein puncture. With increasing experience this has been replaced by ultrasound guidance in most centers [28].

There is now an increasing array of equipment available for transjugular intrahepatic portosytemic shunt (TIPS) insertion. The most widely used needles are a standard transjugular biopsy needle with a straight or reversed bevel (Cook Ltd) or the Richter needle which has a tapered tip and a blunt obturator (Angiomed, Karlsruhe, Germany). Another set with a blunt cannula, through which is passed a sharp style is also available (Cook). There is also a wider choice with regard to the type and dimensions of metal stent. In addition to the original Palmaz and Wall stents, there is the Strecker stent and the Memotherm stent (Angiomed, Karlsruhe, Germany). Claimed advantages for these new stents are increased radioopacity (Strecker stent) and improved delivery systems (Memo stent) [29].

A recent randomized controlled study compared the Palmaz and Wall stent in 90 patients and found little difference in outcome. Early shunt thrombosis was more likely with the Wall stent (9%), whereas stenosis of the hepatic vein was more likely with the Palmaz stent (I3%). Experience with the other stents is limited.

As yet the long-term expectations of TIPS have not been fulfilled in those clinical situations in which long-term efficacy is needed as prevention of variceal rebleeding, ascites, cirrhotic hydrothorax, Budd-Chiari syndrome, and long-term amelioration of clinical status before liver transplantation. All these indications need controlled trials against current best optimal management before TIPS is used routinely even for an individual patient. The high stent obstruction rate is the most important limiting factor, but change in stent shape, coating material or other technical aspects may overcome this [30].

The complications of TIPS are significant if elective and long-term use is considered, thus the need for trials before new therapies are introduced. In an emergency situation the complications due to TIPS are an acceptable risk, but again information from controlled trials is needed. This is particularly true when TIPS is used as a short-term bridge to liver transplantation. TIPS will have a place in the treatment of cirrhotic patients. At present short-term rather than long-term indications appear to be where TIPS will have more beneficial effects [28].

9. Liver transplantation: and hepatic venous obstruction

Liver transplantation for Budd–Chiari syndrome: A European study on 248 patients from 51 centers) [31]: The results of liver transplantation for Budd–Chiari syndrome (BCS) are poorly known and the role and timing of the procedure are still controversial. The aim of this study was to investigate the results of transplantation for BCS, focusing on overall outcome, on prognostic factors and on the impact of the underlying disease. Methods: An enquiry on 248 patients representing 84% of the patients transplanted for BCS in the European Liver Transplantation Registry between 1988 and 1999. Results: Of the 248 patients, 70.4% were female and 29.6% male. The mean age was 35.7 years. The overall actuarial survival was 76% at 1 year, 71% at 5 years and 68% at 10 years. 77% of deaths occurred in the first 3 months: 47% were due to infection and multiple organ failure, and 18% to graft failure or hepatic artery thrombosis. Late mortality (>1 year) occurred in nine patients, due to BCS recurrence in four of them. The only pre-transplant predictors of mortality on multivariate analysis (Cox) were impaired renal function and a history of a shunt.

10. Conclusions

Liver transplantation for BCS is an effective treatment, irrespective of the underlying cause, and should be considered before renal failure occurs [31].

Acknowledgements

We would like to thank all the staff of pediatric department, at National Liver Institute, Menoufya University for supporting our work.

Author details

Elsayed Ibrahim Salama*

Address all correspondence to: elsayedsalama5@yahoo.com

Pediatric Department, National, Menoufia University, Egypt

References

[1] Al, Hasany. M., & Mohamed, A. (1970). Veno occlusive disease of Liver in Iraq. *Archives of disease in childhood*, 45(243), 722-724.

[2] Rollins, B. J. (1989). Hepatic Veno-occlusive Disease. *Am J of Med*, 8, 297.

[3] Bras, G., Jeliffe, D. B., & Stuart, K. L. (1954). *Arch Path, Chicago*, 57, 285.

[4] Stein, H. (1957). Veno-occlusive disease of the liver in African children. *Br Med J*, 1, 1496.

[5] Tandon, B. N., Tandon, R., Tandon, H. D., Narndrunat, L., & Joghi, Y. K. (1976). An epidemic of veno-occlusive disease of liver in central India. *Lancet*, 271-272.

http://dx.doi.org/10.5772/50685

[6] Shirai, M., Nagashima, K., Iwasaki, S., & Mori, W. (1987). A light and scanning electron microscopic study of hepatic veno-occlusive disease. *Acta Path Jpn*, 37(12), 1961-711.

[7] Hashem, M. (1939). Etiology and Pathology of types of liver cirrhosis in Egyptian children. *J Egypt Med Association*, 22, 1-36.

[8] Mohabbat, O., Srivastava, R. N., Younos, M. S., Sedio, G. G., Merzad, A. A., & Aram, G. N. (1967). An outbreak of Hepatic Veno-occlusive Disease due to toxic Alkaloid in herbal tea in north western Afghanistan. *Lancet*, 7950, 269.

[9] Wilmot, F. C., & Robertson, G. W. (1920). Senecio disease and cirrhosis of liver due to senecio boisoning. *Lancet*, 11, 848-849.

[10] El Gholmy, A., El Nabaway, M., Khatab, M., Shukry, Gabr. M., El Sibie, B., Aidaro, S., & Soliman, L. (1956). Infantile liver cirrhosis of Egypt. *Gaz Egypt Ped Assoc*, 4, 320.

[11] Safouh, M. A., Shehata, A., & Elwi, A. (1965). Veno occlusive disease in Egyptian Children. *Arch Path*, 79, 505.

[12] Mc Lean, E. K. (1969). The early sinusoidal lesion in experimental veno occlusive disease of the liver. *British Journal of Experimental Pathology*, 223 -22.

[13] Mellis, C., & Bale, P. M. (1976). Famelial hepatic Veno occlusive disease with probable immune deficiency. *J Pediatrics*, 88, 236-242.

[14] Mc Dermott, W. V., & Ridker, P. M. (1990). The Budd-Chiari syndrome and hepatic veno occlusive. Recognition and treatment. *Archives of surgery*, 125(4), 525-527.

[15] Nattakom, T. V., Charlton, A., & Wilmore, D. W. (1995). Use of Vitamine E. and glutamine in the successful treatment of severe VOD following bone marrow transplantation. *Nutritionin Clinical Practice*, 10(1), 16-18.

[16] Fogteloo, A. J., Smid, W. M., Kok, T., Van Der Meer, J., Van Imhoff, G. W., & Daenen, S. (1993). Successful treatment of veno occlusive disease of the liver with urokinase in a patient with non-hodgkin's lymphoma. *Leukemia*, 7(5), 760-763.

[17] Simpson, D. R., Browett, P. J., Doak, P. B., & Palmer, S. J. (1994). Successful treatment of veno occlusive disease with recombinant tissue plasminogen activator in a patient requiring peritoneal dialysis. *Bone Marrow Transplantation*, 14(4), 635-636.

[18] Cuenoud, P. F., & Mosiman, F. (1992). Surgical treatment of Budd-Chiari syndrome and VOD. *Helvetica Chirurgica Acta*, 58(6), 805-808.

[19] Le Veen, H. H., Christoudias, G., Moon, J. P., et al. (1974). Peritoneovenous shunting for ascites. *Ann Surg*, 180, 580-591.

[20] Le Veen, H. H., Vujic, ., D'Ovidio, N. J., & Hutto, R. B. (1984). Peritoneovenous shunt occlusion: Etiology. diagnosis, therapy. *Ann Surg*, 212-223.

[21] Salemo, F., Badalamenti, S., Incerti, P., et al. (1987). Repeated paracentesis and IV albumin infusion to treat "tense " ascites in cirrhotic patients a safe alternative therapy. *J Hepatol*, 5, 102-108.

[22] Stanley, A. M., Ochi, S., Lee, K. K., et al. (1989). Peritoneovenous shunting as compared with medical treatment in patients with alcoholic cirrhosis and massive ascites. *N Engl J Med*, 321, 1632-1638.

[23] Stanley, M. M. (1985). PVS in patients with cirrhotic ascites and end-stage renal failure. *Am Kidney Dis*, 6, 185-187.

[24] Smajda, C., Tridart, D., & Franco, D. (1986). Recurrent ascites due to central venous thrombosis after peritoneojugular (LeVeen) shunt. *Surgery*, 100, 535-540.

[25] Sale, H. H., Dudley, F. J., Merret, A., et al. (1983). Coagulopathy of peritoneovenous shunt studies on the pathogenic role of ascitic fluid collagen and value of antiplatelet therapy. *Gut*, 24, 412-417.

[26] Rosch, J., Hanafee, W. N., & Snow, H. (1969). Transjugular portal venography and radiological portocaval shunt: an experimental study. *Radiology*, 92, 1112-1114.

[27] Colapinto, R. F., Stonell, R. D., Birch, S. J., et al. (1982). Creation of an intrahepatic portosystemic shunt with a Gruntzig balloon catheter. *Can Med Assoc*, 126, 267-268.

[28] Haag, K., Noldge, G., Sellinger, M., Ochs, A., Gerok, W., & Rossle, M. (1992). Transjugular intrahepatic portosystemic stent shunt (TIPS). Monitoring of function by color duplex sonography. *Gastroenterology*, 102, 817.

[29] Palmaz, I. C., Sibbit, R. R., Reuter, S. R., Garcia, F., & Tio, F. O. (1985). Expandable intraheptic portacaval shunt stents. Early experience in the dog. *Am J Roentgenol*, 145, 821-825.

[30] Conn, H. (1993). Transjugular intrahepatic portal systemic shunts: the state of the art. *Hepatology*, 17, 148-158.

[31] Gilles, Mentha., Giostra, Emiliano, Majno, Pietro E., Bechstein, Wolf. O., Neuhaus, Peter., O'Grady, John., Praseedom, Raaj. K., Burroughs, Andrew. K., Treut, Yves. P., Kirkegaard, Preben., Rogiers, Xavier., Ericzon, Goran -Bo., Hockersted, Krister., Adam, René., & Juergen, Klempnaue. (2005). Liver transplantation for Budd-Chiari syndrome: A European study on 248 patients from 51 centres. *Sciences*, 50(3), 540-546.

Chapter 24

Progressive Familial Intrahepatic Cholestasis

Ahmad Mohamed Sira and Mostafa Mohamed Sira

Additional information is available at the end of the chapter

http://dx.doi.org/10.5772/51769

1. Introduction

Neonatal cholestasis is one of the commonest presentations in the field of pediatric hepatology and gastroenterology and constitutes the major indication for liver transplantation below two years of age. Unfortunately, in spite of being common, fewer categories are amenable to curative or palliative therapy. Moreover, delayed referral to specialized centers is still a problem adding a more difficulty to neonatal cholestasis management. Hepatobiliary surgery is a major line of therapy in some etiologies of neonatal cholestasis. Biliary atresia, choledochal cyst, spontaneous perforation of the bile duct and inspissated bile syndrome are among the commonest known causes for hepatobiliary surgeons. However, there is less orientation about other causes, resulting in progression to cirrhosis and end stage liver disease without being diagnosed. One of these is the progressive familial intrahepatic cholestasis (PFIC) group of diseases [1].

PFIC is an autosomal recessive liver disorder characterized by an intrahepatic cholestasis due to bile canalicular transport defects. It is subdivided into three types with slightly different clinical, biochemical and histological features. PFIC types 1, 2 and 3 are due to mutations in *ATP8B1* (adenosine triphosphatase, type 8B, member 1), *ABCB11* (adenosine triphosphate-binding cassette, subfamily B, member 11) and *ABCB4* (adenosine triphosphate-binding cassette, subfamily B, member 4) genes, respectively. Each of these genes encodes a hepatocanalicular transporter which is essential for the proper secretion and formation of bile [2].

PFIC1 and PFIC2 usually appear in the first months of life, whereas onset of PFIC3 may also occur later in infancy, in childhood or even during young adulthood. The shared main clinical manifestations in all types are cholestasis and pruritus. PFIC represents 10-15 % of causes of cholestasis in children and 10-15% of indications of liver transplantations in children [3].

In this chapter, we want to highlight the etiology, pathophysiology, clinical presentation and the role of surgery in the management of this disease category, especially that medical therapy is of limited value in a magnitude of cases. Moreover, liver transplant is not without significant side effects. So, raising the orientation about this not uncommon condition will help in timely surgical intervention and improving patients' outcome.

2. Historical background

This disorder was first described by Clayton in 1965, and was termed Byler's disease after an American Amish kindred in which it was discovered [4]. Clinical features included severe pruritus, steatorrhea, poor growth and progression to cirrhosis in early childhood. A prominent finding was a low or normal serum gamma glutamyl transpeptidase (GGT), which was discordant with the severe cholestasis. Since its discovery, similar clinical features were described in non-Amish children. Therefore, the more descriptive term, PFIC, is preferred [5].

However, this PFIC nomenclature is not always entirely satisfactory. A preferable term is "bile canalicular transport disorders," especially as it has become apparent that these genetic disorders have numerous clinical phenotypes across all age brackets. For example, benign recurrent intrahepatic cholestasis (BRIC) and intrahepatic cholestasis of pregnancy (ICP) can occur in association with abnormalities in any of the three affected genes [2,6]. However, the PFIC nomenclature is still in use due to its popularity in the literature.

Benign recurrent intrahepatic cholestasis, first described in 1959, is an intermittent form of intrahepatic cholestasis characterized by variable periods of intense pruritus often associated with jaundice [7]. The age of onset is variable, but it typically occurs during childhood or adolescence. The severity and duration of attacks also vary and triggering features are not well known. The benign designation of BRIC refers to the general lack of progressive liver disease, although the pruritus is far from benign during an intense episode [8-10].

As the clinical spectrum between BRIC and PFIC (formerly named Byler's disease) may be a continuum, thus the historical nomenclature of Byler's disease and BRIC may be outdated [11]. So, many clinicians now refer to all these diseases in a general sense as ATP8B1, ABCB11 and ABCB4 deficiency diseases to express the wide continuum of disease severity between the PFIC and BRIC phenotypes [2].

3. Etiology and pathophysiology

3.1. PFIC 1 (ATP8B1 "FIC-1" deficiency)

PFIC1 is an autosomal recessive disease caused by mutations in *ATP8B1* (formerly named *FIC1*) gene on chromosome 18, locus q21-22. This gene encodes a transporter localized on the canalicular membrane of hepatocytes (Figure 1), named FIC1 (ATP8B1), a P-type ATPase [12].

http://dx.doi.org/10.5772/51769

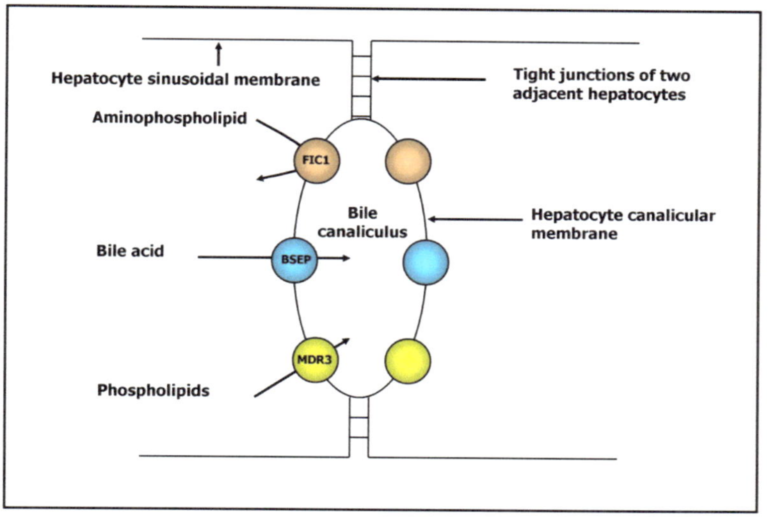

Abbreviations: FIC1: familial intrahepatic cholestasis 1; BSEP: bile salt export pump; MDR3: multidrug resistence protein 3.

Figure 1. A schematic representation of the hepatocyte with its canalicular membrane transporters involved in bile formation. FIC1 is an aminophospholipid flippase, encoded by the *ATP8B1* (*FIC1*) gene. BSEP (bile salt export pump) (formerly sister of P-glycoprotein "SPGP") is a bile acids transporter to the bile canalicular lumen against a high concentration gradient. It is encoded by the *ABCB11* (*BSEP*) gene. The MDR3 is a phospholipid transporter. It is encoded by the *ABCB4* (*MDR3*) gene.

The most widely accepted hypothesis for FIC1 function is that of an aminophospholipid flippase, translocating phospholipids such as phosphatidylserine from the outer to the inner leaflet of the plasma membrane [13]. So, deficiency of FIC1 in the hepatocyte results in the loss of asymmetric distribution of phospholipids in the canalicular membrane, decreasing both membrane stability and function of transmembrane transporters including the bile salt export pump (BSEP) and, as such, causing bile salt retention in hepatocytes with consequent defective bile formation; resulting in cholestasis [14-16].

Different studies have shown that ATP8B1 deficiency is associated with diminished FXR (farnesoid X receptor) activity. The FXR is a nuclear receptor that is highly expressed in the liver and regulates bile acid homeostasis so as to reduce its hepatocyte toxicity. Diminished FXR activity leads to upregulation of bile acid synthesis, reduced expression of the canalicular BSEP, and increased expression of the ileal apical sodium dependent bile acid transporter (ASBT). The net effect of these changes would be increased synthesis of bile acids and diminished its canalicular excretion, coupled with enhanced reabsorption of intestinal bile acids, yielding marked hepatocyte bile acid overload [17,18].

ATP8B1 is abundantly expressed in a wide variety of tissues such as the small intestine, bladder and stomach and to a lesser extent also in the liver and pancreas. This results in the multitude of the extrahepatic manifestations such as the hearing loss, pancreatitis and diarrhea, found in patients with ATP8B1 deficiency [19,20]. Over 50 distinct mutations in

ATP8B1 are described. The mutations G308V found in Amish, D554N found in Inuits and I661T are amongst the most frequently detected [21,22].

In vitro studies showed that ATP8B1 deficiency due to common missense mutations such as G308V, D554N and I661T, can be regarded as a protein folding disease, with different degrees of retention of the mutant protein in the endoplasmic reticulum, resulting in a decreased protein expression at the plasma membrane [23]. The pathophysiologic concept of being a protein folding disease can be used in new therapeutic interventions [24]. Incubation at a reduced temperature could improve proper folding of some of the mutated proteins. Similarly, the pharmacological chaperone 4-phenylbutyrate acid (4-PBA) could stabilize misfolded proteins, partially restoring cell surface expression [25].

Mutations in ATP8B1 are also responsible for:

1. Greenland Eskimo cholestasis (Nielsen syndrome) [26].
2. Benign recurrent intrahepatic cholestasis-1 (BRIC1) [12].
3. Intrahepatic cholestasis of pregnancy-1 (ICP1) [27].
4. Down regulation of CFTR (cystic fibrosis transmembrane regulator): ATP8B1 is highly expressed in biliary epithelial cells, and when it is abnormal in PFIC1, CFTR down regulation in cholangiocytes has been reported which could contribute to impairment of bile secretion [28].

3.2. PFIC 2 (ABCB11 "BSEP" deficiency)

PFIC2 is an autosomal recessive disease caused by mutations in the *ABCB11* (formerly named *BSEP*) gene encoding the BSEP, a liver-specific adenosine triphosphate (ATP)-binding cassette transporter formerly known as sister of P-glycoprotein (SPGP). BSEP is located in the hepatocyte canalicular membrane (Figure 1). *ABCB11* gene is located on chromosome 2, locus q24 [29-31].

The defective canalicular BSEP expression leads to markedly diminished bile salt secretion. This leads to bile secretory failure with secondary retention of bile salts and other biliary constituents in the hepatocytes leading to progressive liver damage and progressive cholestasis. BSEP deficiency represents also a phenotypic continuum between BRIC2 and PFIC2. Different mutations may cause different kinds of BSEP dysfunction, including protein lack, misfolded protein, or protein not delivered from the Golgi to the bile canalicular membrane [31].

Generally missense mutations, e.g. E297G or D482G, lead to a less severe phenotype than mutations that are predicted to result in premature protein truncation or total failure of protein production [31,32]. In vitro, the residual transport function of mutant proteins correlates with the phenotypic differences between BRIC2 and PFIC2, with generally a diminished function in BRIC2 mutants, while complete abolishment is more often seen in PFIC2 mutants [33].

Heterozygous *ABCB11* mutations have also been identified in cases of ICP (ICP2) [34], drug induced cholestasis [35] and transient neonatal cholestasis [36].

3.3. PFIC 3 (ABCB4 "MDR3" deficiency)

PFIC3 is an autosomal recessive disorder due to mutations in the *ABCB4* (formerly named *MDR3*) gene located on chromosome 7, locus q21, which codes for the class III multidrug resistance P-glycoprotein (MDR3). MDR3 is located exclusively on the canalicular membrane of the hepatocyte and serves as a phospholipid translocator (Figure 1) essential for biliary phospholipid (e.g. phosphatidylcholine "PC") secretion [37].

PC in bile normally protects cholangiocytes from bile salt toxicity by forming mixed micelles with it. However, a mutation of the *ABCB4* gene results in decreased biliary PC secretion and high biliary bile salt -to-PC ratio, leading to bile duct injury (cholangitis and ductular proliferation). Also, a decreased biliary PC concentration leads to high biliary cholesterol -to-PC ratio. The high biliary cholesterol saturation promotes crystallization of cholesterol and the lithogenicity of bile [2,38].

Whereas biliary bile salt concentrations are normal in patients with PFIC3, serum bile salt levels are elevated. It is explained by:

1. Downregulation of the bile acid importers to the hepatocyte, NTCP (Na+/taurocholate cotransporting polypeptide) and OATP (organic acid transporting polypeptide) [39].
2. Upregulation of the bile acid exporter from hepatocyte at the sinusoidal membrane, MRP4 (multidrug resistance–related protein 4), mediating bile salt efflux into serum [40].

Over 45 disease-causing mutations in *ABCB4* have been identified [41]. Children with missense mutations seem to have a less severe phenotype, with later onset of disease, slower progression and better response to treatment, as compared to patients with mutations leading to a truncated protein [42]. Possibly this is due to residual transport activity in MDR3 protein affected by missense mutations.

Heterozygous mutations in the *ABCB4* gene can also cause or predispose for a variety of other liver diseases, such as adult biliary cirrhosis, cholelithiasis, transient neonatal cholestasis, drug induced cholestasis and ICP. Mutations can even lead to a cascade of several phenotypes in one patient, indicating the wide phenotypical spectrum of ABCB4 deficiency [43,44].

A small proportion of PFIC phenotypes are not due to mutations in these three genes and therefore additional genes might be involved [2,45].

4. Clinical picture

Mutations in *ATP8B1* and *ABCB11* can result both in progressive cholestatic disease termed PFIC1 and PFIC2, as well as in episodic cholestasis, referred to as BRIC type 1 and 2 respectively. This suggests that PFIC and BRIC are the two ends of a clinical spectrum, with different degrees of severity in between. Therefore, these diseases are preferably referred to as ATP8B1 deficiency and ABCB11 deficiency. While mutations in *ABCB4* can result in progressive cholestatic disease only designated PFIC type 3. Similarly PFIC3 is best designated as *ABCB4* deficiency. Heterozygous mutations in any of these three genes can also be associated with ICP. It is a transient form of cholestasis, characterized by the onset of pruritus during pregnancy, with postnatal resolution [2].

Pruritus is the prominent clinical feature of PFIC; however, until an episode of jaundice intervenes, the diagnosis is often overlooked. Even then, because of the rarity of the condition, children sometimes receive a misdiagnosis of obstructive jaundice caused by the occasionally associated choledocholithiasis in PFIC types 2 and 3 [5].

4.1. PFIC1 "Byler's disease"

- Cholestasis is a major clinical sign in PFIC1 as in all PFIC forms. It usually appears in the first months of life in patients with PFIC1, and is characterized by recurrent episodes of jaundice, which become permanent later in the course of the disease [3]. The variable clinical features are:

1. *Jaundice*: It presents with conjugated hyperbilirubinemia in the first 3–6 months of life. The degree of jaundice may vary [46].
2. *Pruritus*: It is the dominant feature in the majority of patients and is often out of proportion to the level of jaundice [46]. It may initially vary in intensity and may be exacerbated during intercurrent illness. Pruritus may not be noticed until 6 months of age because the neural pathways necessary for concerted scratching are not fully developed. However, affected infants often are irritable and sleep poorly with onset of cholestasis. Scratching is usually evident first as digging at the ears and eyes, which are the first areas to show evidence of excoriation. By one year of age, patients may show generalized mutilation of skin, usually most severe on the extensor surfaces of the arms and legs and on the flanks of the back. The pruritus is very disabling and often responds poorly to medical therapies [12,45].
3. *Hepatomegaly* is present early in life and persists with progression to cirrhosis. The rate of progression to cirrhosis is variable, but usually develops in early childhood without treatment. With progression to cirrhosis splenomegaly develops.
4. *Fat-soluble vitamin deficiencies*, including rickets, may be severe.
5. *Extrahepatic disorders* [19]:
   - Persistent diarrhea with fat malabsorption and protein loss, leading to poor growth and short stature.
   - Bouts of pancreatitis.
   - Recurrent pneumonia may also compromise growth.
   - Sensorineural hearing loss may occur.

- As it has been mentioned before, ATP8B1 deficiency can lead to a continuum of disease severity ranging from the progressive form PFIC1 to the recurrent form, BRIC1. BRIC1 will be discussed briefly in the next paragraphs.

  BRIC is an intermittent form of intrahepatic cholestasis characterized by variable periods of intense pruritus often associated with jaundice, separated by symptom-free intervals. The benign designation of BRIC refers to the general lack of progressive liver disease, although the pruritus is far from benign during an intense episode [10]. Two types of BRIC are present according to the gene defect. BRIC1 is due to a mutation of *ATP8B1* gene and BRIC2, due to *ABCB11* gene mutations.

The age of presentation of the first attack of jaundice ranges from 1–50 years, but jaundice usually occurs before the age of twenty years. Attacks usually are preceded by a minor illness and consist of a preicteric phase of 2–4 weeks (characterized by malaise, anorexia, and pruritus) and an icteric phase that may last from 1–18 months. In some patients, hormonal factors such as the use of oral contraceptives and pregnancy have been associated with precipitation of an attack [10,47]. Patients may have severe coughing during episodes, as is seen sometimes in patients with PFIC1 [48].

During the icteric phase, the concentrations of serum bile acid, bilirubin, and alkaline phosphatase (ALP) are increased. Serum GGT concentration, however, remains low. Liver biopsy results are very benign, often showing no pathologic change even during an episode. Some specimens show hepatocellular cholestasis and cholate injury, mostly centrilobular. During the asymptomatic period, all parameters (clinical, laboratory and liver histology) are normal [49].

4.2. PFIC2 "Byler's syndrome"

- PFIC2 affected children differ from those with PFIC1 in some important respects:

  The initial presentation and the evolution seem to be more severe than PFIC1, with permanent jaundice from the first months of life and rapid appearance of cirrhosis and liver failure within the first years of life [3].

  They do not have extrahepatic involvement such as pancreatitis or diarrhea [45].

  Early hepatocellular carcinoma (before one year of age) may complicate the course of PFIC2 [3]. Up to 15% of the patients with ABCB11 deficiency will develop hepatocellular carcinoma (HCC) or cholangiocarcinoma. Close surveillance for hepatobiliary malignancy is therefore warranted in these patients [31,32,45].

  At diagnosis, the cholestasis in ABCB11 deficiency results in a more detectable fat-soluble vitamin deficiency manifestations [45].

  The development of cholelithiasis in approximately one third of the patients, probably due to the low bile salt concentration in bile, secondary to impaired BSEP function, which might cause supersaturation of cholesterol [32].

- Patients fitting the phenotype of BRIC have been described with mutations in *ABCB11.* They are called BRIC2 and are characterized by:

  The age of onset and total number of recurrent episodes were highly variable. Cholelithiasis occurred in many patients with BRIC2. Several patients had a relatively early onset of the disease and developed permanent cholestasis as adults after initial periods of recurrent attacks.

Occasionally BRIC will progress to the more severe and permanent form of PFIC, indicative of a clinical continuum, with intermediate phenotypes between mild and progressive disease [2,11].

4.3. PFIC3 "MDR3 deficiency"

Mutations in the *ABCB4* gene can cause or predispose to a variety of liver diseases with different age of presentation. Moreover, it can even lead to a cascade of several phenotypes in one patient, indicating the wide phenotypical spectrum of ABCB4 deficiency [43].

1. *PFIC3*: it is characterized by:
   - *Cholestasis* developing within the first year of life in about one third of patients and rarely in the neonatal period. It may also manifest later in infancy, in childhood or even in young adulthood [3,45].
   - *Pruritus* occurs less frequently than in the other types of PFIC and is usually mild.
   - *Jaundice* may be less prominent than pruritus.
   - *Height and weight* may be below normal as the disease progresses.
   - *Hepatomegaly*, and at later stages splenomegaly, as a manifestation of portal hypertension is often observed. Liver disease tends to evolve slowly to biliary cirrhosis with or without overt cholestatic jaundice [42,50].
   - *Cholelithiasis* may develop in older children.
   - *No extrahepatic features* or occurrence of malignancies are described in association with PFIC3 [42,50].
2. *Adult biliary cirrhosis*: gastrointestinal bleeding due to portal hypertension and cirrhosis may be the presenting symptom in adolescent or young adult patients [3].
3. *ICP*: some cases of ICP have been associated with heterozygous mutations in *ABCB4* [43].
4. Heterozygous mutations in the *ABCB4* gene can also cause or predispose for transient neonatal cholestasis and drug induced cholestasis [44].

5. Diagnosis

Diagnosis is dependent firstly on suspicion. The most alarming point making PFIC in the scope of diagnosis is the presence of significant pruritus out of proportion to the level of jaundice especially in the setting of low GGT. However, accurate diagnosis is dependent on a constellation of a clinical, biochemical, radiological, histopathological, immunohistochemical studies and finally can be confirmed by genetic testing for mutations (Table 1).

1. *Biochemical parameters*:

- *Serum GGT* is repeatedly normal or low in PFIC1 & PFIC2, while it is elevated in PFIC3 often more than ten times the normal value. In PFIC1 and PFIC2, the serum GGT concentration may increase to greater than 100 IU/L in patients receiving microsomal inducers such as phenobarbital and rifampicin [51].

  The mechanism for the low serum concentration of GGT in PFIC1 and 2 is not clear. GGT is normally bound to the canalicular membrane by a glycosyl phosphatidyl inositol (GPI) anchor. In obstructive cholestasis, when excessive amounts of bile salts accumulate in the canalicular lumen under increased pressure, GGT is released from the membrane by detergent action and refluxes back into serum, possibly via leaky intercellular junctions. However, in PFIC and BRIC types 1 and 2, the reduced concentrations of biliary bile acids preserve canalicular GGT localization. This explanation is not entirely satisfactory as serum GGT is elevated in most other forms of intrahepatic cholestasis in which biliary bile acid levels are low. Preliminary studies indicate that some canalicular proteins, including GGT and carcinoembryonic antigen (CEA), are poorly expressed at the canaliculus in PFIC1 and 2. It is possible that low serum GGT levels result from the lack of canalicular GGT available for elution as well as from the inadequate concentrations of intracanalicular bile acids to act as detergents [51,52].

- *Serum transaminases*: In PFIC1 serum transaminases are mildly elevated. While in patients with PFIC2, serum transaminases levels are usually elevated to at least five times normal values. In PFIC3, serum aminotransferases, conjugated bilirubin, and ALP are all significantly elevated [2,45].
- *Serum cholesterol*: it is characteristically low or normal in all the three types [3].
- *Serum bile acid concentration*: it is elevated in all the three types [44,45].
- *Alpha-fetoprotein*: it is elevated at diagnosis in PFIC2 than that in PFIC1 [12,45].
- *Absent serum lipoprotein X (LPX) in PFIC3*: because measurement of biliary phospholipids is impractical in the evaluation of most patients, measurement of serum LPX may serve as a surrogate marker for PFIC3. LPX is the predominant lipoprotein in the plasma of cholestatic patients. LPX is absent from the serum of patients with homozygous *ABCB4* mutations. LPX is probably composed of biliary vesicles that are formed at the subapical compartment of the hepatocyte, transcytosed to sinusoidal membrane, and released into plasma. This process is absolutely dependent on MDR3, but the precise mechanism has not been defined [50,53].

2. *Biliary bile analysis*:

Biliary bile analysis is performed on gallbladder bile or on bile collected by duodenal aspiration (pure choledochal bile). In case of gallbladder punction, bile contamination by blood may falsify bile analysis. In case of duodenal aspiration, bile dilution or bile contamination by alimentary phospholipids may falsify bile analysis [3].

The biliary bile salt concentration is dramatically decreased (<1 mmol/L) in PFIC2 patients [54] and only mildly decreased in PFIC1 patients (3–8 mmol/L) [19]. The normal concentration of biliary primary bile salts distinguishes PFIC3 patients from those with PFIC1 and PFIC2 [42].

In PFIC3 patients, the cardinal feature is the dramatically decreased biliary phospholipid level (1–15% of total biliary lipids; normal range 19–24%). Biliary bile salt-to-phospholipid is approximately 5-fold higher than in wild type bile, as is also biliary cholesterol-to-phospholipid [3].

3. *Radiological*:

Initial ultrasonography of the liver is performed to exclude biliary tract disease. Typically, ultrasonography is normal but may reveal a huge gallbladder in PFIC3. Sometimes, biliary stones may be identified in both PFIC2 and PFIC3 [3].

Cholangiography performed in a limited number of patients with PFIC3 showed a normal biliary tree, excluding sclerosing cholangitis, and allowed bile to be collected for biliary lipid analysis [42].

4. *Histopathology: Liver biopsy shows*:

- *In PFIC1*

  Light microscopy (LM): on routine hematoxylin and eosin (H & E) staining, liver biopsy shows bland cholestasis with almost no inflammation. It shows canalicular bile plugs of distinctive color. Small-duct paucity may be present. Fibrosis starts early, with approximately 75 % of patients having some fibrosis by 2 years of age. Fibrosis may appear initially either as pericentral sclerosis or portal fibrosis, or sometimes both. Portal to central bridging then develops in association with lacy lobular fibrosis and eventually leads to cirrhosis. Proliferating bile ductules are observed at the edge of the portal tracts in patients with significant fibrosis. The rate of progression of the fibrosis is highly variable but correlates loosely with the severity of the clinical disease [45].

  On electron microscopy (EM), canalicular bile plugs shows characteristic granular appearance "chunky bile".

- *In PFIC2*

  LM: on H & E stains, there is inflammation with giant cell hepatitis, fibrosis and duct reaction [45].

  On EM, bile appears amorphous [45].

- *In PFIC3*

  LM: on H & E stains, bile ductular proliferation and mixed inflammatory infiltrates are observed in the early stages despite patency of intra- and extrahepatic bile ducts. Cholestasis with slight giant cell transformation and isolated eosinophilic necrotic hepatocytes may also be present. Periductal sclerosis affecting the interlobular bile ducts eventually occurs. Extensive portal fibrosis evolves into biliary cirrhosis in older children [42].

  EM of liver has not been reported in proven cases.

5. *Immunohistochemical staining*:

http://dx.doi.org/10.5772/51769

Commercially available MDR3 and BSEP antibodies allow liver immunostaining to be performed. Absence of canalicular or mild immunostaining is in favor of a gene defect. However, normal staining does not exclude a gene defect as a mutation may induce a loss of function but normal synthesis [31,42].

6. *Genetic testing*:

Molecular analysis remains the definitive diagnostic technique for PFIC. Gene analysis is usually performed by DNA sequencing of the 27 coding exons (coding exons 2-28) of the *ATP8B1*, *ABCB11*, and *ABCB4* genes and their splice junctions [3]. The use of a resequensing chip dedicated to genetic cholestasis could facilitate identification of gene mutation [55].

	PFIC-1	**PFIC-2**	**PFIC-3**
Synonyms	Byler disease ATP8B1 deficiency FIC1 deficiency	Byler syndrome ABCB11 deficiency BSEP deficiency	ABCB4 deficiency MDR3 deficiency
Gene defect	*ATP8B1 (FIC1)*	*ABCB11 (BSEP)*	*ABCB4 (MDR3)*
Locus	18q21-22	2q24	7q21
Transport defect	Aminophospholipid	Bile acid	Phospholipids
Pathophysiology	Impaired inward translocation of aminophospholipids over cellular membranes	Impaired canalicular bile salt transport secondary to malfunction of BSEP	Impaired canalicular translocation of phosphatidylcholine
Clinical picture:			
Onset of cholestasis	Neonatal	Neonatal	Variable
Pruritus	Severe	Severe	Moderate
Extrahepatic manifestations	Present	Absent	Absent
Cholelithiasis	Absent	Increased incidence	Increased incidence
HCC	No	Risk from the 1st year	No
Clinical spectrum of gene defect	PFIC1, BRIC1, and ICP	PFIC2, BRIC2, and ICP	PFIC3, ICP, adult biliary cirrhosis, cholelithiasis, transient neonatal cholestasis, drug induced cholestasis
Biochemical:			
GGT	Normal or low	Normal or low	Elevated
Transaminases	Mildly elevated	More elevated	Elevated
Bile acids	Elevated	More elevated	Elevated
Cholesterol	Normal	Normal	Normal
Alpha fetoprotein	Not significantly elevated	More elevated	--
Histopathological	Bland cholestasis (LM) Coarse granular bile (EM	Giant cell hepatitis (LM) Amorphous bile (EM)	Ductular proliferation (LM)
Immunohistochemical	--	Absent or reduced BSEP staining in the majority of patients	Absent or reduced MDR3 staining in about 50 % of patients

Table 1. Summary of the criteria of different PFIC types.

6. Differential diagnosis

Two groups of diseases are in differential diagnosis with PFIC group of disorders. For PFIC1 and PFIC2, it is to be differentiated from other cholestatic disorders with low GGT. While for PFIC3, when it presents early it, is to be differentiated from cholestatic disorders with high GGT and when it presents in an older age, childhood or adolescence, it is to be differentiated from other causes of chronic liver diseases at respective ages.

- *Cholestasis with low GGT*:
  1. Inborn errors of bile acid metabolism [6].
  2. Familial hypercholanemia: familial hypercholanemia represents a PFIC-like disorder due to a bile canalicular tight junction protein defect combined with a defect of primary bile acid conjugation. Cholestasis is due to impaired transport of unconjugated bile acids into bile and to bile leakage into plasma through abnormal canalicular tight junctions increasing paracellular permeability [56].
  3. Arthrogryposis- renal dysfunction cholestasis (ARC) syndrome is a complex disease due to mutation of *VPS33B* involved in intracellular trafficking and targeting of apical proteins. The gene defect results in a loss of apical protein expression in the liver and kidneys [57].
- *Cholestasis with high GGT*:
  1. Biliary atresia [58].
  2. Neonatal sclerosing cholangitis [59].
  3. Congenital cytomegalovirus (CMV) infection.
  4. Alpha1-antitrypsin deficiency disease [60].
  5. North American Indian Childhood Cirrhosis (NAIC) [61].
  6. Aagenaes syndrome (hereditary cholestasis with lymphedema): a very rare familial cholestatic disorder with cholestasis and lower limb edema [62].
- *Causes of chronic liver disease*:
  1. Chronic viral hepatitis.
  2. Autoimmune liver diseases: autoimmune hepatitis and autoimmune sclerosing cholangitis.
  3. Metabolic liver disorders, e.g., Wilson disease and alpha1-antitrypsin deficiency.

7. Treatment

Initial treatment of PFIC includes the use of cholestyramine, ursodeoxycholic acid, rifampicin, and phenobarbital [63-65]. Until the late 1980s, liver transplantation was the only effective therapy for those who did not respond to medical treatment [66,67]. Later on, less invasive non-transplant surgical approaches were proposed and undertaken early in the course of the disease with promising initial results [68]. In this section, a brief overview about the different lines of management for PFIC patients will be given.

7.1. Medical therapy

Unfortunately, most forms of medical therapy for PFIC types 1, 2, and 3 are of limited effectiveness. Nevertheless, several treatment modalities can be used in specific patients to improve quality of life or prevent progression of the disease [2,69].

- *Cholestyramine* is an anion-exchange resin that binds bile salts, preventing their re-absorption in the enterohepatic circulation. In PFIC, relief of pruritus and normalization of biochemical parameters is only described rarely with cholestyramine. However, in patients with BRIC it can be helpful in shortening episodes [2].
- *Rifampicin*, although it accelerates the hepatic detoxification and excretion of compounds, such as bilirubin and bile salts, it has been used with limited efficacy in patients with PFIC [51]. Nevertheless, in patients with BRIC it can completely abort an episode.
- *Ursodeoxycholic acid (UDCA)* is a relatively hydrophilic bile salt, which is less cytotoxic than endogenous bile salts. Upon oral administration (20 mg/kg/day), it will partially replace endogenous bile salts in the bile salt pool, reducing injury of the hepatocytes during cholestasis. In PFIC3 regular administration of UDCA normalizes liver function tests and improves clinical parameters in up to 50% of the patients. The therapeutic effect appears to be dependent on the type of mutation, with premature stop codons leading to a truncated protein being associated with nearly no response to therapy. UDCA should therefore be the first choice in the initial therapeutic management of patients with ABCB4 deficiency, especially when a missense mutation in the corresponding gene is found [42]. In patients with PFIC1 or PFIC2, the results of UDCA treatment are conflicting, ranging from clear improvement to no effect at all.

In this respect, the recommended treatment strategy is to start with UDCA therapy in all types of PFIC, especially PFIC3. If no appropriate response, especially regarding pruritus, add the other medical lines of therapy. Those who will not respond are shifted to surgical treatment [3,45,65,66].

7.2. Surgical treatment

Surgical treatment for PFIC is an important major line of therapy. If no complete clinical or biochemical improvement is obtained with medical therapy, more invasive therapy such as biliary diversion or even liver transplantation is necessary [2,70].

Interruption of the enterohepatic circulation through biliary diversion has yielded excellent clinical, biochemical, and histologic response in a number of children with PFIC, provided the procedure is performed before the development of significant hepatic fibrosis [46]. It reduces the accumulation of toxic bile salts by decreasing their intestinal re-uptake. It is unclear if these approaches are optimal for specific genetic forms of PFIC rather than others. It is possible that these interventions may be best for severe PFIC1 and milder phenotypic variants of PFIC2. Nasobiliary drainage may help to select potential responders to biliary diversion [71].

There are three major non-transplant surgical techniques to permanently interrupt the enterohepatic circulation, namely partial external biliary diversion (PEBD), ileal bypass (IB) and partial internal biliary diversion (PIBD).

- *Partial external biliary diversion (PEBD)*:

PEBD interrupts the enterohepatic circulation of bile salts by partially diverting bile from the gallbladder through a loop of jejunum connecting the gallbladder to the abdominal skin [72].

In 1988, Whitington and Whitington [68] introduced cholecystojejunocutaneostomy as a PEBD for the surgical treatment of PFIC, to increase the elimination of bile acids accumulated within the body and thus control the intractable pruritus. In this procedure, one end of a loop of jejunum is anastamosed to the dome of the gallbladder, whereas the other is used to form a cutaneous ostomy (Figure 2A). Bile in the gallbladder then flows either out of the ostomy or into the intestine. Typically 30–50% of bile drains out of the ostomy and is discarded. Two variants on the original PEBD have also been described; one using a laparoscopic technique [73] and the other using an appendiceal conduit [74].

Results of PEBD are promising with respect to pruritus, jaundice and histology, both in patients with PFIC1 and PFIC2, with at least partial improvement in more than 75% of the patients [66,72]. Although this seems promising, at present it is unclear whether in patients responding to PEBD liver transplantation can also be avoided at long-term follow-up [75]. Moreover, some patients do not benefit from biliary surgery at all. Obviously in these patients liver transplantation should be considered [72].

The type of mutation seems to be associated with the outcome of PEBD, with better prognosis in disease caused by milder mutations, especially for the ABCB11 mutations E297G and D482G [32,45]. However, when severe fibrosis is already present at the moment of PEBD, prognosis is worse [72]. One patient with PFIC3 who underwent PEBD was described in literature; this patient showed no improvement [67].

No serious PEBD complications are reported, although problems with the stoma (stenosis, recurrent bleeding) (Figure 2) sometimes make a re-operation necessary. In addition excessive stomal losses can cause dehydration and electrolyte imbalance, while cholangitis can also develop [72,75].

The permanent character of the PEBD makes it less suitable for patients with episodic cholestasis (BRIC). In these patients temporary nasobiliary drainage (NBD) to interrupt the enterohepatic circulation can be endoscopically introduced. This procedure is effective in most of these patients, resolving pruritus and normalising bile salts within short time [10,71].

http://dx.doi.org/10.5772/51769

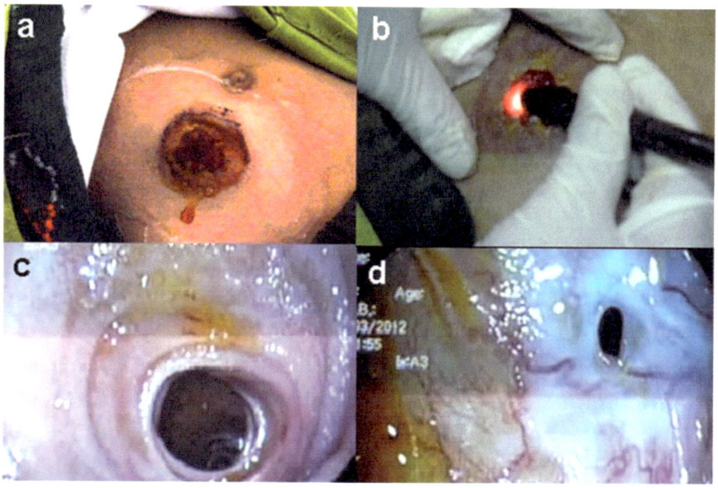

Figure 2. A seven years old child diagnosed as PFIC2 underwent PEBD at the age of 2 years old with good outcome. He had recurrent bleeding from the osteal opening (a). Endoscopy through the osteal opening (b) showed free jejunal loop (c) till its proximal end at the gall bladder (d). The source of bleeding was the stoma itself.

- *Terminal ileal exclusion or ileal bypass (IB)*:

Although most of PFIC patients and their parents tolerate well PEBD with its external biliary fistula and the need for stoma care, sometimes it becomes a real problem, particularly for children of school age and teenagers, who may feel uncomfortable to participate in all activities with their friends. Moreover, there is still a group of patients who cannot undergo PEBD because of a previous cholecystectomy, or who develop postoperative electrolyte inbalance due to the excessive daily amount of bile [5,76].

To deal with these problems, an IB technique was proposed. In IB, the terminal ileum is skipped by an ileocolonic anastomosis. It was developed as an alternative treatment to PEBD, that avoids a long-term stoma complications. In 1994, Whitington et al. described a good initial outcome of IB in two patients after cholecystectomy, but a chronic diarrhea occurred one year later. In 1998, Holland et al. described this procedure in PFIC children after cholecystectomy. All patients were supplemented with vitamin B12 and folic acid. Interestingly, no diarrhea was reported postoperatively. Early results were very promising, with a relief of pruritus and normalization of bilirubin level. Nevertheless, relapse of cholestatsis occurred in half of the patients. The authors underline that IB is not as effective as PEBD and therefore it should not be considered as the primary treatment in children with PFIC [5,51].

The rational of this technique was that the vast majority of intestinal bile salts are reabsorbed in the distal ileum; that is the distal 15% of the small intestine. Therefore, exclusion of this segment of intestine may lead to bile acid wasting. The small intestine is transected at a point that demarcates the distal 15% of the small intestine, and a blind loop is formed with the distal ileal segment. The proximal loop of the intestine is sewn end-to-side to the cecum, completing the internal bypass of the distal ileum. Accurate assessment of the appropriate amount of ileum for bypass is likely to be critical; too little is unlikely to be therapeutic and too much is likely to yield bile acid–induced diarrhea. Mutational analysis may be used eventually to predict which patients are most likely to benefit from surgery. After IB, symptoms may recur within one year requiring conversion to PEBD [5,77].

- *Partial internal biliary diversion (PIBD)*:

PIBD interrupts the enterohepatic circulation of bile salts by partially diverting bile from the gallbladder through a loop of jejunum connecting the gallbladder to the colon [46,76].

This operation combines the advantages of partially diverting the biliary flow from the enterohepatic cycle (such as the PEBD does), while at the same time avoiding an external biliary fistula. In addition, this operation lacks the potential for malabsorption that may result from partially excluding the terminal ileum from the intestinal transit. There is, however, a potential for choleretic diarrhea, which may result from large amounts of bile salts entering the colon. Because of this, it was strongly emphasized that the conduit should be made at least 15 cm long to create a certain resistance to the bile flow; it is believed that this stimulates a certain amount of bile to flow through the normal biliary tract to the duodenum. This problem occurred in a transient way in a few of the patients and it can be controlled with the use of cholestyramine for a limited span of time [46].

Through an upper midline abdominal incision, the gallbladder and the liver are evaluated. An intestinal conduit is constructed using a 15- to 20-cm segment of midjejunum, which is sutured initially to the gallbladder wall and then terminolaterally to the midportion of the ascending colon. The distal end of the jejunum is slightly tapered in a way that the jejunum could reach the colon in an isoperistaltic direction to prevent colonic contents from entering the conduit. The clinical and laboratory results described for PIBD make it a very attractive surgical option for the treatment of PFICs in children with a normal gallbladder. However, long-term follow-up is necessary to evaluate late results and eventual complications associated with this technique [46].

If all previously described therapies fails in controlling pruritus, when there is an end-stage PFIC liver disease, or when the disease is progressive despite treatment; orthotopic liver transplantation (OLT) remains the only alternative [78-80]. Before the development of liver transplantation, therapy for these patients was generally ineffective. With the advent of liver transplantation, many PFIC patients were treated with this life-saving procedure [70,78]. At one time, PFIC was among the 5 most common indications for liver transplantation in children [81,82].

Although OLT is associated with serious surgical risks and lifetime immunosuppressive therapy is necessary, it usually gives complete correction of phenotype in patients with PFIC2 and PFIC3 deficiency in which the disease is hepatocyte specific. However, phenotypic recurrence of severe PFIC2 deficiency post-transplantation can occur as a result of the formation of autoantibodies against BSEP [83,84]. Intensifying immunosuppressive therapy may resolve this problem.

http://dx.doi.org/10.5772/51769

In contrast, in PFIC1, liver transplantation is potentially fraught with a number of potential complications related to the extrahepatic expression of the *ATP8B1* gene. The most prominent posttransplantation problems include intractable diarrhea, hepatic steatosis, poor growth, and recurrent pancreatitis. Worsening diarrhea post liver transplant might be due to an imbalance between bile salt excretion and re-absorption, since the hepatic graft excretes a normal amount of bile salts, whereas the intestine remains functionally impaired. The resulting increased amount of bile salts in the ileum and colon induces or worsens diarrhea, which might respond to cholestyramine treatment [19,85]. Therefore, in PFIC1, non-transplant surgical approaches should be considered the preferred first-line of therapy.

In summary, children with PFIC do better with non-transplant surgical interventions than they do with the natural history of disease, which is uniformly fatal. Successful outcomes have been demonstrated, with marked improvements in clinical symptoms, laboratory values, growth and histology. It appears that the success rate is high enough that many patients may do better with a non-transplant procedure than transplant given the posttransplant morbidities associated with immunotherapy. Those with more advanced disease are most likely to have a poor outcome with non-transplant surgical procedures. This may encourage clinicians to consider a surgical intervention early in the course of disease before significant hepatic scarring develops [76].

Some authors proposed that the treatment strategy is to perform PEBD rapidly after diagnosis in patients with PFIC1 & PFIC2 and to consider OLT when treatment fails. In patients with PFIC3, UDCA treatment is the first-line therapy; if not successful it is followed by liver transplantation. In patients with episodic cholestasis (BRIC) medical treatment with rifampicin with or without cholestyramine can be attempted at the start of an attack. If medication is not successful in aborting the cholestatic episode NBD can be performed [2,69]. In BRIC patients who progress to a more permanent form of cholestasis, or in patients with very frequent or debilitating attacks, a biliary diversion can be considered [69].

7.3. New and future therapies

New and future therapies for PFIC patients include hepatocyte transplantation, the use of nuclear receptor ligands, enhancing the expression of the mutated transporter protein by employing chaperones and mutation specific therapy [2,69].

Hepatocyte transplantation has been successful in partially repopulating the liver, diminishing pathology in a mouse model of ABCB4 deficiency, but unfortunately not yet in patients [86]. In ABCB11 deficiency it is doubtful whether hepatocyte transplantation is a good therapeutic option since possible premalignant cells are left in place.

Certain nuclear receptors regulate bile formation. The key nuclear receptor in bile formation is the bile salt sensor FXR. Activated FXR transactivates a number of genes, resulting in improved bile salt excretion and detoxification. Targeting FXR with synthetic ligands is explored as a possible therapeutic option for cholestasis syndromes [87].

A pharmacological chaperone is defined as a small molecule that specifically binds to its target protein and induces or promotes proper folding and trafficking of the protein [88]. Some researchers have investigated the usefulness of pharmacological chaperones for treatment of diseases caused by folding-defective membrane proteins [24,89,90]. Pharmacological chaperones such as 4-phenylbutyrate acid (4-PBA) have been shown to stabilize proteins misfolded due to missense mutations, thereby preventing degradation in the endoplasmic reticulum. In vitro, 4-PBA enhances cell surface protein expression for some of the missense mutations found in ATP8B1 deficiency and ABCB11 deficiency [25,91]. Misawa et al [24], showed that bile acids do act as pharmacological chaperones of E297G BSEP. They also described the discovery and structural development of non-steroidal compounds with potent pharmacological chaperone activity for E297G BSEP.

Author details

Ahmad Mohamed Sira* and Mostafa Mohamed Sira

*Address all correspondence to: asira@liver-eg.org

Department of Pediatric Hepatology, National Liver Institute, Menofiya University, Egypt

References

[1] De Bruyne, R., Van Biervliet, S., Vande, Velde S., & Van Winckel, M. (2011). Clinical practice: neonatal cholestasis. *Eur J Pediatr*, 170(3), 279-284.

[2] Van der Woerd, W. L., van Mil, S. W., Stapelbroek, J. M., Klomp, L. W., van de Graaf, S. F., & Houwen, R. H. (2010). Familial cholestasis: progressive familial intrahepatic cholestasis, benign recurrent intrahepatic cholestasis and intrahepatic cholestasis of pregnancy. *Best Pract Res Clin Gastroenterol*, 24(5), 541-553.

[3] Davit-Spraul, A., Gonzales, E., Baussan, C., & Jacquemin, E. (2009). Progressive familial intrahepatic cholestasis. *Orphanet J Rare Dis*, 4(1).

[4] Clayton, R. J., Iber, F. L., Ruebner, B. H., & McKusick, V. A. (1969). Byler disease. Fatal familial intrahepatic cholestasis in an Amish kindred. *Am J Dis Child*, 117(1), 112-124.

[5] Hollands, C. M., Rivera-Pedrogo, F. J., Gonzalez-Vallina, R., Loret-de-Mola, O., Nahmad, M., & Burnweit, C. A. (1998). Ileal exclusion for Byler's disease: an alternative surgical approach with promising early results for pruritus. *J Pediatr Surg;*, 33(2), 220-224.

[6] Jankowska, I., & Socha, P. (2012). Progressive familial intrahepatic cholestasis and inborn errors of bile acid synthesis. *Clin Res Hepatol Gastroenterol*, 36(3), 271-274.

[7] Summerskill, W. H., & Walshe, J. M. (1959). Benign recurrent intrahepatic "obstructive" jaundice. *Lancet*, 2(7105), 686-690.

[8] Luketic, V. A., & Shiffman, M. L. (2004). Benign recurrent intrahepatic cholestasis. *Clin Liver Dis*, 8(1), 133-149, vii.

[9] Folvik, G., Hilde, O., & Helge, G. O. (2012). Benign recurrent intrahepatic cholestasis: review and long-term follow-up of five cases. *Scand J Gastroenterol*, 47(4), 482-488.

[10] Toros, A. B., Ozerdenen, F., Bektas, H., & Sari, N. D. (2012). A case report: nasobiliary drainage inducing remission in benign recurrent intrahepatic cholestasis. *Turk J Gastroenterol*, 23(1), 75-78.

[11] Van Ooteghem, N. A., Klomp, L. W., van Berge-Henegouwen, G. P., & Houwen, R. H. (2002). Benign recurrent intrahepatic cholestasis progressing to progressive familial intrahepatic cholestasis: low GGT cholestasis is a clinical continuum. *J Hepatol*, 36(3), 439-443.

[12] Van Mil, S. W., Klomp, L. W., Bull, L. N., & Houwen, R. H. (2001). FIC1 disease: a spectrum of intrahepatic cholestatic disorders. *Semin Liver Dis*, 21(4), 535-544.

[13] Verhulst, P. M., van der Velden, L. M., Oorschot, V., van Faassen, E. E., Klumperman, J., Houwen, R. H., Pomorski, T. G., Holthuis, J. C., & Klomp, L. W. (2010). A flippase-independent function of ATP8B1, the protein affected in familial intrahepatic cholestasis type 1, is required for apical protein expression and microvillus formation in polarized epithelial cells. *Hepatology*, 51(6), 2049-2060.

[14] Cai, S. Y., Gautam, S., Nguyen, T., Soroka, C. J., Rahner, C., & Boyer, J. L. (2009). ATP8B1 deficiency disrupts the bile canalicular membrane bilayer structure in hepatocytes, but FXR expression and activity are maintained. *Gastroenterology*, 1060-1069.

[15] Paulusma, C. C., Groen, A., Kunne, C., Ho-Mok, K. S., Spijkerboer, A. L., Rudi de, Waart. D., Hoek, F. J., Vreeling, H., Hoeben, K. A., van Marle, J., Pawlikowska, L., Bull, L. N., Hofmann, A. F., Knisely, A. S., & Oude, Elferink. R. P. (2006). Atp8b1 deficiency in mice reduces resistance of the canalicular membrane to hydrophobic bile salts and impairs bile salt transport. *Hepatology*, 44(1), 195-204.

[16] Paulusma, C. C., de Waart, D. R., Kunne, C., Mok, K. S., & Elferink, R. P. (2009). Activity of the bile salt export pump (ABCB11) is critically dependent on canalicular membrane cholesterol content. *J Biol Chem*, 284(15), 9947-9954.

[17] Alvarez, L., Jara, P., Sanchez-Sabate, E., Hierro, L., Larrauri, J., Diaz, M. C., Camarena, C., De la Vega, A., Frauca, E., Lopez-Collazo, E., & Lapunzina, P. (2004). Reduced hepatic expression of farnesoid X receptor in hereditary cholestasis associated to mutation in ATP8B1. *Hum Mol Genet*, 13(20), 2451-2460.

[18] Chen, F., Ananthanarayanan, M., Emre, S., Neimark, E., Bull, L. N., Knisely, A. S., Strautnieks, S. S., Thompson, R. J., Magid, M. S., Gordon, R., Balasubramanian, N., Suchy, F. J., & Shneider, B. L. (2004). Progressive familial intrahepatic cholestasis, type 1, is associated with decreased farnesoid X receptor activity. *Gastroenterology*, 126(3), 756-764.

[19] Lykavieris, P., van Mil, S., Cresteil, D., Fabre, M., Hadchouel, M., Klomp, L., Bernard, O., & Jacquemin, E. (2003). Progressive familial intrahepatic cholestasis type 1 and extrahepatic features: no catch-up of stature growth, exacerbation of diarrhea, and appearance of liver steatosis after liver transplantation. *J Hepatol*, 39(3), 447-452.

[20] Stapelbroek, J. M., Peters, T. A., van Beurden, D. H., Curfs, J. H., Joosten, A., Beynon, A. J., van Leeuwen, B. M., van der Velden, L. M., Bull, L., Oude, Elferink R. P., van Zanten, B. A., Klomp, L. W., & Houwen, R. H. (2009). ATP8B1 is essential for maintaining normal hearing. *Proc Natl Acad Sci*, U S A, 106(24), 9709-9714.

[21] Klomp, L. W., Vargas, J. C., van Mil, S. W., Pawlikowska, L., Strautnieks, S. S., van Eijk, M. J., Juijn, J. A., Pabon-Pena, C., Smith, L. B., De Young, J. A., Byrne, J. A., Gombert, J., van der Brugge, G., Berger, R., Jankowska, I., Pawlowska, J., Villa, E., Knisely, A. S., Thompson, R. J., Freimer, N. B., Houwen, R. H., & Bull, L. N. (2004). Characterization of mutations in ATP8B1 associated with hereditary cholestasis. *Hepatology*, 40(1), 27-38.

[22] Liu, L. Y., Wang, X. H., Wang, Z. L., Zhu, Q. R., & Wang, J. S. (2010). Characterization of ATP8B1 gene mutations and a hot-linked mutation found in Chinese children with progressive intrahepatic cholestasis and low GGT. *J Pediatr Gastroenterol Nutr*, 50(2), 179-183.

[23] Folmer, D. E., van der Mark, V. A., Ho-Mok, K. S., Oude Elferink, R. P., & Paulusma, C. C. (2009). Differential effects of progressive familial intrahepatic cholestasis type 1 and benign recurrent intrahepatic cholestasis type 1 mutations on canalicular localization of ATP8B1. *Hepatology*, 50(5), 1597-1605.

[24] Misawa, T., Hayashi, H., Sugiyama, Y., & Hashimoto, Y. (2012). Discovery and structural development of small molecules that enhance transport activity of bile salt export pump mutant associated with progressive familial intrahepatic cholestasis type 2. *Bioorg Med Chem.*

[25] Van der Velden, L. M., Stapelbroek, J. M., Krieger, E., van den Berghe, P. V., Berger, R., Verhulst, P. M., Holthuis, J. C., Houwen, R. H., Klomp, L. W., & van de Graaf, S. F. (2010). Folding defects in P-type ATP 8B1 associated with hereditary cholestasis are ameliorated by 4-phenylbutyrate. *Hepatology*, 51(1), 286-296.

[26] Klomp, L. W., Bull, L. N., Knisely, A. S., van Der Doelen, M. A., Juijn, J. A., Berger, R., Forget, S., Nielsen, I. M., Eiberg, H., & Houwen, R. H. (2000). A missense mutation in FIC1 is associated with greenland familial cholestasis. *Hepatology*, 32(6), 1337-1341.

[27] Mullenbach, R., Bennett, A., Tetlow, N., Patel, N., Hamilton, G., Cheng, F., Chambers, J., Howard, R., Taylor-Robinson, S. D., & Williamson, C. (2005). ATP8B1 mutations in British cases with intrahepatic cholestasis of pregnancy. *Gut*, 54(6), 829-834.

[28] Demeilliers, C., Jacquemin, E., Barbu, V., Mergey, M., Paye, F., Fouassier, L., Chignard, N., Housset, C., & Lomri, N. E. (2006). Altered hepatobiliary gene expressions in PFIC1: ATP8B1 gene defect is associated with CFTR downregulation. *Hepatology*, 43(5), 1125-1134.

[29] Gerloff, T., Stieger, B., Hagenbuch, B., Madon, J., Landmann, L., Roth, J., Hofmann, A. F., & Meier, P. J. (1998). The sister of P-glycoprotein represents the canalicular bile salt export pump of mammalian liver. *J Biol Chem*, 273(16), 10046-10050.

[30] Strautnieks, S. S., Bull, L. N., Knisely, A. S., Kocoshis, S. A., Dahl, N., Arnell, H., Sokal, E., Dahan, K., Childs, S., Ling, V., Tanner, M. S., Kagalwalla, A. F., Nemeth, A., Pawlowska, J., Baker, A., Mieli-Vergani, G., Freimer, N. B., Gardiner, R. M., & Thompson, R. J. (1998). A gene encoding a liver-specific ABC transporter is mutated in progressive familial intrahepatic cholestasis. *Nat Genet*, 20(3), 233-238.

[31] Strautnieks, S. S., Byrne, J. A., Pawlikowska, L., Cebecauerova, D., Rayner, A., Dutton, L., Meier, Y., Antoniou, A., Stieger, B., Arnell, H., Ozcay, F., Al-Hussaini, H. F., Bassas, A. F., Verkade, H. J., Fischler, B., Nemeth, A., Kotalova, R., Shneider, B. L., Cielecka-Kuszyk, J., Mc Clean, P., Whitington, P. F., Sokal, E., Jirsa, M., Wali, S. H., Jankowska, I., Pawlowska, J., Mieli-Vergani, G., Knisely, A. S., Bull, L. N., & Thompson, R. J. (2008). Severe bile salt export pump deficiency: 82 different ABCB11 mutations in 109 families. *Gastroenterology*, 134(4), 1203-1214.

[32] Pawlikowska, L., Strautnieks, S., Jankowska, I., Czubkowski, P., Emerick, K., Antoniou, A., Wanty, C., Fischler, B., Jacquemin, E., Wali, S., Blanchard, S., Nielsen, I. M., Bourke, B., Mc Quaid, S., Lacaille, F., Byrne, J. A., van Eerde, A. M., Kolho, K. L., Klomp, L., Houwen, R., Bacchetti, P., Lobritto, S., Hupertz, V., Mc Clean, P., Mieli-Vergani, G., Shneider, B., Nemeth, A., Sokal, E., Freimer, N. B., Knisely, A. S., Rosenthal, P., Whitington, P. F., Pawlowska, J., Thompson, R. J., & Bull, L. N. (2010). Differences in presentation and progression between severe FIC1 and BSEP deficiencies. *J Hepatol*, 53(1), 170-178.

[33] Kagawa, T., Watanabe, N., Mochizuki, K., Numari, A., Ikeno, Y., Itoh, J., Tanaka, H., Arias, I. M., & Mine, T. (2008). Phenotypic differences in PFIC2 and BRIC2 correlate with protein stability of mutant Bsep and impaired taurocholate secretion in MDCK II cells. *Am J Physiol Gastrointest Liver Physiol*, 294(1), G 58-67.

[34] Pauli-Magnus, C., Lang, T., Meier, Y., Zodan-Marin, T., Jung, D., Breymann, C., Zimmermann, R., Kenngott, S., Beuers, U., Reichel, C., Kerb, R., Penger, A., Meier, P. J., & Kullak-Ublick, G. A. (2004). Sequence analysis of bile salt export pump (ABCB11) and multidrug resistance p-glycoprotein 3 (ABCB4, MDR3) in patients with intrahepatic cholestasis of pregnancy. *Pharmacogenetics*, 14(2), 91-102.

[35] Pauli-Magnus, C., & Meier, P. J. (2006). Hepatobiliary transporters and drug-induced cholestasis. *Hepatology*, 44(4), 778-787.

[36] Hermeziu, B., Sanlaville, D., Girard, M., Leonard, C., Lyonnet, S., & Jacquemin, E. (2006). Heterozygous bile salt export pump deficiency: a possible genetic predisposition to transient neonatal cholestasis. *J Pediatr Gastroenterol Nutr*, 42(1), 114-116.

[37] De Vree, J. M., Jacquemin, E., Sturm, E., Cresteil, D., Bosma, P. J., Aten, J., Deleuze, J. F., Desrochers, M., Burdelski, M., Bernard, O., Oude Elferink, R. P., & Hadchouel, M.

(1998). Mutations in the MDR3 gene cause progressive familial intrahepatic cholestasis. *Proc Natl Acad Sci*, U S A, 95(1), 282-287.

[38] Oude Elferink, R. P., & Paulusma, C. C. (2007). Function and pathophysiological importance of ABCB4 (MDR3 P-glycoprotein). *Pflugers Arch*, 453(5), 601-610.

[39] Noe, J., Kullak-Ublick, G. A., Jochum, W., Stieger, B., Kerb, R., Haberl, M., Mullhaupt, B., Meier, P. J., & Pauli-Magnus, C. (2005). Impaired expression and function of the bile salt export pump due to three novel ABCB11 mutations in intrahepatic cholestasis. *J Hepatol*, 43(3), 536-543.

[40] Keitel, V., Burdelski, M., Warskulat, U., Kuhlkamp, T., Keppler, D., Haussinger, D., & Kubitz, R. (2005). Expression and localization of hepatobiliary transport proteins in progressive familial intrahepatic cholestasis. *Hepatology*, 41(5), 1160-1172.

[41] Degiorgio, D., Colombo, C., Seia, M., Porcaro, L., Costantino, L., Zazzeron, L., Bordo, D., & Coviello, D. A. (2007). Molecular characterization and structural implications of 25 new ABCB4 mutations in progressive familial intrahepatic cholestasis type 3 (PFIC3). *Eur J Hum Genet*, 15(12), 1230-1238.

[42] Jacquemin, E., De Vree, J. M., Cresteil, D., Sokal, E. M., Sturm, E., Dumont, M., Scheffer, G. L., Paul, M., Burdelski, M., Bosma, P. J., Bernard, O., Hadchouel, M., & Elferink, R. P. (2001). The wide spectrum of multidrug resistance 3 deficiency: from neonatal cholestasis to cirrhosis of adulthood. *Gastroenterology*, 120(6), 1448-1458.

[43] Lucena, J. F., Herrero, J. I., Quiroga, J., Sangro, B., Garcia-Foncillas, J., Zabalegui, N., Sola, J., Herraiz, M., Medina, J. F., & Prieto, J. (2003). A multidrug resistance 3 gene mutation causing cholelithiasis, cholestasis of pregnancy, and adulthood biliary cirrhosis. *Gastroenterology*, 124(4), 1037-1042.

[44] Gonzales, E., Davit-Spraul, A., Baussan, C., Buffet, C., Maurice, M., & Jacquemin, E. (2009). Liver diseases related to MDR3 (ABCB4) gene deficiency. *Front Biosci*, 14, 4242-4256.

[45] Davit-Spraul, A., Fabre, M., Branchereau, S., Baussan, C., Gonzales, E., Stieger, B., Bernard, O., & Jacquemin, E. (2010). ATP8B1 and ABCB11 analysis in 62 children with normal gamma-glutamyl transferase progressive familial intrahepatic cholestasis (PFIC): phenotypic differences between PFIC1 and PFIC2 and natural history. *Hepatology*, 51(5), 1645-1655.

[46] Bustorff-Silva, J., Sbraggia Neto, L., Olimpio, H., de Alcantara, R. V., Matsushima, E., De Tommaso, A. M., Brandao, M. A., & Hessel, G. (2007). Partial internal biliary diversion through a cholecystojejunocolonic anastomosis--a novel surgical approach for patients with progressive familial intrahepatic cholestasis: a preliminary report. *J Pediatr Surg*, 42(8), 1337-1340.

[47] Jansen, P. L., & Sturm, E. (2003). Genetic cholestasis, causes and consequences for hepatobiliary transport. *Liver Int*, 23(5), 315-322.

[48] Chatila, R., Bergasa, N. V., Lagarde, S., & West, A. B. (1996). Intractable cough and abnormal pulmonary function in benign recurrent intrahepatic cholestasis. *Am J Gastroenterol*, 91(10), 2215-2219.

[49] Mizuochi, T., Kimura, A., Tanaka, A., Muto, A., Nittono, H., Seki, Y., Takahashi, T., Kurosawa, T., Kage, M., Takikawa, H., & Matsuishi, T. (2012). Characterization of urinary bile acids in a pediatric BRIC-1 patient: Effect of rifampicin treatment. *Clin Chim Acta*, 413(15-16), 1301-1304.

[50] Jacquemin, E. (2001). Role of multidrug resistance 3 deficiency in pediatric and adult liver disease: one gene for three diseases. *Semin Liver Dis*, 21(4), 551-562.

[51] Whitington, P. F., Freese, D. K., Alonso, E. M., Schwarzenberg, S. J., & Sharp, H. L. (1994). Clinical and biochemical findings in progressive familial intrahepatic cholestasis. *J Pediatr Gastroenterol Nutr*, 18(2), 134-141.

[52] Cabrera-Abreu, J. C., & Green, A. (2002). Gamma-glutamyltransferase: value of its measurement in paediatrics. *Ann Clin Biochem*, 39(pt1), 22-5.

[53] Elferink, R. P., Ottenhoff, R., van Marle, J., Frijters, C. M., Smith, A. J., & Groen, A. K. (1998). Class III P-glycoproteins mediate the formation of lipoprotein X in the mouse. *J Clin Invest*, 102(9), 1749-1757.

[54] Jansen, P. L., Strautnieks, S. S., Jacquemin, E., Hadchouel, M., Sokal, E. M., Hooiveld, G. J., Koning, J. H., De Jager-Krikken, A., Kuipers, F., Stellaard, F., Bijleveld, C. M., Gouw, A., Van Goor, H., Thompson, R. J., & Muller, M. (1999). Hepatocanalicular bile salt export pump deficiency in patients with progressive familial intrahepatic cholestasis. *Gastroenterology*, 117(6), 1370-1379.

[55] Liu, C., Aronow, B. J., Jegga, A. G., Wang, N., Miethke, A., Mourya, R., & Bezerra, J. A. (2007). Novel resequencing chip customized to diagnose mutations in patients with inherited syndromes of intrahepatic cholestasis. *Gastroenterology*, 132(1), 119-126.

[56] Carlton, V. E., Harris, B. Z., Puffenberger, E. G., Batta, A. K., Knisely, A. S., Robinson, D. L., Strauss, K. A., Shneider, B. L., Lim, W. A., Salen, G., Morton, D. H., & Bull, L. N. (2003). Complex inheritance of familial hypercholanemia with associated mutations in TJP2 and BAAT. *Nat Genet*, 34(1), 91-96.

[57] Gissen, P., Johnson, C. A., Morgan, N. V., Stapelbroek, J. M., Forshew, T., Cooper, W. N., Mc Kiernan, P. J., Klomp, L. W., Morris, A. A., Wraith, J. E., Mc Clean, P., Lynch, S. A., Thompson, R. J., Lo, B., Quarrell, O. W., Di Rocco, M., Trembath, R. C., Mandel, H., Wali, S., Karet, F. E., Knisely, A. S., Houwen, R. H., Kelly, D. A., & Maher, E. R. (2004). Mutations in VPS33B, encoding a regulator of SNARE-dependent membrane fusion, cause arthrogryposis-renal dysfunction-cholestasis (ARC) syndrome. *Nat Genet*, 36(4), 400-404.

[58] Moreira, R. K., Cabral, R., Cowles, R. A., & Lobritto, S. J. (2012). Biliary atresia: a multidisciplinary approach to diagnosis and management. *Arch Pathol Lab Med*, 136(7), 746-760.

[59] Hadj-Rabia, S., Baala, L., Vabres, P., Hamel-Teillac, D., Jacquemin, E., Fabre, M., Lyonnet, S., De Prost, Y., Munnich, A., Hadchouel, M., & Smahi, A. (2004). Claudin-1 gene mutations in neonatal sclerosing cholangitis associated with ichthyosis: a tight junction disease. *Gastroenterology*, 127(5), 1386-1390.

[60] Stoller, J. K., & Aboussouan, L. S. (2012). A review of alpha1-antitrypsin deficiency. *Am J Respir Crit Care Med*, 185(3), 246-259.

[61] Chagnon, P., Michaud, J., Mitchell, G., Mercier, J., Marion, J. F., Drouin, E., Rasquin-Weber, A., Hudson, T. J., & Richter, A. (2002). A missense mutation (R565W) in cirhin (FLJ14728) in North American Indian childhood cirrhosis. *Am J Hum Genet*, 71(6), 1443-1449.

[62] Bull, L. N., Roche, E., Song, E. J., Pedersen, J., Knisely, A. S., van Der Hagen, C. B., Eiklid, K., Aagenaes, O., & Freimer, N. B. (2000). Mapping of the locus for cholestasis-lymphedema syndrome (Aagenaes syndrome) to a 6.6-cM interval on chromosome 15q. *Am J Hum Genet*, 67(4), 994-999.

[63] Lazaridis, K. N., Gores, G. J., & Lindor, K. D. (2001). Ursodeoxycholic acid 'mechanisms of action and clinical use in hepatobiliary disorders'. *J Hepatol*, 35(1), 134-146.

[64] Cohran, V. C., & Heubi, J. E. (2003). Treatment of Pediatric Cholestatic Liver Disease. *Curr Treat Options Gastroenterol*, 6(5), 403-415.

[65] Jacquemin, E., Hermans, D., Myara, A., Habes, D., Debray, D., Hadchouel, M., Sokal, E. M., & Bernard, O. (1997). Ursodeoxycholic acid therapy in pediatric patients with progressive familial intrahepatic cholestasis. *Hepatology*, 25(3), 519-523.

[66] Ismail, H., Kalicinski, P., Markiewicz, M., Jankowska, I., Pawlowska, J., Kluge, P., Eliadou, E., Kaminski, A., Szymczak, M., Drewniak, T., & Revillon, Y. (1999). Treatment of progressive familial intrahepatic cholestasis: liver transplantation or partial external biliary diversion. *Pediatr Transplant*, 3(3), 219-224.

[67] Wanty, C., Joomye, R., Van Hoorebeek, N., Paul, K., Otte, J. B., Reding, R., & Sokal, E. M. (2004). Fifteen years single center experience in the management of progressive familial intrahepatic cholestasis of infancy. *Acta Gastroenterol Belg*, 67(4), 313-319.

[68] Whitington, P. F., & Whitington, G. L. (1988). Partial external diversion of bile for the treatment of intractable pruritus associated with intrahepatic cholestasis. *Gastroenterology*, 95(1), 130-136.

[69] Stapelbroek, J. M., van Erpecum, K. J., Klomp, L. W., & Houwen, R. H. (2010). Liver disease associated with canalicular transport defects: current and future therapies. *J Hepatol*, 52(2), 258-271.

[70] Kaur, S., Sharma, D., Wadhwa, N., Gupta, S., Chowdhary, S. K., & Sibal, A. (2012). Therapeutic interventions in progressive familial intrahepatic cholestasis: experience from a tertiary care centre in north India. *Indian J Pediatr*, 79(2), 270-273.

[71] Stapelbroek, J. M., van Erpecum, K. J., Klomp, L. W., Venneman, N. G., Schwartz, T. P., van Berge Henegouwen, G. P., Devlin, J., van Nieuwkerk, C. M., Knisely, A. S-, & Houwen, R. H. (2006). Nasobiliary drainage induces long-lasting remission in benign recurrent intrahepatic cholestasis. *Hepatology*, 43(1), 51-53.

[72] Schukfeh, N., Metzelder, M. L., Petersen, C., Reismann, M., Pfister, E. D., Ure, B. M., & Kuebler, J. F. (2012). Normalization of serum bile acids after partial external biliary diversion indicates an excellent long-term outcome in children with progressive familial intrahepatic cholestasis. *J Pediatr Surg*, 47(3), 501-505.

[73] Metzelder, M. L., Bottlander, M., Melter, M., Petersen, C., & Ure, B. M. (2005). Laparoscopic partial external biliary diversion procedure in progressive familial intrahepatic cholestasis: a new approach. *Surg Endosc*, 19(12), 1641-1643.

[74] Rebhandl, W., Felberbauer, F. X., Turnbull, J., Paya, K., Barcik, U., Huber, W. D., Whitington, P. F., & Horcher, E. (1999). Biliary diversion by use of the appendix (cholecystoappendicostomy) in progressive familial intrahepatic cholestasis. *J Pediatr Gastroenterol Nutr*, 28(2), 217-219.

[75] Arnell, H., Bergdahl, S., Papadogiannakis, N., Nemeth, A., & Fischler, B. (2008). Preoperative observations and short-term outcome after partial external biliary diversion in 13 patients with progressive familial intrahepatic cholestasis. *J Pediatr Surg*, 43(7), 1312-1320.

[76] Davis, A. R., Rosenthal, P., & Newman, T. B. (2009). Nontransplant surgical interventions in progressive familial intrahepatic cholestasis. *J Pediatr Surg*, 44(4), 821-827.

[77] Kalicinski, P. J., Ismail, H., Jankowska, I., Kaminski, A., Pawlowska, J., Drewniak, T., Markiewicz, M., & Szymczak, M. (2003). Surgical treatment of progressive familial intrahepatic cholestasis: comparison of partial external biliary diversion and ileal bypass. *Eur J Pediatr Surg*, 13(5), 307-311.

[78] Bassas, A., Chehab, M., Hebby, H., Al, Shahed. M., Al Husseini, H., Al Zahrani, A., & Wali, S. (2003). Living related liver transplantation in 13 cases of progressive familial intrahepatic cholestasis. *Transplant Proc*, 35(8), 3003-3005.

[79] Englert, C., Grabhorn, E., Richter, A., Rogiers, X., Burdelski, M., & Ganschow, R. (2007). Liver transplantation in children with progressive familial intrahepatic cholestasis. *Transplantation*, 84(10), 1361-1363.

[80] Torri, E., Lucianetti, A., Pinelli, D., Corno, V., Guizzetti, M., Maldini, G., Zambelli, M., Bertani, A., Melzi, M. L., Alberti, D., Doffria, E., Giovanelli, M., Torre, G., Spada, M., Gridelli, B., & Colledan, M. (2005). Orthotopic liver transplantation for Byler's disease. *Transplant Proc*, 37(2), 1149-1150.

[81] Esquivel, C. O., Iwatsuki, S., Gordon, R. D., Marsh, W. W., Jr., Koneru, B., Makowka, L., Tzakis, A. G., Todo, S., & Starzl, T. E. (1987). Indications for pediatric liver transplantation. *J Pediatr*, 111(6), Pt 2, 1039-1045.

[82] Whitington, P. F, & Balistreri, W. F. (1991). Liver transplantation in pediatrics: indications, contraindications, and pretransplant management. *J Pediatr*, 118(2), 169-177.

[83] Keitel, V., Burdelski, M., Vojnisek, Z., Schmitt, L., Haussinger, D., & Kubitz, R. (2009). De novo bile salt transporter antibodies as a possible cause of recurrent graft failure after liver transplantation: a novel mechanism of cholestasis. *Hepatology*, 50(2), 510-517.

[84] Jara, P., Hierro, L., Martinez-Fernandez, P., Alvarez-Doforno, R., Yanez, F., Diaz, M. C., Camarena, C., De la Vega, A., Frauca, E., Munoz-Bartolo, G., Lopez-Santamaria, M., Larrauri, J., & Alvarez, L. (2009). Recurrence of bile salt export pump deficiency after liver transplantation. *N Engl J Med*, 361(14), 1359-1367.

[85] Egawa, H., Yorifuji, T., Sumazaki, R., Kimura, A., Hasegawa, M., & Tanaka, K. (2002). Intractable diarrhea after liver transplantation for Byler's disease: successful treatment with bile adsorptive resin. *Liver Transpl*, 8(8), 714-716.

[86] De Vree, J. M., Ottenhoff, R., Bosma, P. J., Smith, A. J., Aten, J., & Oude Elferink, R. P. (2000). Correction of liver disease by hepatocyte transplantation in a mouse model of progressive familial intrahepatic cholestasis. *Gastroenterology*, 119(6), 1720-1730.

[87] Zollner, G., & Trauner, M. (2009). Nuclear receptors as therapeutic targets in cholestatic liver diseases. *Br J Pharmacol*, 156(1), 7-27.

[88] Morello, J. P., Petaja-Repo, U. E., Bichet, D. G., & Bouvier, M. (2000). Pharmacological chaperones: a new twist on receptor folding. *Trends Pharmacol Sci*, 21(12), 466-469.

[89] Chen, Y., & Liu-Chen, L. Y. (2009). Chaperone-like effects of cell-permeant ligands on opioid receptors. *Front Biosci*, 14, 634-643.

[90] Ohgane, K., Dodo, K., & Hashimoto, Y. (2010). Retinobenzaldehydes as proper-trafficking inducers of folding-defective P23H rhodopsin mutant responsible for retinitis pigmentosa. *Bioorg Med Chem*, 18(19), 7022-7028.

[91] Hayashi, H., & Sugiyama, Y. (2007). 4-phenylbutyrate enhances the cell surface expression and the transport capacity of wild-type and mutated bile salt export pumps. *Hepatology*, 45(6), 1506-1516.

[92] Hacein-Bey-Abina, S., von Kalle, C., Schmidt, M., Le Deist, F., Wulffraat, N., Mc Intyre, E., Radford, I., Villeval, J. L., Fraser, C. C., Cavazzana-Calvo, M., & Fischer, A. (2003). A serious adverse event after successful gene therapy for X-linked severe combined immunodeficiency. *N Engl J Med*, 348(3), 255-256.

Chapter 25

Management of Hepatobiliary Trauma

Rajan Jagad, Ashok Thorat and Wei-Chen Lee

Additional information is available at the end of the chapter

http://dx.doi.org/10.5772/52107

1. Introduction:

The liver is the most commonly injured solid abdominal organ, despite its relative protected location [1, 2]. Treatment of traumatic liver injuries is based on patient physiology, mechanism and degree of injury, associated abdominal and extra-abdominal injuries and local expertise. Non-operative management has evolved into the treatment of choice for most patients with blunt liver injuries who are hemodynamically stable and success rates for non-operative management commonly are greater than 95%. With the sweeping shift towards the non-operative management, most hepatic injuries can be treated conservatively [3, 4, 5].

More recently several authors have highlighted an excessive use of non-operative management (NOM), which for some high grade liver injuries is pushed far beyond the reasonable limits, carrying increased morbidity at short and long term, such as bilomas, biliary fistula, early or late haemorrhage, false aneurysm, arterio-venous fistulae, haemobilia, liver abscess, and liver necrosis [5]. Incidence of complications attributed to NOM increases in concert with the grade of injury. In a series of 337 patients with liver injury grades III-V treated non-operatively, those with grade III had a complication rate of 1%, grade IV 21%, and grade V 63% [6].

2. Mechanism of injury and anatomic consideration:

Road traffic accident, antisocial violent behaviours, industrial and farming accidents are the commonest mode of injury to the liver. Though the liver is protected by the rib cage, as the largest solid organ in the abdomen, the liver is particularly vulnerable to the ability of compressive abdominal blows to rupture its relatively thin capsule. The vasculature consists of wide-bore, thin-walled vessels with a high blood flow, and injury is usually associated with significant blood loss. Blunt trauma in a road traffic accident, or fall from a height, may result in a deceleration injury as the liver continues to move on impact. This leads to tears at sites of fixation to the diaphragm and abdominal wall. A well-recognised deceleration injury involves a fracture between the posterior sector (segments VI and VII) and the anterior sector (segments V and VIII) of the right lobe. This type of injury can lead to rupture of right hepatic vein and significant bleeding. In contrast, direct blow on right upper abdomen during vehicular accident or direct blow by a weapon or fist can lead to stellate type of injury to the central liver (segment IV, V and VIII). This type of injury can lead to massive bleeding from portal vein or hepatic vein and can also lead to bile duct injury.

Penetrating injuries may be associated with a significant vascular injury. For example, a stab injury may cause major bleeding from one of the three hepatic veins or the vena cava and also from the portal vein or hepatic artery if it involves the hilum. Gunshots may similarly disrupt these major vessels; this disruption may be much more marked than with stab wounds due to the cavitation effect, particularly with bullets from high-velocity weapons.

The connection between the thin-walled hepatic veins and the inferior vena cava (IVC), at the site where the ligamentous mechanism anchors the liver to the diaphragm and posterior abdominal wall, represents a vulnerable area, particularly to shearing forces during blunt injury. Disruption here leads to the "juxtahepatic" venous injuries, which are usually associated with major blood loss and present a particularly challenging management problem.

3. Grade of liver injury:

The severity of liver injuries ranges from the relatively inconsequential minor capsular tear to extensive disruption of both lobes with associated hepatic vein, portal vein, or vena caval injury. Several classifications have been advised to grade the liver injury and management accordingly. Following table shows the grade of liver injury. Grade I & II are successfully managed non-operatively in most cases. Grade IV and onward injuries will eventually require emergency exploration. Grade III injuries require observation and if such patients are hemodynamically stable will recover with conservative treatment. Such patients should be closely followed in ICU with serial monitoring of hemoglobin and hematocrit level along with cardio-respiratory monitoring. Any fall in hematocrit or hemodynamic instability not responding to fluid resuscitation warrants urgent exploration.

Liver organ injuriy scale

Grade		**description**
I	Hematoma	Subcapsular, <10% surface area
	Laceration	Capsular tear, < 1 cm parenchymal depth
II	Hematoma	Subcapsular, <10%-50% surface area; intraparenchymal, <10 cm in diameter
	Laceration	1-3 cm parenchymal depth, <10 in Length

http://dx.doi.org/10.5772/52107

Liver organ injuriy scale		
III	Hematoma	Subcapsular,>50% surface area or expanding; ruptured subcapsular or parenchymal hematoma
	Laceration	>3cm parenchymal depth
IV	Hematoma	Parenchymal disruption involving 25%-75% of hepatic lobe or 1-3 Couinaud segments within a single lobe
V	Laceration	Parenchymal disruption involving >75% of hepatic lobe >3 Couinaud segments within a single lobe
	Vascular	Juxtahepatic venous injuries; ie, retrohepatic vena cava/central major hepatic vein
VI	Hepatic avulsion	

Table 1. Liver Organ Injury Scale.

4. Early Measures:

4.1. Resuscitation and treatment of Hemodynamic instability:

It is generally accepted that initial resuscitation and management is the same as for any patient with major trauma and should follow the Advanced Trauma Life Support (ATLS) principles of aggressive fluid resuscitation, guided by monitoring of central venous pressure and urinary output [7]. Management should also be directed toward avoidance of any of the sinister triad of hypothermia, coagulopathy, and acidosis, which are associated with significantly increased mortality. Mechanisms to avoid hypothermia are standard now in major centres and include the use of rewarming blankets and heat exchanger pumps for rapid infusion of resuscitation fluids and blood [8].

The next management phase depends largely on the response to resuscitation and the stability of the patient. Liver injury should be suspected in all patients with blunt or penetrating thoracoabdominal trauma but particularly in shocked patients with blunt or penetrating trauma to the right side. There are two major determinants to consider when making decisions in suspected liver trauma: hemodynamic stability and mechanism of injury. In general, hemodynamic instability or peritonism makes decision-making in trauma more straightforward, although ultimately, the surgical procedure required may be complex. Management decisions are more challenging when patients are hemodynamically stable as the array of potential therapeutic modalities are substantial and the patient's future clinical course is unknown [9].

4.2. Advanced Trauma Life Support:

The appropriate evaluation and management of liver injuries results from an organized approach to abdominal trauma. Experience and technical developments over the past several decades make the current approach both logical and effective. It is generally accepted that initial resuscitation and management is the same as for any patient with major trauma and should follow the Advanced Trauma Life Support (ATLS) principles of aggressive fluid resuscitation, guided by monitoring of central venous pressure and urinary output [7]. Management should also be directed toward avoidance of any of the sinister triad of hypothermia, coagulopathy, and acidosis, which are associated with significantly increased mortality.

4.3. Focused assessment by ultrasound for trauma (FAST):

Ultrasonography (USG) is the most important and readily available investigation for any patient with blunt or sharp abdominal injury. It is particularly useful for detecting injury to parenchymal organs and the presence of free intraperitoneal fluid or blood. USG is a quick, non-invasive, inexpensive, and transportable tool, used with increasing frequency in the initial workup of patients with abdominal trauma [10].

The particular relevance to major liver injury is the focused assessment by ultrasound for trauma (FAST), often performed in the emergency department, which involves a rapid examination of several areas, namely, the pericardial region, right upper quadrant (including Morrison's pouch), left upper quadrant, and the pelvis, specifically looking for free fluid. One of the main limitations of USG is that parenchymal injuries, sometimes relevant and requiring surgical or embolization therapy, may be present without combined peritoneal fluid [11,12].

On the basis of detection of free fluid or parenchymal injury, the sensitivity of USG has been found to be 72% to 95% for abdominal organ injuries, 51% to 92% for liver lesions, and 98% for grade III or higher liver injuries [13]. Richards et al reported 56% and 68% sensitivity of FAST and complete USG, respectively, in detecting childhood abdominal trauma [11].

Detection of peritoneal fluid is the first step in FAST. Fluid in the right upper quadrant or in the right upper quadrant and pelvic recess suggests hepatic injury, as opposed to splenic, renal, or enteric injury [14]. Fluid limited to the left upper quadrant or to both upper quadrants is not seen in patients with isolated liver trauma [14]. Hemoperitoneum recognition must prompt further imaging, but its absence does not definitely exclude parenchymal injury. Clinical assessment and observation are also relevant in combination with USG. With special reference to liver trauma, it has been noted that patients with negative USG results but with an aspartate aminotransferase level of greater than 360 IU/L should undergo CT imaging because of potentially overlooked hepatic injury, whereas patients with normal levels can be effectively discharged [15].

Although FAST provides a rapid assessment of liver disruption and intraperitoneal bleeding, it is a limited scan that is highly operator dependent. It is very important to note that a negative FAST scan does not safely rule out injury [12, 16]. Due to the operator dependence of the modality, different end points, and inconsistent comparative gold standards in the studies, the reported specificities, sensitivities, and overall accuracies are variable [17]. It has been demonstrated that up to a quarter of hepatic and splenic injuries, as well as renal, bladder, pancreatic, mesenteric, and gut injuries, can be missed if ultrasound is used as the primary investigative modality in the stable patient. However, while the possibility of false negatives is ever present, the combination of a negative ultrasound scan and normal clinical examination and observations almost excludes liver injury in the event of significant blunt trauma [12, 18].

4.4. Computed Tomography:

The wide availability of high-resolution CT has changed the manner in which blunt abdominal trauma is diagnosed and managed (figure 1). Currently, multi-detector computed tomography (MDCT) scanning with intravenous contrast is the gold standard diagnostic modality in hemodynamically stable patients with intra-abdominal fluid detected with FAST.

CT has a sensitivity of 92% to 97% and a specificity of 98.7% for detection of liver injury. The type and grade of liver injury, the volume of hemoperitoneum, and differentiation between clotted blood and active bleeding can be identified. In addition to increasing the rate of detection of liver lesions following trauma, CT has also helped to improve the understanding of the course of liver injuries [19]. CT scan also allows diagnosis of associated intraperitoneal and retroperitoneal injuries, including splenic, renal, bowel, and chest trauma, and pelvic fractures.

Even though NOM has proven to be of tremendous benefit, a couple of controversies regarding the current management of trauma patients should be discussed. Advances in CT technology have improved the practitioner's ability to determine the degree of injury and to identify patients who are more likely to fail NOM. However, until now, MDCT scanning has not been able to differentiate, in a precise manner, among which patients should be treated conservatively, which would benefit from angio-embolization and which would respond best to a surgical response.

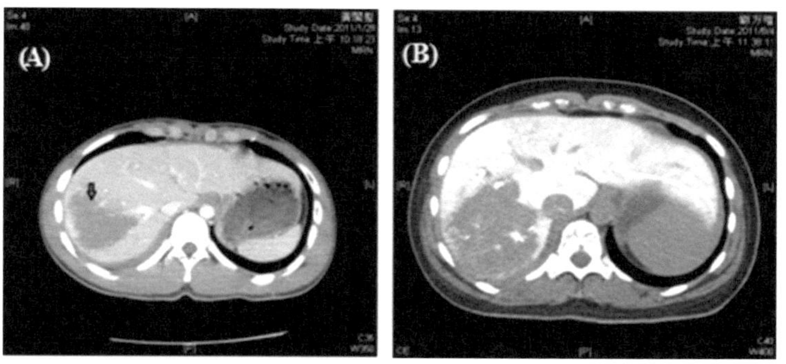

Figure 1. CT scan images of blunt abdominal trauma patients. (A) CT scan of liver showing intraparenchymal hematoma in segment VI. (B) CT scan of liver showing intraparenchymal hematoma in segment VI and extending to segment VII and V.

Although CT is the investigative gold standard, it is important to remember that it involves exposure to high levels of ionising radiation and the use of intravenous contrast may compromise renal function. In the majority of hospitals the use of CT requires movement of the patient away from adequate resuscitation facilities to the X-ray department, highlighting the importance of hemodynamic stability in patients with abdominal trauma being considered for CT examination [16].

4.5. Diagnostic laparoscopy:

The use of laparoscopy for trauma patients has been slower to evolve partly due to factors inherent in the trauma population and some limitations of the laparoscopic technique. Initially, the evaluation of peritoneal violation in hemodynamically stable patients was seen as the greatest benefit of laparoscopy for trauma [20]. Improvements in laparoscopic training and technology have enabled an increase in the use of diagnostic and therapeutic procedures in trauma patients.

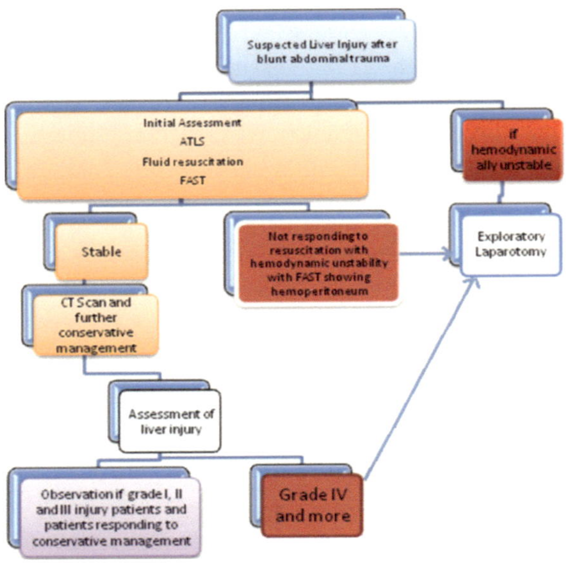

Figure 2. Algorithm - Advanced trauma life support, FAST- focused assessment by ultrasound for trauma. ATLS for managing liver trauma patients.

There are a number of series describing the successful haemostasis of minor liver injuries, in both the civilian [21] and military setting [22], although it is likely that these were self-limiting injuries anyway.

5. Management of hepatic Trauma:

There are two major determinants to consider when making decisions in suspected liver trauma: hemodynamic stability and mechanism of injury. In general, hemodynamic instability or peritonism makes decision-making in trauma more straightforward, although ultimately, the surgical procedure required may be complex (figure 2). Management decisions are more challenging when patients are hemodynamically stable as the array of potential therapeutic modalities are substantial and the patient's future clinical course is unknown [9].

5.1. Non operative management:

Hogarth Pringle, in 1908, provided the first description of operative management of liver trauma. Unfortunately, all eight patients died and Pringle recommended conservative non-operative management of these patients. In the modern surgical literature, non-operative management was first reported in 1972 and has been one of the most significant changes in the treatment of liver injuries over the last two decades [23, 24].

Initiated in pediatric trauma patients [25], nonsurgical management of blunt liver trauma has become recognized as an appropriate treatment option for hemodynamically stable adult patients with blunt hepatic injury [26, 27].

With the wide availability and improved quality of CT scanning, and the more modern, less invasive intervention options, such as angio-embolization, NOM has evolved into the treatment of choice for hemodynamically stable patients. Although angio-embolization has been defined the logical augmentation of damage control techniques for controlling hemorrhage, the overall liver-related complication rate can be as high as 60.6% with 42.2% incidence of major hepatic necrosis [28]. Non-operative management (NOM) consists of close observation of the patient completed with angio-embolization, if necessary. Observational management involves admission to a unit and the monitoring of vital signs, with strict bed rest, frequent monitoring of hemoglobin concentration and serial abdominal examinations [29].

Following factors contribute to conservative management of liver trauma:

i. Realization that more than 50% of liver injuries stop bleeding spontaneously at the time of exploration

ii. Availability of CT scan imaging for better assessment of grade of liver injury and associated injuries

iii. The success of non-operative management in paediatric patients

iv. Knowledge that the liver has tremendous capacity of healing after injury,

v. Improved critical care management in specialized unit

vi. The introduction of angio-embolization which allows patients with specific CT findings to potentially be treated in a minimally invasive manner.

Given the availability of angio-embolization, trauma surgeons are more likely to initiate non-operative treatment, even in higher grade injuries, because, in the event of failure, intervention in the form of angio-embolization is possible and, in the event of angio-embolization failure, surgical intervention is possible. Criteria for non-operative management include foremost, hemodynamic stability, absence of other abdominal injuries that require laparotomy, immediate availability of resources including a fully staffed operating room, and a vigilant surgeon. While non-operative management was initially introduced for minor injuries, it was soon in vogue for more severe injuries (grades III–V) [6, 30]. Close observation and repeated scans are usually recommended to document non-expansion of hematoma and healing of the injuries over time. The shift towards non-operative management of liver injuries has resulted in a lower mortality rate, but still a significant percentage of complications [31]. The current reported success rate of non-operative management of hepatic trauma ranges from 82% to 100%. Twenty-five percent of patients with blunt hepatic injury managed non-operatively, 92% of whom have grade IV or V injury will require an intervention for complications [5].

Despite the reduction of mortality that has been achieved using angio-embolization, some studies describe a rise in severe but treatable complications such as hepatic necrosis, abscesses or bile leakage [6, 28]. Gallbladder ischemia, hepatic parenchymal necrosis and biloma may also occur, and in patients with a high grade liver injury (grade 4 and 5) the incidence of complications can be high [32].

A determinant of the success of NOM is the level of cooperation between different specialists in the hospital. Good teamwork among the trauma surgeon, the anaesthesiologist and the interventional radiologist leads to a quicker understanding of the underlying injuries and thus shortens the time between entering the hospital and the initiation of therapeutic interventions. This seems obvious in level 1 trauma centers, but can be a matter of concern, especially in level II or III trauma centers.

While there has been considerable debate about the grade of liver injury and the acceptable volume of hemoperitoneum, it is now generally accepted that the ultimate decisive factor in favour of non-operative management is the hemodynamic stability of the patient, irrespective of the grade of injury or the volume of hemoperitoneum. It is also essential that appropriate clinical and radiological follow-up is arranged [33].

The rate of liver-related complications is low, and generally ranges from 0% to 7% [31]. Liver-related complication rates in high-grade liver injury patients are 11-13% and can be predicted by the grade of liver injury and the volume of packed red blood cells transfused at 24 hours post-injury [6, 34]. Incidence of complications attributed to NOM increases in concert with the grade of injury. In a series of 337 patients with liver injury grades III-V treated non-operatively, those with grade III had a complication rate of 1%, grade IV 21%, and grade V 63% [6]. Patients with grades IV and V injuries are more likely to require operation, and to have complications of non-operative treatment. Therefore, although it is not essential to perform liver resection at the first laparotomy, if bleeding has been effectively controlled, increasing evidence suggests that liver resection should be considered as a surgical option in patients with complex liver injury, as an initial or delayed strategy, which can be accomplished with low mortality and liver related morbidity in experienced hands [3].

Some of the complications related to conservative management of liver injuries are bile leaks, liver abscess, delayed haemorrhage, false aneurysm, arterio-venous fistulae, haemobilia, liver and gall bladder necrosis. Carrillo described complications in up to 85% of patients with a high (≥4) Abbreviated Injury Score (AIS) in a series of 32 patients who were treated non-operatively [27].

High grade liver injury (>3) treated with NOM and angio-embolization may be associated with severe complications like liver necrosis, bile leaks and severe sepsis. Mortality has been noted in up to 11% of patients in high grade liver injury treated conservatively [35]. Although angio-embolization has been defined the logical augmentation of damage control techniques for controlling hemorrhage, the overall liver-related complication rate can be as high as 60.6% with 42.2% incidence of major hepatic necrosis [28]. Early liver lobectomy in such cases required lesser number of procedures and achieved lower complication rate and lower mortality compared to less aggressive approaches such as serial operative debridements and/or percutaneous drainage [36].

5.2. Transarterial Embolization (TAE):

TAE of blunt hepatic injury was first recognized as a safe and effective treatment for the control of recurrent postoperative hemorrhage, hemobilia and hepatic artery-portal vein fistulas in the late 1970s [37]. Hashimoto et al. [38] also showed the efficacy of emergency TAE in four patients with severe complex hepatic injury and suggested that this method may be useful in nonsurgical management of unstable patients with severe hepatic injury. This multidisciplinary approach to the management of complex hepatic injuries is becoming much more important as the role of interventional radiology expands. Denton et al. [39] reported successful use of a combination of arterial embolization and transhepatic venous stenting in the management of a grade V injury involving the retrohepatic vena cava in a patient whose injury had been temporarily controlled by perihepatic packing. Recent more extensive series of angiography for control of hepatic haemorrhage have reported increasing success, with identification and control of bleeding rates ranging from 68 to 87%. [40] Angiography and embolization or stenting is a very useful adjunctive technique in the stable patient who is being managed non-operatively or in the patient who either has been stabilised by perihepatic packing or has re-bled after a period of initial stability.

The recent literature reveals that the increased use of angio-embolization and decreased mortality rates result in increased frequencies of severe complications, such as liver necrosis, bile leakage and intra-abdominal abscesses [28, 32, 41]. Indications of angiography in hemodynamically stable patients are high grade liver injury in CT scan, evidence of arterial vascular injury, and the presence of hepatic venous injury [41]. Angio-embolization can be used immediately after a damage control laparotomy as part of the primary haemorrhage control strategy [42]. Alternatively, angio-embolization can be used in post-operative patients to manage ongoing bleeding not associated with hemodynamic compromise [32]. This can involve not only angio-embolization, but also the placement of stents to reconstruct vasculature [39].

5.3. Complications of non-operative management:

5.3.1. Biliary complications:

Bile leaks are a frequent complication in the non-operative management of liver injuries, occurring in 6% to 20% of cases. Bile leaks present either as trauma, drainage of bile through surgically placed drain, or percutaneously placed catheter to drain biloma. The time of presentation of biliary leaks is variable. Ultrasound and CT scan are used to diagnose a biloma, whereas a hepatobiliary iminodiacetic acid scan is used to show an active bile leak.

Majority of bile leaks can be treated by ultrasound or CT-guided percutaneous drainage or ERCP and stenting.

5.3.2. Delayed haemorrhage:

The prevalence of delayed haemorrhage following non-operative management of blunt liver injury ranges from 1.7 to 5.9% [27, 43]. The mechanism of delayed hemorrhage may be related to an expanding injury or to a pseudoaneurysm induced by a biloma which eventually causes an expanding hematoma and free rupture into the peritoneal cavity. Early bleeding episodes are attributed directly to the traumatic insult, while late hemorrhage is probably related to infectious hepatic complications. Angio-embolization may prove an useful technique to deal with such complications.

5.4. Operative management:

Patients with associated liver and spleen injuries are twice as likely to fail non-operative therapy as those with only a single organ injured [44]. Missing associated intra-abdominal injury and delayed treatment, significantly affects the outcome. This occurs more often in conjunction with liver than with splenic injury, especially pancreas and bowel injury are significantly associated with liver injury in blunt trauma.

Patients with high grade liver injury who are hemodynamically unstable require surgical management. Failure of NOM also requires urgent exploration and appropriate surgical management.

Anesthesia must ensure that blood products are already in the room. The massive transfusion protocol should be activated so that the blood bank is always ahead of the patient's needs for packed red blood cells, fresh frozen plasma, platelets, and cryoprecipitate. Adequate vascular access and arterial blood pressure monitoring are essential. It is important to preferentially have venous access above the diaphragm. Resuscitation fluids infused under pressure through femoral access will exacerbate hepatic venous bleeding, at times dramatically so. Massive transfusion protocols should be activated early to prevent any delay in resuscitation with blood products.

The most widely adopted incision for the patient with liver trauma is a long midline laparotomy, which can be extended to the right chest if a posterior right lobe injury, major hepatic venous injury, or vena caval injury is encountered. An effective alternative, which gives good exposure and avoids a thoracotomy, is a right subcostal extension. A bilateral subcostal incision is sometimes favoured by hepatobiliary surgeons if there is an obvious penetrating through-and-through liver injury. This allows excellent exposure of the right lobe of the liver, the hepatic veins, and vena cava without having to open the chest or diaphragm; however, it does compromise access to the lower abdomen.

If a major liver injury is encountered, immediate control of bleeding is an absolute priority because the greatest threat to the patient's life at this juncture is exsanguination. Liver should immediately be manually closed and compressed. Patients with massive hemoperitoneum are at risk of coagulopathy, hypothermia and acidosis. Measures should be taken to prevent and treat all these consequences of massive bleeding. If this still does not control the bleeding, pedicle occlusion (Pringle manoeuvre) should be applied using an atraumatic vascular clamp or non-crushing bowel clamp. If bleeding stops after Pringle manoeuvre, the bleeding is from branches of portal vein or hepatic artery. If bleeding continuous after this manoeuvre, the bleeding is likely to be from hepatic vein or IVC. The time of Pringle manoeuvre is controversial, but it can be applied up to 1 hour without compromising the blood supply to the liver.

5.4.1. Damage control surgery:

The concept of damage control was introduced by Stone et al [45] in the 1980s and promulgated by the group at Ben Taub in 1992 [46]. This came after the report by Denver General in patients sustaining fatal hepatic hemorrhage.

After trauma, hemostasis was not possible as patients were hypothermic, acidotic, and receiving large volumes of packed red cells before blood component or fresh blood [47]. This led to the concept of the "bloody vicious cycle." The term "damage control" was popularized by the group at the University of Pennsylvania in the 1993 [48]. They described initial control of haemorrhage and contamination followed by packing and temporary abdominal closure, ICU restoration of normal physiology, and delayed definitive repair of intra-abdominal injuries. The decision for damage control should be made very early in the operation before the onset of severe coagulopathy, acidosis, and hypothermia. Early institution of packing as a damage control technique has been shown to lessen mortality [49].

The damage control concept is very appropriate for the management of major liver injuries. The three key factors that interact to produce a deteriorating metabolic situation are hypothermia, coagulopathy, and acidosis. Patients in this condition are at the limit of their physiological reserve and persistence with prolonged and complex surgical repair attempts will cause exceptionally high mortality [50]. Early recognition of hypo-thermia, coagulopathy, and acidosis is the key to the damage control approach. It is recommended that definitive surgery should cease and a damage control approach be adopted when hypothermia is deteriorating or a temperature of 34°C is reached, when coagulopathy has developed (nonsurgical oozing or prothrombin time greater than 50% above normal), or when acidosis exists ($pH<7.2$ despite adequate volume resuscitation).

Once the patient is stabilized, patient is returned to the operation theatre and definitive surgery is undertaken if needed.

5.4.2. Perihepatic packing:

Tamponade which is achieved by manual compression that can then be maintained by packs, which can also be manually compressed if bleeding continues. Packs placed in an anterio-posterior axis will often distract the injured liver further and worsen the bleeding. The lobes of the liver must be compressed back to normal position, essentially back toward midline. Simultaneously, the liver is pushed toward the diaphragm. Maintenance of this anatomic compression by the first or second assistant is critical to reduce bleeding as the surgeon assesses the liver injury or mobilizes the liver. Perihepatic packing can help to maintain this tamponade. Most minor venous bleeding and small lacerations to the parenchyma can be temporized by this manoeuvre. Haemostatic agents such as surgicell, thrombin-soaked gel foam, or fibrin glue are useful adjuncts.

Packing is not as effective for the injuries to the left hemiliver, because with the abdomen open, there is insufficient abdominal and thoracic wall anterior to the left hemiliver to provide adequate compression. Fortunately, haemorrhage from the left hemiliver can be controlled by dividing the left triangular and left coronary ligaments and compressing the left hemiliver between the hands.

Packs must be placed around the liver to reconstitute its anatomical shape. Packs should never be inserted into the hepatic wound, as it will tear the vessels and will increase the bleeding. It is also important to avoid excessive packing, as compression of IVC can lead to resultant decreased venous return, and reduces left ventricular filling. Excessive packing can also lead to compartment syndrome and multi-organ failure [51]. Conversely under-packing is associated with increased transfusion requirements and unplanned re-look laparotomies [52]. To reduce the risk of abdominal compartment syndrome, some advocate closing the upper part of the wound to enhance the tamponade effect but leaving the lower two-thirds open and temporarily covered with a silastic sheet sutured to the skin edges [53, 54].

Perihepatic packing will control profuse haemorrhage in up to 80% of patients undergoing laparotomy and will allow intraoperative resuscitation (resuscitative packing) [50, 55]. In the management of severe injuries of the liver, packing has emerged as the key to effective damage control [56]. However, more definitive "therapeutic" packing is also a very effective technique, particularly when used judiciously to prevent the cascade of hypothermia, coagulopathy, and acidosis [57].

Once the patient is stabilized, temporary closure of the abdomen is done and patient is shifted to the ICU. Packs can be removed after 36-48 hours. Broad spectrum antibiotics should be started to prevent sepsis. The exact timing of the removal of packs is controversial, but they should not be removed before 24 hours as this is related to re-bleeding and leaving them in place for 24 hours or more does improve outcome [58]. Even delayed removal (up to 1 week) has been reported without increasing the morbidity [59]. During removal, the packs should gently be removed after soaking with saline. Liver should be checked for re- bleeding and if adequate hemostasis is achieved, closure of the abdomen can be done after putting a drain.

5.4.3. Hepatorrhaphy:

This is an older technique which involves passing deep parenchymal sutures to bring disrupted tissue together compressing bleeding vessels and reducing dead space. The major drawback of this procedure is ischemic necrosis and infection of the liver parenchyma. However, some advocate hepatorrhaphy for "hard-to-reach" areas such as the dome and posterior portion of the right lobe.

5.4.3.1. Mesh Wrapping:

Mesh-wrapping is a quick and technically feasible method to achieve definitive hemostasis in severe liver trauma. It can be combined ideally with conventional procedures. Mesh-wrapping technique provides a highly selective, tight compression confined to the liver and does not produce an increased intra-abdominal pressure. Emphasis should be given in two important technical aspects while mesh wrapping. First, the traumatized liver has to be slung with the mesh under enough tension to create a tamponade effect. In addition the mesh should be attached into two anchoring stable points. The diaphragmatic crus and the falciform ligament provide the best options to stabilize the mesh. The mesh is resorbable and therefore reoperation for removal is not necessary. Furthermore, the resulting product of mesh hydrolysis has a bacteriostatic effect, minimizing the risk of infection [60].

5.4.4. Hepatotomy and selective vascular ligation:

Combined hepatotomy and selective vascular ligation has emerged as the preferred method of management for major hepatic venous, portal venous, and arterial injuries in many centres [61]. For control of major vascular injuries, Pachter et al. recommend a rapid and extensive finger fracture, often through normal parenchyma, to reach the site of injury. However, it is important to emphasise that with a major hepatic venous injury, significant haemorrhage may occur while attempting to extend a deep liver laceration and that this bleeding will not be controlled by a Pringle clamp and increased morbidity may be incurred. Hepatotomy is done under Pringle manoeuvre and finger fracture method is used to divide the parenchyma to ligate the bleeding vessels. Pringle clamp is released intermittently to identify bleeding vessels.

5.4.5. Non-anatomical resection of liver:

This refers to removal of devitalised parenchyma using the line of injury as the boundary of the resection rather than standard anatomical planes [62]. Resectional debridement is indicated for peripheral portion of nonviable hepatic parenchyma. Debridement is rarely a technique practised in isolation and is frequently used in conjunction with inflow control and hepatotomy. This allows for haemorrhage control prior to resection of all devitalised tissue while usually involves crossing traditional anatomical boundaries hence the term "non-anatomical resection". All devitalized tissues should be removed without making any attempt to resect normal parenchyma. Operative time should be as short as possible.

Except in rare circumstances, the amount of tissue removed should not be more than 25% of the liver. In some cases simple completion of an extensive parenchymal avulsion may suffice, e.g., when there has been an avulsion of the posterior sector of the right lobe (segments VI and VII). This type of injury is often associated with a right hepatic vein laceration and completion of the "resection" will allow control and suture of this. In such situations, vascular stapling devices are extremely useful for rapid and secure division of major veins.

5.4.6. Anatomical resection of liver:

The final alternative for patients with extensive injury to one hemiliver is anatomic hepatic resection. In elective circumstances, anatomic hemi-hepatectomies can be performed with excellent results; however, in the setting of trauma, the mortality associated with this procedure exceeds 50% in most series [63, 64]. This, plus the fact that the time and magnitude of the surgery goes against the later principles of conservative surgery and damage control, has resulted in anatomical resection being practised rarely and it is now performed in only approximately 2–4% major liver trauma cases [51].

Hepatic resection for an injured segment of the liver definitively controls bleeding, potential bile leak, and removes devitalized tissue. However, the role of hepatic resection in the management of liver injury remains controversial. The traditional poor results and lack of enthusiasm for this technique have been contradicted by the results of some recent series particularly that from Strong et al. who achieved excellent results in a series of 37 patients, 11 of whom (33%) had grade V juxtahepatic venous injuries [61]. These results probably reflect the fact that this procedure was performed in a specialist liver resection and transplantation unit, and while the majority of liver injuries continue to be managed initially in trauma centres or district hospitals, it is likely that more conservative and damage control procedures will remain the most widely practised techniques.

5.4.7. Intrahepatic balloon tamponade:

Intrahepatic balloon tamponade is useful for transhepatic penetrating injury. A device can either be fashioned from a Foley catheter and Penrose drain [65] or a Sengstaken-Blakemore tube. The device is gently delivered into the length of the tract and then inflated, often with a radio-opaque contrast fluid so integrity and position can be later confirmed radiologically if required. Once the patient is stabilized and coagulation and acidosis is corrected, the balloon can be deflated and removed during re-laparotomy.

5.4.8. Total vascular exclusion:

Total vascular exclusion of liver is sometimes used for extensive retrohepatic venous injuries. The technique involves clamping of the portal triad and infra- and supra-hepatic IVC and therefore requires experience with mobilisation of the liver as done in liver resection and transplantation. Excellent results were reported for this technique by Khaneja et al. [66] who used it to manage grade V penetrating injuries with 90% of patients surviving the operation and an overall survival rate of 70%.

The major drawback of this technique is decreased venous return due to clamping of IVC. This will lead to further hypotension in patient who is already in hypothermia and hypotension. This procedure can only be feasible in experienced hand in high volume centres.

5.4.9. Liver transplantation:

This remains a therapy of last resort limited to specialist centres with the literature limited to occasional case reports and series [67]. While liver transplantation may be life-saving for major liver trauma, the logistical problems will mean that it remains a limited option, available only in specialist centres.

6. Postoperative complications and mortality:

Overall mortality for patients with hepatic injuries is approximately 10%. The most common cause of death is exsanguination, followed by MODS and intracranial haemorrhage. Liver trauma is a morbid injury with complication rates from recent series ranges from between 8.1% to 30% [68].

6.1. Postoperative haemorrhage:

Primary exsanguinating haemorrhage is a major source of mortality, but most studies report secondary haemorrhage occurring in 3- 6% of survivors with no significant difference between blunt and penetrating mechanisms [69]. Surgical haemorrhage (ie discrete bleeding) and disseminated intravascular coagulation account for the majority of causes in even proportions. In patients managed by peri-hepatic packing, patients who had packs removed at <36hrs had more episodes of haemorrhage requiring re-packing than those with removal between 36 hours and 72 hours.

In most instances of persistent postoperative haemorrhage, the patient is best served by being returned to the operation room. Angiography with embolization may be considered in selected patients. If the reason for haemorrhage is coagulopathy, it should be corrected first and then patients should be reassessed.

6.2. Sepsis and abscess:

Post-operative sepsis occurs in 12-32% of patients. Minor morbidity occurs with urinary tract, surgical wound and respiratory tract sepsis. More serious are intra-abdominal abscesses which occur in up 24% of patients and are associated with concomitant bowel injury, higher grades of liver injury (IV and V) and massive transfusion [70].

An abdominal CT with intravenous and oral contrast should be performed to diagnose the cause of sepsis. Majority of the abscesses can be drained percutaneously under USG or CT-guidance; however, infected hematoma and infected necrotic liver tissue cannot be expected to respond to percutaneous drainage. Operative drainage may be a better option in such type of patients.

6.3. Biloma:

Bilomas are loculated collection of bile, which is with or without infection. CT-guided percutaneous drainage is the best option for infected bilomas. If the biloma is sterile, it will eventually be resorbed. Biliary ascites is caused by disruption of major bile duct. Reoperation after the establishment of appropriate drainage is the prudent course.

Biliary fistulas occur in approximately 3% of the patients with major liver injury [71]. They are usually of little consequences and generally close without specific treatment.

7. Injuries to the Bile ducts and gall bladder:

Extrahepatic bile ducts are rarely injured during blunt or penetrating abdominal injuries [72, 73]. Diagnosis is usually made during surgery or sometimes postoperatively. Management of bile duct injury detected postoperatively has already been described. If laparotomy is performed for patient with trauma, collection of bile in to the right upper quadrant suggest major bile duct injury. Sometimes it is very difficult to detect the site of bile duct injury, as associated disruption of liver parenchyma and haemorrhage makes detection a challenging task.

Management of bile duct injury is further complicated by small calibre and thin wall of the bile duct. Bile duct injury ranges from small laceration to tissue loss or complete disruption. Primary repair may be attempted when there is small laceration and no tissue loss. When there is a tissue loss or the laceration is larger than 25% to 50% of the diameter of the duct, the treatment option is a Roux-en-Y choledocho-jejunostomy [74, 75]. Isolated injury to left or right hepatic duct is even more challenging and should only be managed by experienced hepatobiliary surgeon. If expertise is not available, large bore tube should be kept and patient should be transferred to higher centre. If both the ducts are injured, both the ducts should be intubated by separate tubes and brought out. Elective repair should be undertaken once the patient is stable and after adequate assessment of injury by cholangiogram.

Injury to the gall bladder is treated either by repair or cholecystectomy.

8. Summary:

The management of injuries of the liver has evolved significantly throughout the last two decades. Non-operative techniques for the management of grade IV–V injuries in stable patients have been established, although there is a higher failure rate for these injuries compared with grade I–III injuries. Because of the progress that has been made in the quality and wide availability of the MDCT scan combined with minimally invasive intervention options like angio-embolization, NOM has evolved to be the treatment of choice for hemodynamically stable patients. In terms of surgical management there has been a definite move away from major, time-consuming procedures toward conservative surgery and damage control. The preferred surgical technique for inaccessible bleeding within a laceration is rapid finger fracture hepatotomy, Kelly –crush hepatic transection and direct suture or ligation. Prolonged attempts at surgical control and repair should be avoided, and definitive perihepatic packing should be employed at an early stage in the persistently unstable patient or at

http://dx.doi.org/10.5772/52107

the first signs of coagulopathy. Formal anatomical resection carries a high morbidity when used for haemorrhage control, although in an experienced centre this may be appropriate. Hepatorrhaphy has become discouraged due to complications of sepsis and bleeding, but may be a useful technique in penetrating trauma where the liver is difficult to access.

Author details

Rajan Jagad*, Ashok Thorat and Wei-Chen Lee

*Address all correspondence to:

Division of Liver and Transplantation Surgery, Department of General Surgery, Chang-Gung Memorial Hospital at Linkou, Chang-Gung University College of Medicine, Taiwan

References

[1] Miller, P. R., Croce, M. A., Bee, T. K., et al. (2002). Associated injuries in blunt solid organ trauma: the implications for missed injury in non-operative management. *J Trauma*, 53, 238-242.

[2] Shanmuganathan, K., Mirvis, S. E., & Chiu, W. C. (2004). Penetrating torso trauma: triple-contrast helical CT in peritoneal violation and organ injury. *A prospective study in 200 patients. Radiology*, 231, 775-784.

[3] Polanco, P., Leon, S., Pineda, J., et al. (2008). Hepatic resection in the management of complex injury to the liver. *J Trauma*, 65(6), 1264-9, 1269-70.

[4] Badger, S. A., Barclay, R., Diamond, T., et al. (2009). Management of liver trauma. *World J Surg*, 33, 2522-37.

[5] Trunkey, D.D. (2004). Hepatic trauma: contemporary management. *Surg Clin North Am*, 84, 437-50.

[6] Kozar, R. A., Moore, J. B., Niles, S. E., et al. (1999). Complications of non-operative management of high-grade blunt hepatic injuries. *J Trauma 2005* 59:1066-1071.

[7] American College of Surgeons. (1997). Advanced Trauma Life Support manual. *American College of Surgeons*, Chicago, IL.

[8] Peng, R. Y., & Bongard, F. S. (1999). Hypothermia in trauma patients. *J Am Coll Surg*, 188, 688-696.

[9] Mac, Kenzie. S., Kortbeek, J. B., Mulloy, R., & Hameed, S. M. (2004). Recent experiences with a multidisciplinary approach to complex hepatic trauma. *Injury*, 35, 869-77.

[10] Dolich, M. O., Mc Kenney, M. G., Varela, J. E., Compton, R. P., Mc Kenney, K. L., & Cohn, S. M. (2001). ultrasounds for blunt abdominal trauma. *J Trauma*, 50, 108-112.

[11] Richards, J. R., Knopf, N. A., Wang, L., & Mc Gahan, J. P. (2002). Blunt abdominal trauma in children: evaluation with emergency US. *Radiology*, 222, 749-754.

[12] Sirlin, C. B., Brown, M. A., Andrade-Barreto, O. A., et al. (2004). Blunt abdominal trauma: clinical value of negative screening US scans. *Radiology*, 230, 661-668.

[13] Poletti, P. A., Kinkel, K., Vermeulen, B., Irmay, F., Unger, P. F., & Terrier, F. (2003). Blunt abdominal trauma: should US be used to detect both free fluid and organ injuries? *Radiology*, 227, 95-103.

[14] Sirlin, C. B., Casola, G., Brown, M. A., Patel, N., Bendavid, E. J., & Hoyt, D. B. (2001). Patterns of fluid accumulation on screening ultrasonography for blunt abdominal trauma: comparison with site of injury. *J Ultrasound Med*, 20, 351-357.

[15] Stassen, N. A., Lukan, J. K., Carrillo, E. H., et al. (2002). Examination of the role of abdominal computed tomography in the evaluation of victims of trauma with increased aspartate aminotransferase in the era of focused abdominal sonography for trauma. *Surgery*, 132, 642-646.

[16] Jansen, J. O., Yule, S. R., & Loudon, M. A. (2008). Investigation of blunt abdominal trauma. *BMJ*, 336, 938-942.

[17] Rozycki, G. S., Ballard, R. B., Feliciano, D. V., et al. (1998). Surgeonperformed ultrasound for the assessment of truncal injuries: lessons learned from 1540 patients. *Ann Surg*, 228, 557-567.

[18] Stengel, D., Bauwens, K., Sehouli, J., et al. (2005). Emergency ultrasound based algorithms for diagnosing blunt abdominal trauma. *Cochrane Database Syst Rev* (2):CD004446.

[19] Taourel, P., Vernhet, H., Suau, A., et al. (2007). Vascular emergencies in liver trauma. *Eur J Radiol*, 64, 73-82.

[20] Smith, R.S. (2001). Cavitary endoscopy in trauma. *Scand J Surg.*, 91, 67-71.

[21] Kawahara, N. T., Alster, C., Fujimura, I., Poggetti, R. S., & Birolini, D. (2009). Standard examination system for laparoscopy in penetrating abdominal trauma. *J Trauma*, 67:589.

[22] Israelit, S. H., & Krausz, M. M. (2006). Laparoscopic management of a combat military injury during the Lebanon War in August., *J Trauma*, 108-10.

[23] Haan, J. M., Bocchicchio, G. V., Kramer, N., et al. (2005). Nonoperative management of blunt splenic injury: a 5-year experience. *J Trauma*, 58, 492-498.

[24] Stein, D. M., & Scalea, T. M. (2006). Nonoperative management of spleen and liver injuries. *J Intensive Care Med*, 21, 296-304.

[25] Cywes, B. S., Rode, H., & Millar, A. J. (1985). Blunt liver trauma in children: nonoperative management. *J Pediatr Surg*, 20, 14-18.

[26] Sherman, H. F., Savage, B. A., Jones, L. M., et al. (1994). Nonoperative management of blunt hepatic injuries: safe at any grade? *J Trauma*, 37, 616-621.

[27] Carrillo, E. H., Spain, D. A., Wohltmann, C. D., et al. (1999). Interventional techniques are useful adjuncts in nonoperative management of hepatic injuries. *J Trauma*, 46, 619-624.

[28] Dabbs, D. N., Stein, D. M., & Scalea, T. M. (2009). Major hepatic necrosis: a common complication after angioembolization for treatment of high-grade liver injuries. *J Trauma*, 66(3), 621-7.

[29] Pachter, H. L., Guth, A. A., Hofstetter, S. R., & Spencer, F. C. (1998). Changing patterns in the management of splenic trauma: the impact of nonoperative management. *Ann Surg*, 227, 708-717.

[30] Meyer, A. A., Crass, R. A., Lim, R. C., et al. (1985). Selective nonoperative management of blunt liver injury using computed tomography. *Arch Surg*, 120, 550-554.

[31] Velamhaos, G. C., Konstantinos, T., Radan, R., Chan, L., Rhee, P., Tillou, A., & Demetriades, D. (2003). High success with nonoperative management of blunt hepatic trauma. *Arch Surg*, 138, 475-81.

[32] Misselbeck, T. S., Teicher, E. J., Cipolle, M. D., Pasquale, M. D., Shah, K. T., Dangleben, D. A., & Badellino, M. M. (2009). Hepatic angioembolization in trauma patients: indications and complications. *J Trauma*, 67, 769-773.

[33] Yaman, I., Nazli, O., Tugrul, T., et al. (2007). Surgical treatment of hepatic injury: morbidity and mortality analysis of 109 cases. *Hepatogastroenterology*, 54, 1507-1511.

[34] Kozar, R. A., Moore, F. A., Cothren, C. C., Moore, E. E., Sena, M., Bulger, E. M., Miller, C. C., Eastridge, B., Acheson, E., Brundage, S. I., Tataria, M., Mc Carthy, M., & Holcomb, J. B. (2006). Risk factors for hepatic morbidity following nonoperative management: multicenter study. *Arch Surg*, 141, 451-8.

[35] Goldman, R., Zilkoski, M., Mullins, R., Mayberry, J., Deveney, C., & Trunkey, D. (2003). Delayed celiotomy for the treatment of bile leak, compartment syndrome, and other hazards of nonoperative management of blunt liver injury. *Am J Surg*, 185(5), 492-7.

[36] Dabbs, D. N., Stein, D. M., Philosophe, B., & Scalea, T. M. (2010). Treatment of major hepatic necrosis: lobectomy versus serial debridement. *J Trauma*, 69(3), 562-7.

[37] Hashimoto, 5., Hiramatsu, K., Ido, K., Yosii, H., et al. (1990). Expanding role of emergency embolization in the management of severe blunt hepatic trauma. *Cardiovasc Intervent Radiol*, 1, 193-199.

[38] Denton, J. R., Moore, E. E., & Coldwell, D. M. (1997). Multimodality treatment for grade 5 hepatic injuries: 'perihepatic packing', arterial embolisation and venous stenting. *J Trauma*, 42, 964-968.

[39] Asensio, J. A., Demetriades, D., Chahwan, S., et al. (2000). Approach to the management of complex hepatic injuries. *J Trauma*, 48, 66-72.

[40] Gaarder, C., Naess, P. A., Eken, T., Skaga, N. O., Pillgram-Larsen, J., Klow, N. E., et al. (2007). Liver injuries- improved results with a formal protocol including angiography., *Injury*, 38, 1075-1083.

[41] Lin, B. C., Wong, Y. C., Lim, K. E., et al. (2010). Management of ongoing arterial haemorrhage after damage control laparotomy: optimal timing and efficacy of transarterial embolisation. *Injury*, 41, 44-9.

[42] Griffen, M., Ochoa, J., & Boulanger, B. R. (2000). A minimally invasive approach to bile peritonitis after blunt liver injury. *Am Surg*, 66, 309-12.

[43] Malhotra, A. K., Latifi, R., Fabian, T. C., et al. (2003). Multiplicity of solid organ injury: influence on management and outcomes after blunt abdominal trauma. *J Trauma*, 54, 925-9.

[44] Stone, H. H., Strom, P. R., & Mullins, R. J. (1983). Management of the major coagulopathy with onset during laparotomy., *Ann Surg.*, 197, 532-535.

[45] Burch, J. M., Ortiz, V. B., Richardson, R. J., Martin, R. R., Mattox, K. L., & Jordan, G. L. (1992). Abbreviated laparotomy and planned reoperation for critically injured patients., *Ann Surg.*, 215, 476-483.

[46] Elerding, S. C., Arragon, G. E., & Moore, E. E. (1979). Fatal hepatic hemorrhage after trauma., *Am J Surg*, 138, 883-888.

[47] Rotondo, M. F., Schwab, C. W., Mc Gonigal, M. D., et al. (1993). Damage control': an approach for improved survival in exsanguinating penetrating abdominal injury., *J Trauma.*, 35, 375-383.

[48] Asensio, J. A., Roldan, G., Petrone, P., et al. (2003). Operative management and outcomes in 103 AAST-OIS grades IV and V complex hepatic injuries: trauma surgeons still need to operate, but angioembolization helps. J Trauma.; , 54, 647-654.

[49] Hoey, B. A., & Schwab, C. W. (2002). Damage control surgery. *Scand J Surg*, 91, 92-103.

[50] Parks, R. W., Chrysos, E., & Diamond, T. (1999). Management of liver trauma. *Br J Surg*, 86, 1121-35.

[51] Aydin, U., Yazici, P., Zeytunlu, M., & Coker, A. (2008). Is it more dangerous to perform inadequate packing?, *World J Emerg Surg*, 3:1.

[52] Sheridan, R., Driscoll, D., & Felsen, R. (1997). Packing and temporary closure in liver injury. *Injury*, 28, 711-712.

[53] Cue, J. I., Cryer, H. G., Miller, F. B., et al. (1990). Packing and planned re-exploration for hepatic and retroperitoneal haemorrhage: critical refinements of a useful technique. *J Trauma*, 30, 1007-1013.

[54] Nicol, A. J., Hommes, M., Primrose, R., et al. (2007). Packing for control of hemorrhage in major liver trauma. *World J Surg*, 31, 569-574.

[55] Krige, J.E.J. (2000). Liver fracture and bleeding. *Br J Surg*, 87, 1615-1616.

[56] Moore, F. A., Moore, E. E., & Seagraves, A. (1985). Non-resectional management of major hepatic trauma. *Am J Surg*, 150, 725-729.

[57] Walt A.J. (1986). Discussion: packing for control of hepatic haemorrhage. *J Trauma*, 26, 741-756.

[58] Balogh, Z., Mc Kinley, B. A., Cox, C. S., et al. (2003). Abdominal compartment syndrome: the cause or the effect of multiple organ failure? *Shock*, 20, 483-492.

[59] Meldrum, D. R., Moore, F. A., Moore, E. E., et al. (1997). Prospective characterisation and selective management of the abdominal compartment syndrome. *Am J Surg*, 174, 667-673.

[60] Dellaportas, D., Nastos, C., Psychogiou, V., Tympa, A., et al. (2011). Iatrogenic liver trauma managed with mesh-wrapping and ligation of portal vein branch: A case report. *Int J Surg Case Rep.*, 2(8), 261-263.

[61] Fang, J. F., Chen, R. J., Lin, B. C., et al. (2000). Blunt hepatic injury: minimal intervention in the policy of treatment. *J Trauma* 49:722-728.

[62] Duane, T. M., Como, J. J., Bochichio, G. V., et al. (2004). Re-evaluating the management and outcomes of severe blunt liver injury. *J Trauma*, 57, 494-500.

[63] Jacobson, L. E., Kirton, O. C., & Gomez, G. A. (1992). The use of an absorbable mesh wrap in the management of major liver injuries. *Surgery* 111:455.

[64] Poggetti, R. S., & Moore, E. E. (1992). Balloon tamponade for bilobar transfixing hepatic gunshot wounds., *J Trauma*, 33:694.

[65] Khaneja, S. C., Pizzi, W. F., Barie, P. S., et al. (1997). Management of penetrating juxtahepatic inferior vena cava injuries under total vascular exclusion. *J Am Coll Surg*, 184, 469-474.

[66] Angstadt, J., Jarrell, B., Moritz, M., et al. (1989). Surgical management of severe liver trauma: a role for liver transplantation., *J Trauma*, 29, 606-8.

[67] Aldrete, J. S., Halpern, N. B., Ward, S., & Wright, J. O. (1979). Factors determining the mortality and morbidity in hepatic injuries. Analysis of 108 cases., *Ann Surg*, 189, 466-74.

[68] Degiannis, E., Levy, R. D., Sa, F. C. S., Velmahos, G. C., Mokoena, T., & Daponte, A. (1995). Gunshot injuries of the liver : The Baragwanath experience. *Surgery I:*, 359-364.

[69] Caruso, D. M., Battistella, F. D., Owings, J. T., Lee, S. L., & Samaco, R. C. (1999). Perihepatic packing of major liver injuries: complications and mortality. *Arch Surg*, 134:958.

[70] Donovan, A. J., Michaelian, M. J., & Yellin, A. E. (1973). Anatomical hepatic lobectomy in trauma to the liver. *Surgery* 73:833.

[71] Fabian, T. C., Croce, M. A., Stanford, G. G., et al. (1991). Factors affecting morbidity after liver trauma. *Ann Surg* 213:540.

[72] Jurkovich, G. J., Hoyt, D. B., Moore, F. A., et al. (1995). Portal triad inuries: a multi-institutional study: *J trauma* 39:426.

[73] Sheldon, G. F., Lim, R. C., Yee, E. S., et al. (1985). Management of injuries to the porta hepatis. *Ann Surg* 202: 539.

[74] Feliciano, D. V., Bitando, C. V., Burch, J. M., et al. (1985). Management of traumatic injuries to the extrahepatic biliary ducts. *Am J Surg* 150:705.

[75] Bade, P. G., Thomson, S. R., Hirshberg, A., et al. (1989). Surgical options in traumatic injury to the extrahepatic biliary tract. *Br J Surg* 76:256.

Chapter 26

Hepatic Trauma

Bilal O. Al-Jiffry and Owaid AlMalki

Additional information is available at the end of the chapter

http://dx.doi.org/10.5772/52793

1. Introduction

The word liver was derived from the old English word "life" [1]. Survival without the liver is impossible for more than a few hours except in very unusual circumstances. The liver is the largest intra-abdominal solid organ; with its friable parenchyma, its thin capsule, and its relatively fixed position in relation to the spine, makes it particularly prone to injury. As a result of its larger size and proximity to the ribs, the right hemi-liver is injured more commonly than the left. It's the second most commonly injured organ in abdominal trauma, but damage to the liver is the most common cause of death after abdominal injury [2], [3]. Management of Liver Trauma may vary widely from non operative management (NOM) with or without angioembolization to Damage Control Surgery (DCS) [4]. DCS is mainly centered on stopping the bleeding by packing, Pringles, and vascular exclusion to totally replacing the liver by a liver transplant [5].

Although blunt liver trauma accounts for 15-20% of abdominal injuries, it is responsible for more than 50% of deaths resulting from blunt abdominal trauma. The mortality rate is higher with blunt abdominal trauma than with penetrating injuries[6]. In Europe, blunt trauma predominates (80-90 per cent of all liver injuries)[6]-[8], while penetrating injuries account for 66 per cent of liver trauma in South Africa [9] and up to 88 per cent in North America [10]-[13]. Unfortunately, we don't have enough data for the Arab countries though we are one of the highest countries in motor vehicle accidents with more than 9000 deaths per year.

As a result of this high mortality rate, emergency surgery was frequently indicated in patients with hepatic injury in the past. However, advances in diagnostic imaging, better monitoring facilities and the introduction of damage control strategy in trauma has influenced our approach in the management of liver trauma [14].

2. Anatomy

In this part we will describe the anatomy of the liver and its attachments in relation to what is needed in liver trauma, to achieve good mobilization with haemorrhage control to reach the first stage of damage control.

2.1. Surface anatomy

It's important to know the location of the liver and its surface anatomy to be able to choose the best incision, to determine if it is involved in a penetrating trauma, and to think of it when you have a chest trauma especially on the right lower chest. When viewed from the front (fig. 1), the normal liver surface markings are [15]:

Upper margin: at the xiphisternal joint arching upwords on both sides. On the left it runs for 7-8cm from the mid-line. On the right, it reaches the fifth rib.

Right boarder: it curves downword from the seventh to the eleventh rib in the mid axillary line.

Inferior boarder: along a line that joins both right lower and upper left points.

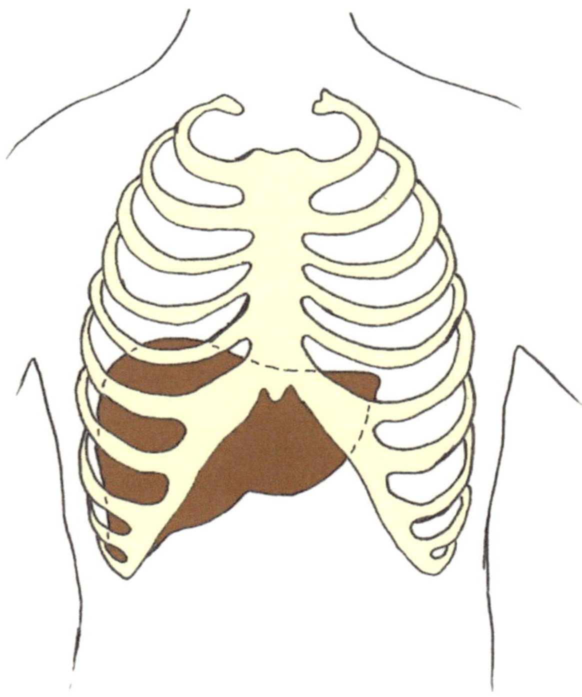

Figure 1. Surface anatomy of the liver

http://dx.doi.org/10.5772/52793

2.2. Gross anatomy

The liver has three surfaces [16]

- Diaphragmatic Surface:

This is covered with peritoneum to act as a sheath around the liver. In the midline the falciform ligament is attached and divides the liver into the right and left anatomical liver, or better descried it runs between the left lateral section (segment 2 and 3) and the left medial section (segment 4).

- Visceral Surface:

The sharp inferior border of the liver joins the diaphragmatic surface with the visceral surface of the liver. The main structures are lined in an H shaped. The cross part is made of the porta hepatis (hilum of the liver). The right limb is made of the inferior vena cava. The left limb is made of the contiuity of the fissures for the ligamentum teres anteriorly and the ligamentum venosum posteriorly. On the left side lies the caudate lobe and on the right lies the bare area of the liver.

- Posterior Surface (fig 2):

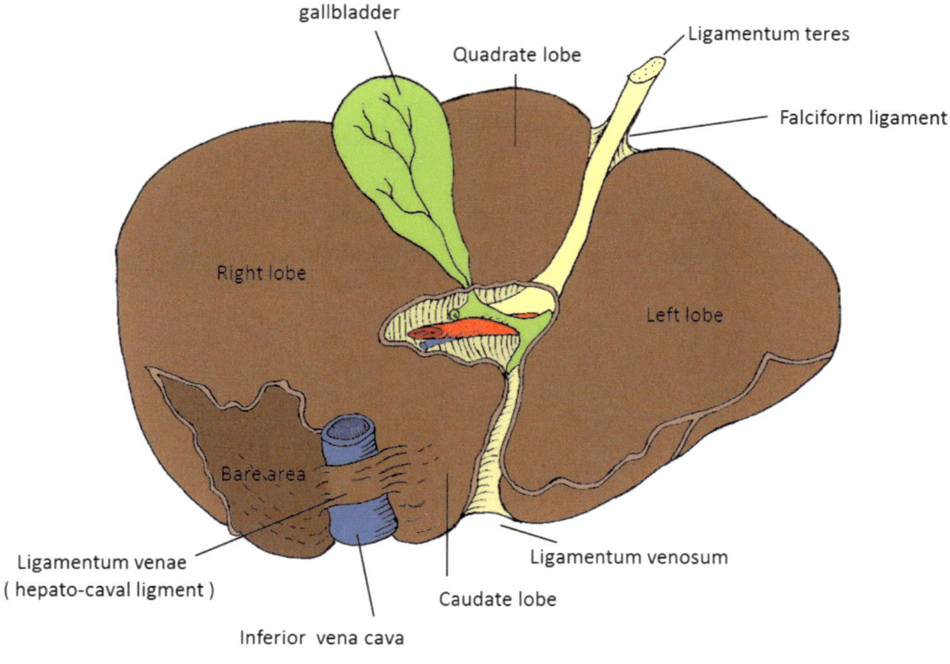

Figure 2. Visceral surface of the Liver

The IVC runs in the centre of the posterior surface. A firous band called the ligamentum venae cavae (hepato-caval ligament) covers part of the IVC posteriorly. The rest of the posterior surface is made of by the ligaments (the left and right triangular ligaments, and the coronary ligament) which attach the liver to the diaphragm.

2.3. Ligaments of the liver

The falciform ligament consists of two closely layers of peritoneum. The ligamentum teres runs on its free edge with a small paraumbilical vein. On the right it forms the upper layer of the coronary ligament, witch continues inferiorly to form the right triangular ligament, then to the lower coronary ligament. On the left, the falciform ligament forms the anterior layer of the left triangular ligament. (fig 3 &4)

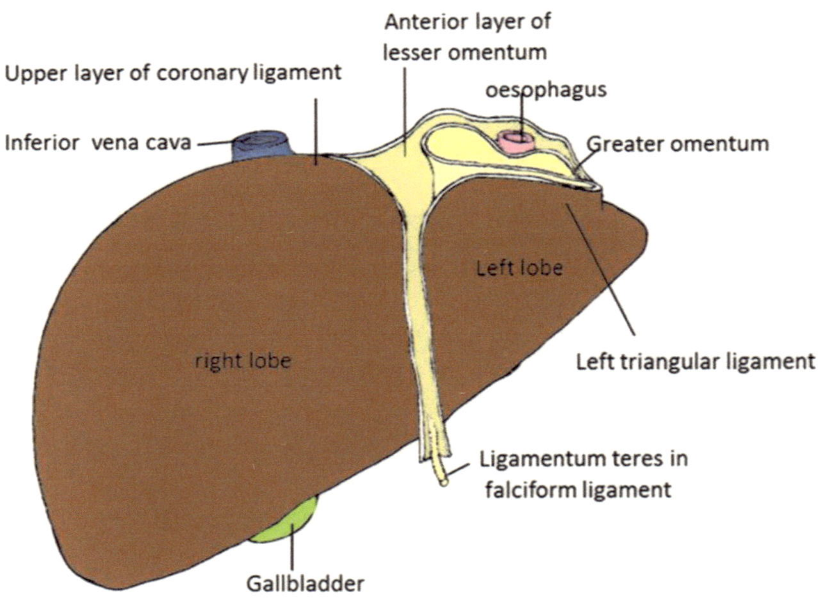

Figure 3. Diaphragmatic surface of the liver and its ligaments

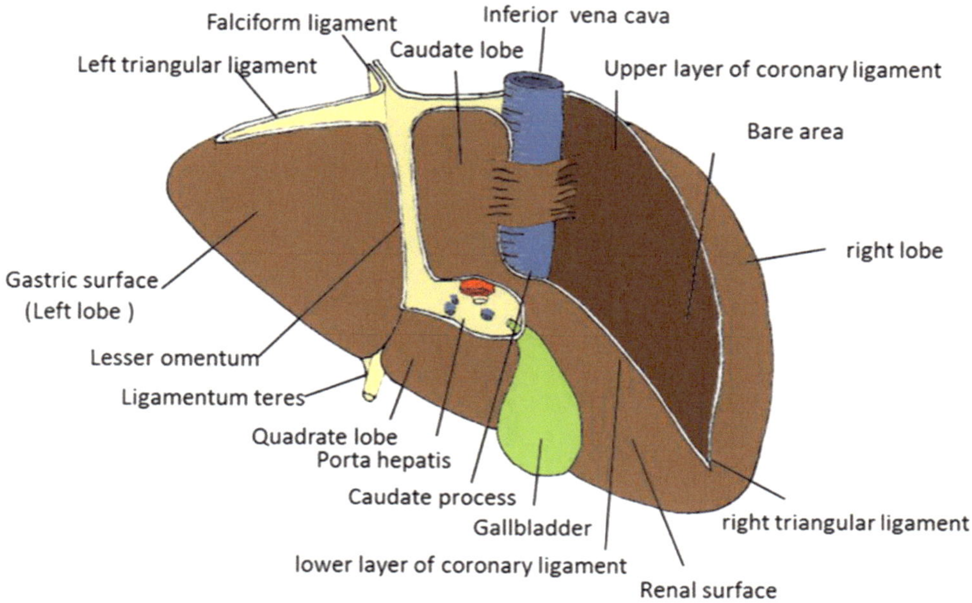

Figure 4. Posterior surface of the liver and its ligaments

2.4. Caudate lobe

The caudate lobe is the dorsal portion of the liver lying posteriorly and embracing the retrohepatic IVC in a semi circumferential fashion. It lies between the IVC posteriorly, the portal triad inferiorly and the hepatic veins superiorly. There is a series of short hepatic veins which drains directly from the caudate lobe to the retrohepatic IVC. Thus it is surrounded by important structures that can be involved in liver trauma 17 (Fig 5).

2.5. The glissonian sheath

Glisson's capsule which covers the liver extends into the liver at the hilus and covers the portal triad were it is called the Glisson's sheath. With relation to liver trauma it is important to know only the extrahepatic portion of the Glissonian pedicle which is called the hepatodudenal ligament. This is very important when a Pringle manoeuvre is needed. It usually composed of connective tissue and peritoneum up to the hepatic hilum. They surround the portal vein posteriorly, the hepatic artery anteriorly and to the left, and the common bile duct anteriorly and to the right (fig 6) 18.

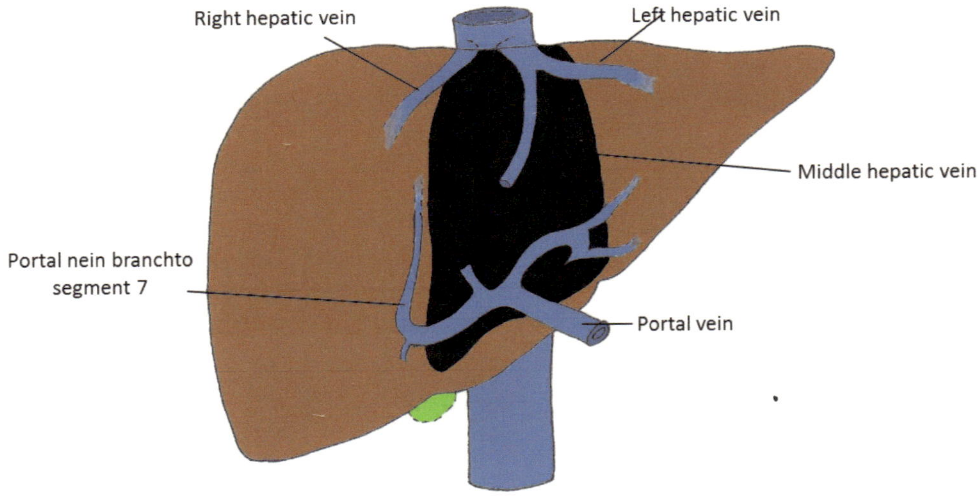

Figure 5. The caudate lobe: front view

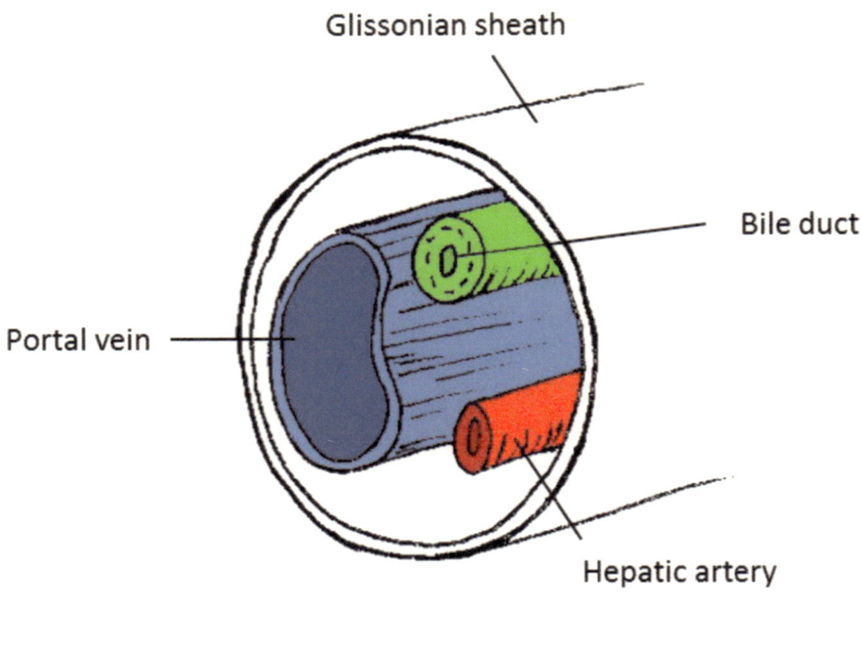

Figure 6. Structures within the glissonian sheath

http://dx.doi.org/10.5772/52793

2.6. Retrohepatic IVC and its branches (fig 7)

In relation to liver trauma we can divide the retrohepatic IVC into four parts:

The suprahepatic group; which is composed of both right and left inferior phrenic veins which drain the right and left diaphragm.

The hepatic veins; which are composed of the right, middle and left hepatic vein. There are multiple variations that can exist and its knowledge is important in liver surgery.

The retrohepatic group; which is composed of short veins that drain part of the right hemi-liver and the caudate lobe directly into the IVC. These veins are short and very fragile and are prone to injury.

Lastly, the infrahepatic group; which consists mainly of both the right and left adrenal veins. These veins are frequently injured in trauma and if not considered during mobilizing the right liver [19].

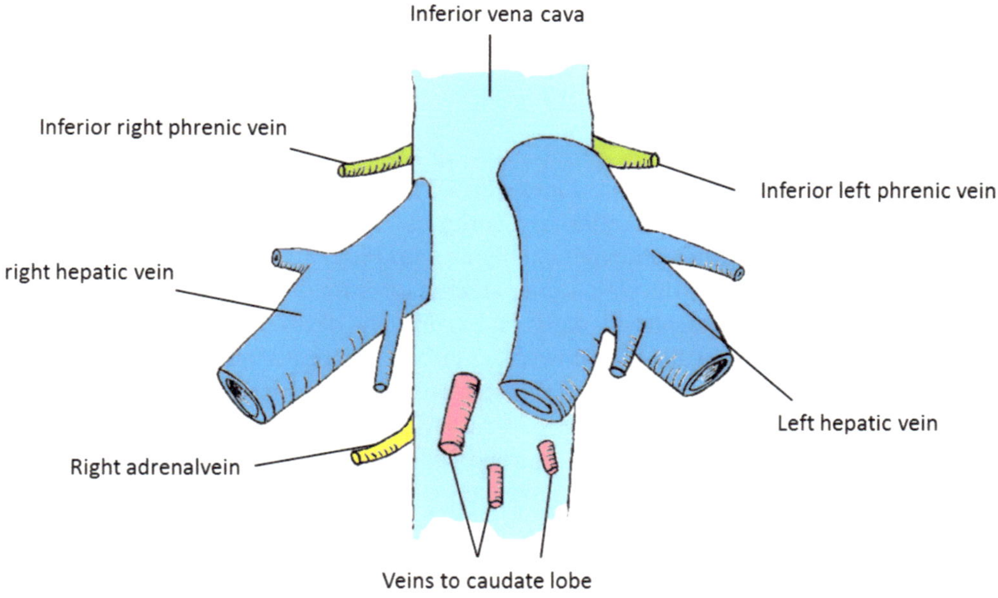

Figure 7. The abdominal inferior vena cava and its suprarenal branches

3. Mechanism

Penetrating and blunt trauma are the two principal mechanisms for liver trauma. Motor vehicle accidents account for the majority of blunt trauma, whereas knife and gunshot wounds constitute the major cause of penetrating injuries

Two types of blunt liver trauma have been described: deceleration (shearing) injuries occur in motor vehicle accidents and in falls from a height where there is movement of the liver in its relatively fixed position, thereby producing a laceration of its relatively thin capsule and parenchyma at the sites of attachment to the diaphragm[13].

The other type of liver injuries is crush injury. Crush injuries follow direct trauma to the abdomen over the liver area. Decelerating injuries typically create lacerations between the right posterior section (segments 6 and 7) and the right anterior section (segments 5 and 8), which can extend to involve major vessels. Crush injuries can lead to damage to the central portion of the liver (segment 4, 5 and 8) and also may cause bleeding from the caudate lobe (segment 1)[12]-[13]. Blunt trauma can cause parenchymal hepatic injury with intact Glisson's capsule, leading to an intraparenchymal or subcapsular haematoma[12]-[13].

Penetrating injuries are usually associated with gunshot or stab wounds, with the former usually resulting in more tissue damage due to the cavitation effect as the bullet traverses the liver substance [13]-[20]. These injuries usually require surgery more often than blunt injuries when the liver is involved.

4. Diagnosis

Signs and symptoms of hepatic injuries are related to the amount of blood loss, peritoneal irritation, right upper quadrant tenderness, and guarding. Rebound abdominal tenderness is common but nonspecific. Occasionally, patients with blunt abdominal trauma do well initially, but they subsequently develop a liver abscess, presumably due to unrecognized liver damage. These patients present with signs and symptoms of deep-seated infection [21]. Patients may present with severe peritonism due to bile peritonitis resulting from bile leaks. Signs of blood loss, such as shock, hypotension, and a falling hematocrit level, may dominate the picture [21] As resuscitation proceeds, a detailed physical examination is carried out. Most conventional texts emphasis the need for a careful history and physical examination of the abdomen. While this is undoubted importance, it is extremely difficult to assess the abdomen in the trauma situation as the history may not be available and all the existing physical signs are misleading. Fresh blood is not a peritoneal irritant [22]. The mechanism of injury is critically important in assessing the potential for abdominal injury. This information may be obtained from the patient, relatives, police or emergency care personnel [22]

Following initial assessment, a conscious patient, who is haemodynamically unstable following blunt trauma and has generalized peritonism, should undergo immediate laparotomy without further investigation [13]. Urgent laparotomy is also indicated in patients who have sustained a stab wound to the abdomen and are haemodynamically unstable. If the patient is stable and a liver injury is suspected, imaging studies should be performed [21]-[23] However, haemodynamically stable patients with suspected liver injury can be investigated at this stage to define the nature of the injury.

Ultrasonography (FAST) has gained increased acceptance, particularly in the emergency department, for the rapid evaluation of patients with blunt or penetrating abdominal trauma [24]-[29]. It is cheap, portable and noninvasive, compare to peritoneal lavage and it does not use radiation or iodinated contrast media [30]-[32]. Its sensitivity for the presence of intra-abdominal fluid in patients with trauma ranges from 75 to 93.8% and the specificity from 97 to 100% [24]-[25]. However, some pitfalls remain in abdominal ultrasonography. Injuries at the dome or lateral segments of the liver can easily by missed with ultrasound, especially in the presence of ileus or if the patient cannot cooperate because of pain. Hepatic laceration or hematomas are usually difficult to distinguish, especially in the acute phase, because they are isoechoic to the normal liver [33]-[34].

Kalogeropoulu and colleagues (2006) demonstrated the usefulness of contrast enhanced ultrasonography in penetrating liver trauma [35]. It increases the sensitivity and the specificity of ultrasound in evaluation of abdominal trauma not only in detection of free peritoneal fluid but also in the visualization of the parenchymal lacerations. The use of contrast in addition to the conventional ultrasound scanning does not significantly prolong the examination time, compared with a contrast enhanced CT scan. Furthermore repeated doses of the contrast can be injected to scan the rest of the solid abdominal organs such spleen and kidneys if a more complex trauma is suspected [35]. However, US is operator dependent, were you may not find an expert ultrasonographer in the middle of the night. In addition, US contrast is not wildly available in every casualty.

Computed tomography (CT) is the gold standard investigation for the evaluation of a stable patient with suspected liver trauma [36]-[39]. CT has high sensitivity and specificity for detecting liver injuries which increase as the time between injury and scanning increases, evidently because haematomas and lacerations become better defined [40]. Contrast-enhanced CT, is accurate in localizing the site and extent of liver and associated injuries, providing vital information for treatment in patients. CT without intravenous contrast enhancement is of limited value in hepatic trauma, but it can be useful in identifying or following up a hemoperitoneum [41]-[43].

CT scanning allows reasonably accurate grading of liver injuries and provides crude quantitation of the degree of hemoperitoneum. CT scanning is mandatory for patients with blunt trauma whose liver injury is to be managed nonoperatively. CT has also been useful for detecting missile tracts in penetrating trauma patients. Such information is imperative for surgeons who want to attempt nonoperative management of penetrating wounds [44]-[47]

Although CT is very useful in the evaluation of stable patients with abdominal trauma, most authors agree that unstable patients, with either blunt or penetrating trauma, are unlikely to benefit from this investigation because of the valuable time that it requires [44] (Fig 8)

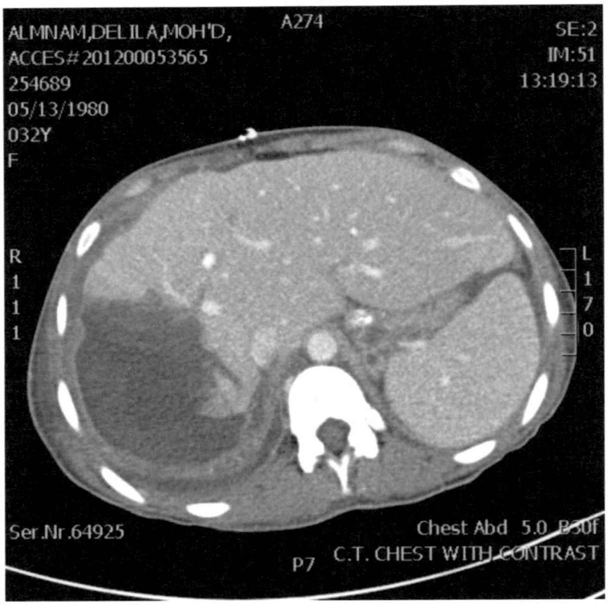

Figure 8. A CT demonstrating a grade 4 liver injury that was treated surgically

False-positive errors in the diagnosis of liver injury with CT scans may occur as a result of beam-hardening artifacts from adjacent ribs, which can mimic contusion or hematoma. An air-contrast level within the stomach in a patient with a nasogastric tube can produce streak artifacts throughout the left lateral section of the liver; these may mimic intrahepatic lacerations and/or hemorrhage. The nature of these artifacts can be confirmed if the patient is scanned in a decubitus position [48].

False-negative findings may occur in the setting of a fatty liver only when contrast-enhanced CT scan are obtained. On these images, the enhanced fatty liver may become isoattenuating relative to the laceration or hematoma. In this situation, a nonenhanced CT scan may provide useful information regarding hepatic injury. Focal fatty infiltration may also mimic hepatic hematoma, laceration, or infarction. Hepatic lacerations with a branching pattern can mimic unopacified portal or hepatic veins or dilated intrahepatic bile ducts. Careful evaluation of all branching intrahepatic structures is important and the diagnosis is made with serial images to differentiate the various structures [48]-[49]

MRI has a limited role in the evaluation of blunt abdominal trauma, and it has no advantage over CT scanning. Theoretically, MRI can be used in follow-up monitoring of patients with blunt abdominal trauma, and MRI may be useful in young and pregnant women with abdominal trauma in whom the radiation dose is a concern [6], [50].

MRCP has been used in the assessment of pancreatic duct trauma and its sequelae, and it can be used to image biliary trauma. Another potential use of MRI is in patients with renal failure and in patients who are allergic to radiographic contrast medium. MRI offers no significant advantage over CT scanning for routine evaluation of acute abdominal trauma. Experience is insufficient for assessing the value of the special circumstances mentioned above. Sufficient experience has not been gained in the use of MRI to establish false-positive and false-negative findings [6]

Angiography has no role in the evaluation of unstable patients. However, if the patient is stable, cross-sectional imaging may provide sufficient detail to treat the patient conservatively. A dynamic angiographic study may demonstrate the site of active bleeding. This when combined with angiographic embolization, especially in high-grade liver injury is of significant value and may be the only treatment required [51]-[52]. Although angiography is useful in selected patients, both false-positive and false-negative results occur in patients with hepatic trauma [6]

Endoscopic retrograde cholangiopancreatography (ERCP) may help in the delineation of the biliary tree in patient with liver trauma, and stents may be used to treat biliary Leaks [53]-[54] (Fig 9).

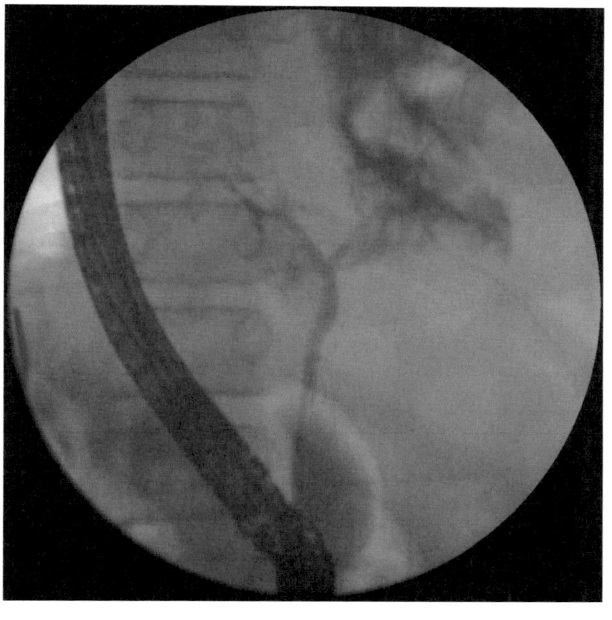

Figure 9. ERCP demonstrating a bile leak from the main right duct

Diagnostic laparoscopy has been used successfully in patients with abdominal trauma [55]-[58], and laparoscopic fibrin glue in managing liver injuries has also been reported [60].The benefits of laparoscopic assessment include reducing negative and non-therapeutic laparotomy rates, patient morbidity rates, hospital stay and treatment costs [56]-[57]. Raphael and colleagues(1999) reviewed 37 studies with more than 1,900 trauma patients (including those with liver trauma), and laparoscopy was analyzed as a screening, diagnostic, or therapeutic tool. They came out with the conclusion that "Laparoscopy has been applied safely and effectively as a screening tool in stable patients with acute trauma. Because of the large number of missed injuries when used as a diagnostic tool, its value in this context is limited. Laparoscopy has been reported infrequently as a therapeutic tool in selected patients, and its use in this context requires further study.[61].

5. Classification of liver injury

Liver trauma ranges from a minor capsular tear, with or without parenchymal injury, to extensive disruption involving both hemi liver with associated hepatic vein or vena caval injury. In 1989, the Organ Injury Scaling Committee of the American Association for the Surgery of Trauma produced a Hepatic Injury Scale [62] by which hepatic injuries are described in most major trauma centers (Table 1). Grade I or II injuries are considered minor; they represent 80-90 per cent of all cases and usually require minimal or no operative treatment [1], [63]. Grade III-V injuries are generally considered severe and often require surgical intervention, while grade VI injuries are regarded as incompatible with survival.

Grade	Type of Injury	Description of injury
I (fig 10)	Hematoma Laceration	Subcapsular, < 10% surface area Capsular tear, < 1cm parenchymal depth
II (Fig 11)	Hematoma Laceration	Subcapsular, 10% to 50% surface area Capsular tear, 1-3cm parenchymal depth and < 10cm in length
III (Fig 12)	Hematoma Laceration	Subcapsular, > 50% surface area or expanding Intraparenchymal hematoma > 2cm or expanding Capsular tear, >3cm parenchymal depth
IV (Fig 13)	Hematoma Laceration	Ruptured intraparenchymal hematoma with active bleeding Parenchymal disruption involving 25-50% of hepatic lobe
V	Laceration Vascular	Parenchymal disruption involving >50% of hepatic lobe Juxtahepatic venous injuries
VI	Vascular	Hepatic avulsion

Table 1. Classification of liver injury

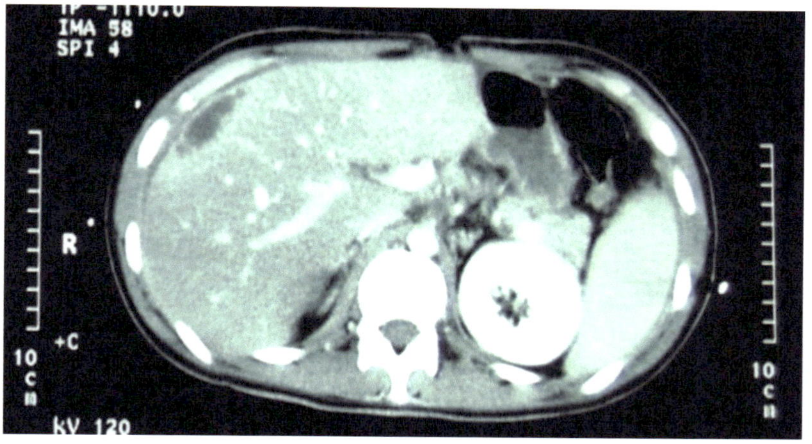

Figure 10. Grade 1 liver injury treated non surgically

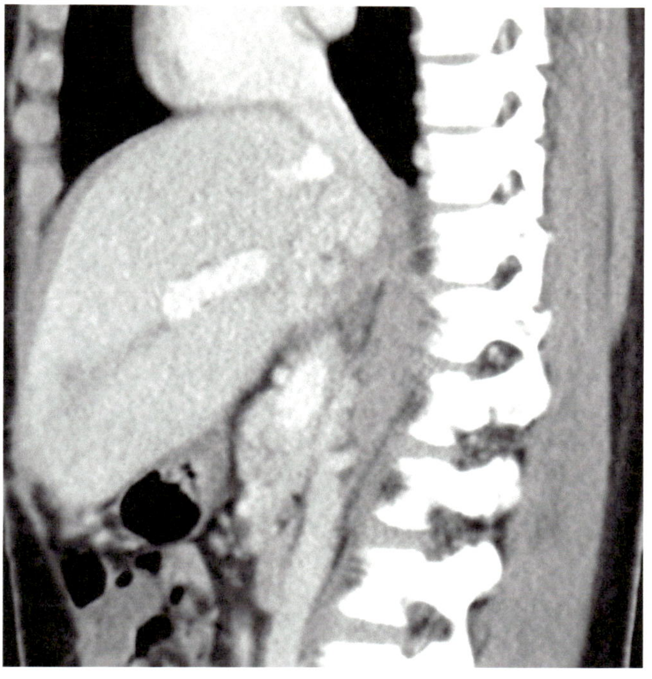

Figure 11. Grade 2 liver injury

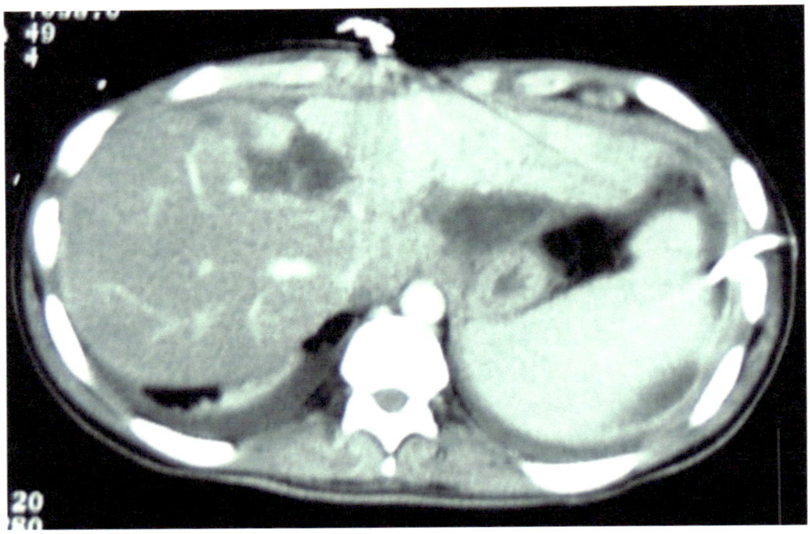

Figure 12. Grade 3 liver injury that was treated non surgically

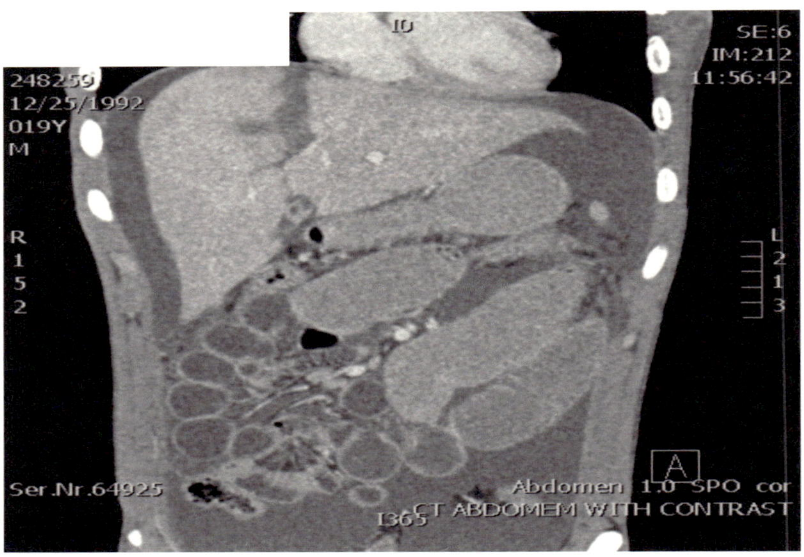

Figure 13. Grade 4 liver injury that was treated non surgically

6. Management

6.1. Non operative

The countercurrent argument was that nonoperative treatment (NOM) was associated with virtually a 100% mortality rate, so all patients with suspected or diagnosed liver injuries must have an operation. Improved mortality rates during and after World War II assured the primacy of operative treatment [64].

Three observations prompted the move towards nonoperative treatment. First, the practice of nonoperative treatment was initially advocated for splenic injuries and then extended to the liver. The success in children led to attempts of nonoperative treatment in adults [65]-[66] Second, the high rate of nontherapeutic operations in many patients with blunt hepatic injuries was not in patients' best interest. Third, the advent of CT scanning greatly facilitated both diagnosis and grading of injuries and gave some reassurance that the intestinal injuries had not occurred.

There has been several reports started since 1985, were Trunkey *etal* [67], defined the criteria for NOM:

- haemodynamic stability
- absence of peritoneal sign
- Availability of CT
- Monitor in ICU
- Facility of immediate surgery
- Absence of other organ injuries

These criteria has become more and more less strict, were multiple reports are trending more to NOM [3]. There is no time limit for NOM, continues monitoring is the only key to take the patient to the operating room [68]. Other reports even went to the extreme as if the patient had risk factors by the injury severity score (ISS) [69] and all patients should be treated first by NOM regardless of their trauma [70]. However, all of these reports mentioned that this is possible with the addition of angiography and embolization that made the NOM more feasible and more successful.

The success rate of nonoperative treatment has been remarkably high. The necessity for operations for ongoing hemorrhage has been reported to be from 5% to 15%. There remains a concern over missed bowel injuries that have been reported from 1% to 3%.[71]-[75].

Nonoperative treatment of abdominal stab wounds has been practiced successfully in numerous centers and is on the rise. NOM of gunshot wounds has been more controversial, however, many reports are calling to add these group of patients to the NOM group [76]-[79] Demetriades and colleagues(2006) reported 152 patients with penetrating solid organ injuries. 28.4% of all liver injuries were successfully managed nonoperatively [80]. However, in the last few years NOM has emerged a huge mile stone. Appropriately selected patients with liver gunshot injuries deemed feasible, safe, and effective, regardless of the liver injury severity [77]. However, they all mentioned that CT scan was mandatory before adopting the NOM. Another report stated that regardless of the grade of liver trauma, NOM is safe and effective in appropriately selected patients with liver gun shoot injuries treated in centers with suitable facilities [79].

6.2. Operative

6.2.1. Damage control surgery

As the first intention when taking the patient to the operating room is to do damage control surgery (DCS). This usually implies saving the patient's life and stopping the bleeding. This will make the patient more stable and in a better physiologically and hemodynamically state to be able to have the definitive treatment.

Skin preparation should allow for extension of a midline abdominal incision to a median sternotomy or right thoracotomy, if necessary, for adequate exposure of posterior liver injuries [81]-[82]. If the indication for surgery is an obvious penetrating through-and-through liver injury, or the patient failed the NOM and is clear liver injury only a bilateral subcostal incision is a useful alternative and has been adopted by some to have better liver exposure (fig 14).

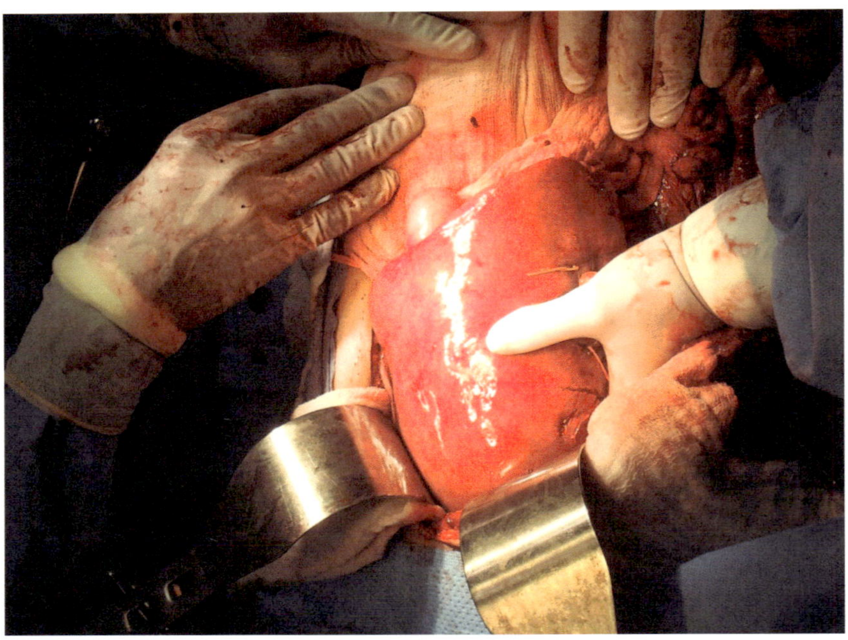

Figure 14. Mobilization of the right hemi-liver to achieve excellent exposure of the injury

http://dx.doi.org/10.5772/52793

DCS includes perihepatic packing and partial abdominal closure or Bogota bag. Usually an average of six laparotomy pads can be packed to get the tamponade effect between the liver and the abdominal wall. The timing of re-exploration is controversy but usually 12-24 hours is safe time for re-exploration were the patients condition permits (fig 15).

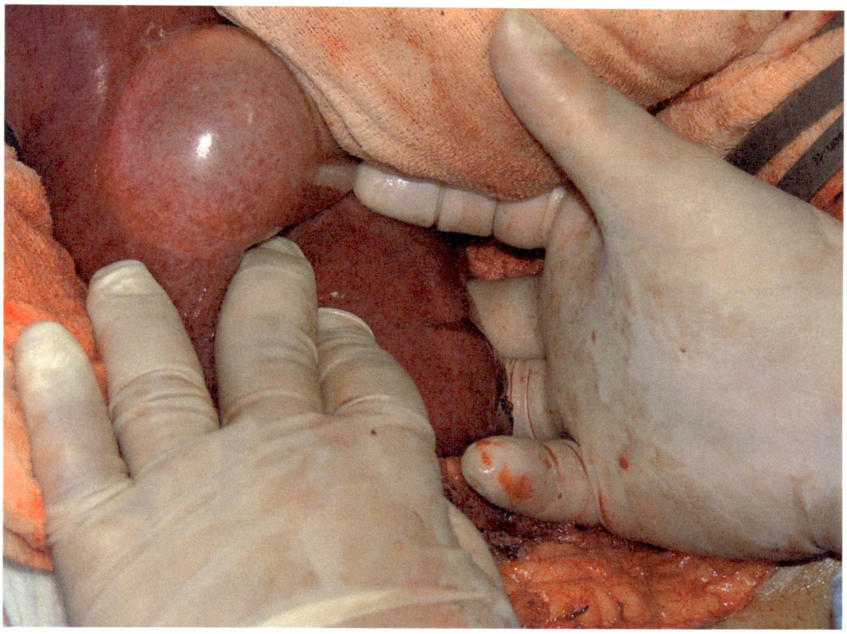

Figure 15. Packs as it was done in the first DCS were the bleeding stopped, fingers demonstrating the liver laceration

Even 30 years after the resurrection of packing as a treatment alternative, it remains an important part of the armamentarium of surgeons in managing difficult hepatic injuries. It is always better to have a patient with packs to come and deal with on another day, than trying to stop the bleeding with no success, especially if the surgeon has limited experience, which usually happens in the first operation. As many hospitals have a general surgeon on-call with limited liver or trauma experience.

If a major liver injury is encountered, initial control of bleeding can be achieved with temporary tamponade of the right upper quadrant using packs, portal triad occlusion (Pringle manoeuvre) (Fig 16a &b), bimanual compression of the liver or even manual compression of the abdominal aorta above the coeliac trunk [83]-[84]. Attempts to evaluate the liver injury before adequate resuscitation may result in further blood loss and worsening hypotension.

(a)

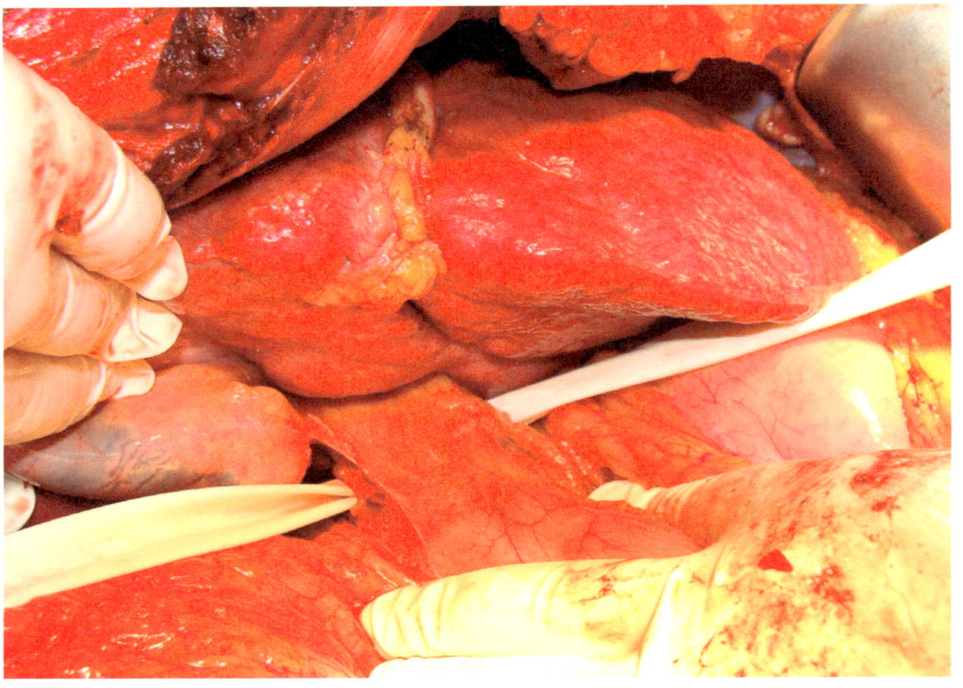

(b)

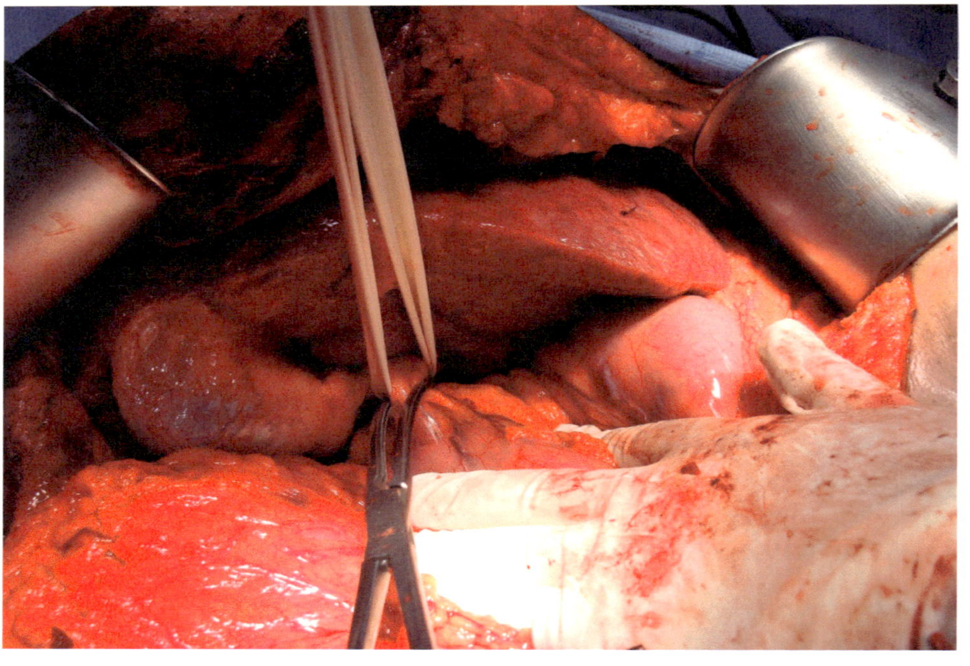

Figure 16. a. Tape inserted around the portal triad. b. Pringles manouver were the clamp is gently applied to occlude the portal triad

Digital compression of the portal triad (Pringle manoeuvre) can be used diagnostically and compression can be maintained with an atraumatic vascular clamp if haemorrhage decreases [85]. The clamp should be occluded only to the degree necessary to compress the blood vessels in order not to injure the common bile duct. If haemorrhage is unaffected by portal triad occlusion, major vena cava injury or atypical vascular anatomy should be suspected 86-87 Although the permitted occlusion time of the portal triad is controversial, most authors now agree that clamping of the hepatic pedicle for up to 1h is well tolerated with no adverse effects on liver function [81],[88]

After initial intraoperative resuscitation, the liver must be mobilized adequately to allow a thorough examination of the damaged area, unless the injury is already accessible through the incision [81,84,89] The liver is mobilized by dividing the falciform, triangular and coronary ligaments, and by placing abdominal packs posteriorly to maintain this position [90]. This manoeuvre allows the surgeon to determine the nature and severity of the injury and to decide on the necessary surgical technique. Care should be taken to avoid impairing venous return, by either excessive lifting and/or rotation of the mobilized liver, or excessive packing causing caval compression [90].

There are several tricks to stop the bleeding other than the one mentioned before, however we advise that most of these should be done by experienced surgeons in a stable patient or if the patient is still bleeding after trying the previous methods mentioned. Several specific modalities began to be used more often to treat arterial bleeding. Hepatorrhaphy was used with increased frequency. When the arterial bleeding occurred deep within the hepatic parenchyma, a tractotomy was advocated to expose and suture ligate the arterial flow. But control of deep arterial bleeding was often technically difficult to accomplish.[91]-[93]

In response to futile attempts to directly suture ligate arterial bleeding, Dr Aaron's group performed ligation of the hepatic artery.[94] Initially performed at the Louisville General Hospital to control arterial hemorrhage from a ruptured hepatic adenoma, Mays found this technique useful to control arterial bleeding in trauma patients. A literal explosion in its use occurred in Louisville, and surgeons there proposed it to prevent rebleeding.[95]-[96] A high rate of infection led to reconsideration of its use, and it was subsequently used less frequently [103], although it remained an operation that could occasionally be life-saving.97-98

Major venous bleeding was recognized as a major source of mortality, particularly in patients who had been in high-speed motor vehicle crashes. The nearly uniform lethality of retrohepatic vena caval injuries with attempt at direct repair led to the development of the atriocaval shunt. This technique, developed by Schrock and associates, [99] theoretically bypassed the caval injury and allowed direct suture repair of the cava itself and main hepatic veins. The operation required opening the chest to expose the atria. This bicavitary exposure accelerated hypothermia and coagulopathy in many patients. Consequently, the mortality rate remained high, but the concept of direct repair of this deadly injury was very important.

Both previously mentioned bleeding problems often were treated initially with temporary inflow occlusion by clamping the portal triad. The concept of inflow occlusion actually predated Pringle, [85] but his work published in 1908 was rediscovered and popularized in the 1960s after rarely being mentioned in the literature for more than 50 years.

Diffuse bleeding from damaged or devitalized liver increasingly required surgical treatment. Reports on civilian liver injuries from the 1950s generally cautioned against debridement of damaged liver for fear it would worsen preexisting hemorrhage. Absorbable gauze packing and drainage were mostly used for this problem. As the forces of injury increased, other techniques were required.

Resectioned debridement was increasingly used. There was a brief flurry of activity with use of major anatomic resections, but the high mortality rate of this procedure led to discontinuing its use in most centers.[100]-[101] The omental pedicle described for liver injury in 1910 and mentioned occasionally through the years was reintroduced by Stone and Lamb[102] and gained widespread popularity.

In summary; as a general surgeon facing a major hepatic injury in the middle of the night think of NOM and try not to rush to the operating room unless clearly indicated. However, if you were forced to the operating room do the minimal to stop the bleeding (DCS). If major procedure is required, the decision must be made early in the operation were technical /clinical expertise and speed are critical. Plan definitive surgeries in a stable patient were optimal condition ably.

6.2.2. *Definitive surgery*

This is usually carried out in a stable patient by an experienced surgeon at a second stage to deal with a certain problem (Fig 17). One of the commonest problem is bile leak and collection with an incidence of 6-20 %. This is usually after the patient recovered, were they develop an intra-abdominal collection that is best treated by a radiological applied drain. Then it can be investigated by MRCP or ERCP. The MRCP is non invasive, however with the collection it can have very little input. ERCP is advocated by some to be much better were the leak is identified and can be treated by sphinctrotomy and a stent [104] with very high success rate [105]. However, some of these patients fail and require surgical ligation of the leak which is much easier when the location is identified pre-operatively and a stent is in place to increase the success rate.

Another reason to go to the operating room is liver necrosis and abscess formation that occurs when bleeding stoops and demarcation of the live is obvious. Liver necrosis might increase with attempts to stop the bleeding with angioembolization in NOM or by arterial ligation and packing in DCS.The best option will be to drain the abscess radiologically were this might be sufficient. However, if not we advise operative drainage and an anatomical liver resection to maintain adequate live tissue and maintain a good vascular supply. This should be carried out by an experienced liver surgeon to get the best result (Fig 18).

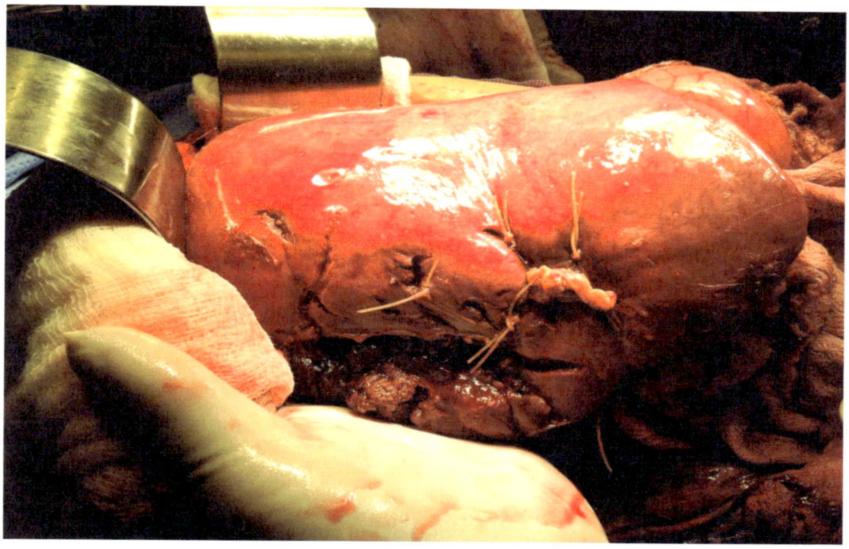

Figure 17. Full mobilization in a second look operation to stop the bleeding and to do definitive surgery.

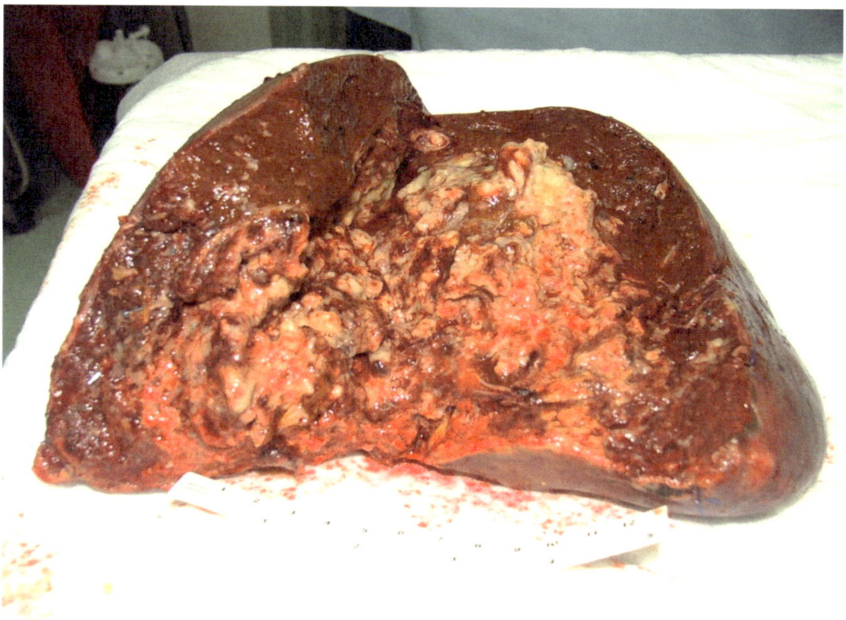

Figure 18. Liver necrosis following embolization with NOM for bleeding. The patient was treated by right hemi hepatectomy because the necrosis could not be drained radiologically.

Liver resection might be necessary with reported frequency of 2% to 5% in most series, with an overall mortality of 17.8% and morbidity around 30%.[106-108] (Fig 19).

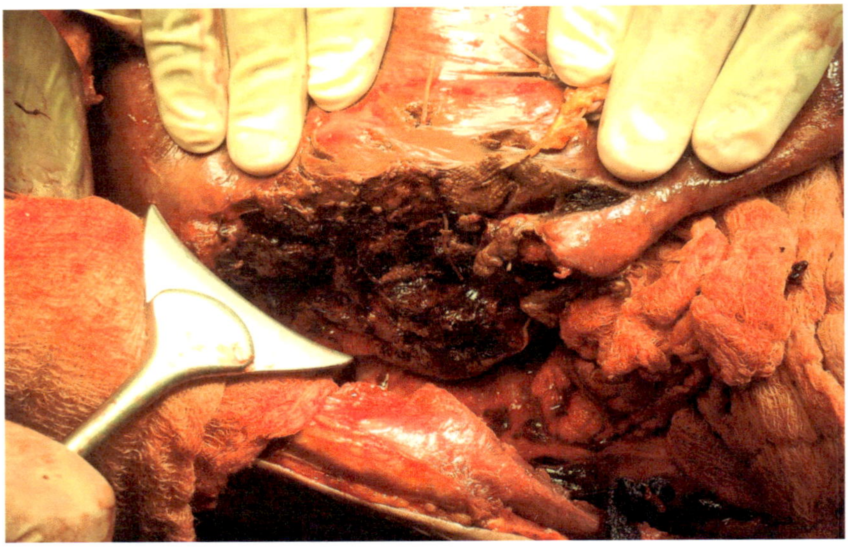

Figure 19. Liver trauma which was treated with a right posterior sectionectomy (seg 6&7)

Liver transplantation has been reported in the literature as an extreme intervention in cases of severe and complicated hepatic trauma. The main indications for liver transplant in such cases were uncontrollable bleeding and postoperative hepatic insufficiency. Liver transplant for trauma is a rare condition with 20 cases described in the literature [109]. Esquivel *et al.* first reported the use of liver transplantation in two patients with progressive hepatic failure and uncontrollable bleeding. [110]. The transplant decision is difficult because usual criteria are not validated, liver's potential recovery is difficult to evaluate and sepsis and head injuries often associated, complicating the decision because of their own prognosis. [111].

7. Complications

7.1. Non operative

The most common complication of NOM is failure, ending with the patient in the operating room. This is even more serious, because the patient most of the time is in a worse state than what he was and bleeding (the leading cause) is still ongoing. This also is more profound if it occurs in the middle of the night or with a surgeon of limited liver expertise. It should be borne in mind that this most common complication usually arises as a result of inappropriate selection of a patient for conservative management [23]. The failure rate ranges from 6-10% [68, 112] especially when it was combined with arterial emobolization, however, the incidence of liver necrosis was higher [113] (Fig 20a &b).

http://dx.doi.org/10.5772/52793

(a)

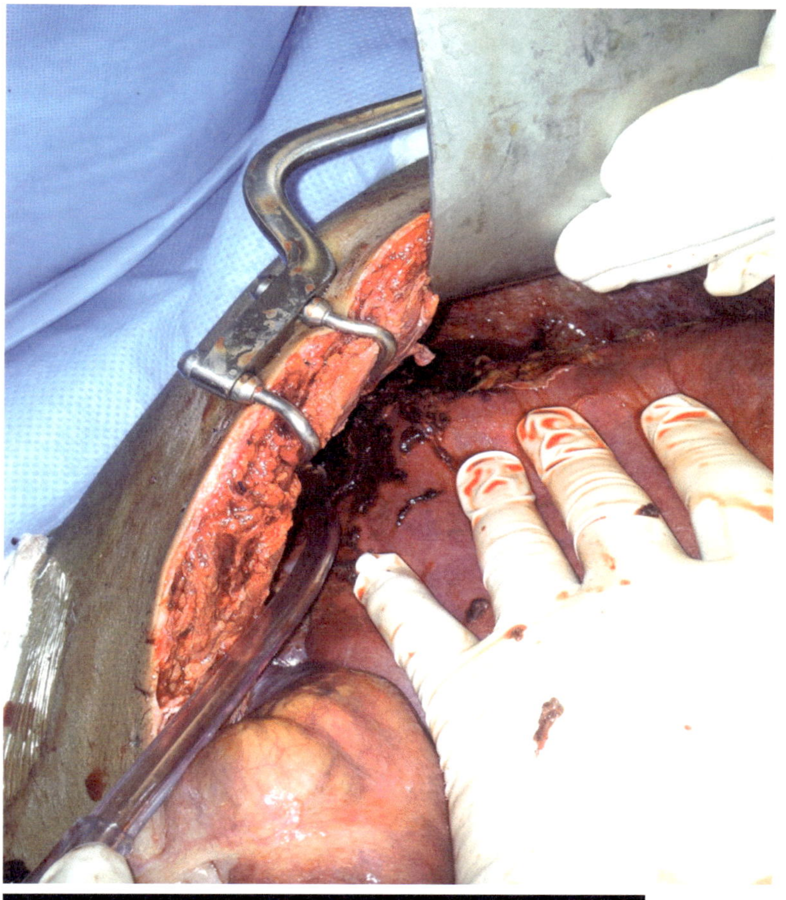

(b)

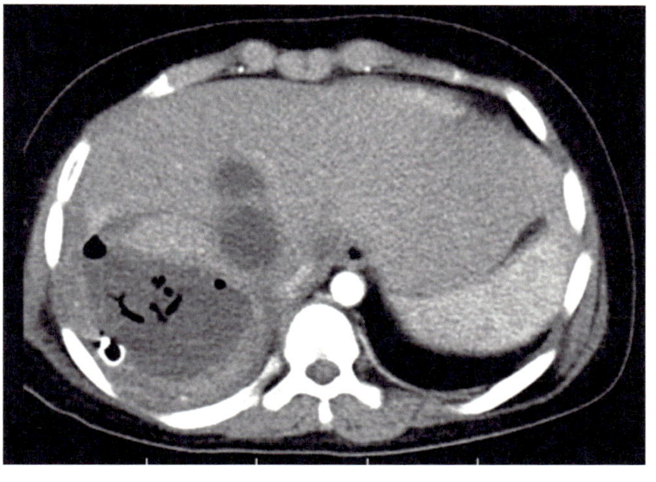

Figure 20. a. Failed NOM showing the bleeding from the liver dome. b. Same patient with grade 4 liver injury that failed NOM, drain left in place.

Complications can arise from injuries that have not been recognized at the time of initial presentation or /and become apparent after initial delay. Associated injuries seem to be the most important factors predisposing to postoperative problems [114]-[117].

In a recent multicenter study, hepatic complications developed in 5% (13 of 264) of patients with grade 3 injuries, 22% (36 of 166) of patients with grade 4 injuries, and 52% (12 of 23) of patients with grade 5 injuries. Univariate analysis revealed 24-hour crystalloid, total and first 24-hour packed red blood cells, fresh frozen plasma, platelet, and cryoprecipitate requirements and liver injury grade to be significant, but only liver injury grade and 24-hour transfusion requirement predicted complications by multivariable analysis. They came out with the Conclusion that NOM of high-grade liver injuries is associated with significant morbidity and correlates with grade of liver injury. Screening patients with transfusion requirements and high-grade injuries may result in earlier diagnosis and treatment of hepatic-related complications [118]. We have discussed in the previous section the management of each of these complications as a part of the operative management to liver trauma.

7.2. Operative

Rebleeding in the postoperative period is a challenging problem. Delayed haemorrhage is the most common complication of the non-operative management of hepatic injuries and is the usual indication for a delayed operation [119]. Coagulopathy, inadequate initial surgical repair and missed retrohepatic venous injury may result in further haemorrhage. Confirmed coagulation defects should be corrected as rapidly as possible with fresh frozen plasma and platelet transfusions.

Some authors recommend reoperation after transfusion of 10 units of blood in 24 h [120], however the limit of 6 units in the first 12 h seems to be more reasonable [121]-[122]. In cases with slow rebleeding when the limit of 6 units has not been exceeded, embolization of the bleeding vessels may be helpful [122]. Multiple bleeding vessels is usually the cause of failure because the vascular lesions distal to the area of embolization with rich collateral circulation, or bleeding from the portal or hepatic veins [123]-[125]

Late complications like sepsis, bile leak and liver failure occur at a later stage. Intra-abdominal sepsis in the postoperative period occurs in approximately 7-12 per cent of patients 126 Predisposing factors include the presence of shock and increased transfusion requirements, increased severity of liver injury, associated injuries such as small bowel or colonic perforation, the use of perihepatic packs, superficial suturing of deep lacerations with intrahepatic haematoma formation, and the presence of devitalized parenchyma. Adequate initial surgical management in an effort to reduce transfusion requirements, with debridement of all devitalized tissue and early removal of perihepatic packs, has been recommended to reduce the incidence of septic complications [81],.

Arteriovenous fistula is not an uncommon complication with an incidence of less than 3%. It can manifest after liver injury as an arterioportal fistula that can result in portal hypaertension and is usually treated by embolization [127].

http://dx.doi.org/10.5772/52793

8. Outcome

The mortality rate from liver trauma has fallen from 66 per cent in World War I, to 27 per cent in World War II, to current levels of 10-15 per cent [8],[10],[12],[128]-[129]. Better knowledge of liver pathophysiology and anatomy, and enhanced resuscitation, anaesthesia and intensive care, have contributed to this improvement. Schweizer et al,(1993) compared outcome to grade of injury. The overall mortality was 12% [9], specially with the livers excellent regeneration capability (Fig 21).

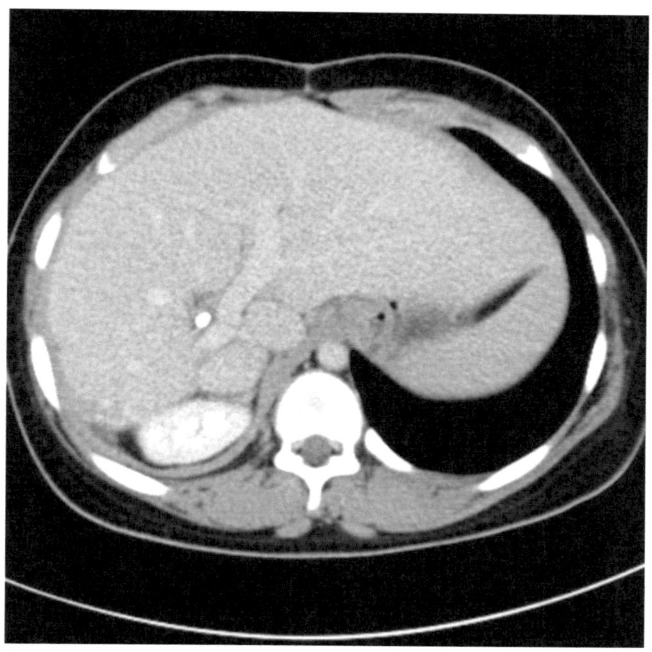

Figure 21. Liver regeneration post resection of the right liver

The mechanism of injury has an important bearing on mortality rate with blunt trauma carrying a higher mortality rate (10-30 per cent)[130]. than penetrating liver trauma (0-10 per cent)[10-11].

While most early deaths in patients with liver trauma seem to be due to uncontrolled haemorrhage and associated injuries, most late deaths result from head injuries and sepsis with multiple organ failure [131].

Author details

Bilal O. Al-Jiffry[1,2] and Owaid AlMalki[1]

1 Surgery, Taif University, Taif, Saudi Arabia

2 Surgery, AlHada Military Hospital, Taif, Saudi Arabia

References

[1] Wachtel T. Critical care concepts in the management of abdominal trauma. Crit Care Nurs Q. 1994;17(2):34-50.

[2] Feliciano DV. Surgery for liver trauma. Surg Clin North Am 1989; 69: 273-84.

[3] Cox EF. Blunt abdominal trauma. A five 5-year analysis of 870 patients requiring celiotomy. Ann Surg 1984; 199: 467-74.

[4] Clemente N, Di Saverio S, Giorgini E, Biscardi A, Villani S, Senatore G, Filicori F, Antonacci N, Baldoni F, Tugnoli G. Management and outcome of 308 cases of liver trauma in Bologna Trauma Center in 10 years. Ann Ital Chir. 2011 Sep-Oct;82(5):351-9

[5] Li Petri S, Gruttadauria S, Pagano D, Echeverri GJ, Di Francesco F, Cintorino D, Spada M, Gridelli B. Surgical management of complex liver trauma: a single liver transplant center experience. Am Surg. 2012 Jan;78(1):20-5

[6] A. Nawaz Khan H. Vadeyar Liver Trauma emedicine September 2005

[7] Matsch T, Begquist D, Hedelin M, Findblack B. Leberverletzungen nachstumpfem Bauchtrauma. Unfallchirurgie 1982; 85: 524-8.

[8] Schweizer W, Tanner S, Baer HU, Huber A, Berchtold R, Blumgart LH. Diagnostik und Therapie von Leberverletzungen beim polytraumatisierten Patienten. Helv Chir Acta 1989; 55: 597-612.

[9] Schweizer W, Tanner S, Baer HU, Lerut J, Huber A, Gertsch P et al. Management of traumatic liver injuries. Br J Surg 1993; 80: 86-8.

[10] Krige JE, Bornman PC, Terblanche J. Liver trauma in 446 patients. South Afr J Surg 1997; 35: 10-15.

[11] Feliciano DV, Mattox KL, Jordan GL Jr, Burch JM, Bitando CG, Cruse PA. Management of 1000 consecutive cases of hepatic trauma (1979-1984). Ann Surg 1986; 204: 438-45.

[12] Cogbill TH, Moore EE, Jurkovich GJ, Feliciano DV, Morris JA, Mucha P. Severe hepatic trauma: a multi-center experience with 1335 liver injuries. J Trauma 1988; 28: 1433-8.

[13] Park RW, Chrysos E, Diamond T, Management of liver trauma. Br J Surg 1999;86:1121-35.

[14] Parray FQ, Wani ML, Malik AA, Thakur N, Wani RA, Naqash SH, Chowdri NA, Wani KA, Bijli AH, Irshad I, Nayeem-Ul-Hassan. Evaluating a conservative approach to managing liver injuries in Kashmir, India. J Emerg Trauma Shock. 2011 Oct;4(4):483-7

[15] Liver resection and liver transplantation: the anatomy of the liver and associated structures. Jamieson Glyn, Launois B. In: The Anatomy of General Surgical Operation, Ed. Jamieson GG. Elsevier Churchill Livingstone, Edinburgh 2nd Ed. 2006. Chapter2, pp 8-23

[16] Gray`s anatomy of the human body, twentieth edition, Philadelphia , 2000.

[17] Peng SY. Isolated caudate lobe resection. In: Hepatocellular Carcinoma, Ed. Law WY, world Scientific Singapore2008. Chapter 26, pp 465-489

[18] Kawarada Y, Das BC, Taoka H. Anatomy of the hepatic hilar area: the plate system. Journal of HBP surgery 2000; 7: 580-586.

[19] Scheuerlein H, Kockerling F. The anatomy of the liver. In: liver surgery, Operative techniques and Avoidance of Complications. J.A. Barth, Heidelberg.2001, pp 9-38.

[20] Sherlock DJ, Bismuth H. Secondary surgery for liver trauma. Br J Surg 1991; 78: 1313-17.

[21] Arrillo EH, Wohltmann C, Evolution in the treatment of complex blunt liver injuries. Curr Probl Surg 2,001 Jan; 38(1): 1-60.

[22] Paterson-Brown, Core topics in general and emergency surgery; third edition 2005. Elsevier 239-257

[23] Garden, hepatobiliary and pancreatic surgery; third edition 2003. Elsevier 331-347

[24] . Bain IM, Kirby RM, Tiwary P, et al. Survey of abdominal ultrasound and diagnostic peritoneal lavage for suspected intra-abdominal injury following blunt trauma. Injury. 1999;29:65–71.

[25] Bode PJ, Edwards MJR, Kruit MC, van Vugt AB. Sonography in a clinical algorithm for early evaluation of 1671 patients with blunt abdominal trauma. Am J Radiol. 1999;172:905–911.

[26] Kimura A, Otsuka T. Emergency center ultrasonography in the evaluation of hemoperitoneum: a prospective study. J Trauma 1991; 31: 20-3.

[27] Hoffmann R, Nerlich M, Muggia-Sullam M, Pohlemann T, Wippermann B, Regel G et al. Blunt abdominal trauma in cases of multiple trauma evaluated by ultrasonography: a prospective analysis of 291 patients. J Trauma 1992; 32: 452-8.

[28] Pachter HL, Feliciano DV. Complex hepatic injuries. Surg Clin North Am 1996; 76: 763-82.

[29] Carrillo EH, Platz A, Miller FB, Richardson JD, Polk HC Jr. Non-operative management of blunt hepatic trauma. Br J Surg 1998; 85: 461-8.

[30] Goletti O, Ghiselli G, Lippolis PV, Chiarugi M, Braccini G, Macaluso C et al. The role of ultrasonography in blunt abdominal trauma: results in 250 consecutive cases. J Trauma 1994; 36: 178-81.

[31] Rozycki GS, Ochsner MG, Schmidt JA, Frankel HL, Davis TP, Wang D et al. A prospective study of surgeon-performed ultrasound as the primary adjuvant modality for injured patient assessment. J Trauma 1995; 39: 492-500.

[32] McKenney MG, Martin L, Lentz K, Lopez C, Sleeman D, Aristide G et al. 1000 consecutive ultrasounds for blunt abdominal trauma. J Trauma 1996; 40: 607-12.

[33] Richards JR, McGahan JP, Pali MJ, Bohnen PA. (1999) Sonographic detection of blunt hepatic trauma: hemoperitoneum and parencymal patterns of injury. J Trauma. 1999;47:1092–1097.

[34] Soto JA, Morales C, Murena F, Sanabria A, Guevara JM, Suarez T. Penetrating stab wounds to the abdomen: use of serial US and contrast enhanced CT in stable patients. Radiology. 2001;220:365–371.

[35] Hochmuth A, Fleck M, Hauff P, et al. First experience in using a new ultrasound mode and ultrasound contrast agent in the diagnosis of blunt renal trauma: a feasibility study in an animal model. [Preliminary report]. Invest Radiol. 2000;35:205–211.

[36] Adam A, Roddie ME. CT of the liver and biliary tract. In:Blumgart LH (ed.) surgery of the liver and the biliary tract, 2nd edn. Edinburgh: Churchil Livingstone, 1994;pp 243-70.

[37] Safi F, Weiner S, Poch B et al. surgical management of liver rupture. : Chirurgie 1999,70:253-8.

[38] Cachecho R, Clas D, Gersin K et al. Evolution in the management of the complex liver injury at a level 1 trauma center. J Trauma 1998; 45:79-82.

[39] Strong RW. The management of blunt liver injuries. Aust NZ J Surg 1999; 69:609-16.

[40] Toombs BD, Sandler CM, Rauschkolb EN, Strax R, Harle TS. Assessment of hepatic injuries with computed tomography. J Comput Assist Tomogr 1982; 6: 72-5.

[41] Carrillo EH, Wohltmann C, Evolution in the treatment of complex blunt liver injuries. Curr Probl Surg 2001 Jan; 38(1): 1-60.

[42] Casillas VJ, Amendola MA, et al, Imaging of nontraumatic hemorrhagic hepatic lesions. Radiographics 2000 Mar-Apr; 20(2): 367-78.

[43] Fang JF, Chen RJ, Wong YC, et al: Classification and treatment of pooling of contrast material on computed tomographic scan of blunt hepatic trauma. J Trauma 2000 Dec; 49(6): 1083-8.

[44] Meredith JW, Trunkey DD. CT scanning in acute abdominal injuries. Surg Clin North Am. 1988;68:255–268.

[45] Federle MP, Jeffrey RB. Hemoperitoneum studied by computed tomography. Radiology. 1983;148:187–192.

[46] Federle MP, Goldberg HI, Kaiser JA, et al.. Evaluation of abdominal trauma by computed tomography. Radiology. 1981;138:637–644.

[47] Toombs BD, Lester RC, Ben-Menachem Y, et al.. Computed tomography in blunt trauma. Rad Clin North Am. 1981;19:17–35.

[48] McGehee M, Kier R, Cohn SM, McCarthy SM: Comparison of MRI with postcontrast CT for the evaluation of acute abdominal trauma. J Comput Assist Tomogr 1993 May-Jun; 17(3): 410-3.

[49] Shuman WP. CT of blunt abdominal trauma in adults. Radiology 1997; 205: 297-306.

[50] Vock P, MRI. In: Blumgart LH (ed.) Surgery of the liver and biliary tract, 2nd edn. Edinburgh: Churchill Livingstone, 1994; pp271-82.

[51] Poletti PA, Mirvis SE, Shanmuganathan K, et al: CT criteria for management of blunt liver trauma: correlation with angiographic and surgical findings. Radiology 2000 Aug; 216(2): 418-27

[52] Hagiwara A, Yukioka T, Ohta S et al. non-surgical management of patients with blunt hepatic injury; efficacy of transcatheter arterial embolization. Am J Roentgenol 1997; 169:1151-6.

[53] Carrillo EH, Spain DA, Wohltmann CD et al.Interventional techniques are useful adjuncts in the non-operative management of hepatic injuries. J Trauma 1999;46:619-22.

[54] Sugimoto K, Asari Y, Sakaguchi T et al. ERCP in the non-surgical management o blunt liver trauma. J Trauma 1993;35:192-9.

[55] Sosa JL, Markley M, Sleeman D, Puente I, Carrillo E. Laparoscopy in abdominal gunshot wounds. Surg Laparosc Endosc 1993; 3: 417-19.

[56] Sosa JL, Arrillaga A, Puente I, Sleeman D, Ginzburg E, Martin L. Laparoscopy in 121 consecutive patients with abdominal gunshot wounds. J Trauma 1995; 39: 501-6.

[57] Ditmars ML, Bongard F. Laparoscopy for triage of penetrating trauma: the decision to explore. J Laparoendosc Surg 1996; 6: 285-91

[58] Hallfeld KK, Trupka AW, Erhard J et al. Emergency laparoscopy for abdominal stab wounds. Surg Endosco 1998; 12:907-10.

[59] Chen RJ, Fang JF,Lin BC et al. selective application of laparoscopy and fibrin glue in the failure of non-operative management of blunt hepatic trauma. J Trauma1998;44:691-5.

[60] Pilcher CJ, Wesolowski MS, Jawad MA. Laparoscopic applications for abdominal trauma injuries. AORN J 1996; 64: 366-75.

[61] Raphael T, Villavicencio , John A.Aucar. Analysis of laparoscopy in trauma. JACS 1999;189:pp11-20.

[62] Moore EE, Shackford SR, Pachter HL, McAninch JW, Browner BD, Champion HR et al. Organ injury scaling: spleen, liver and kidney. J Trauma 1989; 29: 1664-6.

[63] 14 Ochsner MG, Jaffin JH, Golocovsky M, Jones RC. Major hepatic trauma. Surg Clin North Am 1993; 73: 337-52.

[64] David Richardson, changes in the management of injuries to the liver and spleen. JACS May 2005 pages 648-669

[65] Richie JP, Fonkalsrud EN. Subcapsular hematoma of the liver. Arch Surg. 1972;104:781–784

[66] Karp MP, Cooney DR, Pros GA, et al.. The non-operative management of pediatric hepatic trauma. J Pediatr Surg. 1983;18:512–518.

[67] Meyers AA, Crass RA, Lim RA, et al.. Selective non-operative management of blunt liver injury using computed tomography. Arch Surg. 1985;120:550–554

[68] Parks NA, Davis JW, Forman D, Lemaster D. Observation for nonoperative management of blunt liver injuries: how long is long enough? J Trauma. 2011 Mar;70(3):626-9

[69] Norrman G, Tingstedt B, Ekelund M, Andersson R. Non-operative management of blunt liver trauma: feasible and safe also in centres with a low trauma incidence. HPB (Oxford). 2009 Feb;11(1):50-6

[70] Letoublon C, Chen Y, Arvieux C, Voirin D, Morra I, Broux C, Risse O. Delayed celiotomy or laparoscopy as part of the nonoperative management of blunt hepatic trauma. World J Surg. 2008 Jun;32(6):1189-93

[71] Marx JA, Moore EE, Jordan RC, et al.. Limitations of computed tomography in the evaluation of acute abdominal trauma—prospective randomized study. J Trauma. 1985;25:933–938.

[72] Buckman RF, Piano G, Dunham CM, et al.. Major bowel and diaphragmatic injuries associated with blunt spleen or liver rupture. J Trauma. 1988;28:1317–1321.

[73] Fischer RP, Miller-Crotchet P, Reed RL. The hazards of non-operative management of adults with blunt abdominal injury. J Trauma. 1988;28:1445–1449.

[74] Kemmeter PR, Hoedema RE, Foote JA, et al. Concomitant blunt enteric injuries with injuries of the liver and spleen (a dilemma for trauma surgeons). Am Surg. 2001;267:221–226.

[75] Sherk JP, Oakes DD. Intestinal injuries missed by computed tomography. J Trauma. 1990;30:1–7.

http://dx.doi.org/10.5772/52793

[76] Schnüriger B, Talving P, Barbarino R, Barmparas G, Inaba K, Demetriades D. Current practice and the role of the CT in the management of penetrating liver injuries at a Level I trauma center. J Emerg Trauma Shock. 2011 Jan;4(1):53-7

[77] Navsaria PH, Nicol AJ, Krige JE, Edu S. Selective nonoperative management of liver gunshot injuries. Ann Surg. 2009 Apr;249(4):653-6

[78] Velmahos GC, Constantinou C, Tillou A, Brown CV, Salim A, Demetriades D. Abdominal computed tomographic scan for patients with gunshot wounds to the abdomen selected for nonoperative management. J Trauma. 2005 Nov;59(5):1155-60; discussion 1160-1

[79] Omoshoro-Jones JA, Nicol AJ, Navsaria PH, Zellweger R, Krige JE, Kahn DH. Selective non-operative management of liver gunshot injuries. Br J Surg. 2005 Jul;92(7): 890-5

[80] Demetriades,Demetrios, Selective nonoperative management of penetrating abdominal solid organ injuries. Ann. Surg 2006;244:pp620-28

[81] Wilson RH, Moorehead RJ. Hepatic traumaand its management. Injury 1991;22:439-45.

[82] Stain SC, Yellin AE, Donovan AJ. Hepatic trauma. Arch Surg 1988; 123: 1251-5.

[83] Feliciano DV, Pachter HL. Hepatic trauma revisited. Curr Probl Surg 1989; 26: 453-524

[84] Canizaro PC, Pessa ME. Management of massive hemorrhage associated with abdominal trauma. Surg Clin North Am 1990; 70: 621-34.

[85] Pringle JH. Notes on the arrest of hemorrhage due to trauma. Ann Surg. 1908;48:546–566.

[86] Moore EE, Edgar J. Poth Lecture. Critical decisions in the management of hepatic trauma. Am J Surg 1984; 148: 712-16.

[87] Walt AJ, Bender JS. Injuries of the liver. In: Schwartz SI, Ellis H, eds. Maingot's Abdominal Operations. Vol. 2. Norwalk, Connecticut: Appleton-Century-Crofts, 1985: 1577-90.

[88] Shuman WP. CT of blunt abdominal trauma in adult . radiology 1997; 205: 297-306.

[89] Smadja C, Traynor O, Blumgart LH. Delayed hepatic resection for major liver injury. Br J Surg 1982; 69: 361-4.

[90] Ochsner MG, Jaffain JH, Golocovsky M. Jones RC. Major hepatic trauma. Surg clin north am 1993;73:337-52.

[91] Lucas CE, Ledgerwood AM. Prospective evaluation of hemostatic techniques for liver injuries. J Trauma. 1976;16:442–451.

[92] Feliciano DV, Mattox KL, Jordan GL, et al.. The management of 1000 consecutive cases of hepatic trauma. Ann Surg. 1988;204:438–495.

[93] Trunkey DD, Shires GT, McClellan R. Management of liver trauma in 811 consecutive patients. Ann Surg. 1974;179:722–728.

[94] Morris JA, Eddy VA, Blinman TA, et al.. The staged celiotomy for trauma (issues in unpacking and reconstruction). Ann Surg. 1993;217:576–586.

[95] Aaron WS, Fulton RL, Mays ET. Selective ligation of the hepatic artery for trauma of the liver. Surg Gynecol Obstet. 1975;141:187–189.

[96] Mays ET, Conti S, Fallahzadkh H, et al.. Hepatic artery ligation. Surgery. 1979;86:536–543

[97] Mays ET. Hepatic trauma. Curr Prob Surg. 1976;13:1–86.

[98] Flint LM, Polk HC. Selective hepatic artery ligation (limitations and failures). J Trauma. 1979;19:319–323.

[99] Schrock T, Blaisdell FW, Mathewson C, et al.. Management of blunt trauma to the liver and hepatic veins. Arch Surg. 1968;96:698–704.

[100] FA, Moore EE, Seagraves A. Non-resectional management of major hepatic trauma. Amer J Surg. 1985;150:725–729.

[101] Walt AJ. The mythology of hepatic trauma or babel revisited. Amer J Surg. 1978;135:1218.

[102] Stone HH, Lamb JM. Use of pedicled omentum as an autogenous pack for control of hemorrhage in major injuries of the liver. Surg Gynecol Obstet. 1975;141:92–94.

[103] Carmona RH, Peck D, Lim RC. The role of packing and re-operation in severe hepatic trauma. J Trauma. 1984;24:779–784.

[104] Wahl WL, Brandt MM, Hemmila MR, Arbabi S. Diagnosis and management of bile leaks after blunt liver injury. Surgery. 2005 Oct;138(4):742-7; discussion 747-8

[105] Sugimoto K, Asari Y, Sakaguchi T et al. ERCP in the non-surgical management o blunt liver trauma. J Trauma 1993;35:192-9.

[106] Pachter HL, Spencer FC, Hofstetter SR, et al. Significant trends in the treatment of hepatic injuries. Experience with 411 injuries. Ann Surg 1992;215:492–500.

[107] Polanco P, Leon S, Pineda J, et al. Hepatic resection in the management of complex injury to the liver. J Trauma 2008;65(6):1264–9 [discussion: 1269–70].

[108] Richardson JD, Franklin GA, Lukan JK, et al. Evolution in the management of hepatic trauma: a 25-year perspective. Ann Surg 2000;232:324–30.

[109] Honore C, et al. Liver transplantation for hepatic trauma: Discussion about a case and its management. J Emerg Trauma Shock. 2011 Jan;4(1):137-9.

[110] Liver replacement after massive hepatic trauma. Esquivel CO, Bernardos A, Makowka L, Iwatsuki S, Gordon RD, Starzl TE. J Trauma. 1987 Jul;27(7):800-2

[111] Delis SG, Bakoyiannis A, Selvaggi G, Weppler D, Levi D, Tzakis AG. Liver transplantation for severe hepatic trauma: experience from a single center. World J Gastroenterol 2009;15:1641-4.

[112] Clemente N, Di Saverio S, Giorgini E, Biscardi A, Villani S, Senatore G, Filicori F, Antonacci N, Baldoni F, Tugnoli G. Management and outcome of 308 cases of liver trauma in Bologna Trauma Center in 10 years. Ann Ital Chir. 2011 Sep-Oct;82(5):351-9

[113] Beuran M, Nego I, Ispas AT, Păun S, Runcanu A, Lupu G, Venter D. Nonoperative management of high degree hepatic trauma in the patient with risk factors for failure: have we gone too far? J Med Life. 2010 Jul-Sep;3(3):289-96

[114] Fabian TC, Croce MA, Stanford GG, Payne LW, Mangiante EC, Voeller GR et al. Factors affecting morbidity following hepatic trauma. A prospective analysis of 482 injuries. Ann Surg 1991; 213: 540-8.

[115] 126 Flint LM, Mays ET, Aaron WS, Fulton RL, Polk HC. Selectivity in the management of hepatic trauma. Ann Surg 1977; 185: 613-18.

[116] Bender JS, Geller ER, Wilson RF. Intra-abdominal sepsis following liver trauma. J Trauma 1989; 29: 1140-5.

[117] Menegaux F, Langlois P, Chigot JP. Severe blunt trauma of the liver: study of mortality factors. J Trauma 1993; 35: 865-9.

[118] Rosemary A. Kozar, Frederick A. Moore, C. Clay Cothren, ; Risk Factors for Hepatic Morbidity Following Nonoperative Management Multicenter Study Arch Surg. 2006;141:451-459.

[119] Carrillo EH, Platz A, Miller FB, Richardson JD, Polk HC Jr. Non-operative management of blunt hepatic trauma. Br J Surg 1998; 85: 461-8.

[120] Cue JI, Cryer HG, Miller FB, Richardson JD, Polk HC Jr. Packing and planned reexploration for hepatic and retroperitoneal hemorrhage: critical refinements of a useful technique. J Trauma 1990; 30: 1007-13

[121] Beal SL. Fatal hepatic hemorrhage: an unresolved problem in the management of complex liver injuries. J Trauma 1990; 30: 163-9.

[122] De Toma G, Mingoli A, Modini C, Cavallaro A, Stipa S. The value of angiography and selective hepatic artery embolization for continuous bleeding after surgery in liver trauma: case reports. J Trauma 1994; 37: 508-11.

[123] Brick SH, Taylor GA, Potter BM, Eichelberger MR. Hepatic and splenic injury in children: role of CT in the decision for laparotomy. Radiology 1987; 165: 643-6.

[124] Krige JEJ, Bornman PC, Terblanche J. Therapeutic perihepatic packing in complex liver trauma. Br J Surg 1992; 79: 43-6.

[125] Tisnado J, Beachley MC, Cho SR. Control of intrahepatic bleeding by superselective embolization of the middle hepatic artery. South Med J 1982; 75: 70-1.

[126] Morimoto RY, Birolini D, Junqueira AR Jr, Poggetti R, Horita LT. Balloon tamponade for transfixing lesions of the liver. Surg Gynecol Obstet 1987; 164: 87-8.

[127] Oishi AJ, Nagorney DM Portl hypertension, variceal bleeding and high output cardiac failure secondary to an intrahepatic arterioportal fistula. HPB surg 1993;7:53-9.

[128] Pachter HL, Liang HG, Hofstetter SR. Liver and biliary tract trauma. In: Moore EE, Mattox KL, Feliciano DV, eds. Trauma. 2nd ed. Norwalk, Connecticut: Appleton and Lange, 1991: 441-63.

[129] Helling TS, Morse G, McNabney WK, Beggs CW, Behrends SH et al. Treatment of liver injuries at level I and level II centres in a multi-institutional metropolitan trauma system. The Midwest Trauma Society Liver Trauma Study Group. J Trauma 1997; 42: 1091-6.

[130] Sherman HF,Savage BA, Jones LM et al. non-operative management of blunt hepatic injuries: safe at any grade? J Trauma 1994; 37:616-21.

[131] Cox EF, Flancbaum L, Dauterive AH, Paulson RL. Blunt trauma to the liver. Analysis of management and mortality in 323 consecutive patients. Ann Surg 1988; 207: 126-34